Malignant Brain Tumors

Jennifer Moliterno Günel
Joseph M. Piepmeier
Joachim M. Baehring
Editors

Malignant Brain Tumors

State-of-the-Art Treatment

Springer

Editors
Jennifer Moliterno Günel
Department of Neurosurgery
Section of Neurosurgical Oncology, Yale University School of Medicine
New Haven, CT
USA

Joachim M. Baehring
Department of Neurology and Neurosurgery
Yale University School of Medicine
New Haven, CT
USA

Joseph M. Piepmeier
Department of Neurosurgery
Section of Neurosurgical Oncology, Yale University School of Medicine
New Haven, CT
USA

ISBN 978-3-319-84259-2 ISBN 978-3-319-49864-5 (eBook)
DOI 10.1007/978-3-319-49864-5

Softcover reprint of the hardcover 1st edition 2017

Printed on acid-free paper

This Springer imprint is published by Springer Nature
The registered company is Springer International Publishing AG
The registered company address is: Gewerbestrasse 11, 6330 Cham, Switzerland

Preface

Malignant gliomas remain one of the most difficult types of tumors to treat, with a relatively poor prognosis with current standard of care. Thus, treatment paradigms rely on a multidisciplinary clinical effort that encompasses the expertise of dedicated neurosurgeons, neuro-oncologists, radiation oncologists, neuropathologists, and radiologists. This combined clinical focus from a number of specialties reflects the importance of the combined effort from each of these disciplines for providing patients with the latest advances in care.

More recent observations from translational research have underscored the difficulty with treatment of these tumors due to their profound heterogeneity at the biological level and have identified specific genomic and pathological characteristics that correlate with responses to treatment. These findings are not only changing the way tumors are classified, but also ultimately treated, both on initial care and at the time of recurrence. While malignant gliomas remain a therapeutic challenge, the importance of these research findings in shaping treatment options has changed the way clinicians are addressing patients' options.

The aims and scope of this study is to address all the aspects of patient evaluation and care. This includes new findings in imaging that provide a better understanding of the extent of the lesion as well as its relationship with critical neuroanatomic function. The evolution of intraoperative imaging, functional brain mapping, and technology to identify tumor from brain has significantly improved the ability of surgeons for safer and more aggressive tumor removal. More importantly, a better understanding of tumor biology and genomics has created an opportunity to significantly revise tumor classification and better select optimal therapy for individual patients. These more recent findings have directed changes in patient management and have stimulated novel and innovative treatment options including immunotherapy, tumor vaccines, antiangiogenic agents, and personalized cancer treatment. In addition, novel agent delivery techniques offer the potential for increasing the effectiveness of treatment by delivering active agents directly where they are needed most. Radiation therapy has been a standard of care for malignant brain tumors, and recent attempts to improve the efficacy of this modality are helping to reduce morbidity while improving outcomes.

Therefore, a comprehensive overview of the state-of-the-art treatment for malignant gliomas, organized by subspecialized discipline, will prove useful by updating physicians on new therapeutic paradigms and what is on the horizon for the near future. This study will be informative for surgeons, oncologists, neurologists, residents, and students who treat these patients and those who are training for a career in managing patients with these challenging tumors.

New Haven, CT, USA

Jennifer Moliterno Günel, MD
Joseph M. Piepmeier, MD
Joachim M. Baehring, MD, D.Sc.

Contents

Contributors

Manmeet Ahluwalia Department of Hematology and Oncology, Cleveland Clinic Foundation, Cleveland, OH, USA

Joachim M. Baehring Department of Neurology and Neurosurgery, Yale University School of Medicine, New Haven, CT, USA

Tracy T. Batchelor Department of Neurology, Department of Radiation Oncology, Department of Division of Hematology/Oncology, Stephen E. and Catherine Pappas Center for Neuro-Oncology, Massachusetts General Hospital, Boston, MA, USA

Kevin P. Becker Department of Neurology, Yale School of Medicine, New Haven, CT, USA

Ranjit S. Bindra Department of Therapeutic Radiology, Yale University School of Medicine, New Haven, CT, USA

S. Bulent Omay Department of Neurosurgery, Yale University School of Medicine, New Haven, CT, USA

Marc R. Bussiére Department of Radiation Oncology, Massachusetts General Hospital, Boston, MA, USA

Veronica L.S. Chiang Department of Neurosurgery, Yale University School of Medicine, New Haven, CT, USA

Owen Clark Human Oncology and Pathogenesis Program (HOPP), Memorial Sloan Kettering Cancer Center, New York, NY, USA

Christopher D. Corso Department of Therapeutic Radiology, Yale University School of Medicine, New Haven, CT, USA

Hugues Duffau Department of Neurosurgery, Gui de Chauliac Hospital, Montpellier, France

E. Zeynep Erson-Omay Department of Neurosurgery, Yale School of Medicine, New Haven, CT, USA

Elena Fomchenko Department of Neurosurgery, Yale University school of Medicine, New Haven, CT, USA

Christian Grommes Department of Neurology, Memorial Sloan Kettering Cancer Center, New York, NY, USA

Murat Günel Department of Neurosurgery, Genetics and NeuroBiology, Yale School of Medicine, New Haven, CT, USA

David S. Hersh Department of Neurosurgery, Marlene and Stewart Greenebaum Comprehensive Cancer Center, University of Maryland School of Medicine, Baltimore, MD, USA

Andrei I. Holodny Department of Radiology, Memorial Sloan Kettering Cancer Center, New York, NY, USA

Anita Huttner Department of Pathology, Yale University School of Medicine, New Haven, CT, USA

Rakesh K. Jain Department of Radiation Oncology, Massachusetts General Hospital, Boston, USA

Santosh Kesari Department of Translational Neuro-Oncology and Neurotherapeutics, John Wayne Cancer Institute, Santa Monica, CA, USA

Jonas Kloepper Department of Radiation Oncology, Massachusetts General Hospital, Boston, USA

Gregory Kuzmik Department of Neurosurgery, Yale University School of Medicine, New Haven, CT, USA

Charles Marc Leyrer Department of Radiation and Oncology, Cleveland Clinic Foundation, Cleveland, OH, USA

Anne Long Department of Neurosurgery, Yale University School of Medicine, New Haven, CT, USA

Jacob Mandel Department of Neurology and Neurosurgery, Baylor College of Medicine, Houston, TX, USA

Emmanuel Mandonnet Department of Neurosurgery, Lariboisière Hospital, Paris, France

Jennifer Moliterno Günel Department of Neurosurgery, Yale University School of Medicine, New Haven, CT, USA

Erin Murphy Cleveland Clinic Foundation, Department of Radiation Oncology, Cleveland, OH, USA

Nicole M. Petrovich Brennan Department of Radiology, Memorial Sloan Kettering Cancer Center, New York, NY, USA

John H. Sampson Department of Neurosurgery, Duke University Medical Center, Durham, NC, USA

Teilo H. Schaller Department of Neurosurgery, Duke University Medical Center, Durham, NC, USA

Helen A. Shih Department of Radiation Oncology, Massachusetts General Hospital, Boston, MA, USA

Walter Stummer Department of Neurosurgery, University of Münster, Münster, Germany

Ghazaleh Tabatabai Interdisciplinary Division of Neuro-Oncology, Departments of Neurology & Stroke and Neurosurgery, Hertie Institute for Clinical Brain Research, University Hospital Tübingen, Eberhard Karls University Tübingen, Tübingen, Germany

Aniket S. Wadajkar Department of Neurosurgery, Marlene and Stewart Greenebaum Comprehensive Cancer Center, University of Maryland School of Medicine, Baltimore, MD, USA

Nancy Wang Department of Neurology, Massachusetts General Hospital, Boston, USA

Laura E.G. Warren Department of Radiation Oncology, Massachusetts General Hospital, Boston, MA, USA

Michael Weller Department of Neurology, University Hospital Zurich, Zurich, Switzerland

Hans-Georg Wirsching Department of Neurology, University Hospital Zurich, Zurich, Switzerland

Graeme F. Woodworth Department of Neurosurgery, Department of Anatomy and Neurobiology, Marlene and Stewart Greenebaum Comprehensive Cancer Center, University of Maryland School of Medicine, Baltimore, MD, USA

Mark W. Youngblood Department of Neurosurgery, Yale School of Medicine, New Haven, CT, USA

Part I

Molecular and Clinical Characterization of Gliomas

1 Use of Advanced Neuroimaging (fMRI, DTI/Tractography) in the Treatment of Malignant Gliomas

Nicole M. Petrovich Brennan and Andrei I. Holodny

Functional MRI

Task-Based fMRI

Task-based blood oxygen-dependent (BOLD) fMRI measures relative changes in regional blood oxygenation during a behavioral task. Increases in net neuronal activity in a cortical or subcortical region lead to increased regional blood flow through specific metabolic signals that dilate local arterioles. This increase in perfusion of oxygenated blood to typically exceeds the increased metabolic demand, resulting in a paradoxical rise in oxygen saturation (the fraction of hemoglobin carrying oxygen) within the capillary bed and draining veins of brain regions that are neuronally active. Because oxyhemoglobin and deoxyhemoglobin differ in their magnetic susceptibility, rising oxygen saturation alters the local magnetic field: As oxyhemoglobin arrives in the capillary beds, the local magnetic field becomes more homogeneous, MR T2* relaxation becomes longer, and MR signal intensity increases. It is this contrast in T2* signal between baseline and task periods that is the basis of the BOLD fMRI mapping. The activity-driven fMRI signal (or hemodynamic response function) is transient on the order of seconds and is small: only approximately a 5% change from baseline in the healthy brain [1]. A proportionally longer resting epoch is often used to allow the hemodynamic response to recover more completely, and task/rest epochs are repeated and the results averaged in order to increase the contrast between the two behavioral states and increase detection of the fMRI signal.

The most common applications of task-based functional neuroimaging for presurgical planning of glioma surgery are sensorimotor mapping and language mapping, with more limited use for vision and memory systems. Each modality measured in the brain tumor patient has a unique set of challenges that will be addressed in detail. While there are many ways to collect fMRI data, a typical block-designed clinical scanning paradigm consists of a baseline resting epoch alternating with a task epoch repeated multiple times each. In this way, a task-based fMRI scan demands timed participation from the patient in behavioral and cognitive tasks that can range from simple finger tapping to picture naming or sentence completion.

Resting State fMRI

Where task-based fMRI shows regions of the brain that are active during a specific task, resting state fMRI (RS-fMRI) measures spontaneous low-frequency fluctuations in the BOLD signal at rest in order to discern patterns of cortical participation in spontaneous brain activity [2]. It reveals regions or networks with temporally

N.M. Petrovich Brennan (✉) · A.I. Holodny
Department of Radiology, Memorial Sloan Kettering Cancer Center, 1275 York Avenue, New York, NY 10065, USA
e-mail: brennann@mskcc.org

J. Moliterno Günel et al. (eds.), *Malignant Brain Tumors*,
DOI 10.1007/978-3-319-49864-5_1

correlated variations in BOLD signal. Many intrinsic networks have been described using this technique including a somatosensory network [2], a visual network, an auditory network, a language network, and a dorsal and ventral attention network among others [3]. RS-fMRI not only localizes members of a network, but also provides a quantitative measure of the degree of correlation which may relate to the degree of network participation or "connectedness." This measure has been recently exploited in a number of pathologies including brain tumors to study the effects of a tumor on intrinsic connectivity [4]. While the reliability of these networks has been demonstrated in control subjects [5], the clinical utility of RS-fMRI is still in the process of being validated. What follows is a discussion of both task-based fMRI and RS-fMRI as they demonstrate different but complimentary components of brain function in the presurgical planning toolbox.

Motor Mapping Using fMRI

Among noninvasive brain mapping techniques, task-based motor mapping by BOLD fMRI has been subject to the most experimental validation of sensitivity, predictive value, and reliability [6, 7]. Hirsch et al found 97% sensitivity for the identification of the primary motor gyrus [8] and Roessler et al found 100% concordance between DCS and fMRI motor localization within 10 mm [9]. Motor mapping using fMRI has proven to reliably identify rolandic structures even in the presence of edema and malignant tumor [10] and has supplanted the need for invasive functional mapping by direct cortical stimulation or somatosensory evoked potentials in some instances [11]. The high reliability of fMRI in sensorimotor mapping, when compared to language or other cognitive functions, may reflect the relatively large BOLD signals elicited by sensorimotor tasks [12].

Typical regions requested for motor mapping in brain tumor patients include the hand, foot, tongue, and the supplementary motor area (SMA). In most cases, the central sulcus can be identified by landmarks on standard anatomic images and the cortical expansion of the precentral gyrus subtending hand motor function is discernible (the "omega sign"). When landmarks appear clear, fMRI may provide confirmation or may even alert the clinician to a discrepancy in functional cortical organization. fMRI is most useful when patients presented with intrinsically ambiguous anatomical landmarks and/or when anatomy is distorted by mass effect from tumor and edema—a common circumstance among the patient population referred to functional imaging of motor function [13, 14] (Fig. 1.1).

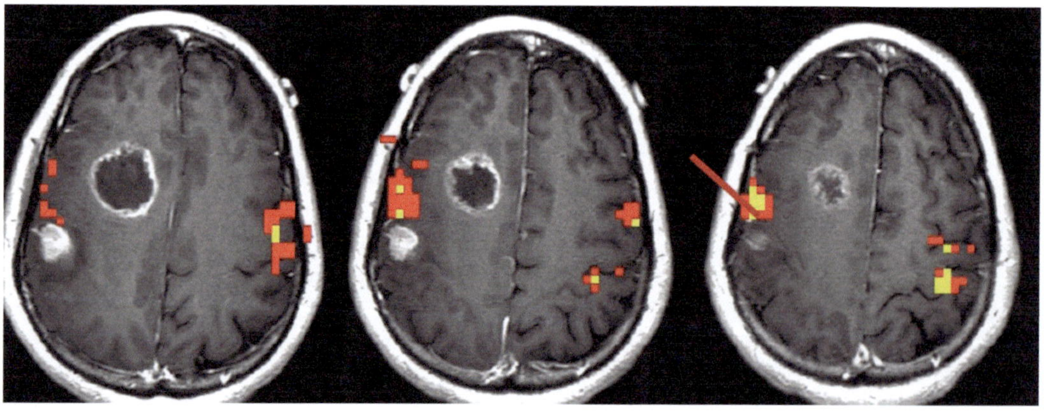

Fig. 1.1 Hand motor fMRI activation in a patient with two contrast enhancing tumors that both displace the motor gyrus and efface the central sulcus. The *red line* indicates the position of the central sulcus

An area where functional imaging for neurosurgical planning excels is foot motor localization. In contrast to the more lateral hand representation, the foot motor region is less well defined anatomically (as the central sulcus sometimes meets the midline and sometimes does not). As such, foot motor can be difficult to predict precisely using anatomy alone, more so in the presence of tumor. Further, mapping of foot motor cortex by intraoperative direct cortical stimulation within the interhemispheric fissure is often infeasible due to limited access beneath the sagittal sinus. Functional MRI is therefore well suited to aid the surgeon in pretreatment planning when a tumor involves or is in the proximity to the foot motor area. A recent study showed that raters who were experienced with fMRI were significantly better at predicting the location of the foot motor area than raters without [15]. This study suggests that even when anatomical landmarks are present, they are not always sufficient to predict more medial motor regions.

The tongue motor region is located in the lateral extremity of the motor homunculus. Anatomically, the central sulcus truncates as it moves inferiorly and can be difficult to extrapolate from more superior/medial localizations (Fig. 1.2). Thus, if a tumor approaches the inferior aspect of the motor gyrus, tongue motor mapping with fMRI may be informative. Because tongue motor cortex is positioned just posterior to Broca's area in the dominant hemisphere, it is often mapped in combination with language and in anticipation of confirmation by direct cortical stimulation intraoperatively. In this context, preoperative tongue motor localization may be useful to guide this portion of intraoperative mapping by providing a starting point where clear speech arrest is expected.

In addition, the tongue motor region is bilaterally represented. So, while resection of the tongue and face motor region will result in central facial paresis and/or dysarthria, these deficits are often transient and recoverable [16]. Therefore, if fMRI can demonstrate that a tumor is relatively confined to the tongue motor region, it may help guide the decision for surgery.

Sensorimotor areas have been successfully localized using RS-fMRI in the brain tumor patient. Kokkonen et al. localized sensorimotor cortices in both brain tumor patients and control subjects using RS-fMRI and found no differences in volume, spatial correlation, or temporal correlation [17]. And yet other studies have also validated RS-fMRI with direct cortical stimulation [4]. Mitchell et al. developed an algorithm to identify language and motor networks, validated in tumor patients undergoing both presurgical fMRI and intraoperative direct cortical stimulation [18]. The RS-fMRI AUC for motor networks when analyzed pairwise with electrocortical stimulation positive sites was 89. This

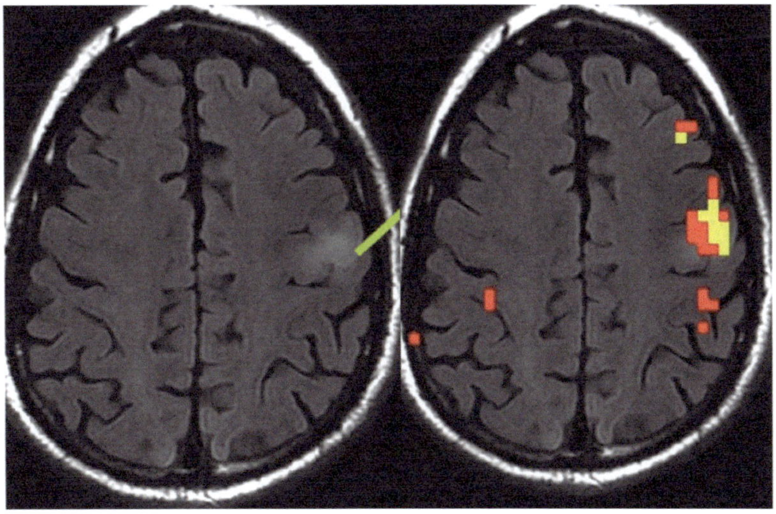

Fig. 1.2 Tongue motor fMRI in a patient with a low-grade glioma. It can be difficult using anatomy on MRI alone to determine the location of inferior motor regions such as face/tongue

finding has been supported by other studies suggesting that motor gyrus localization for presurgical planning is particularly feasible using resting state fMRI [19]. As such there is little argument that RS-fMRI may prove useful in localizing primary sensory networks even in the presence of a brain tumor. Of note, there is literature to suggest that motor mapping using fMRI can be performed with accuracy in the anesthetized patient as well, offering a potentially valuable adjunct for functional mapping in pediatrics and in adult populations with limited capacity for task participation [20].

Supplementary Motor Area

fMRI is commonly used to localize the SMA a functional designation attributed to the postero-medial superior frontal region in both hemispheres. This region is particularly amenable to fMRI localization for glioma surgery as there are no well-defined anatomical boundaries. The SMA is segregated into functionally specific regions with the anterior aspect planning the motor output of language function and the more posterior region subserving motor planning. Evidence has also suggested both somatotopy within the SMA [21] and a central region between the language and motor components of the SMA with shared functionality [22]. The preoperative localization of tumors in relation to both SMA and the motor gyrus may be useful in order to predict and interpret postoperative deficits. SMA injury is associated with a syndrome of temporary paresis and dysphasia that can mimic effects of injury to primary motor and language cortices, but which is distinguished by a high potential for recovery within weeks [23]. The mechanisms underlying SMA syndrome (and its transient nature) are not clear. A recent study using RS-fMRI suggested that interhemispheric connectivity decreases in the immediate postoperative period and ultimately interhemispheric SMA connectivity rises to higher levels than preoperative measurements. This gives rise to the possibility that SMA syndromes may result from disrupting interhemispheric connectivity [24].

Language fMRI

Applications of fMRI language mapping in the brain tumor patient can be segregated into evaluations of language laterality and language localization.

Language Lateralization

Using fMRI to lateralize language was historically seen as a welcome alternative to the intracarotid amobarbital procedure (IAP or "Wada" test). During the IAP, the patient is tested for language and memory task performance while each hemisphere of the brain is anesthetized separately via angiographically directed injection of individual carotids or selected arteries. This invasive test carries a small risk of significant complications including stroke [25]. Multiple studies have investigated the concordance between fMRI and IAP language lateralization. A meta-analysis of twenty-three studies showed that the sensitivity and specificity of fMRI for atypical language dominance (using IAP as the standard of reference) were 83.5–88.1%, respectively [26]. This study also showed that fMRI and IAP showed at least 80% concordance between the two tests in 21 of 23 studies. A separate study reported 10 patients who underwent anterior temporal lobectomy for epilepsy in whom preoperative fMRI and IAP lateralization were discordant. Postoperative language deficits were more accurately predicted by the fMRI result in 7 of the patients, and IAP more predictive in 2 [27].

Discordance between IAP and task-based fMRI is not surprising, given the significant variability in both IAP and fMRI task selection, and MRI image acquisition, analysis, and interpretation. In an attempt to address fMRI task variability, Rutten et al. have proposed a combined task analysis wherein multiple language task runs are concatenated and only activations in common with all language tasks are represented in the output [28]. In this procedure, task-dependent activations fall away and, arguably, only language essential regions remain.

Combined task analyses were more concordant with IAP than their individual counterparts in all cases in this study.

A second cause for discrepancy between fMRI and IAP results is the relatively high granularity of fMRI mapping and its sensitivity to nondominant hemispheric activation leading to more cases of fractional laterality indices [29]. It remains to be seen whether fractional laterality indices are predictive of deficits.

Lastly, differences between techniques may partly account for the discordance that is seen not only between WADA and fMRI, but also between DCS and fMRI. For example, most language fMRI is acquired with the patient performing tasks silently in order to avoid head motion, whereas intraoperative mapping involves the arrest of vocalized speech. Our group showed that when tongue movement is added to the silent speech fMRI mapping protocol, the region of speech arrest found using DCS encompasses the fMRI prediction in a way that it does not with silent speech tasks alone [11]. Mismatches like this have driven refinement of intermodality testing protocols.

Language Localization

Localization of peritumoral activations comes with its own set of caveats. Localizing language may assist the neurosurgeon in planning a trajectory to a tumor. This can be helpful information because both intra-axial and extra-axial tumors can displace function.

It is important and appropriate here to note that fMRI activations are thought to represent local field potentials that include both excitatory and inhibitory components [30]. Some have even argued that the LFP is a combination of local and distant sources [31]. Related, a language fMRI map (and any other fMRI signal) is comprised of both essential and supportive activations. An essential activation can be defined as a region critical for a task and cannot be resected without significant deficit. A supportive function, if resected, may impart a minor deficit or none at all. fMRI maps of language cannot distinguish between the two, and as a result, DCS is often performed in order to confirm which fMRI localizations are critical and which are expendable in the service of the most complete resection possible (Fig. 1.3).

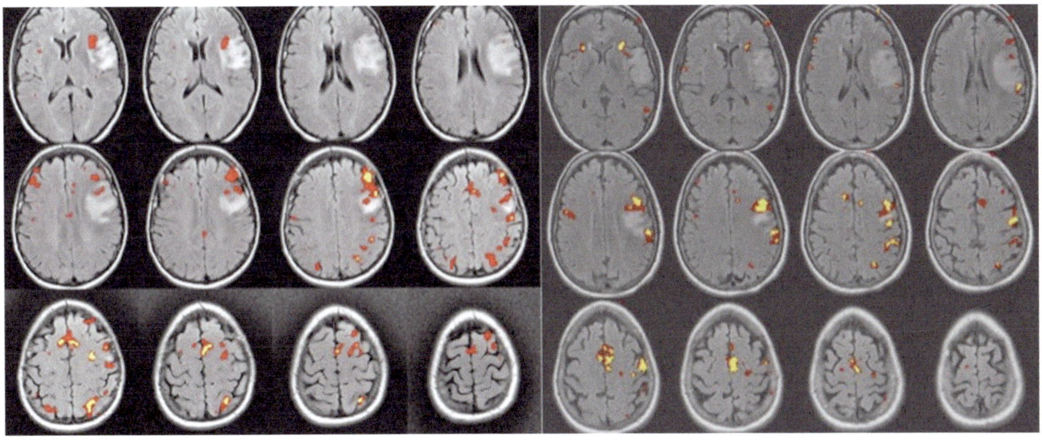

Fig. 1.3 Language fMRI (Phonemic Fluency) in two patients with very similar low-grade gliomas. The patients are similar both in the anatomical location of their tumors and in the fMRI activation patterns in the middle frontal gyrus. The patient on the left demonstrated speech disruption upon direct cortical stimulation of the middle frontal gyrus fMRI activation loci in the operating room and the patient on the right did not. This is a key example of how what is essential fMRI activation for one patient is not for another

Technical Considerations

There are many technical considerations in the use of fMRI in malignant glioma patients. Of these, abnormal neovasculature that is inherent to many glial tumors is one of the most significant. High-grade gliomas in particular have been shown to decouple the BOLD fMRI signal from behavior through dysautoregulation [32]. In such cases, the measured BOLD response lags the expected response when compared to the timing of the stimulus presentation. If not carefully identified, such an error can lead to false negatives.

Additionally, dysautoregulation poses a particular risk to language lateralization studies as lateralization is based on a ratio measure (# Left Hemisphere Voxels-# Right Hemisphere voxels/# Left Hemisphere Voxels + # Right Hemisphere voxels). Ulmer et al show that tumor suppression of the language-related BOLD signal could make contralateral fMRI speech signals take on more significance in the ratio determination of hemispheric dominance for language and can erroneously lead to what the authors' term pseudodominance [33]. Further, decoupling has been shown to affect RS-fMRI as well as it is derived from the same vascular signal [34]. The use of perfusion imaging to identify patients with tumors that are highly perfused may contribute by identifying those fMRI scans that are at high risk for false negatives in regions that are hyperperfused. Therefore, fMRI in low-grade tumors where abundant abnormal neovasculature is less burdensome may be more reliable.

Another technical consideration worth mentioning is vascular density. Vascular density differs between brain regions and will affect spatial specificity. For example, the temporal lobe shows regions of both rich and sparse capillary bed density. This variable distribution of capillaries will affect spatial specificity and may yield false-negative estimates of function [35]. To the authors' knowledge, this physiologic limitation has not been shown to have direct consequences clinically but it is worth noting as a potential limitation.

While head motion is an issue for any fMRI study, it is of particular concern in impaired patients. Anything that changes the gray-scale value of the fMRI volume registers as a statistical difference to most analysis software programs if it occurs at the right time. If a patient were to move their head every time, they attempted to move a paretic limb; for example, the resultant fMRI map may represent that stimulus-locked motion and not BOLD perfusion itself. Additional concern is warranted to use of RS-fMRI clinically as multiple studies have suggested that poor motion correction can lead to false-positive network correlations [36, 37].

Diffusion Tractography

Whereas fMRI measures changes in gray matter perfusion, diffusion tractography (DTI) uses water diffusion to estimate white matter tract directionality. Water diffuses parallel to axonal fibers and is restricted in the perpendicular direction. This directionality is termed anisotropy [38]. With six or more MR gradient measurements, a diffusion tensor (a vector measure) can be calculated. From the diffusion tensor, the fractional anisotropy (FA) (a scalar measure) ranging from zero to one represents the degree of directionality of a tract. FA is used to infer tract density and demonstrates anatomical connectivity (as opposed to functional connectivity that we saw with RS-fMRI). FA maps are color-coded 2D visual representations of directional water diffusion (Fig. 1.4), whereas tensor maps are their 3D counterparts (Fig. 1.5). Some of the most common tracts mapped in the treatment of gliomas are the cortico-spinal tracts (motor), the arcuate fasciculus (language), and the visual projections. DTI provides more sensitivity to tract disruption than routine MR imaging where white matter tracts can appear normal [39].

Cortico-Spinal Tract

Connecting the different regions of the motor gyrus to the spinal cord, these upper motor neurons form a large descending bundle that courses from the medial and lateral cortex

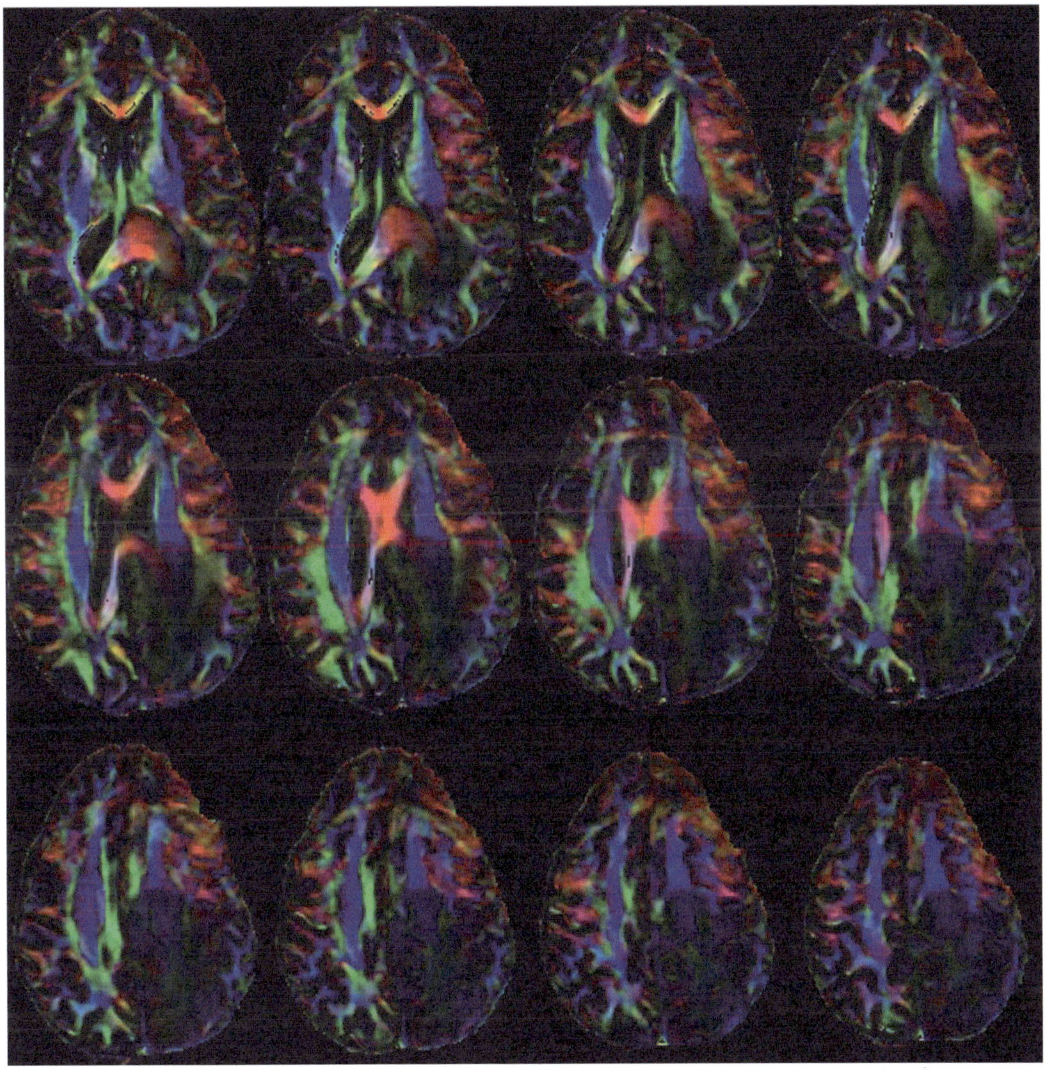

Fig. 1.4 Directionally encoded color FA map in a glioma patient. *Red left* to *right*, *Green* anterior to posterior, *Blue* inferior to superior (courtesy of Dr. Kyung Peck, MSKCC)

through the anterior limb of the internal capsule, into the medulla and ultimately into the spinal cord. Tumors that impinge upon the cortico-spinal tract (CST) can cause weakness or paresis at multiple levels in the descending pathway. DTI, as a result, may be helpful in demonstrating displacement relative to a tumor or when combined with intraoperative DTI and may be used to update relative positioning of the CST and the tumor dynamically during surgery using intraoperative MRI [40, 41].

Arcuate Fasciculus

The Arcuate Fasciculus (AF) is a bidirectional white matter tract that connects the frontal (Broca's area), temporal (Wernicke's area), and parietal lobes (Fig. 1.6). Because it spans much of the language dominant hemisphere, there are many opportunities for a tumor to interact with it causing language symptoms ranging from conduction aphasias to comprehension deficits depending on the region of the AF affected [42].

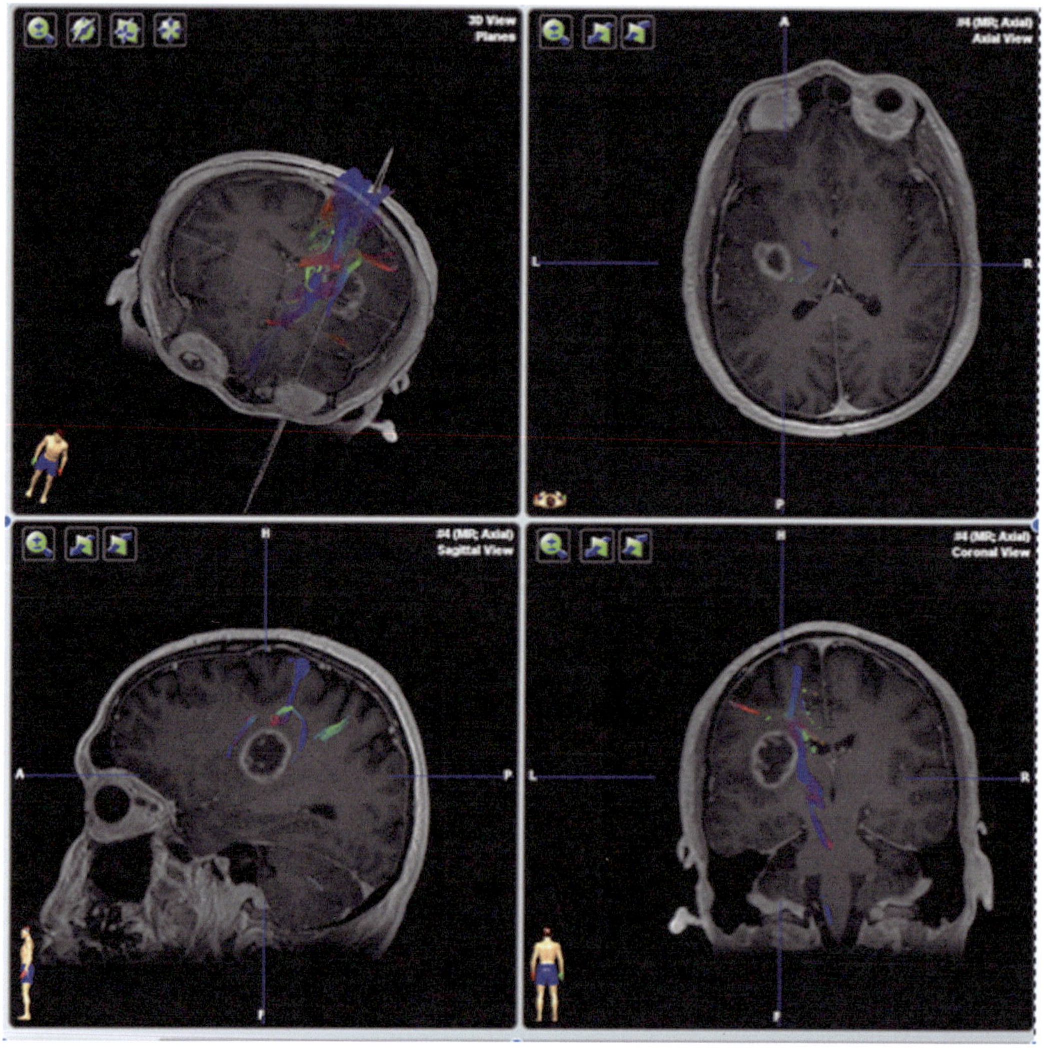

Fig. 1.5 Cortico-spinal tractography in a glioma patient imported into the neurosurgical navigation system. In this case, the cortico-spinal tract is estimated and converted to a 3D object for intraoperative dynamic navigation

High angular resolution diffusion-weighted imaging (HARDI), a higher order DTI algorithm was recently used in brain tumor patients to map the AF to successfully predict long-term language dysfunction. They found that patients whose language was intact had the preservation of the AF in common as well as the temporo-parietal component of the superior longitudinal fasciculus ($P < 001$) [43]. As DTI becomes more refined, the subcomponents of the AF may be a particularly interesting application for the use of DTI to predict ever more subtle iatrogenic speech deficits.

Visual Projections

Visual impairments are common after suprasellar tumor resections. DTI has been used to determine the distance between optic tract fibers that in turn may predict visual outcomes. In a study of 25 patients with suprasellar tumors, the mean

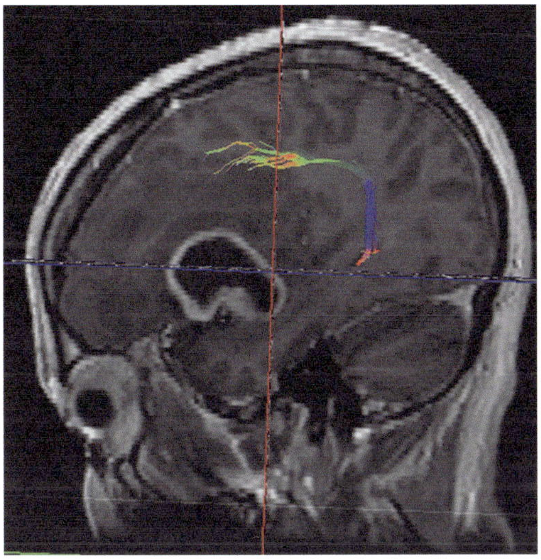

Fig. 1.6 DTI tractogram of the arcuate fasciculus (courtesy of Dr. Robert Young, MSKCC)

distance between optic tracts positively correlated with visual improvement 1 week and 3 months after surgery [44]. DTI has also been used to localize the optic radiations in an effort to predict or spare function but this is a more common approach during epilepsy rather than tumor resection [45].

Limitations

Just as BOLD fMRI is a proxy measure for neuronal functional so is water diffusion a proxy measure for white matter bundles. DTI does not measure white matter bundles directly and its output is dependent upon the algorithm chosen. A study investigated the generation of the cortico-spinal tract using multiple algorithms (deterministic and probabilistic) and validated them against subcortical stimulation [46]. This study showed that HARDI was significantly more sensitive than standard DTI and probabilistic approaches were more sensitive than deterministic. Therefore, many centers opt to use the 2D FA maps over the 3D algorithm-dependent tractograms unless they have a methodology that they have extensive experience using.

Validation has proven more difficult for DTI than for fMRI. Whereas DCS can easily confirm or refute fMRI localizations of function, DCS of subcortical white matter tracts is technically more challenging with monopolar electrical stimulation often showing more reliable white matter tract signs than the bipolar stimulation that is used for cortical mapping [47, 48]. Further, white matter bundles are not easily visualized during brain tumor resection without a radiographic aid and shift of anatomical structures during tumor resection has hindered validation efforts.

Anything that affects water diffusion will affect the DTI measurement. Accordingly, edema is a common hindrance to accurate measures of diffusivity necessary for DTI tracking in brain tumor patients. Technical attempts are being made to enhance current algorithms to be able to better distinguish between gray matter, white matter, tumor, and surrounding edema [49].

Lastly, there are efforts to use DTI quantitatively to determine whether tumor involves a tract as evidenced by a drop in relative FA values in the infiltrated versus the noninfiltrated contralateral tract. One study used FA values in ipsilateral versus contralateral tracts according to the equation FA change (DeltaFA(%) = [FA(lesion) − FA(normal)]/FA(normal) 100%) [50]. In this study, a positive ratio measure was likely to be associated with edema and DeltaFA (%) between 0 and 30% was likely to be associated with infiltration. However, field strength and interscan instability in diffusion measurements have hindered use of quantitative FA values for diagnostic purposes [51].

References

1. Biswal BB, Kannurpatti SS, Rypma B. Hemodynamic scaling of fMRI-BOLD signal: validation of low-frequency spectral amplitude as a scalability factor. Magn Reson Imaging. 2007;25(10):1358–69.
2. Biswal B, et al. Functional connectivity in the motor cortex of resting human brain using echo-planar MRI. Magn Reson Med. 1995;34(4):537–41.
3. Lee MH, Smyser CD, Shimony JS. Resting-state fMRI: a review of methods and clinical applications. AJNR Am J Neuroradiol. 2013;34(10):1866–72.

4. Zhang D, et al. Preoperative sensorimotor mapping in brain tumor patients using spontaneous fluctuations in neuronal activity imaged with functional magnetic resonance imaging: initial experience. Neurosurg. 2009;65(6 Suppl):226–36.
5. Shehzad Z, et al. The resting brain: unconstrained yet reliable. Cereb Cortex. 2009;19(10):2209–29.
6. Mahdavi A, et al. Functional MRI in clinical practice: assessment of language and motor for pre-surgical planning. Neuroradiol J. 2015;28(5):468–73.
7. Gorgolewski KJ, et al. A test-retest fMRI dataset for motor, language and spatial attention functions. Gigascience. 2013;2(1):6.
8. Hirsch J, et al. An integrated functional magnetic resonance imaging procedure for preoperative mapping of cortical areas associated with tactile, motor, language, and visual functions. Neurosurgery. 2000;47(3):711–21; discussion 721–2.
9. Roessler K, et al. Evaluation of preoperative high magnetic field motor functional MRI (3 Tesla) in glioma patients by navigated electrocortical stimulation and postoperative outcome. J Neurol Neurosurg Psychiatry. 2005;76(8):1152–7.
10. Fraga de Abreu VH, et al. Brain tumors: the influence of tumor type and routine mr imaging characteristics at BOLD functional MR imaging in the primary motor gyrus. Radiology. 2016:151951.
11. Petrovich N, et al. Discordance between functional magnetic resonance imaging during silent speech tasks and intraoperative speech arrest. J Neurosurg. 2005;103(2):267–74.
12. Tyndall AJ, et al. Presurgical motor, somatosensory and language fMRI:technical feasibility and limitations in 491 patients over 13 years. Eur Radiol. 2016.
13. Yetkin FZ, et al. Location of the sensorimotor cortex: functional and conventional MR compared. AJNR Am J Neuroradiol. 1995;16(10):2109–13.
14. Rodrigues T, et al. Is the omega sign a reliable landmark for the neurosurgical team? an anatomical study about the central sulcus region. Arq Neuropsiquiatr. 2015;73(11):934–8.
15. Fisicaro RA, et al. Challenges in identifying the foot motor region in patients with brain tumor on routine MRI: advantages of fMRI. AJNR Am J Neuroradiol. 2015;36(8):1488–93.
16. Teunissen F,Verheul J, Rutten.G. Functionality of glioma-infiltrated precentral gyrus: experience from 14 patients. J Neurosurg Sci. 2015.
17. Kokkonen SM, et al. Preoperative localization of the sensorimotor area using independent component analysis of resting-state fMRI. Magn Reson Imaging. 2009;27(6):733–40.
18. Mitchell TJ, et al. A novel data-driven approach to preoperative mapping of functional cortex using resting-state functional magnetic resonance imaging. Neurosurgery. 2013;73(6):969–82; discussion 982–3.
19. Breshears JD, et al. Mapping sensorimotor cortex with slow cortical potential resting-state networks while awake and under anesthesia. Neurosurgery. 2012;71(2):305–16; discussion 316.
20. Ives-Deliperi VL, Butler JT. Functional mapping in pediatric epilepsy surgical candidates: functional magnetic resonance imaging under sedation with chloral hydrate. Pediatr Neurol. 2015;53(6):478–84.
21. Fontaine D, Capelle L , Duffau H. Somatotopy of the supplementary motor area: evidence from correlation of the extent of surgical resection with the clinical patterns of deficit. Neurosurgery. 2002;50(2): 297–303; discussion 303–5.
22. Peck KK, et al. Joint activation of the supplementary motor area and pre supplementary motor area during simultaneous motor and language functional MRI. NeuroReport. 2009;20(5):487–91.
23. Russell SM, Kelly PJ. Incidence and clinical evolution of postoperative deficits after volumetric stereotactic resection of glial neoplasms involving the supplementary motor area. Neurosurgery. 2003;52 (3):506–16; discussiom 515–6.
24. Vassal M, et al. Recovery of functional connectivity of the sensorimotor network after surgery for diffuse low-grade gliomas involving the supplementary motor area. J Neurosurg. 2016;1–10.
25. Loddenkemper T, Morris HH, Moddel G. Complications during the Wada test. Epilepsy Behav. 2008;13(3):551–3.
26. Dym RJ, et al. Is functional MR imaging assessment of hemispheric language dominance as good as the Wada test? A meta-analysis. Radiology. 2011;261 (2):446–55.
27. Janecek JK, et al. Naming outcome prediction in patients with discordant Wada and fMRI language lateralization. Epilepsy Behav. 2013;27(2): Ć399–403.
28. Rutten GJ, et al. FMRI-determined language lateralization in patients with unilateral or mixed language dominance according to the Wada test. Neuroimage. 2002;17(1):447–60.
29. Janecek JK, et al. Language lateralization by fMRI and Wada testing in 229 patients with epilepsy: rates and predictors of discordance. Epilepsia. 2013;54 (2):314–22.
30. Einevoll GT, et al. Modelling and analysis of local field potentials for studying the function of cortical circuits. Nat Rev Neurosci. 2013;14(11):770–85.
31. Mitzdorf U. Properties of the evoked potential generators: current source-density analysis of visually evoked potentials in the cat cortex. Int J Neurosci. 1987;33(1–2):33–59.
32. Hou BL, et al. Effect of brain tumor neovasculature defined by rcbv on BOLD fMRI activation volume in the primary motor cortex. Neuroimage. 2006;32 (2):489–97.
33. Ulmer JL, et al. Lesion-induced pseudo-dominance at functional magnetic resonance imaging: implications for preoperative assessments. Neurosurgery. 2004;55 (3):569–79; discussion 580–1.
34. Agarwal S, et al. Neurovascular uncoupling in resting state fMRI demonstrated in patients with primary brain gliomas. J Magn Reson Imaging. 2016;43 (3):620–6.

35. Harrison RV, et al. Blood capillary distribution correlates with hemodynamic-based functional imaging in cerebral cortex. Cereb Cortex. 2002;12(3):225–33.
36. Laumann TO, et al. On the stability of BOLD fMRI correlations. cereb cortex, 2016.
37. Van Dijk KR, Sabuncu MR, Buckner RL. The influence of head motion on intrinsic functional connectivity MRI. Neuroimage. 2012;59(1):431–8.
38. Chenevert TL, Brunberg JA, Pipe JG. Anisotropic diffusion in human white matter: demonstration with MR techniques in vivo. Radiology. 1990;177 (2):401–5.
39. Breier JI, et al. Language dysfunction after stroke and damage to white matter tracts evaluated using diffusion tensor imaging. AJNR Am J Neuroradiol. 2008;29(3):483–7.
40. Romano A, et al. Pre- and intraoperative tractographic evaluation of corticospinal tract shift. Neurosurgery. 2011;69(3):696–704; discussion 704–5.
41. Shahar T, et al. Preoperative imaging to predict intraoperative changes in tumor-to-corticospinal tract distance: an analysis of 45 cases using high-field intraoperative magnetic resonance imaging. Neurosurgery. 2014;75(1):23–30.
42. Catani M, Thiebaut de Schotten M. A diffusion tensor imaging tractography atlas for virtual in vivo dissections. Cortex. 2008;44(8):1105–32.
43. Caverzasi E, et al. Identifying preoperative language tracts and predicting postoperative functional recovery using HARDI q-ball fiber tractography in patients with gliomas. J Neurosurg. 2016;125(1): 33–45.
44. Hajiabadi M, Samii M, Fahlbusch R. A preliminary study of the clinical application of optic pathway diffusion tensor tractography in suprasellar tumor surgery: preoperative, intraoperative, and postoperative assessment. J Neurosurg. 2016;125(3):759–65.
45. Winston GP, et al. Optic radiation tractography and vision in anterior temporal lobe resection. Ann Neurol. 2012;71(3):334–41.
46. Bucci M, et al. Quantifying diffusion MRI tractography of the corticospinal tract in brain tumors with deterministic and probabilistic methods. Neuroimage Clin. 2013;3:361–8.
47. Shiban E, et al. Intraoperative subcortical motor evoked potential stimulation: how close is the corticospinal tract? J Neurosurg. 2015;123(3):711–20.
48. Szelenyi A, et al. Intra-operative subcortical electrical stimulation: a comparison of two methods. Clin Neurophysiol. 2011;122(7):1470–5.
49. Mekkaoui C, et al. Diffusion tensor imaging in patients with glioblastoma multiforme using the supertoroidal model. PLoS ONE. 2016;11(1): e0146693.
50. Yen PS, et al. White matter tract involvement in brain tumors: a diffusion tensor imaging analysis. Surg Neurol. 2009;72(5):464–9; discussion 469.
51. Grech-Sollars M, et al. Multi-centre reproducibility of diffusion MRI parameters for clinical sequences in the brain. NMR Biomed. 2015;28(4):468–85.

Molecular Neuropathology and the Ontogeny of Malignant Gliomas

2

Anita Huttner

Introduction

Gliomas are the most common primary parenchymal central nervous system (CNS) neoplasms and form a complex and heterogeneous group of tumors. The classification, grading, and treatment of this diverse group of tumors have been primarily based on morphological criteria, which introduced a certain degree of interpretative subjectivity and moreover provided only suboptimal accuracy for the prediction of treatment response [1]. The discovery of distinct genetic and epigenetic profiles for various glioma subtypes not only contributed to improved understanding of glioma pathogenesis, but also revealed that certain molecular changes are linked to therapeutic response and prognosis. The emergence of molecular signatures challenged the prognostic value of classic morphological grading. Consequently, it became a major goal for contemporary glioma diagnostics to incorporate molecular advances into routine tumor classification, which led to the 'ISN (International Society of Neuropathology) Haarlem consensus guidelines' and a revised World Health Organization (WHO) classification for tumors of the central nervous system in 2016. The new guidelines propose a 'layered' approach, which combines histological classification, WHO grading, and molecular biomarkers to establish an 'integrated' diagnostic assessment of gliomas [2, 3].

This chapter discusses the classification, grading, and molecular features of diffuse malignant gliomas as defined in the revised 2016 WHO classification. It focuses on some of the practical aspects of integrated glioma classification and provides an overview of prognostic and predictive molecular biomarkers, and their importance for the diagnosis and management of malignant gliomas.

A. Huttner (✉)
Department of Pathology, Yale University School of Medicine, 310 Cedar Street, BML167, New Haven, CT 06520-8023, USA
e-mail: anita.huttner@yale.edu

2016 WHO Classification—Integrated Diagnostics

Bailey and Cushing's first systematic approach to the classification of gliomas, which was published in 1928, laid the foundation for a classification scheme that was based on the 'histogenesis' of brain tumors [4]. The guiding principle was centered on morphological similarities between tumor cells and various normal constituent glial cell types under the assumption that these would give rise to the different types of glial neoplasms. Subsequent classifications, including the classifications devised by the WHO [5], continued to rely on the assessment of light microscopic criteria for tumor typing and histological grading and presented the 'gold standard' for the diagnosis and management of brain tumor patients [1, 6]. However, over time, it became apparent that the pure morphological classification of gliomas was associated with considerable

J. Moliterno Günel et al. (eds.), *Malignant Brain Tumors*,
DOI 10.1007/978-3-319-49864-5_2

subjectivity and inter-observer variability, particularly in the context of tumor heterogeneity [7]. Furthermore, there is considerable biological and clinical variability, even within morphologically well-defined tumor entities, and it becomes difficult to predict response to therapeutic regimens. Although the morphological classification has its advantages, there are significant limitations. Over the past decade, numerous molecular and translational studies have led to the identification of critical genetic and epigenetic abnormalities in various glioma types [8–11]. They not only provide insight into glioma pathogenesis and allow for a more accurate classification, but also show significant associations with biological behavior, response to therapy, and prognosis. As a result, the 'ISN Haarlem guidelines' and the 2016 WHO classification break with the traditional morphologic approach and institute a new diagnostic concept that merges classic histology with molecular diagnostic testing to create a 'layered' diagnosis (see Fig. 2.1). The layers are formed by histologic classification (tumor type), WHO grading ('malignancy level'), and

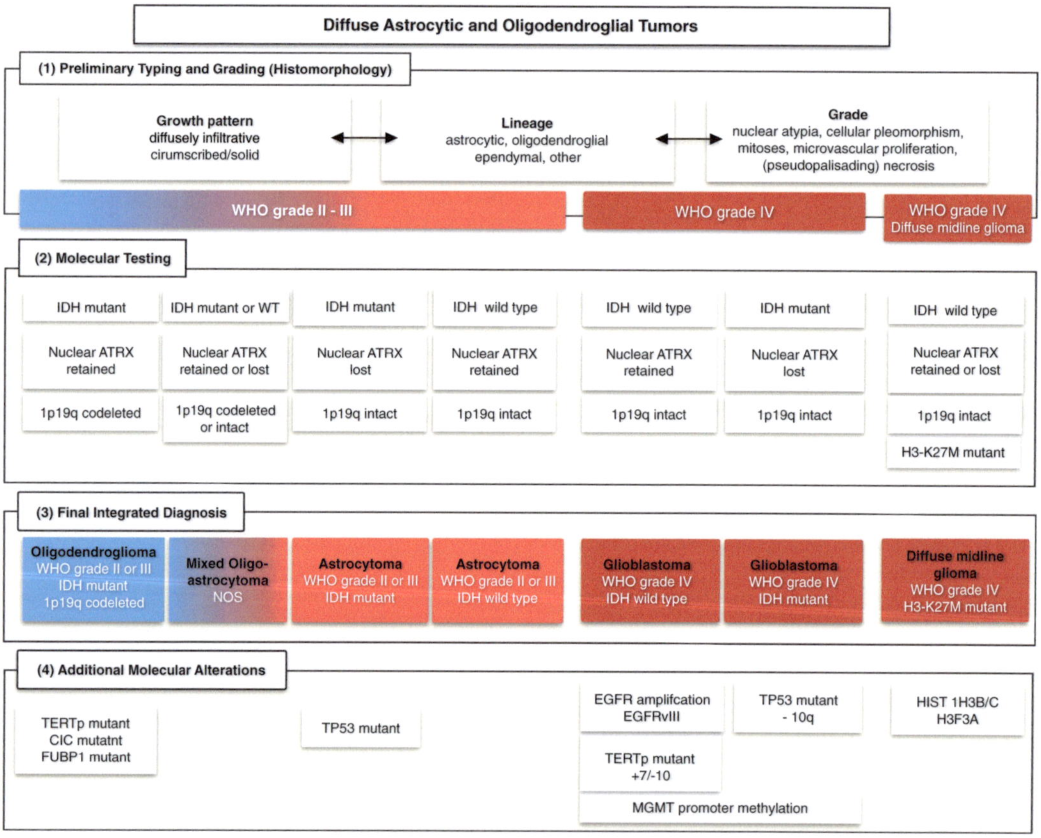

Fig. 2.1 The panels display the new 'layered' approach to the diagnosis of malignant gliomas as suggested by the 'ISN (International Society of Neuropathology) Haarlem consensus guidelines' and revised World Health Organization (WHO) classification. The light microscopic evaluation of gliomas begins the process of glioma classification and grading according to 2016 WHO standards (Preliminary Typing and Grading). Included are lineage-specific immunohistochemical stains such as GFAP. A second step involves molecular testing/biomarker detection for further subclassification and stratification. The results of both, morphology and biomarker analysis, are combined into a 'final integrated diagnosis'. Certain mutational profiles appear to be mutually exclusive and define tumor lineages: The combination of IDH1/1p19q/TERT defines oligodendrogliomas, whereas the combination of IDH1/p53/ATRX is typical for astrocytic tumors. Additional molecular tests are included to add further prognostic and predictive value (e.g., MGMT)

molecular biomarker information, which are combined into the final 'integrated diagnosis'. The purpose of this layered approach is to define individual entities as precisely as possible and to increase and optimize inter-observer diagnostic accuracy. This in turn will optimize predictions for the clinical–pathological behavior of tumors and allow for better prognostic stratification and therapeutic planning [2].

Diffuse Astrocytic and Oligodendroglial Gliomas

The inclusion of molecular markers led to significant changes in the 2016 classification system of gliomas. In prior editions, astrocytic gliomas, oligodendrogliomas, and mixed oligoastrocytic gliomas each formed a separate entity within the larger category of neuroepithelial neoplasms [1]. The 2016 WHO classification (see Table 2.1) merges these gliomas into a single group as '*Diffuse astrocytic and oligodendroglial tumors*' [3]. Aside from their infiltrative growth pattern, diffuse gliomas share frequent isocitrate dehydrogenase (IDH) mutations, a hallmark genetic alteration, which plays a significant role for the stratification of gliomas (please see below). Seminal studies could demonstrate that IDH-mutant gliomas are biologically and clinically distinct from IDH-wild-type gliomas [12, 13].

Diffuse gliomas form the vast majority of glial neoplasms and are primarily classified according to their histopathological appearance as astrocytic, oligodendroglial, or mixed oligoastrocytic

Table 2.1 2016 WHO Classification of Gliomas

Tumor entity/variant	WHO grade
Diffuse astrocytic and oligodendroglial tumors	
Diffuse astrocytoma, IDH-mutant	II
Gemistocytic astrocytoma, IDH-mutant	II
Diffuse astrocytoma, IDH-wild type	II
Diffuse astrocytoma, NOS	II
Anaplastic astrocytoma, IDH-mutant	III
Anaplastic astrocytoma, IDH-wild type	III
Anaplastic astrocytoma, NOS	III
Glioblastoma, IDH-wild type	IV
Giant cell glioblastoma	IV
Gliosarcoma	IV
Epithelioid glioblastoma	IV
Glioblastoma, IDH-mutant	IV
Glioblastoma, NOS	IV
Diffuse midline glioma, H3K27M-mutant	IV
Oligodendroglioma, IDH-mutant and 1p/19q-co-deleted	II
Oligodendroglioma, NOS	II
Anaplastic oligodendroglioma, IDH-mutant and 1p/19q-co-deleted	III
Anaplastic oligodendroglioma, NOS	III
Oligoastrocytoma, NOS	II
Anaplastic oligoastrocytoma, NOS	III
Other astrocytic tumors	
Pilocytic astrocytoma	I
Pilomyxoid astrocytoma	II
Subependymal giant cell astrocytoma	I
Pleomorphic xanthoastrocytoma	II
Anaplastic pleomorphic xanthoastrocytoma	III
Ependymal tumors	
Subependymoma	I
Myxopapillary ependymoma	I
Ependymoma	II
Papillary ependymoma	II
Clear cell ependymoma	II
Tanycytic ependymoma	II
Ependymoma, RELA fusion-positive	II or III
Anaplastic ependymoma	III
Other gliomas	
Chordoid glioma of the third ventricle	II
Angiocentric glioma	I
Astroblastoma	

(continued)

tumors. Although the cellular origin is still under investigation, the histological classification (cell lineage) relies on morphological similarities of tumor cells with their presumed non-neoplastic counterpart. Diffuse gliomas are graded in a tiered system as WHO grade II (low-grade), WHO grade III (anaplastic), or WHO grade IV (glioblastoma and variants). The grade is based on histological criteria such as cell density, nuclear atypia, cellular pleomorphism, mitotic activity, vascular proliferation, and necrosis. It can be viewed as 'malignancy scale' that is used to predict the biological behavior of neoplasms [1, 3].

As the name implies, diffuse gliomas display a diffusely infiltrative growth pattern with tumor cells invading brain parenchyma as single cells or small groups of cells. The ability to diffusely disseminate in a single-cell fashion throughout the brain is a rather unique feature among tumor cells and typical of glioma cells. They have the remarkable ability to migrate over long distances along myelinated fiber tracts and not infrequently cross the corpus callosum to infiltrate the contralateral hemisphere ('butterfly glioma') or follow descending fiber tracts. The accumulation of glioma cells around neurons ('perineuronal satellitosis'), around blood vessels and under the pial membrane ('secondary structures of Scherer') are additional classic features [14].

Histological Profiles of Diffuse Astrocytic and Oligodendroglial Tumors

Diffuse Astrocytic Tumors

The incidence of diffuse astrocytomas differs somewhat regionally, but recent estimates suggest an incidence rate of 0.4 per 100,000 people for WHO grade II astrocytomas and an incidence rate of 3.2 per 100,000 people for glioblastomas. The histological grade shows a direct correlation with the age at presentation, as WHO grade II tumors tend to present in younger adults in their 4th or 5th decades, while glioblastomas (WHO grade IV) peak in the elderly (mean age at diagnosis 61 years). Males appear to be more affected than females with a male:female ratio of 1.5:1.0 for all astrocytic tumors [15].

WHO grade II diffuse astrocytomas are morphologically heterogeneous and characterized by a higher degree of cellular differentiation, relatively slow growth, low mitotic activity, diffuse infiltration, and spread into adjacent brain structures (Fig. 2.2a). Tumor cells express GFAP (glial fibrillary acidic protein), a protein typically found in astrocytomas. WHO grade II diffuse astrocytomas can be found at any site within the CNS, but preferentially within the cerebral hemispheres, particularly within the subcortical and deep white matter of frontotemporal lobes. Although these lesions are rare in children, the main site in pediatric patients is the brain stem (so-called brain stem glioma). The 2016 WHO classification removed two variants, *fibrillary* and *protoplasmic* astrocytoma, due to lack of reproducible definition. The *gemistocytic* variant, which shows a very distinct appearance with eccentrically placed nuclei and dense cytoplasm, remains. Further, *gliomatosis cerebri*, previously defined by the diffuse involvement of several cerebral lobes, was also removed as separate entity, and it is simply viewed as an extreme example of widespread dissemination of tumor cells [3, 16].

Anaplastic astrocytomas (WHO grade III) are defined as diffuse astrocytomas with focal or dispersed anaplasia. These tumors are grossly more discernible since they are more cellular and form a more readily identifiable tumor mass. The infiltrative nature tends to create an overall increase in tissue volume without inducing a destructive effect. They are seen to arise from low-grade astrocytomas, but are also frequently diagnosed at first biopsy, without indication of a less malignant precursor lesion. In comparison with low-grade tumors, these neoplasms are microscopically remarkable for increased cellularity and enlarged, irregular hyperchromatic nuclei (Fig. 2.2b). Capillaries are lined by a single layer of endothelium, and frank vascular proliferation and necrosis are not present. Immunoreactivity for GFAP is less consistent than that for grade II lesions. In contrast to low-grade astrocytomas, these lesions display

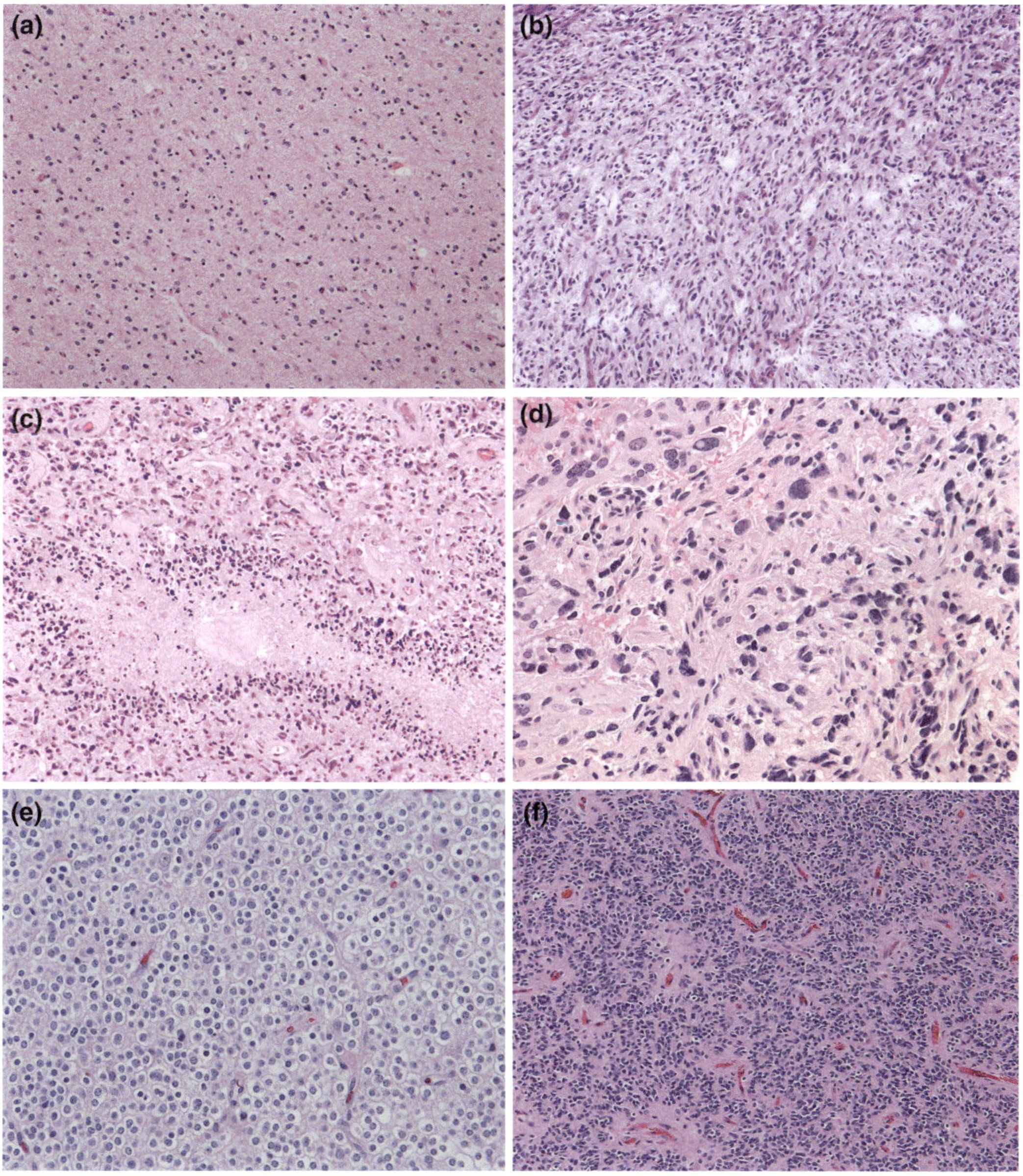

Fig. 2.2 Morphologic appearance of gliomas (hematoxylin- and eosin-stained sections). **a** Diffuse astrocytoma, WHO grade II, characterized by low cellularity and mild nuclear pleomorphism; **b** Anaplastic astrocytoma, WHO grade III with increased cellularity and anaplastic nuclei; **c** Glioblastoma, WHO grade IV with pleomorphic tumor cells, mitoses, and pseudo-palisading necrosis; **d** Diffuse midline glioma with a high degree of pleomorphism; **e** Oligodendroglioma, WHO grade II, with relatively round to oval cell nuclei and typical cytoplasmic clearing ('fried-egg' appearance); **f** Ependymoma, WHO grade II, relative monomorphous appearance of small tumor cells which form perivascular pseudorosettes

increased mitotic activity with a proliferative index (Ki-67/MIB-1 labeling) of 5–10% [3].

Glioblastomas (WHO grade IV) are the most malignant tumors within the spectrum of diffuse astrocytomas and account for up to 60% of all astrocytic tumors [15]. They affect mainly adults with a peak incidence between 40 and 70 years. Less than 10% of glioblastomas arise from a lesion of lower malignancy grade (secondary glioblastoma) and manifest in younger patients (mean age of 45 years). Most are found de novo (primary glioblastoma) after a short clinical history and are seen in older individuals (mean age 62 years). The majority of tumors are located within the cerebral hemispheres and show a tendency to infiltrate deep nuclei and spread along white matter tracts to the contralateral hemisphere. Brain stem involvement is rare and mainly present in children. Sites such as spinal cord or cerebellum are infrequently involved. Microscopically, glioblastomas are extremely heterogeneous and show a higher degree of cellularity, nuclear atypia, cellular pleomorphism, and mitotic activity, in addition to microvascular proliferation and (palisading) necrosis (Fig. 2.2c). The latter two features are the cardinal diagnostic features of glioblastomas and help distinguish them from grade III astrocytomas. Three distinct glioblastoma variants are part of the 2016 classification, which are giant cell glioblastoma, gliosarcoma, and the recently added variant of epithelioid glioblastoma. [3].

Giant cell glioblastoma is a variant remarkable for the presence and predominance of many markedly large and bizarre appearing, multinucleated giant cells, within an abundant stromal reticulin network. In spite of their unusual appearance, the consistent expression of GFAP in conjunction with data from genetic profiling confirmed their astrocytic nature.

Gliosarcomas are defined as high-grade astrocytomas with an intermixed sarcomatous component. Gliosarcomas are relatively rare and represent about 2% of all glioblastomas. The clinical features are similar to those of classic glioblastomas. Critical diagnostic parameters are a biphasic growth pattern with areas of glial and mesenchymal differentiation. Molecular changes are variable, but similar to those occurring in glioblastoma; however, tumor histogenesis is still controversial.

Epithelioid glioblastoma is a newly accepted and rare variant, which is characterized by the presence of predominantly epithelioid or focally rhabdoid morphology. This entity poses a diagnostic challenge due to its resemblance to poorly differentiated carcinomas [3, 17].

Diffuse Oligodendroglial Tumors

Oligodendrogliomas form a group of diffusely infiltrative glial tumors with features reminiscent of oligodendrocytes. Oligodendrogliomas account for approximately 5–6% of all glial neoplasms, and overall for 2–3% of all primary brain tumors. The annual estimated incidence rate lies within a range of 0.27–0.35 per 100,000 individuals. Although oligodendrogliomas can develop at any age, the majority of tumors arise within the 4th–5th decade, and less than 2% of oligodendrogliomas are found in children younger than 14 years. Males are more affected than females [15]. Oligodendrogliomas can arise anywhere within the central nervous system, but the majority of tumors are found within the frontal and temporal lobes of the cerebral hemispheres. Other cortical regions are less involved and oligodendrogliomas are rare within deep nuclei or spinal cord. Microscopically, these tumors are composed of a relatively monomorphous population of cells with round-to-oval nuclei with delicate chromatin pattern, and surrounded by perinuclear ‘halos’ (cytoplasmic clearing), an artifact seen in formalin-fixed and paraffin-embedded sections. The vasculature is typically thin-walled and described by some authors as ‘chicken-wire’ vasculature (Fig. 2.2e).

The WHO classification assigns two grades to oligodendrogliomas: well-differentiated relatively slow-growing tumors correspond to WHO grade II, whereas oligodendrogliomas with anaplastic features are assigned WHO grade III. Anaplastic oligodendrogliomas are characterized by an increase in cellularity and nuclear atypia, increased cellular pleomorphism, in addition to increased mitotic activity, endothelial proliferation, and necrosis. In contrast to other gliomas, such as astrocytomas and ependymomas, oligodendrogliomas show a more slowly progressive clinical course [3].

Diffuse Oligoastrocytomas

Oligoastrocytomas are defined as diffusely infiltrative glial neoplasms consisting of a mixture of two distinct cell types, which morphologically resemble the tumor cells of diffuse astrocytomas as well as oligodendrogliomas. These two components coexist either side by side or in a diffusely intermingled fashion. Definitive criteria for identification and classification of these lesions, however, remain somewhat controversial. Oligoastrocytomas are graded as WHO grade II lesions, and the acquisition of anaplastic features will increase the grade to WHO grade III.

Although oligoastrocytomas appear to have a mixed phenotypic appearance, they seem to demonstrate either an astrocytic or oligodendroglial genotype. This indicates that these tumors do not form a separate entity. The new WHO classification recommends molecular testing to assign these tumors a definitive lineage. Therefore, the new WHO classification discourages the diagnoses of oligoastrocytoma and anaplastic oligoastrocytoma. The term 'oligoastrocytoma, NOS' and 'anaplastic oligoastrocytoma, NOS' should be used in cases when gliomas are morphologically mixed or ambiguous and cannot be resolved using molecular testing [2, 18].

Molecular Profiles of Diffuse Astrocytic and Oligodendroglial Tumors

Isocitrate Dehydrogenase (IDH) Mutations

The hallmark genetic alterations in diffuse gliomas are somatic mutations in the gene encoding human cytosolic NADPH-dependent isocitrate dehydrogenase 1 (IDH1), a citric acid cycle component. Less frequently involved are mutations of *IDH2*. The IDH1 enzyme normally catalyzes the oxidative carboxylation of isocitrate to alpha-ketoglutarate (α-KG), resulting in the reduction of nicotinamide adenine dinucleotide phosphate (NADP) to NADPH. Numerous studies uncovered several mechanisms to explain the tumorigenic potential of IDH proteins. There is convincing evidence that mutant IDH, such as IDH1 (R132H), acquires neomorphic activity that converts alpha-ketoglutarate (α-KG) to 2-hydroxygluturate (2-HG) [19]. 2-HG in turn inhibits α-KG-dependent dioxygenases, including the members of the TET family of 5-methylcytosine hydroxylases and Jumonji-C domain-containing histone lysine demethylases. It has been shown that inhibition of these enzymes increases DNA and histone methylation, which eventually triggers the aberrant methylation of multiple cytosine–phosphate–guanine (CpG) dinucleotide-rich islands across the genome [20]. This 'glioma CpG-island methylator phenotype (G-CIMP)' is a characteristic profile seen in diffuse gliomas [21, 22] and likely contributes to the neoplastic transformation of neural stem or progenitor cells. Additional studies have shown that the production of 2-HG stimulates the activity of prolyl-hydroxylase domain isoform 3 (PHD3/EGLN) and prolyl 4-hydroxylases, which leads to reduced levels of hypoxia-inducible factor (HIF) and consequently to the enhanced proliferation of human astrocytes [23]. Increased oxidative stress due to decreased intracellular NADPH levels as a result of IDH mutations additionally promotes tumorigenesis [24].

It has been postulated that IDH mutations likely represent an initiating event, but that they are probably not sufficient to induce tumor growth on their own, instead they have to be accompanied by additional genetic mutations. Mutations involving tumor protein 53 (TP53) and ATRX genes play a role in diffuse and anaplastic astrocytomas. Co-deletions of 1p/19q and mutations involving the promoter region of telomerase reverse transcriptase (TERT) have been described for oligodendrogliomas [25].

These mutational profiles appear to be mutually exclusive and define tumor lineages: The combination of IDH1/p53/ATRX and IDH1/1p19q/TERT are mutational signatures for astrocytic tumors and oligodendrogliomas, respectively [26] (see Fig. 2.1). The new WHO classification requires the demonstration of both IDH1 mutation and 1p19q co-deletion for the diagnosis of oligodendroglioma and anaplastic oligodendroglioma. Similarly, the diagnosis of diffuse or anaplastic astrocytoma requires molecular testing for IDH mutations, with additional demonstration of ATRX mutation or loss of nuclear ATRX expression confirming an astrocytic lineage [27, 28].

Numerous studies established that IDH1 mutations are present at high frequency in secondary glioblastomas that originate from prior low-grade gliomas (~85%), which is contrasted by the fact that these mutations rarely occur in primary or de novo glioblastomas (<1%), which are found in the absence of low-grade precursor lesion. IDH1 mutations are further identified in the vast majority of diffuse low-grade (WHO grade II) and anaplastic (WHO grade III) astrocytomas (~70–80%), oligodendrogliomas (80%), anaplastic oligodendrogliomas (85%), and mixed oligoastrocytomas (100%). The IDH1 mutation frequency appears to be similar for WHO grade II and WHO grade III tumors [29]. Interestingly, the mutation rate in pilocytic astrocytomas (WHO grade I), ependymal tumors, or other less common glial tumors is extremely low or absent [13]. It was further demonstrated that IDH1 mutations do not exist in reactive conditions related to cerebral ischemia or infarctions, viral infections, or radiation change [30]. These findings are of particular diagnostic value as they enable the distinction of reactive gliosis from low-grade diffuse astrocytoma, a diagnostically challenging task, especially in the context of small biopsy samples.

It is of clinical importance that IDH 1 and IDH 2 mutations are found to be associated with a favorable prognosis and overall prolonged survival time independent of treatment. The survival of patients with the mutant form of IDH1 in astrocytomas or oligodendrogliomas (WHO grade II-III) and glioblastoma is longer than that of their IDH1 wild-type counterparts. Interestingly, patients with IDH1-mutated glioblastomas (WHO grade IV) show better survival than patients with wild-type anaplastic astrocytomas (WHO grade III). The IDH status, however, does not predict treatment-specific responses of patients with glioma [31].

In 2010, an antibody (Fig. 2.3a) was developed which is able to specifically recognize the mutant IDH1-R132H protein, which represents the majority (90%) of glioma-associated hotspot mutations [32, 33]. In the case of IDH1-R132H-negative immunostaining, testing for other IDH1 or IDH2 mutations is required for WHO grade II and III gliomas as well as glioblastomas from young patients and secondary glioblastomas [34]. This is usually accomplished by direct DNA sequencing or pyrosequencing using DNA extracted either from frozen tissue or more commonly formalin-fixed tissue [35, 36].

Co-deletion of 1p/19q

The combined deletion of the short arm of chromosome 1 (1p) and the long arm of chromosome 19 (19q) together with IDH1 mutations defines oligodendrogliomas and anaplastic oligodendrogliomas [37]. Mechanistically, this co-deletion results from of an unbalanced centromeric translocation and leads to loss of entire chromosomal arms t(1;19) (q10;p10). The frequency of 1p/19q co-deletions has been estimated to be 80–90% in WHO grade II oligodendrogliomas and 50–70% in WHO grade III oligodendrogliomas. In spite of a strong association between 1p/19q loss and classic oligodendroglioma morphology, morphology alone cannot predict the 1p/19q status. Interestingly, the chromosomal regions of 1p and 19q have been mapped in great detail; however, no definitive candidate genes have been identified which could explain the tumorigenic effect. Although the genes on 1p/19q remain enigmatic, numerous correlations have been established demonstrating that many tumors with 1p/19q co-deletions also show IDH1/IDH2 mutations; however, 1p/19q loss appears to be absent in cases with tumor protein p53 (TP53) mutations or EGFR amplifications. Notably, the combined loss of 1p/19q is also found in mixed glial tumors (oligoastrocytomas), but extremely rare in non-glial malignancies.

In the 2016 classification, co-deletion of 1p/19q serves a diagnostic biomarker. It was originally described in oligodendrogliomas in 1994, and a few years later, it was noted that a high proportion of oligodendrogliomas with 1p/19q loss demonstrated a favorable response to chemotherapeutic agents, in addition to substantially improved survival times [38]. Long-term follow-up data from the RTOG 9402 and EORTC 26951 phase III trials also pointed toward a role of 1p/19q loss in predicting long-term survival following aggressive

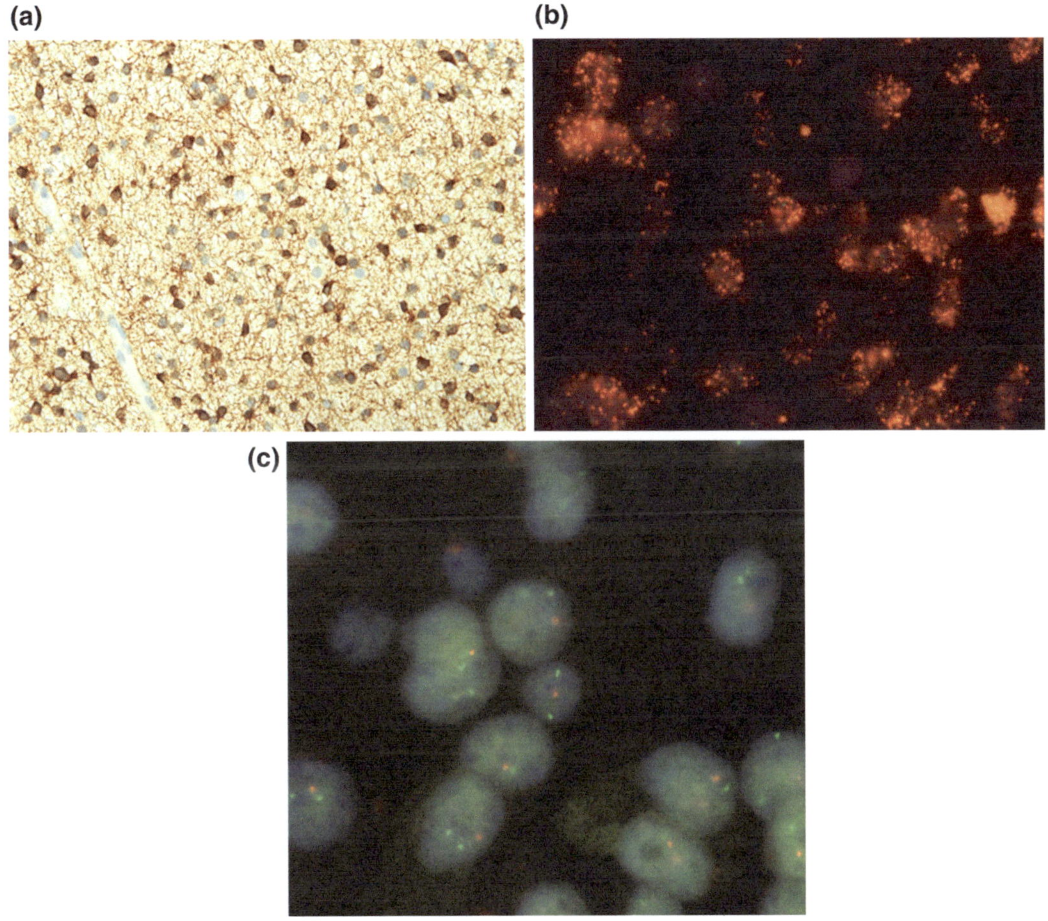

Fig. 2.3 Molecular biomarkers detected in FFPE (formalin-fixed paraffin-embedded) tissue **a** Immunohistochemistry for IDH1 shows mainly cytoplasmic, to a lesser extent nuclear, staining. This mutation-specific antibody against the most common IDH1 mutation, R132H, allows the identification of more than 90% of all IDH-mutant diffuse gliomas. **b** FISH (fluorescent in situ hybridization) for EGFR amplification is recognized by innumerable interphase FISH signals in red (probe set for gene region 7p11). The green signal is a SE7 gene region probe to facilitate chromosome identification. **c** FISH (fluorescent in situ hybridization) to demonstrate loss of the short arm of chromosome 1 (1p loss) as indicated by the presence of only *one red signal* (probe binds to gene region on 1p). The *green signal* serves as control and is a centromeric enumeration probe for chromosome 1 (CEP1). The presence of *2 green signals* indicates both chromosomes (paternal and maternal) are present

multimodal treatment (surgery and upfront combined radio- and chemotherapy with procarbazine, CCNU, and vincristine). In contrast, patients with 1p/19q deleted tumors, who undergo tumor resection alone without receiving any adjuvant chemotherapy or radiation, do not show longer progression-free survival, suggesting that 1p/19q loss characterizes a group of tumors with greater sensitivity to genotoxic agents. Subgroup analyses have further shown that cases of anaplastic oligodendrogliomas with 1p/19q co-deletion and IDH mutation had significantly longer median survival times when treated upfront with radiotherapy and vincristine as compared to treatment with radiotherapy alone. The lack of 1p/19q co-deletion in anaplastic oligodendrogliomas, in contrast, led to a significantly shorter survival times and showed no difference between radio-chemotherapy and radiotherapy-only arms [39]. These findings have been replicated numerous times over the past decade and extended to the use of additional chemotherapeutic drugs such as temozolomide in conjunction with radiation therapy. The molecular mechanisms, however, that underlie the association between 1p/19q loss, chemosensitivity and favorable prognosis remain to be elucidated.

Due to the well-accepted prognostic significance of 1p/19q loss in conjunction with adjuvant chemotherapy, testing for 1p/19q has become routine many institutions. Commonly used methods for 1p/19q co-deletion testing include fluorescent or chromogenic in situ hybridization (FISH/CISH) (Fig. 2.3c), microsatellite analysis for loss of heterozygosity (LOH), and multiplex ligation-dependent probe amplification (MLPA).

Importantly, 1p/19q co-deletion refers to whole-arm deletions of both chromosome arms that are typically due to an unbalanced translocation [t(1;19)(q10;p10)]. If testing for IDH mutation and 1p/19q co-deletion is not possible or remains inconclusive, tumors with classic oligodendroglial histology should be diagnosed as 'oligodendroglioma, NOS' or 'anaplastic Oligodendroglioma, NOS'.

MGMT Methylation Status

The gene encoding the O^6-methylguanine-DNA methyltransferase (*MGMT*) at 10q26 has become one of the most widely studied molecular markers in neurooncology, because it has the potential to counteract the efficacy of chemotherapy with temozolomide (TMZ). MGMT is a suicide DNA repair enzyme that protects cells against damage from ionizing radiation and alkylating agents [40]. Alkylating chemotherapeutic drugs, such as temozolomide, have been used for years in the treatment of patients with glioblastoma. Mechanistically, these drugs methylate the O^6 position of the DNA nucleotide guanine leading to cell death. MGMT is constitutively expressed in cells and part of an inherent DNA repair mechanism that can counteract the effects of alkylating agents. It catalyzes DNA repair by transferring this methyl group from the O^6 position of the DNA nucleotide guanine to a cysteine residue of the MGMT protein, acting against the cytotoxic effects of chemotherapy [41].

A significant proportion of glioblastomas have been found to express decreased levels of MGMT, which makes these tumors more susceptible to the effects of alkylating agents. The primary mechanism of MGMT downregulation is via aberrant DNA methylation of the promoter of the MGMT gene at its 5′-associated CpG-island. The MGMT promoter methylation represents an epigenetic regulatory mechanism, which consequently leads to transcriptional silencing and is found in 40% of IDH-wild-type glioblastomas as well as the vast majority of IDH-mutant and G-CIMP-positive gliomas. Consequently, glioblastoma cells with MGMT promoter (hyper) methylation respond better to temozolomide, as they lack the ability to efficiently repair the damage introduced by alkylation.

Numerous studies found an association between MGMT promoter hypermethylation and response of malignant gliomas to alkylating agents. In the EORTC/NCIC trial, Hegi et al. found that patients with hypermethylated MGMT promoters who were treated with temozolomide and radiation showed significantly increased survival times when compared to patients whose tumors were hypomethylated [42]. Interestingly, when treated with radiation alone, there was no significant extension of survival times, emphasizing a predictive role for MGMT hypermethylation and a favorable response to chemotherapy. The MGMT promoter methylation status is at the moment viewed as one of the most significant predictors of clinical outcome and response to treatment with temozolomide. Analyses by Gorlia et al. go as far as to suggest a stratification of all patients according to MGMT status as soon as they are enrolled in glioblastoma trials that use alkylating agents [43]. Also, a retrospective analysis could show that MGMT promoter methylation patterns can change between initial tumor diagnosis and later recurrence, particularly in MGMT-methylated cases [44]. This implies that MGMT methylation is only of prognostic value for the initial assessment, and it is not predictive of outcome for recurrences [45].

Further, MGMT promoter methylation is detectable in the vast majority of IDH-mutant gliomas, including both, astrocytic and oligodendroglial tumors, and associated with longer survival, independent of chemo- or radiation therapy. MGMT methylation appears to be frequent in low grade and anaplastic gliomas (up to 90%), which show 1p/19q co-deletion. Treatment with temozolomide correlated positively with longer progression-free survival in those patients. It should be pointed out that in the absence of alternative treatments, temozolomide is often applied as first-line agent, even without a methylated MGMT promoter, as these patients appear to benefit from this drug [46].

The MGMT status is most commonly being tested by methylation-specific PCR (MSP) (Fig. 2.4) or methylation-specific pyrosequencing, whereby both approaches are based on bisulfite conversion of unmethylated cytosines

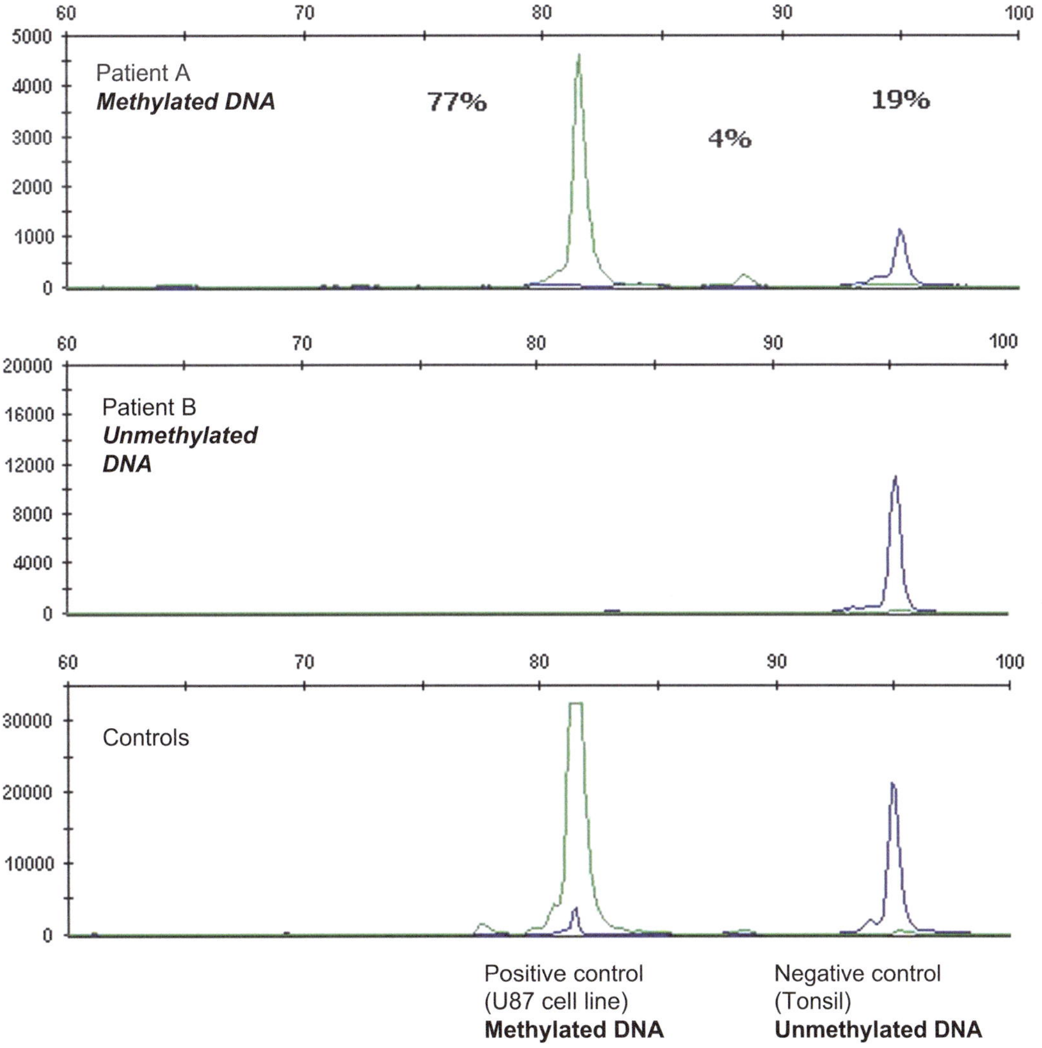

Fig. 2.4 O^6-methylguanine-DNA methyltransferase (MGMT) promoter methylation status. The graphs represent the result of capillary gel electrophoresis after sodium bisulfite conversion and methylation-specific multiplex PCR. The DNA was extracted from FFPE (formalin-fixed paraffin-embedded) tumor tissue. The *upper panel* shows a patient whose tumor DNA is methylated, and the *middle panel* shows a different patient whose tumor DNA is unmethylated. The *bottom panel* shows the controls for reference

into uracil [47]. Other techniques, like methylation-specific multiplex ligation-dependent probe amplification (MS-MLPA), combined bisulfite restriction analysis (COBRA), or methylation-specific high-resolution melting (HRM) analysis, are less commonly used [48, 49].

Role of Epidermal Growth Factor Receptor (EGFR) Pathway Aberrations

Malignant glial neoplasms, particularly glioblastomas, have been found to upregulate several growth factors and their receptors. The epidermal growth factor receptor (EGFR) gene at 7p12 has been described as the most frequently amplified and overexpressed gene in about 60% of glioblastomas and has been associated with shorter survival times. Further, about one-half of glioblastomas that overexpress wild-type EGFR also express EGFR mutant alleles, such as the EGFR variant III (EGFRvIII), which constitutes an 801-bp-in-frame deletion of exons 2–7 and leads to a truncated receptor protein that lacks the ligand-binding domain. This mutation ultimately leads to a constitutively activated EGFR-phosphoinositide 3-kinase pathway and appears to be unique to glial cells [50, 51].

The identification of EGFR amplifications and mutations, especially EGFRvIII, has been associated with poorer prognosis and in general are considered indicative of high-grade malignancy. However, the prognostic value of this information is somewhat ambiguous as several studies produced rather contradictory results. The EGFRvIII mutation, however, might be helpful in the identification of a subgroup of tumors with more malignant behavior than suggested by their histopathology alone. Further, gene expression profiling approaches for glioblastomas with EGFR amplifications enabled a subclassification of morphologically indistinguishable tumors based on their gene expression signatures [52].

Although EGFR pathway aberrations represent attractive therapeutic targets for molecular inhibition, the clinical benefits thus far have been rather disappointing. Attempts to impact tumor growth with the use of EGFR inhibitors, such as erlotinib and gefitinib, failed in spite of sufficient bioavailability and activity to dephosphorylate the EGFR in the tumor tissue. The overall progression-free survival was not prolonged, and only a subset of patients showed some response. Additional missense mutations have been identified in exons that encode extracellular EGFR domains, which appear to drive oncogenesis in vitro and potentially could convey sensitivity to small molecule tyrosine kinase inhibitors [53].

In general, a network of complex and redundant signal transduction pathways that bridge cell surface bound epidermal growth factor receptors with its oncogenic effects in the nucleus likely prevents rather simplistic therapeutic approaches from being successful. In addition, glioblastoma cells often show activation of multiple growth factor pathways, suggesting that a panel of targeting drugs might be necessary to interfere with tumor growth. At this stage, assessments of EGFR signaling pathways for glioblastomas is academically interesting, but clinically not indicated due to a lack of standard drug regimens that specifically target these pathways.

The characterization of EGFR amplification in glioblastoma is typically based on the detection of double-minute chromosomes, which are small fragments of extrachromosomal DNA by fluorescent in situ hybridization (FISH) (Fig. 2.3b). Other techniques such as real-time PCR and MLPA are also used to identify EGFR amplification. MLPA may also detect EGFRvIII rearrangement in EGFR-amplified tumors but appears to be less sensitive.

Diffuse Midline Glioma

Diffuse Midline Glioma is a high-grade glioma with predominantly astrocytic differentiation (Fig. 2.2d), which is mainly seen in children, but can also occur in young adults [3]. The most common locations are brain stem, thalamus, and spinal cord. The diffuse midline glioma was previously known as 'brain stem glioma' and 'diffuse intrinsic pontine glioma (DIPG)'. Histologically, it shows divergent patterns. Approximately, 10% of cases have a histologically low-grade appearance, whereas the remainder is of higher grade with features of anaplasia such as mitoses, vascular proliferation, and necrosis [54]. Sequencing studies have demonstrated that diffuse midline gliomas typically carry the H3F3A K27M mutation, which correlates with poor prognosis independent of histologic grade. Consequently, the K27M-mutated diffuse midline gliomas are now introduced as a separate entity in the WHO 2016 classification [55, 56].

Ependymal Tumors

Ependymomas are defined as slowly growing glial neoplasms, which can arise anywhere along the walls of the cerebral ventricles or within the spinal canal. The group of ependymal tumors is comprised of the classic ependymoma (plus variants) and anaplastic ependymoma (malignant variant). The benign variants subependymoma and myxopapillary ependymoma will not be discussed in this chapter.

Ependymomas (Fig. 2.2f) account for approximately 5–6% of all gliomas, and for 2.5% of all primary intracranial neoplasms in adults. In children below 14 years, these tumors play a significant role and form about 7–8% of all primary intracranial neoplasms with an adjusted annual incidence rate of 5–6 per 1 million individuals [15]. Overall, ependymomas are the third most common pediatric tumor after astrocytomas and medulloblastomas. Ependymomas can develop at any age; however, there are two distinct incidence peaks: one in children before the age of 14 years and a second one in adults between 35 and 45 years. These tumors can arise anywhere along the ventricular system within brain and spinal canal, but approximately 60% of lesions are located in the 4th ventricle, particularly in pediatric patients. In the spinal cord, it is the most common type of glial neoplasm affecting adults. Males are in general slightly more affected than females.

Morphologically, classic ependymomas are composed of a relatively monotonous population of cells, which tend to form characteristic rosette-like structures, so-called perivascular pseudo-rosettes and ependymal rosettes that have been recognized as diagnostic hallmark features (Fig. 2.4). Recent studies suggest that they might arise from radial glial cells [57].

The WHO classification [3] separates ependymal tumors into three grades, whereby subependymoma and myxopapillary ependymoma correspond to WHO grade I, and classic ependymoma and related variants (cellular, papillary, clear cell, and tanycytic ependymoma) correspond to WHO grade II, and anaplastic ependymomas are WHO grade III.

Anaplastic ependymomas are the malignant variant of classic ependymomas, characterized by high cell density, high mitotic activity, microvascular proliferation, and necrosis. Anaplastic ependymomas are associated with rapid disease progression and unfavorable outcome.

Molecular Profiles of Ependymal Tumors

Until recently, there was very limited information of molecular pathogenesis of ependymal tumors. Frequent NF2 gene mutations and chromosome arm 22q deletion had been described in spinal intramedullary ependymomas [58]. Recent studies led to the discovery of a highly recurrent fusion gene involving the NF-kB downstream intermediate transcription factor p65 (RELA) and an anonymous gene (C11 or f95) in a significant number of supratentorial ependymomas [59, 60]. These RELA fusion-positive supratentorial ependymomas are associated with unfavorable prognosis and form a new entity in the WHO classification of 2016.

A smaller subgroup of supratentorial ependymomas is characterized by gene fusions involving the YES-associated protein 1 gene (YAP1). DNA methylation profiling revealed further subtypes in an evolving field [61].

Disclosures Anita Huttner has no relationship with any commercial company that has a direct financial interest in the subject matter or the materials discussed in the article or with any company making a competing product.

References

1. Louis DN, et al. The 2007 WHO classification of tumours of the central nervous system. Acta Neuropathol. 2007;114(2):97–109.
2. Louis DN, et al. International Society Of Neuropathology-Haarlem consensus guidelines for nervous system tumor classification and grading. Brain Pathol. 2014;24(5):429–35.
3. Louis DN, et al. The 2016 World Health Organization classification of tumors of the central nervous system: a summary. Acta Neuropathol. 2016;131 (6):803–20.
4. Bailey P, Cushing H. A classification of the tumors of the glima group on a histogenetic basis with a correlated study of prognosis. JB Lippincott, 1928.
5. Scheithauer BW. Development of the WHO classification of tumors of the central nervous system: a historical perspective. Brain Pathol. 2009;19(4):551–64.
6. Scheithauer BW, Fuller GN, VandenBerg SR. The 2007 WHO classification of tumors of the nervous system: controversies in surgical neuropathology. Brain Pathol. 2008;18(3):307–16.
7. van den Bent MJ. Interobserver variation of the histopathological diagnosis in clinical trials on glioma: a clinician's perspective. Acta Neuropathol. 2010;120(3):297–304.
8. Suzuki H, et al. Mutational landscape and clonal architecture in grade II and III gliomas. Nat Genet. 2015;47(5):458–68.
9. Ceccarelli M, et al. Molecular profiling reveals biologically discrete subsets and pathways of progression in diffuse glioma. Cell. 2016;164(3):550–63.
10. Brat DJ, et al. Comprehensive, integrative genomic analysis of diffuse lower-grade gliomas. N Engl J Med. 2015;372(26):2481–98.
11. Brennan CW, et al. The somatic genomic landscape of glioblastoma. Cell. 2013;155(2):462–77.
12. Zou P, et al. IDH1/IDH2 mutations define the prognosis and molecular profiles of patients with gliomas: a meta-analysis. PLoS ONE. 2013;8(7): e68782.
13. Hartmann C, et al. Type and frequency of IDH1 and IDH2 mutations are related to astrocytic and oligodendroglial differentiation and age: a study of 1,010 diffuse gliomas. Acta Neuropathol. 2009;118 (4):469–74.
14. Peiffer J, Kleihues P. Hans-Joachim Scherer (1906–1945), pioneer in glioma research. Brain Pathol. 1999;9(2):241–5.
15. Ostrom QT, et al. CBTRUS Statistical Report: Primary Brain and Central Nervous System Tumors Diagnosed in the United States in 2008–2012. Neuro Oncol. 2015; 17 Suppl 4:iv1–62.
16. Herrlinger U, et al. Gliomatosis cerebri: no evidence for a separate brain tumor entity. Acta Neuropathol. 2016;131(2):309–19.
17. Sugimoto K, et al. Epithelioid/rhabdoid glioblastoma: a highly aggressive subtype of glioblastoma. Brain Tumor Pathol. 2016;33(2):137–46.
18. Sahm F, et al. Farewell to oligoastrocytoma: in situ molecular genetics favor classification as either oligodendroglioma or astrocytoma. Acta Neuropathol. 2014;128(4):551–9.
19. Xu W, et al. Oncometabolite 2-hydroxyglutarate is a competitive inhibitor of alpha-ketoglutarate-dependent dioxygenases. Cancer Cell. 2011;19 (1):17–30.
20. Lu C, et al. IDH mutation impairs histone demethylation and results in a block to cell differentiation. Nature. 2012;483(7390):474–8.
21. Turcan S, et al. IDH1 mutation is sufficient to establish the glioma hypermethylator phenotype. Nature. 2012;483(7390):479–83.
22. Noushmehr H, et al. Identification of a CpG island methylator phenotype that defines a distinct subgroup of glioma. Cancer Cell. 2010;17(5):510–22.
23. Sun W, Jelkmann W, Depping R. Prolyl-4-hydroxylase 2 enhances hypoxia-induced glioblastoma cell death by regulating the gene expression of hypoxia-inducible factor-alpha. Cell Death Dis. 2014;5:e1322.
24. Pistollato F, et al. Molecular mechanisms of HIF-1alpha modulation induced by oxygen tension and BMP2 in glioblastoma derived cells. PLoS ONE. 2009;4(7):e6206.
25. Molenaar RJ, et al. The driver and passenger effects of isocitrate dehydrogenase 1 and 2 mutations in oncogenesis and survival prolongation. Biochim Biophys Acta. 2014;1846(2):326–41.
26. Eckel-Passow JE, et al. Glioma groups based on 1p/19q, IDH, and TERT promoter mutations in tumors. N Engl J Med. 2015;372(26):2499–508.
27. Reuss DE, et al. ATRX and IDH1-R132H immunohistochemistry with subsequent copy number analysis and IDH sequencing as a basis for an "integrated" diagnostic approach for adult astrocytoma, oligodendroglioma and glioblastoma. Acta Neuropathol. 2015;129(1):133–46.
28. Liu XY, et al. Frequent ATRX mutations and loss of expression in adult diffuse astrocytic tumors carrying IDH1/IDH2 and TP53 mutations. Acta Neuropathol. 2012;124(5):615–25.
29. Hartmann C, et al. Patients with IDH1 wild type anaplastic astrocytomas exhibit worse prognosis than IDH1-mutated glioblastomas, and IDH1 mutation status accounts for the unfavorable prognostic effect of higher age: implications for classification of gliomas. Acta Neuropathol. 2010;120(6):707–18.
30. Camelo-Piragua S, et al. Mutant IDH1-specific immunohistochemistry distinguishes diffuse astrocytoma from astrocytosis. Acta Neuropathol. 2010;119 (4):509–11.
31. Olar A, et al. IDH mutation status and role of WHO grade and mitotic index in overall survival in grade II-III diffuse gliomas. Acta Neuropathol. 2015;129 (4):585–96.

32. Capper D, et al. Characterization of R132H mutation-specific IDH1 antibody binding in brain tumors. Brain Pathol. 2010;20(1):245–54.
33. Capper D, et al. Monoclonal antibody specific for IDH1 R132H mutation. Acta Neuropathol. 2009;118 (5):599–601.
34. Ohgaki H, Kleihues P. The definition of primary and secondary glioblastoma. Clin Cancer Res. 2013;19 (4):764–72.
35. Preusser M, Capper D, Hartmann C. IDH testing in diagnostic neuropathology: review and practical guideline article invited by the Euro-CNS research committee. Clin Neuropathol. 2011;30(5):217–30.
36. Tanboon J, Williams EA, Louis DN. The diagnostic use of immunohistochemical surrogates for signature molecular genetic alterations in gliomas. J Neuropathol Exp Neurol. 2016;75(1):4–18.
37. Smith JS, et al. Alterations of chromosome arms 1p and 19q as predictors of survival in oligodendrogliomas, astrocytomas, and mixed oligoastrocytomas. J Clin Oncol. 2000;18(3):636–45.
38. Jenkins RB, et al. A t(1;19)(q10;p10) mediates the combined deletions of 1p and 19q and predicts a better prognosis of patients with oligodendroglioma. Cancer Res. 2006;66(20):9852–61.
39. Wick W, et al. Temozolomide chemotherapy alone versus radiotherapy alone for malignant astrocytoma in the elderly: the NOA-08 randomised, phase 3 trial. Lancet Oncol. 2012;13(7):707–15.
40. Esteller M, et al. Inactivation of the DNA-repair gene MGMT and the clinical response of gliomas to alkylating agents. N Engl J Med. 2000;343 (19):1350–4.
41. Hegi ME, et al. MGMT gene silencing and benefit from temozolomide in glioblastoma. N Engl J Med. 2005;352(10):997–1003.
42. Stupp R, et al. Effects of radiotherapy with concomitant and adjuvant temozolomide versus radiotherapy alone on survival in glioblastoma in a randomised phase III study: 5-year analysis of the EORTC-NCIC trial. Lancet Oncol. 2009;10(5):459–66.
43. Gorlia T, et al. Nomograms for predicting survival of patients with newly diagnosed glioblastoma: prognostic factor analysis of EORTC and NCIC trial 26981-22981/CE.3. Lancet Oncol. 2008;9(1):29–38.
44. Brandes AA, et al. O(6)-methylguanine DNA-methyltransferase methylation status can change between first surgery for newly diagnosed glioblastoma and second surgery for recurrence: clinical implications. Neuro Oncol. 2010;12(3):283–8.
45. Wick W, et al. MGMT testing–the challenges for biomarker-based glioma treatment. Nat Rev Neurol. 2014;10(7):372–85.
46. Lalezari S, et al. Combined analysis of O6-methylguanine-DNA methyltransferase protein expression and promoter methylation provides optimized prognostication of glioblastoma outcome. Neuro Oncol. 2013;15(3):370–81.
47. Wiestler B, et al. Assessing CpG island methylator phenotype, 1p/19q codeletion, and MGMT promoter methylation from epigenome-wide data in the biomarker cohort of the NOA-04 trial. Neuro Oncol. 2014;16(12):1630–8.
48. Hsu CY, et al. Prognosis of glioblastoma with faint MGMT methylation-specific PCR product. J Neurooncol. 2015;122(1):179–88.
49. Xie H, Tubbs R, Yang B. Detection of MGMT promoter methylation in glioblastoma using pyrosequencing. Int J Clin Exp Pathol. 2015;8(1):636–42.
50. Furnari FB, et al. Heterogeneity of epidermal growth factor receptor signalling networks in glioblastoma. Nat Rev Cancer. 2015;15(5):302–10.
51. Gessi M, et al. High frequency of H3F3A (K27 M) mutations characterizes pediatric and adult high-grade gliomas of the spinal cord. Acta Neuropathol. 2015;130(3):435–7.
52. Pelloski CE, et al. Epidermal growth factor receptor variant III status defines clinically distinct subtypes of glioblastoma. J Clin Oncol. 2007;25(16):2288–94.
53. Vivanco I, et al. Differential sensitivity of glioma-versus lung cancer-specific EGFR mutations to EGFR kinase inhibitors. Cancer Discov. 2012;2 (5):458–71.
54. Solomon DA, et al. Diffuse midline gliomas with histone H3-K27M mutation: a series of 47 cases assessing the spectrum of morphologic variation and associated genetic alterations. Brain Pathol. 2016;26 (5):569–80.
55. Bechet D, et al. Specific detection of methionine 27 mutation in histone 3 variants (H3K27M) in fixed tissue from high-grade astrocytomas. Acta Neuropathol. 2014;128(5):733–41.
56. Ryall S, et al. Targeted detection of genetic alterations reveal the prognostic impact of H3K27M and MAPK pathway aberrations in paediatric thalamic glioma. Acta Neuropathol Commun. 2016;4(1):93.
57. Andreiuolo F, et al. Neuronal differentiation distinguishes supratentorial and infratentorial childhood ependymomas. Neuro Oncol. 2010;12(11):1126–34.
58. Ebert C, et al. Molecular genetic analysis of ependymal tumors. NF2 mutations and chromosome 22q loss occur preferentially in intramedullary spinal ependymomas. Am J Pathol. 1999;155(2):627–32.
59. Parker M, et al. C11orf95-RELA fusions drive oncogenic NF-kappaB signalling in ependymoma. Nature. 2014;506(7489):451–5.
60. Nambirajan A, et al. C11orf95-RELA fusion present in a primary intracranial extra-axial ependymoma: Report of a case with literature review. Neuropathology. 2016;36(5):490–5.
61. Pajtler KW, et al. Molecular Classification of Ependymal Tumors across All CNS Compartments, Histopathological Grades, and Age Groups. Cancer Cell. 2015;27(5):728–43.

3 Personalized Medicine Through Advanced Genomics

Mark W. Youngblood, E. Zeynep Erson-Omay and Murat Günel

Introduction

Advances in genomic technologies have revolutionized clinical approaches to the diagnosis and treatment of various disorders. Over the past decade, a drastic reduction in the cost and technical infrastructure needed for next-generation sequencing has enabled routine clinical testing at many large medical centers. Data from these studies are processed by bioinformatic teams, and the results are leveraged by the patient's physician to deliver precise molecular therapies with minimal morbidity. Multidisciplinary teams composed of geneticists, oncologists, pharmacologists, and other experts are often consulted to decide the optimal treatment for complex cases. Insights gained from these collaborations can have considerable impact on the course and quality of patient care. Cases that might previously remain undiagnosed can now be characterized using unbiased methods. Additionally, well-established diagnoses have also benefited from genomic analysis, often through subclassification that informs prognosis and effective treatment options.

The proliferation of next-generation sequencing has also benefited the research community, with rapid integration of this technique as a standard method of characterization. As a result, a growing body of genomic literature has described the pathologic effects of disease-causing genomic alterations, providing a crucial foundation for clinicians to draw upon when interpreting patient data. These studies have also directed commercial investment in promising molecular targets, increasing the arsenal of therapies available for precision medicine. The establishment of standard treatment protocols for the application of these medications remains an ongoing challenge that will be addressed over the coming years.

Among medical disciplines, cancer has particularly benefited from the proliferation of genomic techniques [1]. Large-cohort sequencing studies by consortiums such as The Cancer Genome Atlas (TCGA) (http://cancergenome.nih.gov/) and International Cancer Genome Consortium (ICGC) [2] (https://www.icgc.org/icgc) have described the molecular landscape of the most common tumor types [3], with others underway. Additionally, public resources such as the Catalogue of Somatic Mutations in Cancer (COSMIC) have compiled sequencing data from hundreds of studies into databases that are readily searchable [4]. In many cases, downstream studies have capitalized on these genomic findings by characterizing the molecular mechanisms involved in initiation and

M.W. Youngblood · E.Z. Erson-Omay · M. Günel (✉)
Department of Neurosurgery, Genetics and NeuroBiology, Yale School of Medicine, 333 Cedar St., Tompkins 4, New Haven, CT 06510, USA
e-mail: murat.gunel@yale.edu

J. Moliterno Günel et al. (eds.), *Malignant Brain Tumors*,
DOI 10.1007/978-3-319-49864-5_3

progression of cancer. These studies have reported targetable pathways that are frequently involved in multiple cancer types, leading some to suggest that genomic alterations could play an important role in the classification of tumors [5–7].

This chapter will discuss personalized medicine through the use of genomic techniques, focusing on the underlying technology that has created this new field as well as important studies that inform clinical decision-making. A series of recent studies will illustrate how this technology is being used to better understand disease mechanisms and ultimately guide treatment.

Advanced Genomic Technologies

Following the completion of the Human Genome Project in 2003, advances in technologies (such as short read sequencing) and computational methods (including alignment and assembly tools) started the era of "next-generation sequencing" (NGS) [8–10]. As NGS technologies evolved, the cost of sequencing an individual human genome dropped from ninety-five million dollars in 2001 to ten thousand dollars in 2011, and to close to a thousand dollars in 2015 [11] (Fig. 3.1). With the exponential cost decrease after 2008, sequencing individual genomes to better identify the genomic background of individual maladies, such as cancer, became a reality and paved the way for precision medicine.

Before looking in depth at how NGS technologies have improved our understanding of the complexity of cancer and made personalized treatments possible, we will review commonly used NGS techniques.

Whole-Genome Sequencing (WGS) and Whole-Exome Sequencing (WES)

The emergence of precision medicine is a direct result of technical advances in genomic sequencing platforms. While the human genome was largely assembled using automated Sanger technology (commonly referred to as "first generation") [12], this approach was incapable of scaling to provide personalized data in routine clinical practice. The emergence of next-generation approaches has drastically reduced the cost and complexity of genomic analysis, such that enormous amounts of data can now be acquired in a relatively short period of time. Due to the availability of several excellent review articles on this topic [13–15], we will give only a brief overview of the technical steps involved in exome and genome sequencing.

NGS technologies rely on massive parallelization of sequencing tasks, allowing for rapid collection of data that scales with increasing sample numbers. The process begins with library preparation, in which a patient sample is fragmented into smaller genomic regions that can be sequenced continuously. The optimal size of fragments varies based on sequencing platform (i.e., Illumina, Pacific Biosciences, and Solexa); however, longer reads are generally preferred to reduce ambiguities in bioinformatics analysis, such as alignment. Platform-specific, universal adaptors are ligated to the ends of each fragment that permit hybridization to a flow cell, a substrate upon which sequencing will take place. These adaptors also allow for amplification to create a localized colony of each fragment, which increase the signal during the sequencing stage. With the flow cell prepared, sequencing commences with the stepwise addition of labeled nucleotides to each colony. After addition of each base, an image snapshot of the flow cell is collected that will be assembled chronologically to infer the fragment's sequence. Because many colonies are imaged simultaneously, sequencing is performed in parallel and scale is only limited by the surface area and colony density of the flow cell. With the sequences collected, bioinformatics approaches are then used to align each read to its corresponding genomic region (further discussed below).

In exome sequencing, only the protein-coding region of the genome is sequenced (less than 2%), significantly reducing the expense of data

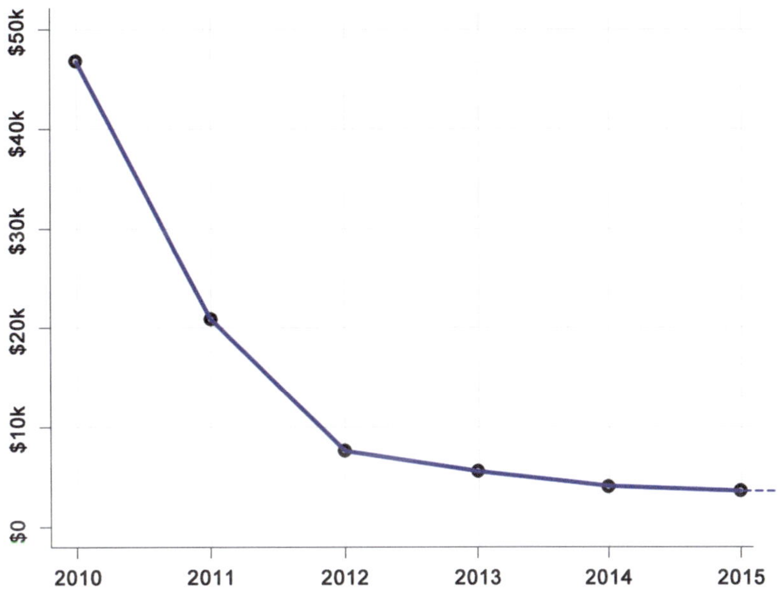

Fig. 3.1 Cost of sequencing a single human genome. Sequencing costs have fallen rapidly over the past five years as next-generation technologies become increasingly efficient. Graph is reproduced using data from the National Human Genome Research Institute [11]

acquisition and complexity of analysis [16]. The vast majority of human disease is driven by mutations in these regions, making this approach an efficient method for the detection of most pathogenic variants. From a technical standpoint, the biggest difference from whole-genome sequencing occurs during library preparation, in which an additional capture step is performed. This most often occurs through hybridization of adaptor-ligated fragments to biotinylated DNA baits, followed by selective pull-down, amplification, and sequencing [17]. Several commercially available kits provide bait coverage of the entire coding genome or selective regions, depending on the application.

Bioinformatic Analysis of NGS

Computational components of genomic data can be grouped into three stages: primary, secondary, and tertiary analyses [18] (Fig. 3.2). Primary analysis includes the conversion of raw image data captured from the flow cell in sequencing machines into human-readable representations of the input (i.e., sequences of nucleotides). A secondary analysis then compares this sequence to the reference genome, which was made available with the completion of the Human Genome Project. This step includes alignment of read sequences to the reference genome and identification of variations between the datasets, which represent possible disease-causing mutations. The alignment step tries to identify the genomic origin of each sequencing read; however, ambiguous alignments can sometimes occur in regions containing similar DNA sequences. Technologies that produce longer sequencing reads help to solve this problem by reducing ambiguity. Following the alignment step, variant calling identifies regions in the aligned read that differ from the reference genome, called mismatches. However, stochastic machine errors introduced during sequencing and image capture can introduce noise, which complicates this step. These kinds of errors are handled computationally by the use of redundancy in data, achieved by oversampling of the DNA [8]. Over the years, many programs have been developed for various components of the secondary analysis step, including quality control, alignment/assembly, and variant calling. Some of these tools are for specific technologies, such as CASAVA and ELAND for Illumina sequencing machines and Newbler/GS Reference Mapper for Roche/454 machines. However, it was the open access tools, providing standard and streamlined analysis of genomic and transcriptomic data, which paved the way for collaborative and large-scale studies such as TCGA and ICGC. Some of these tools include BWA [19], MAQ [20], and Bowtie [21] for short DNA sequence alignment, as well as toolsets such as SAMtools [22] and GATK [23] which create a streamlined analysis pipeline platform.

In tertiary analysis, variations identified in the secondary analysis step are analyzed individually to assess the biological impact and ultimately decide whether an alteration is disease-causing, specifically a driver event for cancer cases. Whether it is genomic or transcriptomic data, identification of a driver event is computationally and biologically a challenging step due to the large plethora of variations that are called in most studies. To overcome this challenge, information from various sources is aggregated to improve understanding of the impact of the alteration on disease biology. These annotation steps include evaluating the functionality of the genomic region in which the alteration occurs, by leveraging data from projects such as the Encyclopedia of DNA Elements project (ENCODE) [24] and the encyclopedia of genes and gene variants project (GENCODE) [25]. Additional annotations use computational prediction algorithms to assess the impact of an alteration on the DNA residue based on 3D structure of the protein, or the conservation of the amino acid residue where the alteration occurs [26, 27]. In addition to the structural and functional annotation schemes, the occurrence frequency of the alteration in healthy populations such as 1000 Genomes [28] and disease cohorts such as COSMIC [29] is also used to separate the disease-causing alterations from passenger alterations or noise. Once a set of candidate variations are identified by downstream bioinformatics analysis, the next step is the biological validation of the candidates and clinical interpretation that will ultimately lead the way to a precise treatment of the individual case.

Gene Expression Studies

Gene expression studies have provided insight on the molecular mechanisms underlying malignancy and aided in subclassification of seemingly homogeneous tumors into clinically distinct entities [30]. In this approach, messenger RNA (mRNA) is extracted and purified from a tumor sample and undergoes transcript quantification

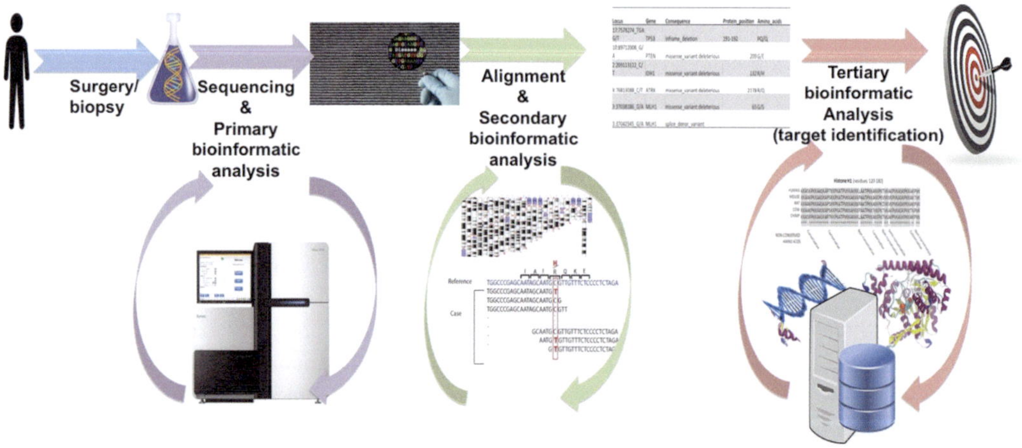

Fig. 3.2 Lifecycle of genomic analysis guided personalized medicine. Genomic or transcriptomic material extracted from each patient's tumor is sequenced in NGS machines to produce raw sequence data. Bioinformatic algorithms are used to align the raw data to the reference genome, and variations in each tumor are identified. Lastly, candidate alterations that may cause tumorogenesis are identified as targets and appropriate treatment regimens selected

using either expression microarray or RNA-sequencing (Fig. 3.3). In the former case, mRNA is washed over a substrate covered with complementary probes, with each probe emitting florescence that is proportional to the amount of RNA hybridized to it. The abundance of each transcript can then be calculated by measuring the signal of each probe [31]. In the case of RNA-sequencing, purified mRNA undergoes reverse transcription to produce a complementary DNA (cDNA) library. This library undergoes NGS, and the amount of reads that align to each gene is used to estimate the transcript's abundance. In both approaches, careful normalization must be performed to ensure that accurate comparisons can be made between samples. This is often performed with respect to the overall number of RNA-sequencing reads, as well as the size of each gene (i.e., larger genes are expected to have higher number of reads mapping to them).

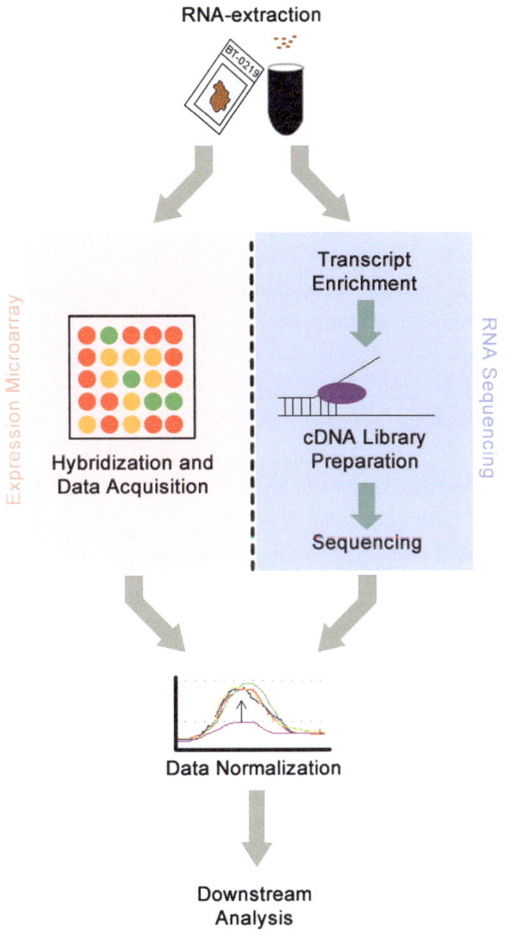

Fig. 3.3 Gene expression analysis pipeline. Gene expression analysis is most often performed using either expression microarray, or RNA-sequencing. Each technique offers benefits depending on the application and project goals

Proteomics

An emerging approach in precision medicine is the application of insights from systems biology to an individual's disease [32]. DNA-sequencing and gene expression studies give an indirect view of cellular activity, since they measure activity upstream of the molecular effectors. By providing a complete picture of the functional status within a cell, proteomics has become an important tool in personalized treatment. While technological approaches in protein quantification lag behind equivalent tools in RNA and DNA measurement, recent progress has been promising. The most widely used methods are based on mass spectrometry, in which ionized protein fragments are detected according to their mass and charge. In many cases, an additional selection technique such as chromatography is used to limit the spectrum of proteins that undergo detection. While assessment of the complete proteome remains a technical challenge, measuring the status and abundance of individual biomarkers can be a valuable tool for clinicians. One such example is prostate-specific antigen (PSA), which can be differentially detected in patients with prostate cancer using proteomic techniques [33]. The packaging of multiple biomarkers can also be used to construct an oncogenic signature that is detectable using patient serum. A previous study used this technique in combination with machine learning to achieve a positive predictive value of 94% for the detection of ovarian cancer [34].

Genomic Approaches to Personalized Medicine

Precision or personalized medicine, a concept that existed long before the emergence of NGS technologies, is defined as the prevention and treatment strategies developed based on an individual's biological and physiological variabilities [35]. With the application of NGS technologies, genomic variations that underlie disease mechanisms have been better characterized, leading the way to improved targeted treatments. Specifically for cancer, personalized treatment is the precise planning of treatment regimens based on the molecular, genomic, and transcriptomic profile of the individual tumor in addition to the pathological and physiological features.

Before the emergence of personalized medicine using NGS technologies, the first targeted cancer treatment developed for a specific genetic alteration was for chronic myelogenous leukemia (CML). Development of the drug imatinib, which targets the tyrosine kinase fusion protein BCR-ABL, has increased the 5-year survival for CML to 89% of patients [36]. This result ushered in a period of expectant optimism regarding the promise of targeted therapies, with many hoping that cancer might some day be eliminated using precision approaches. Unfortunately, most malignant cancer types, such as gliomas, have been found to be genomically heterogeneous, making treatments that target a single genetic alteration obsolete [37] (Fig. 3.4). The emergence of cost-effective genomic and transcriptomic profiling of tumors through NGS technologies helped to identify this complexity within most malignant cancer types, particularly in malignant tumors such as gliomas [38–40], medulloblastomas [41], and neuroblastomas [42] and also in more benign types such as meningiomas [43]. While these findings have diminished hope for a "silver bullet" to selectively melt away tumors, they have laid the groundwork for personalized combination targeted therapies that will increase survival.

Insights on Malignant Brain Tumors from Genomic Studies

As genomic tools have become increasingly accessible for clinical use, attention has shifted to developing protocols for interpretation of patient results. Until recently, the genomic landscape of many cancers was poorly described, leaving the significance of variants found in a clinical dataset unclear. However, global efforts over the past decade have elucidated the oncogenic drivers underlying most tumor types, including genetic mutations, changes in gene expression, chromatin accessibility, and other molecular features. These efforts have largely occurred through national or international consortiums that sequence hundreds of tumors from large patient populations. By comparing the genome of each tumor to a matching non-tumor sample from the same patient, researchers can identify genetic changes that may drive oncogenesis. The variant databases that are generated from these studies provide an invaluable resource for clinicians, allowing direct annotation of patient results with aggregated data from across the spectrum of cancer, such as COSMIC [4]. In addition to confirming the presence of known oncogenic variants, prognostic and therapeutic insights can also be gleaned by studying the clinical course of patients harboring similar mutations in previous studies. The availability of large-cohort genomic studies has provided critical context necessary to carry out personalized medicine.

This section will briefly review several genomic studies that have made seminal contributions to understanding the molecular drivers of brain tumors. The discussion is not intended to be an exhaustive list of identified mutations for each tumor type, but instead will focus on a small number of pathways identified by researchers that hold clinical promise. For almost all tumor types, excellent review articles are available that extensively describe the landscape of genomic findings (Table 3.1).

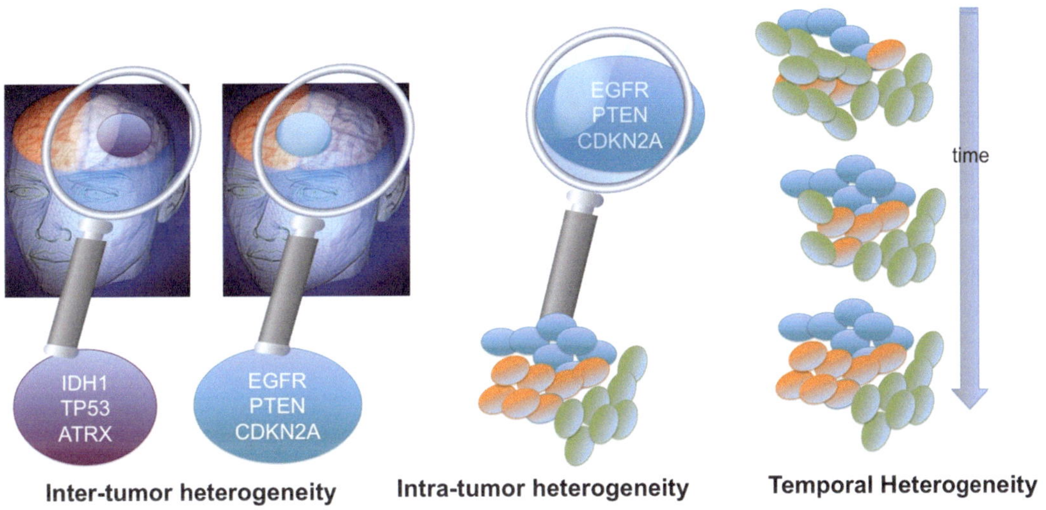

Fig. 3.4 Types of tumor heterogeneity. The presence of several forms of tumor heterogeneity makes treatment of malignant brain tumors a challenge. Schematics of inter-tumor heterogeneity, intra-tumor heterogeneity, and temporal heterogeneity are shown

Table 3.1 Common driver events associated with malignant brain tumors

Tumor type	Cell of origin	Driver events
Ependymoma	Radial glial cells [103]	*Spinal*: Chr7 amplification, Chr22 deletion, NF2 mutation [104], *Intracranial*: Chr1q amplification [105], genomic imbalance [106], CDKN2A deletion, C11orf95-RELA fusion [107] Epigenomic alterations with CIMP-positive [108]
Schwannoma	Schwann cells	Bi-allelic NF2 loss with Chr22 deletion and NF2 mutation [109]
Pituitary adenoma	Lactotroph Somatotroph Corticotroph Gonadotroph	*Prolactionoma*: Deletion of Chr 11p [110] *Acromegaly*: GNAS [111], GPR101 mutations [112] *Cushing syndrome*: USP8 mutation [113], PRKACA for ACTH independent cases [114] *Non-functioning adenomas*: Chr 9p deletion [115]
Meningioma	Arachnoid cap cells	Bi-allelic NF2 loss with Chr22 deletion and NF2 mutation, mutations in WD40 repeat region of TRAF7, DNA-binding domain of KLF4, activating mutations in PI3K, and sonic hedgehog signaling [67, 68]
Medulloblastoma	Cerebellar lineage	Activating mutations in WNT or SHH signaling [54–56], amplification of MYC and CDK6, and super-enhancer hijacking [116]
Glioblastoma	Glial lineage	*Primary GBM:* Dysregulation of RTK/Ras/PI3K signaling, p53, and Rb pathways [44, 117] *Secondary GBM:* Mutations in IDH1 with comutation of ATRX and TP53, or deletions in RB1, CDKN2A, and PTEN [52, 118, 119]

While considerable overlap exists in the molecular mechanisms underlying transformation, each tumor type also harbors unique genomic vulnerabilities based on its cell of origin and microenvironment

Glioblastoma Multiforme

Perhaps the best studied of malignant brain tumors is glioblastoma (GBM), which was selected by TCGA as the first type of cancer to undergo extensive genomic characterization [44]. While previous studies had uncovered recurrent genetic events in these tumors, their approaches were largely hypothesis-driven and therefore did not investigate the full landscape of GBM using unbiased methods. The TCGA study was notable for establishing a systematic framework for the characterization of tumors, including standardization of biospecimen collection and integration of data modalities to draw actionable conclusions. They reported on alterations in DNA copy number, gene expression, DNA methylation, and somatic variants in a total of 206 GBM samples. In addition to confirming several suspected pathways underlying GBM, they also identified an association between promoter methylation of the DNA-repair gene O-6-*Methylguanine-DNA Methyltransferase* (*MGMT*) and hypermutation in treated samples. Methylation of this gene was previously correlated with response to the alkylating agent temozolomide [45], and subsequent studies have established this event as an important biomarker for prognosis and therapeutic course [46].

Collectively, genomic studies of this tumor have led identification of numerous molecular targets as well as classification schemes. Based on gene expression studies, GBM can be divided into proneural, neural, classical, and mesenchymal subtypes, each with distinct mutational profiles [47, 48]. Genomic evidence, including specific marker expression patterns, has suggested that these subtypes may arise from distinct cellular origins, although a common neural stem cell hypothesis has also been proposed [49]. The classification of a patient's tumor may guide treatment decisions, as classical tumors tend to respond to aggressive therapy, while proneural tumors are often refractory. Altered expression and genomic events involving the epidermal growth factor receptor (*EGFR*) are associated with the classical subtype and are seen in a majority of cases. The most common variant in this gene involves deletion of exons 2–7 (termed "*EGFRvIII*"), which is a negative prognostic indicator in patients surviving greater than one year [50]. In addition to *EGFR* amplification, deletion of *p16INK4a* and mutations in the tumor suppressor phosphatase and tensin homolog (*PTEN*) are other common events seen in primary GBM. By contrast, secondary GBMs are associated with mutations in the gene *isocitrate dehydrogenase 1* (IDH1), with frequent comutation of *alpha-thalassemia/mental retardation syndrome, X-linked* (*ATRX*) or *tumor protein P53* (*TP53*) and deletion of *cyclin-dependent kinase inhibitor 2A* (*CDKN2A*), and *PTEN*, or *retinoblastoma 1* (*RB1*) [51].

In addition to GBM, other malignant gliomas such as anaplastic astrocytoma and oligodendroglioma have also been genomically characterized. *IDH1* mutations are common in these grade III tumors, which is consistent with their high prevalence in secondary GBMs. The malignant progression of oligodendroglioma, which initially harbors losses on chromosomes 1p and 19q as well as mutations in the growth regulators *capicua transcriptional repressor* (*CIC*) and *far upstream element binding protein 1* (*FUBP1*), may be propelled by the loss of *CDKN2A* and *PTEN* [52, 53]. As discussed above, malignant astrocytoma (including grade III lesions) is more likely to be driven by mutations in *ATRX* and *TP53*, in addition to Rb pathway mutations.

Medulloblastoma

Like glioma, medulloblastoma has undergone extensive genomic and transcriptomic characterization [54, 55]. These studies have led to the classification of medulloblastoma into four molecular subgroups, including WNT, SHH, Group 3, and Group 4. While the WNT and SHH subgroups harbor overactivity of their associated pathways, Group 3 and Group 4 tumors are characterized by MYC and CDK6 amplification, respectively. Importantly, each of these groups carries specific clinical and demographic features as well as implications for prognosis and therapeutic options. For example, WNT medulloblastomas are more commonly found in older children and are almost always of the classic histological subtype [56]. By contrast, SHH tumors often present during infancy and are associated with the desmoplastic subtype (although all histologies are possible in this group). Until recently, the major drivers of Group 3 and Group 4 subgroup medulloblastomas were mostly unknown, as there were only a few recurrent somatic mutations identified. This changed with the publication of a large whole-genome sequencing project that identified recurrent structural variations in 33% of Group 3 and 5–10% of Group 4 medulloblastomas, leading to the juxtaposition of the growth factor independent-1 family proto-oncogenes, GFI1 and GFI1B, with upstream *cis*-acting regulatory elements such as super-enhancers [57]. Such genomic structural alterations, defined as the super-enhancer hijacking, lead to overexpression of the proto-oncogenes, GFI1 and GFI1B, and were shown to be oncogenic in mouse models in the same study [57].

Importantly, medulloblastoma subgroups also carry prognostic implications, with Group 3 medulloblastomas having a particularly poor prognosis, while WNT tumors are relatively favorable [58]. Interestingly, genomic approaches have suggested that these subgroups may arise from different cells of origin in the cerebellum, perhaps explaining the differences in features and presentations [59, 60].

The identification of medulloblastoma subgroups has opened novel treatment approaches that target specific pathways. The most notable of these is the use of antagonists that block activation of the SHH pathway. Previous administration of the SMO inhibitor GDC-0449 in an adult patient with metastatic disease caused a rapid regression of the tumor; however, resistant clones soon arose and the tumor returned [61]. Clinical trials are ongoing for pharmaceuticals that block SHH, and this subgroup may be the first to benefit from routine targeted therapy [62]. Owing to the favorable prognosis of WNT-driven tumors, most attention has focused on the optimization of current treatment approaches (i.e., radiation, non-specific chemotherapy, and surgery). With continued characterization of Group 3 and Group 4 tumors, new genomic targets may become available in coming years.

Meningioma

For decades, the only genetic alteration associated with meningioma was biallelic loss of the tumor suppressor *neurofibromin 2* (*NF2*), which is found in approximately 50% of sporadic cases [63]. Prior to 2013, numerous studies had investigated the gene expression patterns and copy number events in these tumors or used candidate approaches to elucidate possible oncogenic mechanisms [64–66]. However, the recent use of unbiased methods has led to important insights about meningioma pathogenesis, identifying five pathways that are altered in over 80% of cases [67–69]. Besides *NF2* loss, exome sequencing of tumor–normal paired samples has revealed recurrent activating mutations in the PI3K signaling molecule *V-akt murine thymoma viral oncogene homolog 1* (*AKT1*) and sonic hedgehog (SHH) mediator *smoothened* (*SMO*). Additionally, mutations in genes not previously associated with cancer have been identified. Somatic mutations affecting the WD40-repeat domain of *TNF receptor-associated factor 7* (*TRAF7*) were found in approximately one-quarter of sporadic meningioma. Interestingly, these mutations frequently co-occur with either *AKT1* activating mutations, or a recurrent K409Q alteration in the DNA-binding domain of *Kruppel-like factor 4* (*KLF4*). *KLF4* is one of four Yamanaka factors sufficient to induce pluripotency from somatic cells [70]. Recent work has also identified recurrent mutations in the dock domain of RPB1, the largest and catalytic subunit of RNA polymerase II [69].

While activating mutations in PI3K and SHH signaling are involved in numerous forms of cancer, the mechanisms underlying other identified meningioma genes remain unclear. Downstream molecular studies, similar to those undertaken in glioma and medulloblastoma, will provide important insights over the coming years and may reveal pharmacologic targets. Despite the identification of genomic drivers in the vast majority of sporadic meningioma, the primary treatment modality remains neurosurgical excision. While this procedure is curative in most cases and carries relatively low risk, it is an invasive procedure that is not without complications [71]. Medical therapies for meningioma have been investigated previously, but this occurred prior to the identification of recurrent somatic events in these tumors and therefore targeted general candidate pathways [72, 73]. Higher-grade meningiomas (World Health Organization grades II and III) in particular may benefit from targeted therapies, as they are associated with aggressive features and carry relatively poor prognosis [74]. As the oncogenic mechanisms of *TRAF7*, *POLR2A*, and *KLF4* remain largely unknown, clinicians have focused on leveraging treatments from other tumor types to target the well-established PI3K and SHH pathways in meningioma. Notably, clinical trials have started for the treatment of recurrent meningiomas that harbor activating *SMO* mutations using SHH pathway inhibitors [75].

Tumor Heterogeneity and the Need for Personalized Approaches

As the cost of NGS exponentially dropped after 2008, further analysis of individual tumors with higher resolution revealed another level of complexity: intra-tumoral heterogeneity (Fig. 3.4). Heterogeneity within a single tumor is caused by the presence of different genetic alterations in distinct subclones that carry separate biological functions for the tumor to survive and proliferate [76]. The complexity caused by both intra- and inter-tumoral heterogeneity is sufficient to make the classic "one-size-fits-all" impractical for most patients. Therefore, detailed genomic characterization of individual tumors is essential to tailor the most effective treatment regimen, making the treatment personalized.

In this section, we will use a series of studies to depict why conventional one-size-fits-all approaches for cancer treatment have not been consistently successful in malignant brain tumors and how advanced genomic technologies promise to improve outcomes. We will specifically focus on the causes of treatment resistance, how these resistance mechanisms have been revealed with genomic technologies, and how genomic information can be utilized to overcome these mechanisms.

Gliomas, the most common malignant brain tumor, are an excellent model to discuss the clinical use of advanced genomics. Genomic data from this tumor have revealed the reasons for variability in not only the treatment response, but also for prognostic markers. Temozolomide (TMZ) is an alkylating chemotherapeutic agent commonly used in gliomas as a standard of care treatment. As discussed earlier, a prognostic marker in gliomas for assessing the response to TMZ treatment is the methylation status of the MGMT promoter region [77]. However, it has also been shown that prognostic value of this marker is dependent on the genomic background of the tumor, such as existence of an IDH1 mutation [78]. In another prognostic marker study, the tumors with mutant TP53 were shown to be less sensitive to TMZ treatment. Even though there are no other chemotherapy agents as effective as TMZ that can be used as an alternative in gliomas, it is clear that genomic profiling of individual tumor improves the prognostic assessment for each patient.

As detailed above, EGFR is one of the frequently altered genes in GBMs, either through mutation, rearrangement, alternative splicing, or amplification in 57% of all cases [38]. Since EGFR is also frequently altered in other cancer types, it has been intensely studied as a pharmacologic target using tyrosine kinase inhibitor (TKI), antibody-based therapies, immunotherapies, and RNA therapies. TKI studies resulted in the development of successful inhibitors for certain types of cancer, such as non-small lung cancer. In these patients, those receiving targeted treatment had a 1-year progression free survival rate of 42.9%, compared to 9.7% for patients receiving standard chemotherapy [79, 80]. However, similar trials targeting EGFR with agents such as gefitinib and erlotinib in gliomas have not been as promising [81, 82]. One of the reasons for this variability is the intra-tumor heterogeneity presented with other alterations that co-occur with EGFR in the same tumor.

Another reason may be the location of EGFR alterations in glioma, which occur primarily at extracellular sites of the protein. As opposed to the kinase domain mutations frequently observed in lung cancer, extracellular EGFR mutations such as A289V and EGFRvIII are more common in gliomas and are known to be resistant to kinase domain inhibitors such as erlotinib [83]. The most common EGFR mutation, EGFRvIII, is found in 50% EGFR-amplified tumors [84] and is known to create a constitutively active EGFR by forming a complex with STAT3 and activating downstream signaling [81]. It is also shown that EGFRvIII mutations create a different conformation than EGFR kinase domain mutations, leading to TKI resistance. There are, however, studies showing that certain extracellular domain mutations respond relatively better to second generation of EGFR inhibitors such as lapatinib [83], aimed at targeting the conformational change caused by the EGFRvIII mutation. Besides the TKIs, there are also immunotherapy approaches developed specifically for EGFRvIII mutations with promising results. A multicenter phase II trial using EGFRvIII peptides induced patient immune systems to target the tumor cells with this mutation, resulting in an improved overall survival of 26 months compared to 14 months with standard therapy [85].

The other reason for the failure of targeting EGFR mutations in gliomas is due to pathway redundancy created by the co-occurrence of other growth factor genes such as PDGFR and receptor tyrosine kinase mutations [81]. With such redundancy introduced by multiple hits in activating growth pathways, the use of a single-target treatment only leads to the selection of alternative clones, ultimately leading to treatment resistance. Indeed, the co-occurrence of multiple receptor tyrosine kinase mutations (EGFR, PDGFRA, and MET) in distinct subclones originating from a single founder clone was shown in 4.5% of GBMs in a study depicting the intra-tumoral heterogeneity of gliomas [86]. One of the alterations that frequently co-occur with EGFR mutation in gliomas is the loss of function alterations in PTEN (36% of all gliomas), which results in the activation of the PI3K/AKT/mTOR pathway downstream of EGFR. Interestingly, single-target treatments for EGFR have been shown to cause treatment resistance in cases where there are clones with PTEN phosphorylation (Y240) [87]. Therefore, even if the EGFR activation status is determined in a tumor, the mechanisms through which this activation occurs (amplification, EGFRvIII mutation, EGFR kinase domain mutation, etc.) and also other alterations that co-occur with EGFR activation should be considered when designing personalized therapies.

Another factor introducing complexity to the management of malignant tumors is related to the temporal evolution of tumors under the pressure of treatment and progression (Fig. 3.4). Tumors with increased heterogeneity may evolve by selection of a subclone during a targeted treatment, leading to a completely new genomic profile of the relapsed or progressed tumor compared to the primary tumor. Indeed, it has been shown that IDH1 mutant gliomas evolve and progress to high grade through acquiring new genetic and epigenetic alterations on MYC, RTK/RAS/PI3K pathways and FOXM1/EZH2-mediated cell cycle transitions [88]. Interestingly, a nonlinear progression pattern has been observed, whereby mutations on certain genes such as CIC and TP53 are lost and replaced by new mutations on these genes during progression. This shows the dynamic potential of progression. Since longitudinal analyses display immense heterogeneity, it is also expected to see heterogeneity topologically within tumors. This is confirmed in a related study investigating specimens from different sections of primary and recurrent gliomas, which demonstrated intra-tumoral heterogeneity in genomic mutations [89]. By comparing information from multiple regions of the primary and recurrent tumors, two distinct models for tumor evolution (linear and nonlinear) were observed in this study. In the linear model, the recurrent tumors evolved from a founding clone that can be traced to a specific sector in the primary tumor by gaining additional mutations. In the cases displaying a nonlinear evolution model, however, the recurrent tumor emerged from an early branch in the primary tumor and shared very few alterations with the primary tumor and its clones. Similar phenomenon of topologic genomic heterogeneity has been shown with deep sequencing techniques in other various solid tumors such as prostate cancer [90] and non-small cell lung cancer [91]. Moreover, in a study investigating the genomic profiles of various primary tumors and their brain metastases, a similar pattern was also observed. This study presented the branching evolution of the primary tumor into the metastatic tumor by gaining new alterations in addition to the founding clone. Strikingly, 53% of cases presented potentially targetable alterations in the brain metastasis, which were not observed in the matching primary tumor [92].

In addition to glioma, clonal separation is also observed in metastatic medulloblastomas, despite a long-held belief that primary and metastatic tumors were biologically very similar. Recent work has shown in both human cases and mouse models that metastatic tumors can emerge from a subclone in the primary tumor and gain additional genetic alterations. To test the impact of this clonal separation on therapy, a previous study compared therapeutic responses in primary and matching metastatic tissues. Interestingly, the results showed different response measures between primary and metastatic tumors in 58% of cases (however, the authors stated that there might be different exposure rates between both tissues) [93]. Genomic responses to therapy have also been recorded in human medulloblastoma cases. A previous case report described the treatment of a *PTCH1*-mutated SHH-driven tumor using the *SMO* inhibitor GDC-0449. Even though the tumor initially showed remission, the disease progressed after 3 months. Interestingly, upon genomic analysis of the recurred tumor, a new somatic mutation was found in *SMO* that blocked the therapeutic effect of GDC-0449 [94]. In a more comprehensive study, the genomic profile of primary and recurrent medulloblastomas was analyzed both in human samples and in murine models. This work found that only 12 and 5% of genetic events were preserved in recurrent tumor that was observed in the primary tumor, in human samples, and in murine models, respectively [95].

Besides intra-tumoral heterogeneity that is observed temporally or topologically, another component causing heterogeneity in malignant brain tumors may be related to the cancer stem cell (CSC) hypothesis. In this theory, a subset of cells with long-term growth potential gives rise to more differentiated, progenitor cells with limited proliferation potential, similar to the classic stem cell paradigm. This hypothesis can be extrapolated to explain to the clonal evolution of tumors leading to heterogeneity [96]. To support the CSC hypothesis, the neural stem cell marker CD133 is found to be strongly correlated with tumor initiation and resistance to radiotherapy in gliomas [97]. It is also known that similar to normal stem cells, CSCs depend on a specific microenvironment where the signals and nourishment requirements are satisfied. Specifically, CSCs leading to brain tumors are located in subgranular and subventricular zones where these requirements can be supplied [98].When all these attributes of CSC hypothesis are analyzed, it is clear that the CSCs and their ability to create new cancer progenitor cells, together with their dependence to microenvironment, should be addressed for successful targeted treatments. Therefore, targeted treatments designed for CSCs must have multiple facets, such as targeting the surface markers (such as CD133), microenvironment elements, and downstream biological pathways such as Notch, AKT, Hedgehog, Wnt, and NF-KB [99].

These studies, which reveal multiple mechanisms of genomic heterogeneity and tumor plasticity, largely explain the varying response rates of standard and targeted treatments. Therefore, personalized treatments for malignant brain tumors should consider (i) intra-tumoral heterogeneity where multiple targets must be addressed, (ii) temporal heterogeneity where selective pressure of treatment or progression affects and alters the genomic profile of the tumor, and also (iii) the CSC-like structure where new resistant clones are continuously being generated. Hence, not only do genomic profiles of individual tumors need to be analyzed, but repeated profiling should also be performed upon progression and recurrence. Only with detailed longitudinal data produced by advanced genomic technologies can more successful personalized treatments be realized based on adaptive regimens.

Future Directions and Challenges

As our genomic understanding of cancer continues to grow, it has become clear that the molecular events underlying tumor biology are more complex than we previously imagined. We have long abandoned the idea that a single tumor profile can be informative across all types of cancer, nor can a single agent be efficacious in all cases. It is this insight that has necessitated the development of precision treatment approaches. Years of detailed genomic profiling of individual tumors have revealed that there are often multiple oncogenic clones within even a single tumor, such that adequate treatment requires high-resolution profiling and organization of a personalized regimen.

Despite recent advances, there remains room for improvement in the technical and clinical foundations of precision medicine. Current NGS technologies such as whole-exome and whole-genome sequencing use bulk DNA as input, which is useful to assess the overall genomic profile of individual tumors. However, even if applying deeper sequencing increases the resolution (i.e., through increased data redundancy), critical information about subclones can be lost due to pooling of all DNA from a tumor. Therefore, recent advances in single-cell DNA/RNA-sequencing technologies stand as promising technologies. Although still in development, preliminary studies have demonstrated the potential to better resolve and understand intra-tumor heterogeneity at cell-level resolution. For example, a population-based single-cell study of GBM found that seemingly coexisting alterations of EGFR were in fact mutually exclusive in distinct clones of cells [100]. This finding suggests the idea that there are actually many tumors within a single lesion [76], emphasizing the importance of high-resolution genomic profiling for personalized treatments.

Another challenge facing precision medicine is the emergence of treatment-resistant clones within a tumor, effectively making it a moving target. As presented above, there are mainly two paths for therapeutic resistance: selection of a preexisting clone that is resistant to the treatment and de novo formation of treatment-resistant genetic alterations in new clones. There have been many studies concerning the selection of preexisting clones; however, a recent study not only showed the possibility of de novo mutations causing resistance during treatment, but also demonstrated that the two paths to drug resistance have different mechanisms [101]. The dynamic nature of clonal evolution has been demonstrated repeatedly in longitudinal studies of treated tumors. In one interesting study, extrachromosomal DNA amplicons harboring EGFRvIII alterations in GBMs were treated with the tyrosine kinase inhibitor erlotinib. While the clones with EGFRvIII were lost during treatment, EGFRvIII-mutated clones re-emerged and reached the original ratio upon removal of the drug [102]. Such biologic and mechanistic variations in resistance will require dynamic treatment regimens, introducing another challenge for personalized treatments.

Ongoing technical and bioinformatic studies will tackle these challenges in the coming years. In the meantime, the role of precision approaches will continue to grow in the treatment of brain tumors. As our understanding of the molecular pathways underlying these lesions becomes more complete, we expect to see new generations of targeted pharmaceuticals that leverage genomic insights. The combination of increasingly sophisticated genomic analyses, development of efficient clinical paradigms for interpreting patient results, and availability of targeted medications will provide optimal therapy for the treatment of malignant brain tumors.

References

1. Feero WG, Guttmacher AE, McDermott U, Downing JR, Stratton MR. Genomics and the continuum of cancer care. N Engl J Med. 2011;364(4):340–50.

2. International network of cancer genome projects. Nature. 2010;464(7291):993–8.
3. Weinstein JN, Collisson EA, Mills GB, Shaw KRM, Ozenberger BA, Ellrott K, et al. The cancer genome atlas pan-cancer analysis project. Nat Genet. 2013;45(10):1113–20.
4. Forbes SA, Bindal N, Bamford S, Cole C, Kok CY, Beare D, et al. COSMIC: mining complete cancer genomes in the catalogue of somatic mutations in cancer. Nucleic Acid Res. 2010:gkq929.
5. Song Q, Merajver SD, Li JZ. Cancer classification in the genomic era: five contemporary problems. Hum Genomics. 2015;9(1):1.
6. Bunn PA, Franklin W, Doebele RC. The evolution of tumor classification: a role for genomics? Cancer Cell. 2013;24(6):693–4.
7. Weigelt B, Horlings HM, Kreike B, Hayes MM, Hauptmann M, Wessels LF, et al. Refinement of breast cancer classification by molecular characterization of histological special types. J Pathol. 2008;216(2):141–50.
8. Meyerson M, Gabriel S, Getz G. Advances in understanding cancer genomes through second-generation sequencing. Nat Rev Genet. 2010;11(10):685–96.
9. Shendure J, Ji H. Next-generation DNA sequencing. Nat Biotech. 2008;26(10):1135–45.
10. Metzker ML. Sequencing technologies [mdash] the next generation. Nat Rev Genet. 2010;11(1):31–46.
11. NHGRI. DNA sequencing costs: data 2016 Available from: https://www.genome.gov/sequencingcosts.
12. Consortium IHGS. Finishing the euchromatic sequence of the human genome. Nature. 2004;431(7011):931–45.
13. Metzker ML. Sequencing technologies—the next generation. Nat Rev Genet. 2010;11(1):31–46.
14. Mardis ER. Next-generation DNA sequencing methods. Annu Rev Genomics Hum Genet. 2008;9:387–402.
15. Shendure J, Ji H. Next-generation DNA sequencing. Nat Biotechnol. 2008;26(10):1135–45.
16. Mamanova L, Coffey AJ, Scott CE, Kozarewa I, Turner EH, Kumar A, et al. Target-enrichment strategies for next-generation sequencing. Nat Methods. 2010;7(2):111–8.
17. Bamshad MJ, Ng SB, Bigham AW, Tabor HK, Emond MJ, Nickerson DA, et al. Exome sequencing as a tool for Mendelian disease gene discovery. Nat Rev Genet. 2011;12(11):745–55.
18. Moorthie S, Hall A, Wright CF. Informatics and clinical genome sequencing: opening the black box. Genet Med. 2013;15(3):165–71.
19. Li H, Durbin R. Fast and accurate short read alignment with Burrows-Wheeler transform. Bioinformatics. 2009;25(14):1754–60.
20. Li H, Ruan J, Durbin R. Mapping short DNA sequencing reads and calling variants using mapping quality scores. Genome Res. 2008;18(11):1851–8.
21. Langmead B, Trapnell C, Pop M, Salzberg SL. Ultrafast and memory-efficient alignment of short DNA sequences to the human genome. Genome Biol. 2009;10(3):1–10.
22. Li H, Handsaker B, Wysoker A, Fennell T, Ruan J, Homer N, et al. The sequence alignment/map format and SAMtools. Bioinformatics. 2009;25(16):2078–9.
23. McKenna A, Hanna M, Banks E, Sivachenko A, Cibulskis K, Kernytsky A, et al. The genome analysis toolkit: a MapReduce framework for analyzing next-generation DNA sequencing data. Genome Res. 2010;20(9):1297–303.
24. The EPC. A user's guide to the encyclopedia of DNA elements (ENCODE). PLoS Biol. 2011;9(4):e1001046.
25. Harrow J, Denoeud F, Frankish A, Reymond A, Chen C-K, Chrast J, et al. GENCODE: producing a reference annotation for ENCODE. Genome Biol. 2006;7(Suppl. 1):S4.1–9.
26. Adzhubei IA, Schmidt S, Peshkin L, Ramensky VE, Gerasimova A, Bork P, et al. A method and server for predicting damaging missense mutations. Nat Methods. 2010;7(4):248–9.
27. Kumar P, Henikoff S, Ng PC. Predicting the effects of coding non-synonymous variants on protein function using the SIFT algorithm. Nat Protoc. 2009;4(7):1073–81.
28. The Genomes Project C. A global reference for human genetic variation. Nature. 2015;526(7571):68–74.
29. Forbes SA, Beare D, Gunasekaran P, Leung K, Bindal N, Boutselakis H, et al. COSMIC: exploring the world's knowledge of somatic mutations in human cancer. Nucleic Acids Res. 2015;43(D1):D805–11.
30. Golub TR, Slonim DK, Tamayo P, Huard C, Gaasenbeek M, Mesirov JP, et al. Molecular classification of cancer: class discovery and class prediction by gene expression monitoring. Science. 1999;286(5439):531–7.
31. Slonim DK, Yanai I. Getting started in gene expression microarray analysis. PLoS Comput Biol. 2009;5(10):e1000543.
32. Weston AD, Hood L. Systems biology, proteomics, and the future of health care: toward predictive, preventative, and personalized medicine. J Proteome Res. 2004;3(2):179–96.
33. Wu G, Datar RH, Hansen KM, Thundat T, Cote RJ, Majumdar A. Bioassay of prostate-specific antigen (PSA) using microcantilevers. Nat Biotechnol. 2001;19(9):856–60.
34. Petricoin EF, Ardekani AM, Hitt BA, Levine PJ, Fusaro VA, Steinberg SM, et al. Use of proteomic patterns in serum to identify ovarian cancer. Lancet (London, England). 2002;359(9306):572–7.
35. Collins FS, Varmus H. A new initiative on precision medicine. N Engl J Med. 2015;372(9):793–5.
36. Druker BJ, Guilhot F, O'Brien SG, Gathmann I, Kantarjian H, Gattermann N, et al. Five-year

follow-up of patients receiving imatinib for chronic myeloid leukemia. N Engl J Med. 2006;355 (23):2408–17.

37. Ene CI, Holland EC. Personalized medicine for gliomas. Surg Neurol Int. 2015;6(Suppl. 1):S89–95.
38. Brennan Cameron W, Verhaak Roel GW, McKenna A, Campos B, Noushmehr H, Salama Sofie R, et al. The somatic genomic landscape of glioblastoma. Cell.155(2):462–77.
39. Comprehensive genomic characterization defines human glioblastoma genes and core pathways. Nature. 2008;455(7216):1061–8.
40. Verhaak RGW, Hoadley KA, Purdom E, Wang V, Qi Y, Wilkerson MD, et al. Integrated genomic analysis identifies clinically relevant subtypes of glioblastoma characterized by abnormalities in PDGFRA, IDH1, EGFR, and NF1. Cancer Cell. 2010;17(1):98–110.
41. Taylor MD, Northcott PA, Korshunov A, Remke M, Cho Y-J, Clifford SC, et al. Molecular subgroups of medulloblastoma: the current consensus. Acta Neuropathol. 2012;123(4):465–72.
42. Pugh TJ, Morozova O, Attiyeh EF, Asgharzadeh S, Wei JS, Auclair D, et al. The genetic landscape of high-risk neuroblastoma. Nat Genet. 2013;45 (3):279–84.
43. Clark VE, Erson-Omay EZ, Serin A, Yin J, Cotney J, Özduman K, et al. Genomic analysis of non-NF2 meningiomas reveals mutations in TRAF7, KLF4, AKT1, and SMO. Science. 2013;339(6123):1077–80.
44. McLendon R, Friedman A, Bigner D, Van Meir EG, Brat DJ, Mastrogianakis GM, et al. Comprehensive genomic characterization defines human glioblastoma genes and core pathways. Nature. 2008;455(7216):1061–8.
45. Hegi ME, Diserens A-C, Gorlia T, Hamou M-F, de Tribolet N, Weller M, et al. MGMT gene silencing and benefit from temozolomide in glioblastoma. N Engl J Med. 2005;352(10):997–1003.
46. Thon N, Kreth S, Kreth F-W. Personalized treatment strategies in glioblastoma: MGMT promoter methylation status. Onco Targets Ther. 2013;6:1363–72.
47. Verhaak RG, Hoadley KA, Purdom E, Wang V, Qi Y, Wilkerson MD, et al. Integrated genomic analysis identifies clinically relevant subtypes of glioblastoma characterized by abnormalities in PDGFRA, IDH1, EGFR, and NF1. Cancer Cell. 2010;17(1):98–110.
48. Mischel PS, Shai R, Shi T, Horvath S, Lu KV, Choe G, et al. Identification of molecular subtypes of glioblastoma by gene expression profiling. Oncogene. 2003;22(15):2361–73.
49. Galli R, Binda E, Orfanelli U, Cipelletti B, Gritti A, De Vitis S, et al. Isolation and characterization of tumorigenic, stem-like neural precursors from human glioblastoma. Cancer Res. 2004;64 (19):7011–21.
50. Heimberger AB, Hlatky R, Suki D, Yang D, Weinberg J, Gilbert M, et al. Prognostic effect of epidermal growth factor receptor and EGFRvIII in glioblastoma multiforme patients. Clin Cancer Res. 2005;11(4):1462–6.
51. Ohgaki H, Kleihues P. Genetic pathways to primary and secondary glioblastoma. Am J Pathol. 2007;170 (5):1445–53.
52. Jiao Y, Killela PJ, Reitman ZJ, Rasheed BA, Heaphy CM, de Wilde RF, et al. Frequent ATRX, CIC, FUBP1 and IDH1 mutations refine the classification of malignant gliomas. Oncotarget. 2012;3 (7):709–22.
53. Reifenberger J, Reifenberger G, Liu L, James CD, Wechsler W, Collins VP. Molecular genetic analysis of oligodendroglial tumors shows preferential allelic deletions on 19q and 1p. Am J Pathol. 1994;145(5):1175.
54. Thompson MC, Fuller C, Hogg TL, Dalton J, Finkelstein D, Lau CC, et al. Genomics identifies medulloblastoma subgroups that are enriched for specific genetic alterations. J Clin Oncol. 2006;24 (12):1924–31.
55. Northcott PA, Shih DJ, Peacock J, Garzia L, Morrissy AS, Zichner T, et al. Subgroup-specific structural variation across 1000 medulloblastoma genomes. Nature. 2012;488(7409):49–56.
56. Northcott PA, Korshunov A, Pfister SM, Taylor MD. The clinical implications of medulloblastoma subgroups. Nat Rev Neurol. 2012;8(6):340–51.
57. Northcott PA, Lee C, Zichner T, Stutz AM, Erkek S, Kawauchi D, et al. Enhancer hijacking activates GFI1 family oncogenes in medulloblastoma. Nature. 2014;511(7510):428–34.
58. Clifford SC, Lusher ME, Lindsey JC, Langdon JA, Gilbertson RJ, Straughton D, et al. Wnt/wingless pathway activation and chromosome 6 loss characterise a distinct molecular sub-group of medulloblastomas associated with a favourable prognosis. Cell Cycle. 2006;5(22):2666–70.
59. Lin CY, Erkek S, Tong Y, Yin L, Federation AJ, Zapatka M, et al. Active medulloblastoma enhancers reveal subgroup-specific cellular origins. Nature. 2016.
60. Gibson P, Tong Y, Robinson G, Thompson MC, Currle DS, Eden C, et al. Subtypes of medulloblastoma have distinct developmental origins. Nature. 2010;468(7327):1095–9.
61. Rudin CM, Hann CL, Laterra J, Yauch RL, Callahan CA, Fu L, et al. Treatment of medulloblastoma with hedgehog pathway inhibitor GDC-0449. New Engl J Med. 2009;361(12):1173–8.
62. Low JA, de Sauvage FJ. Clinical experience with Hedgehog pathway inhibitors. J Clin Oncol. 2010;28(36):5321–6.
63. Ruttledge MH, Sarrazin J, Rangaratnam S, Phelan CM, Twist E, Merel P, et al. Evidence for the complete inactivation of the NF2 gene in the

majority of sporadic meningiomas. Nat Genet. 1994;6(2):180–4.
64. Arslantas A, Artan S, Oner U, Durmaz R, Muslumanoglu H, Atasoy MA, et al. Comparative genomic hybridization analysis of genomic alterations in benign, atypical and anaplastic meningiomas. Acta Neurol Belg. 2002;102(2):53–62.
65. Carlson KM, Bruder C, Nordenskjöld M, Dumanski JP. 1p and 3p deletions in meningiomas without detectable aberrations of chromosome 22 identified by comparative genomic hybridization. Genes Chromosom Cancer. 1997;20(4):419–24.
66. Lee Y, Liu J, Patel S, Cloughesy T, Lai A, Farooqi H, et al. Genomic landscape of meningiomas. Brain Pathol. 2010;20(4):751–62.
67. Clark VE, Erson-Omay EZ, Serin A, Yin J, Cotney J, Özduman K, et al. Genomic analysis of non-NF2 meningiomas reveals mutations in TRAF7, KLF4, AKT1, and SMO. Science. 2013;339(6123):1077–80.
68. Brastianos PK, Horowitz PM, Santagata S, Jones RT, McKenna A, Getz G, et al. Genomic sequencing of meningiomas identifies oncogenic SMO and AKT1 mutations. Nat Genet. 2013;45 (3):285–9.
69. Clark VE, Harmancı AS, Bai H, Youngblood MW, Lee TI, Baranoski JF, et al. Recurrent somatic mutations in POLR2A define a distinct subset of meningiomas. Nat Genet. 2016.
70. Takahashi K, Yamanaka S. Induction of pluripotent stem cells from mouse embryonic and adult fibroblast cultures by defined factors. Cell. 2006;126 (4):663–76.
71. van Alkemade H, de Leau M, Dieleman EM, Kardaun JW, van Os R, Vandertop WP, et al. Impaired survival and long-term neurological problems in benign meningioma. Neuro-Oncology. 2012:nos013.
72. Wen PY, Quant E, Drappatz J, Beroukhim R, Norden AD. Medical therapies for meningiomas. J Neurooncol. 2010;99(3):365–78.
73. Kaley T, Barani I, Chamberlain M, McDermott M, Panageas K, Raizer J, et al. Historical benchmarks for medical therapy trials in surgery-and radiation-refractory meningioma: a RANO review. Neuro-Oncology. 2014;16(6):829–40.
74. Durand A, Labrousse F, Jouvet A, Bauchet L, Kalamaridès M, Menei P, et al. WHO grade II and III meningiomas: a study of prognostic factors. J Neurooncol. 2009;95(3):367–75.
75. Bi WL, Mei Y, Agarwalla PK, Beroukhim R, Dunn IF. Genomic and epigenomic landscape in meningioma. Neurosurg Clin N Am. 2016;27(2):167–79.
76. Ene Chibawanye I, Fine Howard A. Many tumors in one: a daunting therapeutic prospect. Cancer Cell. 20(6):695–7.
77. Hegi ME, Diserens A-C, Gorlia T, Hamou M-F, de Tribolet N, Weller M, et al. MGMT gene silencing and benefit from temozolomide in glioblastoma. N Engl J Med. 2005;352(10):997–1003.
78. Wick W, Meisner C, Hentschel B, Platten M, Schilling A, Wiestler B, et al. Prognostic or predictive value of MGMT promoter methylation in gliomas depends on IDH1 mutation. Neurology. 2013;81(17):1515–22.
79. Yang X, Yang K, Kuang K. The efficacy and safety of EGFR inhibitor monotherapy in non-small cell lung cancer: a systematic review. Curr Oncol Rep. 2014;16(6):1–10.
80. Liang W, Wu X, Fang W, Zhao Y, Yang Y, Hu Z, et al. Network meta-analysis of erlotinib, gefitinib, afatinib and icotinib in patients with advanced non-small-cell lung cancer harboring EGFR mutations. PLoS ONE. 2014;9(2):e85245.
81. Padfield E, Ellis HP, Kurian KM. Current therapeutic advances targeting EGFR and EGFRvIII in glioblastoma. Front Oncol. 2015;5:5.
82. Gan HK, Kaye AH, Luwor RB. The EGFRvIII variant in glioblastoma multiforme. J Clin Neurosci. 2009;16(6):748–54.
83. Vivanco I, Robins HI, Rohle D, Campos C, Grommes C, Nghiemphu PL, et al. Differential sensitivity of glioma- versus lung cancer-specific EGFR mutations to EGFR kinase inhibitors. Cancer Discovery. 2012;2(5):458–71.
84. Pelloski CE, Ballman KV, Furth AF, Zhang L, Lin E, Sulman EP, et al. Epidermal growth factor receptor variant III status defines clinically distinct subtypes of glioblastoma. J Clin Oncol. 2007;25 (16):2288–94.
85. Schuster J, Lai RK, Recht LD, Reardon DA, Paleologos NA, Groves MD, et al. A phase II, multicenter trial of rindopepimut (CDX-110) in newly diagnosed glioblastoma: the ACT III study. Neuro-Oncology. 2015;17(6):854–61.
86. Snuderl M, Fazlollahi L, Le Long P, Nitta M, Zhelyazkova Boryana H, Davidson Christian J, et al. Mosaic amplification of multiple receptor tyrosine kinase genes in glioblastoma. Cancer Cell. 2011;20(6):810–7.
87. Fenton TR, Nathanson D, Ponte de Albuquerque C, Kuga D, Iwanami A, Dang J, et al. Resistance to EGF receptor inhibitors in glioblastoma mediated by phosphorylation of the PTEN tumor suppressor at tyrosine 240. Proc Natl Acad Sci. 2012;109 (35):14164–9.
88. Bai H, Harmanci AS, Erson-Omay EZ, Li J, Coskun S, Simon M, et al. Integrated genomic characterization of IDH1-mutant glioma malignant progression. Nat Genet. 2015 (advance online publication).
89. Kim H, Zheng S, Amini SS, Virk SM, Mikkelsen T, Brat DJ, et al. Whole-genome and multisector exome sequencing of primary and post-treatment glioblastoma reveals patterns of tumor evolution. Genome Res. 2015.
90. Hong MKH, Macintyre G, Wedge DC, Van Loo P, Patel K, Lunke S, et al. Tracking the origins and drivers of subclonal metastatic expansion in prostate cancer. Nat Commun. 2015;6.

91. de Bruin EC, McGranahan N, Mitter R, Salm M, Wedge DC, Yates L, et al. Spatial and temporal diversity in genomic instability processes defines lung cancer evolution. Science. 2014;346 (6206):251–6.
92. Brastianos PK, Carter SL, Santagata S, Cahill DP, Taylor-Weiner A, Jones RT, et al. Genomic characterization of brain metastases reveals branched evolution and potential therapeutic targets. Cancer Discovery. 2015.
93. Wu X, Northcott PA, Dubuc A, Dupuy AJ, Shih DJH, Witt H, et al. Clonal selection drives genetic divergence of metastatic medulloblastoma. Nature. 2012;482(7386):529–33.
94. Yauch RL, Dijkgraaf GJP, Alicke B, Januario T, Ahn CP, Holcomb T, et al. Smoothened mutation confers resistance to a hedgehog pathway inhibitor in medulloblastoma. Science. 2009;326(5952):572–4.
95. Morrissy AS, Garzia L, Shih DJH, Zuyderduyn S, Huang X, Skowron P, et al. Divergent clonal selection dominates medulloblastoma at recurrence. Nature. 2016;529(7586):351–7.
96. Beck B, Blanpain C. Unravelling cancer stem cell potential. Nat Rev Cancer. 2013;13(10):727–38.
97. Singh SK, Clarke ID, Terasaki M, Bonn VE, Hawkins C, Squire J, et al. Identification of a cancer stem cell in human brain tumors. Cancer Res. 2003;63(18):5821–8.
98. Huse JT, Holland EC. Targeting brain cancer: advances in the molecular pathology of malignant glioma and medulloblastoma. Nat Rev Cancer. 2010;10(5):319–31.
99. Chen K, Huang Y-H, Chen J-L. Understanding and targeting cancer stem cells: therapeutic implications and challenges. Acta Pharmacol Sin. 2013;34 (6):732–40.
100. Francis JM, Zhang C-Z, Maire CL, Jung J, Manzo VE, Adalsteinsson VA, et al. EGFR variant heterogeneity in glioblastoma resolved through single-nucleus sequencing. Cancer Discovery. 2014.
101. Hata AN, Niederst MJ, Archibald HL, Gomez-Caraballo M, Siddiqui FM, Mulvey HE, et al. Tumor cells can follow distinct evolutionary paths to become resistant to epidermal growth factor receptor inhibition. Nat Med. 2016 (advance online publication).
102. Nathanson DA, Gini B, Mottahedeh J, Visnyei K, Koga T, Gomez G, et al. Targeted therapy resistance mediated by dynamic regulation of extrachromosomal mutant EGFR DNA. Science. 2014;343 (6166):72–6.
103. Taylor MD, Poppleton H, Fuller C, Su X, Liu Y, Jensen P, et al. Radial glia cells are candidate stem cells of ependymoma. Cancer Cell. 2005;8(4):323–35.
104. Ebert C, von Haken M, Meyer-Puttlitz B, Wiestler OD, Reifenberger G, Pietsch T, et al. Molecular genetic analysis of ependymal tumors: NF2 mutations and chromosome 22q loss occur preferentially in intramedullary spinal ependymomas. Am J Pathol. 1999;155(2):627–32.
105. Mendrzyk F, Korshunov A, Benner A, Toedt G, Pfister S, Radlwimmer B, et al. Identification of gains on 1q and epidermal growth factor receptor overexpression as independent prognostic markers in intracranial ependymoma. Am Assoc Cancer Res. 2006;12(7):2070–9.
106. Modena P, Lualdi E, Facchinetti F, Veltman J, Reid JF, Minardi S, et al. Identification of tumor-specific molecular signatures in intracranial ependymoma and association with clinical characteristics. J Clin Oncol. 2006;24(33):5223–33.
107. Parker M, Mohankumar KM, Punchihewa C, Weinlich R, Dalton JD, Li Y, et al. C11orf95-RELA fusions drive oncogenic NF-[kgr]B signalling in ependymoma. Nature. 2014;506(7489):451–5.
108. Mack SC, Witt H, Piro RM, Gu L, Zuyderduyn S, Stutz AM, et al. Epigenomic alterations define lethal CIMP-positive ependymomas of infancy. Nature. 2014;506(7489):445–50.
109. Evans D, Huson S, Donnai D, Neary W, Blair V, Newton V, et al. A clinical study of type 2 neurofibromatosis. QJM. 1992;84(1):603–18.
110. Melmed S. Mechanisms for pituitary tumorigenesis: the plastic pituitary. J. Clin Invest.112(11):1603–18.
111. Landis CA, Masters SB, Spada A, Pace AM, Bourne HR, Vallar L. GTPase inhibiting mutations activate the [alpha] chain of Gs and stimulate adenylyl cyclase in human pituitary tumours. Nature. 1989;340(6236):692–6.
112. Trivellin G, Daly AF, Faucz FR, Yuan B, Rostomyan L, Larco DO, et al. Gigantism and acromegaly due to Xq26 microduplications and GPR101 mutation. N Engl J Med. 2014;371(25):2363–74.
113. Reincke M, Sbiera S, Hayakawa A, Theodoropoulou M, Osswald A, Beuschlein F, et al. Mutations in the deubiquitinase gene USP8 cause Cushing's disease. Nat Genet. 2015;47(1):31–8.
114. Sato Y, Maekawa S, Ishii R, Sanada M, Morikawa T, Shiraishi Y, et al. Recurrent somatic mutations underlie corticotropin-independent Cushing's syndrome. Science. 2014;344(6186):917–20.
115. Farrell WE, Simpson DJ, Bicknell JE, Talbot AJ, Bates AS, Clayton RN. Chromosome 9p deletions in invasive and noninvasive nonfunctional pituitary adenomas: the deleted region involves markers outside of the MTS1 and MTS2 genes. Cancer Res. 1997;57(13):2703–9.
116. Northcott PA, Lee C, Zichner T, Stütz AM, Erkek S, Kawauchi D, et al. Enhancer hijacking activates GFI1 family oncogenes in medulloblastoma. Nature. 2014;511(7510):428–34.
117. Brennan CW, Verhaak RG, McKenna A, Campos B, Noushmehr H, Salama SR, et al. The somatic genomic landscape of glioblastoma. Cell. 2013;155 (2):462–77.

118. Dunn GP, Rinne ML, Wykosky J, Genovese G, Quayle SN, Dunn IF, et al. Emerging insights into the molecular and cellular basis of glioblastoma. Genes Dev. 2012;26(8):756–84.

119. Parsons DW, Jones S, Zhang X, Lin JC-H, Leary RJ, Angenendt P, et al. An integrated genomic analysis of human glioblastoma multiforme. Science. 2008;321(5897):1807–12.

Part II

Surgery: Maximizing the Extent of Tumor Resection

4 The Usefulness of Stereotactic Neuronavigation Along with Intraoperative Imaging in Malignant Brain Tumor Surgery

Gregory Kuzmik, Anne Long, S. Bulent Omay and Jennifer Moliterno Günel

Introduction

Neurosurgeons plan surgical approaches for the initial stages of brain tumor surgery based on preoperative magnetic resonance imaging (MRI). Registering this imaging with astereotactic guidance (i.e., neuronavigation) system allows for more precise localization of the tumor, with more focused craniotomies centered over the area of interest. After the initial approach, however, navigation based on preoperative imaging that was once accurate and useful can become less reliable due to the well-defined phenomenon of brain shift following hyperosmotic therapy, cerebrospinal fluid (CSF) release, and initial tumor resection [1]. Similarly, for certain types of tumors in particular, such as gliomas, distinguishing between tumor and infiltrative, gliotic brain during resection can prove difficult for even the most experienced brain tumor surgeon. Thus, the neurosurgeon could benefit from a more updated representation of the remaining tumor on more current imaging to guide the completion of resection. Moreover, the surgeon's understanding of the tumor's vascular supply, with the possibility of decreasing it with intraoperative embolization of particularly vascular malignant brain tumors, can be important.

G. Kuzmik · A. Long · S. Bulent Omay · J. Moliterno Günel (✉)
Department of Neurosurgery, Yale University School of Medicine, 15 York Street LLCI 810, P.O. Box 208082, New Haven, CT 06510, USA
e-mail: jennifer.moliternogunel@yale.edu

Intraoperative imaging is a powerful and valuable tool in brain tumor surgery that has come a long way since Walter Dandy pioneered pneumoencephalography [2]. Modern intraoperative imaging modalities, with the potential for real-time information and more advanced neuronavigation systems, including intraoperative ultrasound (iUS) and intraoperative magnetic resonance imaging (iMRI), as well as intraoperative angiography (iA), can improve patient safety and minimize surgical morbidity by allowing the surgeon to more accurately localize pathology and avoid eloquent neural and vascular structures. At the same time, it facilitates more complete resection of tumors by demonstrating to the surgeon the location of residual tumor which is particularly salient in the setting of glioma resection because these tumors, due to their infiltrative nature, can be difficult to differentiate from normal brain tissue intraoperatively, particularly at the time of reoperation.

Thorough surgical resection when possible, followed by adjuvant chemotherapy and radiation, represents the standard approach to treatment of malignant brain tumors, such as high-grade gliomas (HGG), including glioblastoma (GBM) [3]. A more complete extent of tumor resection (EOR), and achieving a gross total resection (GTR) when possible, has been shown to improve outcomes in patients with gliomas [3–7] and is associated with improved progression-free and overall survival [4]. In one multivariate analysis comprising data from over 400 patients with GBM, EOR was found to be an independent predictor of survival [6]. In another recent meta-analysis encompassing over

J. Moliterno Günel et al. (eds.), *Malignant Brain Tumors*,
DOI 10.1007/978-3-319-49864-5_4

12,000 patients studying the impacts of EOR of high-grade malignant gliomas HGG, the authors found that GTR was superior to subtotal resection (STR) with regard to overall survival (mean difference 3.8 months), progression-free survival (mean difference 2.2 months), and postoperative Karnofsky performance status (mean difference 4.9% points) [3]. The authors also noted that there was no significant difference in surgical morbidity or mortality between the GTR and STR groups [3]. Another study found that even in the case of recurrent GBM, extent of repeat resection was an independent predictor of survival and that patients who had initially undergone a STR had significantly improved overall survival when GTR was achieved on their recurrent tumor compared to STR [5]. Data from meta-analyses of patients with malignant gliomas provide evidence that increasing extent of resection leads to improvements in survival time, functional recovery, and tumor recurrence rate [3, 6]. Studies similarly suggest that safe extent of resection is associated with improved outcomes in patients with low-grade gliomas [8–10]. Achieving a greater extent of resection has also been shown to improve survival in patients with recurrent GBM [5]. It is also important to note that achieving GTR may also be an important and necessary step in fulfilling the criteria for clinical trial enrollment.

In this chapter, we will discuss the utility of stereotactic neuronavigation, iUS and iMRI, as well as the potential usefulness of iA, and their role in improving the success of surgery for malignant brain tumors.

Stereotactic Neuronavigation

The precise localization of a tumor within the brain and its relationship to critical neurovascular structures is of significant importance and fundamental to every malignant brain tumor surgery.

Stereotactic neuronavigation systems use three-dimensional (3D) digitizers to register anatomical landmarks with preoperative imaging [11]. The result is effectively a GPS for localizing the tumor through the use of a tracking system that links to a detector (optical or electromagnetic) with a probe [12]. While these systems previously required the use of a frame and thus quite cumbersome, more modern, frameless neuronavigation has become standard at major tumor centers in the last two decades and offers comparable accuracy.

Neuronavigation is incredibly effective with targeting specific areas within a tumor for more accurate biopsy and diagnosis. For instance, areas of restricted diffusion or contrast enhancement seen within a tumor on preoperative MRI can serve as a stereotactic target to help establish a more representative diagnosis of a malignant brain tumor and therefore appropriately influence treatment decisions. With regard to surgical resection, more focused, smaller craniotomies can be performed and reliably centered over the tumor epicenter when stereotactic neuronavigation guides the surgical planning. Smaller craniotomies are associated with reduced blood loss, decreased operating time, and minimum trauma and brain retraction [11, 13]. Furthermore, during tumor resection, particularly for deep tumors, neuronavigation can serve as a useful adjunct for understanding the relationship with critical structures nearby (i.e., ventricular system), allowing for avoidance of complications and potential morbidity.

More modern multimodal systems can incorporate functional data with regard to eloquent cortex (i.e., motor or speech areas) and white matter tracts (i.e., corticospinal tract), with co-registration of functional MRI (fMRI) and diffusion tensor imaging (DTI), further improving the safety of surgery. This allows for navigation while taking these important structures into consideration, providing a better understanding of their anatomical relationship in general and with respect to the tumor. This is paramount as important anatomy can be displaced and altered by malignant brain tumors. Moreover, it allows to facilitate the identification of eloquent cortex and subcortical tracts, enabling direct stimulation for confirmation of their locations. Taken together, this can help minimize the risk of injury to highly functional brain with improved preservation of function. Indeed, studies have suggested the combination of using multimodal neuronavigation with fMRI- and DTI-integrated systems, coupled with cortical and subcortical mapping techniques, enhances surgical safety by reducing surgical time, identifying tracts for stimulation, preserving function, and facilitating maximal surgical resection [14–18].

The major limitations of the use of stereotactic neuronavigation include patient-to-image registration inaccuracies and brain shift, resulting in loss of anatomic accuracy. With regard to the former, there is an inherent error in frameless stereotactic navigation systems related to the accuracy of probe tracking, the quality of the images, and the method of image-to-patient registration [19]. In addition, numerous routine steps of an operation have been shown to negatively impact the accuracy of frameless stereotactic neuronavigation [1]. These include the placement of surgical drapes, the placement of skin retractors, and the process of performing a craniotomy [1]. These factors may add up to an overall spatial registration error of 5 mm [1]. The duration of an operation has also been shown to be a significant factor in loss of frameless stereotactic neuronavigation accuracy; one study demonstrated that 5 h of operating time can result in a registration error of up to 3 mm [1]. Nonetheless, studies using pre- and postoperative MRI suggest that more modern frameless methods for localization have accuracy within 2–3 mm during surgery, similar to the accuracy of previously used frame-based stereotaxy [20]. As for brain shift, it is a well-described phenomenon that can occur when such common events during surgery, such as the resultant effects of hyperosmolar therapy on the brain, cerebrospinal fluid loss, cyst decompression, tumor resection, and cerebral edema, can effectively change the anatomy from the preoperative imaging and thus decrease navigational accuracy [21]. State-of-the-art operating rooms with iUS and iRMI capabilities can help overcome this with the re-registration of intraoperative ultrasound and MRI images. This allows for the ability to navigate from a more accurate representation of the current anatomical state. Finally, decrease in navigational accuracy can also be introduced by registering preoperative images obtained too far in advance (i.e., weeks, months) from the time of surgery. Malignant brain tumors, in particular, can grow quite rapidly, and thus, obtaining preoperative imaging as close to the time of surgery is recommended and can change surgical planning based on neuronavigation [12, 22].

Intraoperative Ultrasound (iUS)

iUS is commonly used as a noninvasive adjunct in brain tumor surgery and can help evaluate normal anatomical relationships, providing information about location and size of brain tumors with regard to the brain parenchyma [23]. Additionally, iUS with Doppler can provide valuable information on the overall vascularity of a tumor, where the main feeders are located, as well as the location of normal cerebral vasculature [24, 25]. Intraoperatively, the transducer probe of the ultrasound is wrapped in a sterile sheath with sterile lubrication on the tip and thus can be readily available to the surgeon on the operative field throughout the entirety of the case. The use of saline is important when using the iUS on the brain in an effort to improve acoustic coupling, and the operator has the ability to increase or reduce the intonation depth to provide more anatomical detail. CSF within the lateral ventricles is anechoic (i.e., dark), while the falx is hyperechoic (i.e., bright); thus, these structures can serve as landmarks for orientation purposes. In general, hyperechoic lesions have decreased water content, a rich capillary network, and stromal components [26]. Brain tumors can be heterogeneous in appearance, often appearing hyperechoic to normal brain tissue (Fig. 4.1), and can mostly be differentiated from a resection cavity. However, the variable appearance of the surrounding brain due to edema and tumor infiltration can sometimes render this interpretation confusing.

The most important advantage of iUS is that it provides the neurosurgeon with *real-time* information, including accurate localization and

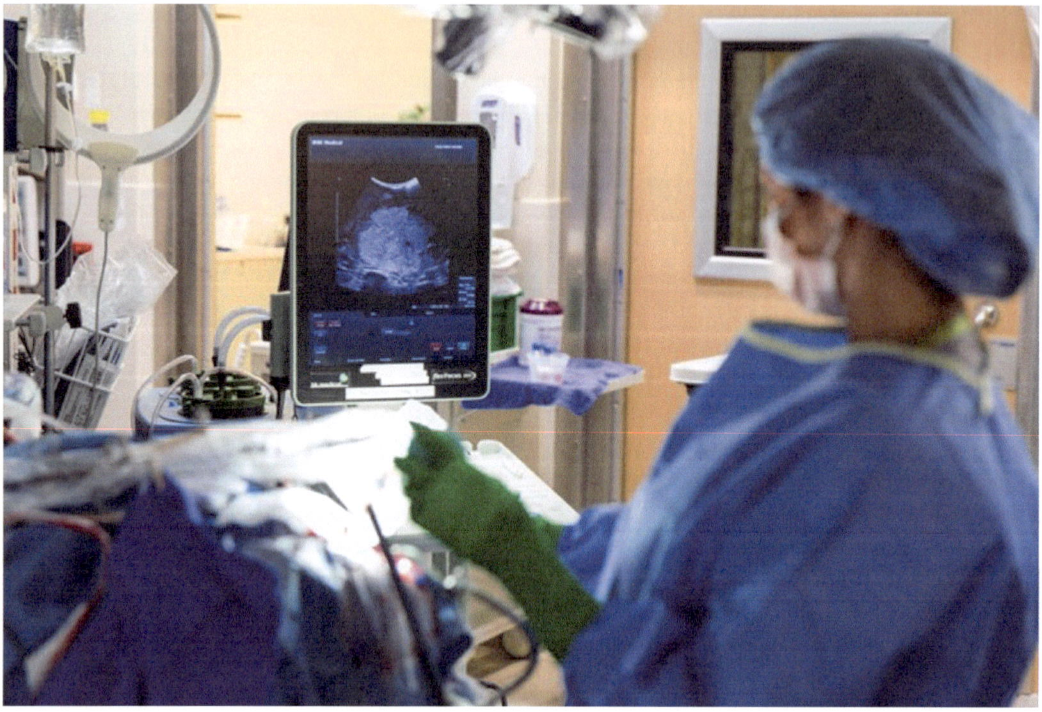

Fig. 4.1 Intraoperative use of ultrasound revealing a hyperechoic lesion representing tumor prior to resection. A hypoechoic area in the center is the carotid artery. The apparatus remains on the field allowing for relatively quick, real-time feedback about extent of resection

characterization of a lesion, compensation for brain shift that can be problematic for stereotactic neuronavigation systems, and detection of unforeseen surgical sequelae, such as intraoperative hemorrhage or hydrocephalus, therefore decreasing surgical time and potential morbidity [25]. iUS can better define critical tumor margins and decrease the likelihood of leaving residual tumor [14, 27]. It can easily locate and help evacuate cystic components, as well as define tumor tissue planes. iUS can be readily available with a relatively low cost when used routinely in an established tumor practice [25, 28]. The time it takes to perform an intraoperative ultrasound is very short (i.e., seconds to minutes) and can be performed numerous times, and no additional personnel is needed if the surgeon has sufficient experience with its use and interpretation.

Evidence indeed suggests that the imaging provided by iUS is seemingly advantageous to the success of brain tumor surgery. Saether et al. studied the use of 3D iUS in GBM surgery, and their findings suggest improvement in survival with this technology even after adjusting for known prognostic factors [14, 29]. In this retrospective study, Seather et al., reviewed 193 GBM patients and analyzed the effect of the use of 3D ultrasound and neuronavigation on overall survival [29]. They observed an increase in survival (9.6 vs. 11.9 months; $HR = 0.7$; $p = 0.034$) after adjusting for age, WHO performance status, and type of radiotherapy and chemotherapy [29]. Moiyadi et al. in a retrospective series studied the effects of the use of 3D iUS and revealed that combining 3D iUS data with MR guided neuronavigation resulted in further resection attempts and gross total resection (GTR) levels comparable to the use of iMRI [14, 30]. In the senior author's practice, the use of iUS, along with stereotactic neuronavigation, is standard on all tumor cases. The use of iMRI is reserved as an adjunct to iUS in more infiltrative tumors, such as malignant gliomas, where it can be more difficult to interpret residual tumor versus edematous brain on the border of the resection cavity.

Though undeniably useful, versatile, and readily available, it should be noted, however, the sensitivity and specificity of iUS is far less as compared with iMRI (see below) and interpretation of findings requires training and experience [31]. For example, a hyperechoic rim can be observed around the resection cavity which may be interpreted as tumor, although this is a nonspecific finding [32]. One of the other common artifactual problems of iUS is acoustic enhancement artifact (AEA). These artifacts appear at the bottom of the resection cavity after some tumor debulking when ultrasound penetrates through a higher column of saline. The appearance of AEAs is due to a large difference between a very low attenuation of acoustic waves in saline and high attenuation of acoustic waves in brain tissue, and they may block detection of tumor remnants at the depth of resection cavity [33, 34]. Using a mini US probe within the cavity may decrease the column of saline between the probe area of interest and then reduce the AEAs at the depth of the resection cavity [34, 35].

Novel technological advancements in ultrasonography can help overcome some of the shortcomings of more traditional, two-dimensional (2D) iUS. Over the last two decades, for instance, 3D iUS systems have become available and such multiplanar imaging capabilities can help overcome some of the limitations with regard to orientation of 2D US, leading to improved quality of imaging [30]. As mentioned, navigated iUS can use tracked ultrasound images (both 2D and 3D) for guidance and improvement in orientation [36]. The ultrasound can be used along with the preoperative MRI for the purpose of navigation and can help eliminate any inherent potential registration inaccuracies [37]. Co-registering with functional imaging [i.e., functional MRI (fMRI) and diffusion tensor imaging (DTI)] can further enhance the safety of the resection. Finally, contrast-enhanced iUS techniques can help improve tumor visualization with the intraoperative administration of contrast [38].

Intraoperative Magnetic Resonance Imaging (iMRI)

While MRI imaging has long been a fundamental component in the diagnosis and treatment of malignant brain tumors for its ability to provide surgeons with high-resolution multiplanar anatomic detail of the brain, it has more recently become an important intraoperative tool [39]. The ability to image the brain during surgery facilitates superior neuronavigation and can help overcome the limitations of stereotactic neuronavigation systems, rendering them more effective throughout the entirety of the surgery. More specifically, the use of iMRI can correct for these inherent neuronavigation inaccuracies that accrue over the course of an operation by allowing re-registration of the stereotactic neuronavigation with the intraoperative scan that is obtained after many of these steps of the operation that contribute to neuronavigation inaccuracy are completed. iMRI also has substantial benefit in verifying the extent of tumor resection and location of residual tumor after resection has begun, although it should be noted that this pertains primarily to intra-axial tumors that can be difficult to distinguish from normal brain tissue and holds less benefit from easily delineated extra-axial masses (Fig. 4.2). Intraoperative imaging has the additional capabilities that it can be used to confirm the correct positioning of a biopsy needle in the case of stereotactic biopsies or demonstrate the presence of early complications such as hemorrhage or ischemia that can be addressed intraoperatively [40].

Intraoperative MRI first became available in the 1990s with the advent of open bore magnets [39]. The first intraoperative magnets had low field strength (0.2–0.5T), which required longer scan times, limited anatomic resolution, and had lower signal-to-noise ratios compared to modern conventional high field strength MRIs [41, 42]. Furthermore, low field strength MRIs did not provide the ability to perform more advanced imaging techniques such as diffusion-weighted imaging (DWI), DTI, magnetic resonance angiography (MRA), magnetic resonance spectroscopy (MRS), and functional (fMRI) imaging [43]. More recent advancements with higher field

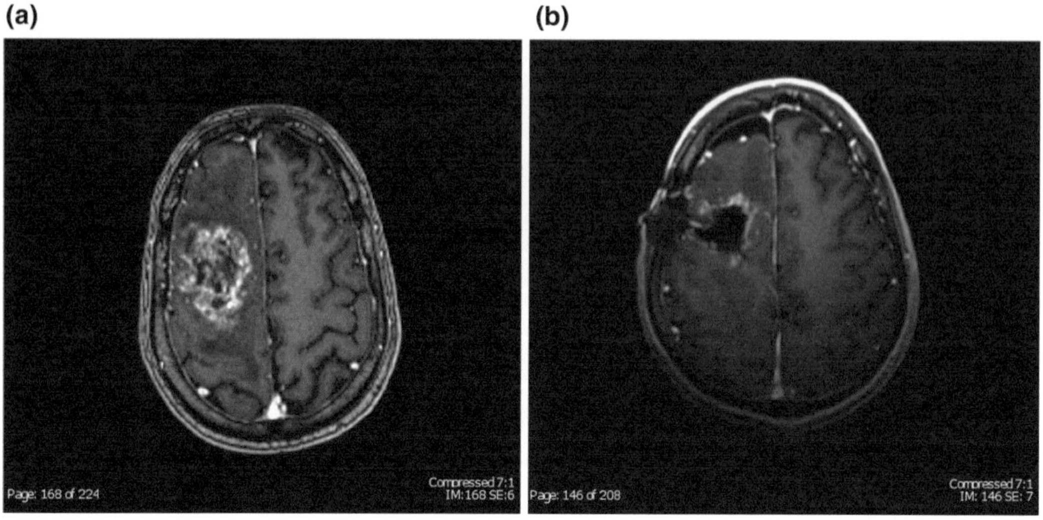

Fig. 4.2 A 47-year-old man with recurrent GBM after treatment with radiation and chemotherapy. Preoperative T1-weighted post gadolinium MRI (**a**) reveals a right frontoparietal mass. Intraoperative T1-weighted post gadolinium MRI (**b**) shows some residual treatment effects with tumor along the anterior resection cavity that appeared like gliotic brain grossly under the microscope

strength (1.5–3.0T) MRI systems address these shortcomings and have subsequently become an emerging tool in malignant brain tumor resection. The benefits of such an iMRI system not only provide for high-resolution multiplanar anatomic detail of intracranial tissues (and the same caliber as preoperative imaging), but also allow for these advanced imaging techniques.

iMRI has been shown to be an effective tool in improving neurosurgical outcomes while minimizing complications [44]. In one recent randomized controlled trial of adults with enhancing gliomas, 49 patients were analyzed after randomization to undergo conventional surgical resection or resection with the aid of intraoperative MRI [44]. Patients in the iMRI group had a significantly higher rate of complete tumor resection than the control group, while the rates of postoperative neurological deficits did not significantly differ [44]. Notably, in patients who underwent additional tumor resection based on the iMRI findings, none suffered neurological complications. Various case series have shown that iMRI results in improved rates of tumor resection [10, 31, 45–57]. For example, Senft and colleagues demonstrated that in patients undergoing surgery for intended GTR of GBM, the use of iMRI leads to a significantly increased rate of complete tumor resection (100%), compared to patients who underwent resection without iMRI (61%) [54]. One study investigating the role of iMRI in GBM resection found that achieving a >98% resection was significantly associated with improved overall survival compared to resection of <98% of the tumor (median survival 14 months vs. 9 months) [10]. Hatiboglu et al. found that in a subset of their patients undergoing glioma resection, the use of iMRI followed by additional tumor resection improved the average extent of resection from 76 to 96% [45]. Likewise, in a series of nearly 300 patients, Kuhnt and colleagues found that the use of iMRI with subsequent additional tumor resection guided by the intraoperative images significantly improved the rate of GTR of gliomas. Additionally, they found using volumetric analysis that additional resection following iMRI leads to a significantly lower volume of residual tumor [46]. Others, however, have not shown similar benefits of iMRI. A recent but small randomized controlled trial comparing resection with standard neuronavigation to resection aided by low

(a) (b)

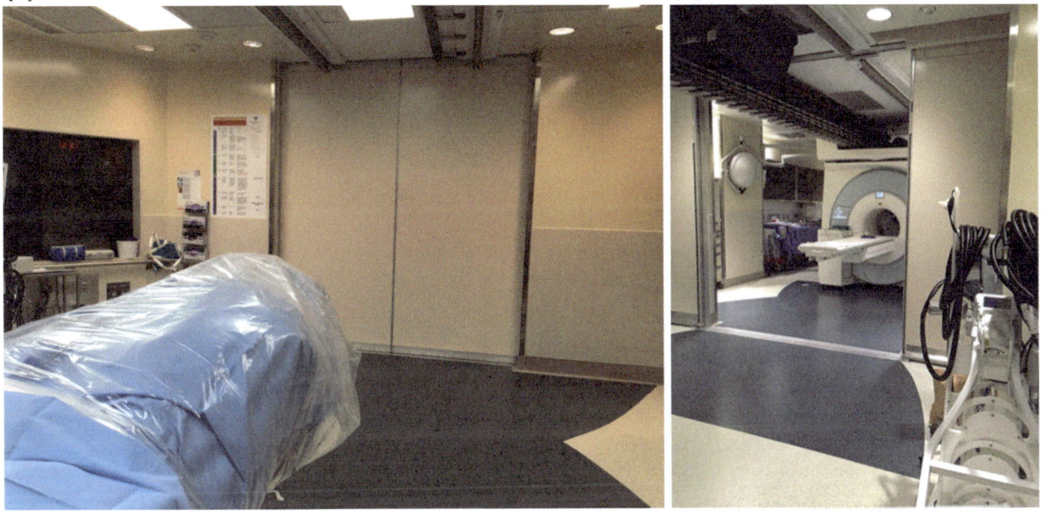

Fig. 4.3 iMRI suite at Yale New Haven Hospital. Photograph taken from the operating room looking toward the garage that houses the iMRI (**a**). The patient has been sterilely draped, and the metal objects have been moved to safety. The magnet moves into the operating room, along a track system, allowing its use in two separate rooms. The magnet is centered over the patient's head and ready for use (**b**)

field iMRI found no significant differences with respect to extent of resection, clinical performance, and survival. However, the benefits of iMRI in this study may have been limited by the low-strength (0.15T) magnet used [58].

Despite these advantages, an iMRI system presents a number of logistical and safety challenges that must be addressed prior to clinical implementation. The first among these is the design and construction of a suitable operating room. iMRI systems require rooms with adequate radiofrequency shielding in order to prevent image artifact and magnetic shielding to protect equipment and patients outside the iMRI suite. Additionally, the rooms must be equipped with dedicated MR-compatible surgical and anesthesia equipment and must be large enough so that non-MRI-compatible equipment can be stored at a safe distance from the magnet while it is in use. Non-MRI-compatible equipment must be kept at a distance beyond the 5-gauss field line of the magnet while it is in use [59]. While the magnets themselves may be too deep to allow easy surgical access while the patient is positioned in the scanner, mobile systems, in which the MRI bore can be brought in and out of the operating room, circumvent this drawback [41]. Many modern iMRI suites house the MRI magnet in a separate room connected to the main operating area, and the magnet can be brought into the main operating room via tracks on the ceiling to center over the patient's head (Fig. 4.3).

Drawbacks to an iMRI system include the significant upfront expense of the MRI systems and constructing an MRI-compatible operating suite, not to mention availability of space to be specifically allocated to the suite which may not be possible at certain centers. Apart from the initial costs, and unlike iUS, these systems also require additional personnel, including MRI technicians, as well as additional traditional surgical staff to operate the MRI during an operation. Special anesthesia monitors are required. Older models of MRI-compatible head holders can be quite cumbersome and can prohibit positioning in the lateral or prone position, but newer iMRI systems and head holders have improved considerably to where this is amenable (Fig. 4.4). It is also important to note that the use of an iMRI system may be limited by metallic implants in the patient, such as old aneurysm clips or implanted defibrillators. An additional

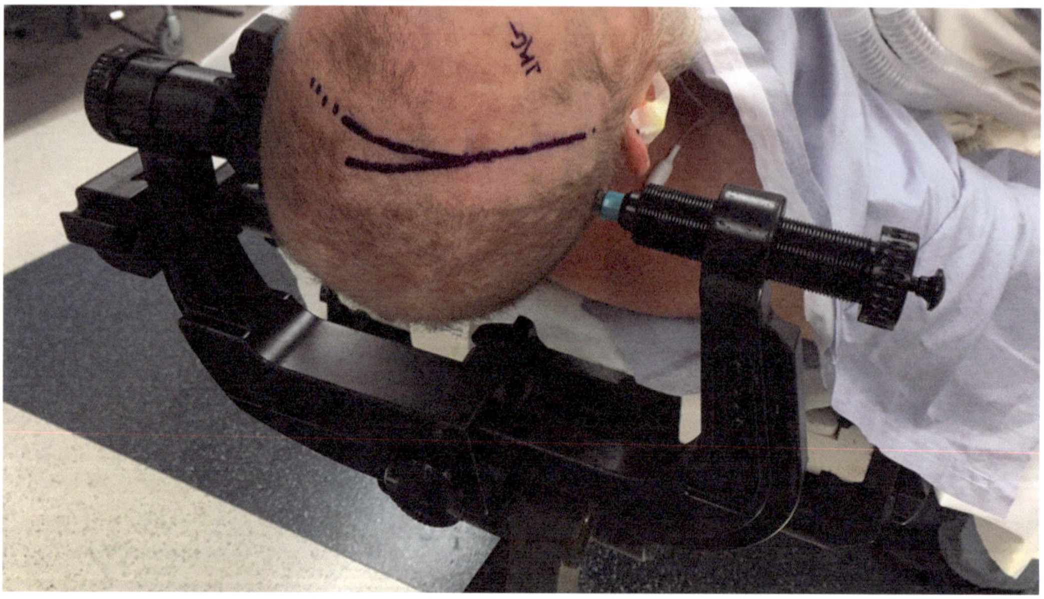

Fig. 4.4 A more current version of the nonmetal, 3.0T iMRI-compatible head holder

safety consideration is that obtaining an iMRI requires suspension of the surgical procedure in order to place the patient within the MRI scanner. The sterility of the surgical field must also be maintained throughout the imaging process. Relatively slow image acquisition time, coupled with the time it takes to prepare the patient and the room, results in relatively longer operating times than without imaging and, therefore, longer time under anesthesia. In the senior author's experience, this time is typically approximately forty minutes. In patients with medical comorbidities, the benefits of obtaining intraoperative imaging must be weighed against the risks of additional operating and anesthesia time. In some patients, depending on the type and extent of their tumor in addition to their overall health and prognosis, it may be best to complete tumor resection without obtaining iMRI.

Intraoperative Angiography (iA)

The use of cerebral angiography for brain tumors may be indicated when more detailed vascular information is needed to evaluate arteriovenous shunting, the relationship with major arterial and venous structures, coexisting vascular pathology within or in close vicinity of malignant tumors [60, 61]. Moreover, embolization of tumors can prove invaluable in tumor cases with a robust vascular supply that may be difficult to otherwise control during surgery. The one caveat with preoperative embolization of tumors, however, is that the sudden cutoff of the tumor's blood supply can lead to an acute worsening of cerebral edema, rendering an immediate life-threatening situation for the patient. Tumor embolization may also cause hemorrhage in large tumors, also leading to acute herniation syndromes [62]. Thus, the removal of the skull flap and resection of the tumor immediately after embolization can be critical to relieve pressure, but these procedures are often performed at two separate locations in the most hospitals.

State-of-the-art operating rooms, however, allow for multiple modalities of diagnostic and intervention capabilities, namely iA and iMRI to coexist in the same room (i.e., hybrid rooms), thus allowing for the opportunity to maximize the success of surgery and patient safety. The accessibility of a biplanar imaging technology

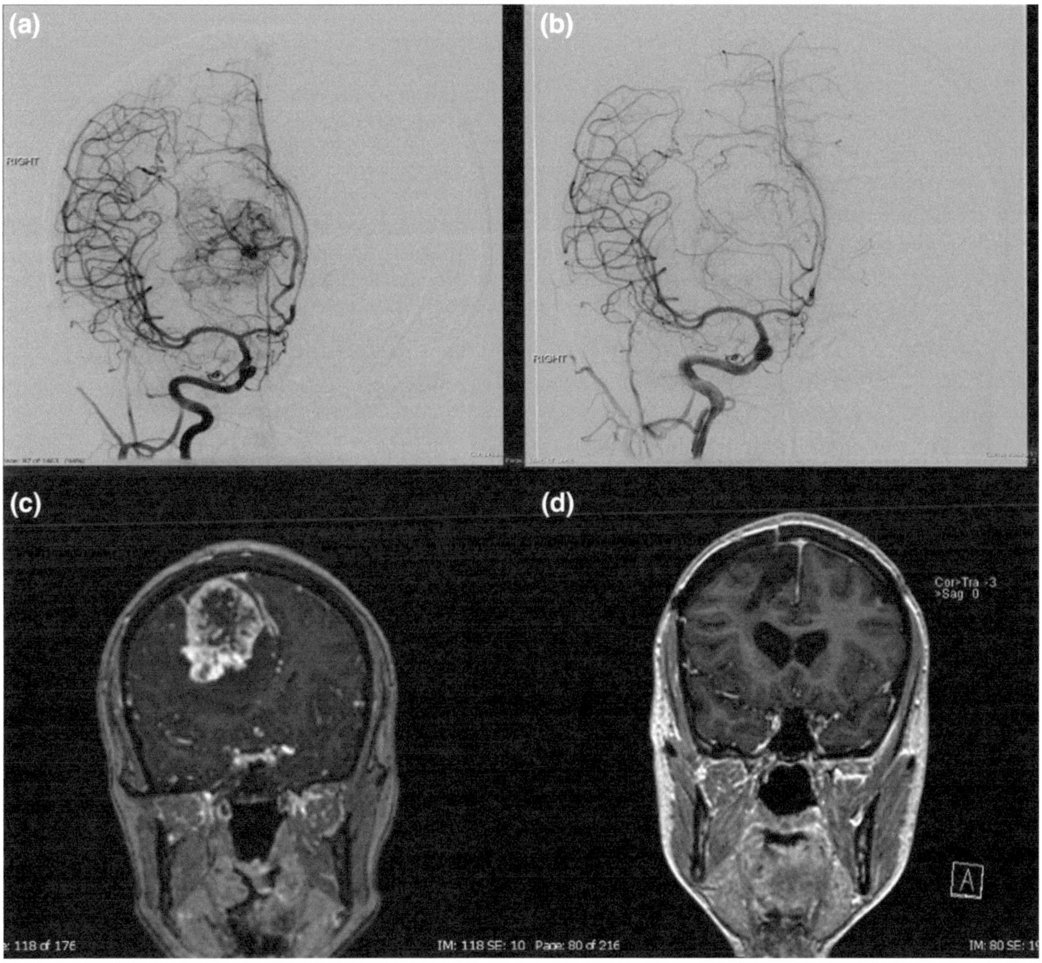

Fig. 4.5 29-year-old patient with a malignant hemangiopericytoma found to have a feeding artery aneurysm on CT angiogram. She was treated in a hybrid operating room with intraoperative angiography capabilities, allowing for embolization (**a**, **b**) in the same setting as craniotomy and resection (**c**, **d**), minimizing the risk of malignant cerebral edema

within a neurosurgical operating suite allows the neurosurgeon to have the ability to perform a diagnostic or therapeutic cerebral angiogram during or immediately before or after tumor resection. Patients may be anesthetized in the same operation suite, in the same setting, where life-threatening cerebral edema and risks of herniation can be controlled and prevented. Hybrid rooms provide the infrastructure to begin the craniotomy and tumor resection immediately after an embolization procedure, therefore reaping the benefits of eradicating the tumor blood supply, without the consequences. These adjuncts increase the safety, accuracy, and success of each procedure. One example of the success of such a hybrid room is exemplified in Fig. 4.5 in which a feeding artery aneurysm was found deep within a malignant brain tumor. Such an aneurysm would have been difficult to gain access to and control with conventional open surgery, and thus, the use of iA with embolization in a hybrid suite allowed for treatment of the aneurysm and removal of the tumor in the same operative setting.

Summary

Stereotactic neuronavigation is critical for more precise surgery for malignant brain tumors and for establishing diagnosis at the minimum, when surgical resection is not possible. iUS and iMRI are increasingly useful adjuncts in brain tumor surgery and, when coupled with navigation, can help push the extent of surgical resection, while minimizing morbidity, resulting in improved survival and decreased recurrence for patients with malignant brain tumors. The upfront investment of both can be costly and is usually found at large medical centers with a high-volume brain tumor surgical service and specialized brain tumor surgeons. iUS can provide quick, real-time information regarding the extent of resection, as well as critical relationships of the remaining tumor with critical neurovascular structures of the brain. Expertise in interpreting the ultrasound imaging is paramount to its usefulness. While the iMRI requires a longer pause in the surgical procedure, more logistical considerations and preparations for its use, and a greater expense and dedication of space, the improved imaging quality can be invaluable. The complementary use of both iUS and iMRI, when appropriate, along with the ability to re-register neuronavigation can make a significant difference in the state-of-the-art neurosurgical management of patients with malignant brain tumors. iA also serves as a critically useful adjunct in select cases where the benefits of preoperative embolization of particularly vascular tumors in hybrid operative suites can be performed and can immediately mediate any negative effects of resultant increased cerebral edema.

References

1. Stieglitz LH, Fichtner J, Andres R, Schucht P, Krähenbühl AK, Raabe A, et al. The silent loss of neuronavigation accuracy: a systematic retrospective analysis of factors influencing the mismatch of frameless stereotactic systems in cranial neurosurgery. Neurosurgery. 2013;72(5):796–807.
2. Sutherland GRG. A mobile high-field magnetic resonance system for neurosurgery. J Neurosurg. 1999;91(5):804–13.
3. Almenawer SASA. Biopsy versus partial versus gross total resection in older patients with high-grade glioma: a systematic review and meta-analysis. Neuro-oncology (Charlottesville, Va). 2015;17(6):868–81.
4. Almeida JPJP. The value of extent of resection of glioblastomas: clinical evidence and current approach. Curr Neurol Neurosci Rep. 2015;15 (2):517.
5. Bloch OO. Impact of extent of resection for recurrent glioblastoma on overall survival: clinical article. J Neurosurg. 2012;117(6):1032–8.
6. Lacroix MM. A multivariate analysis of 416 patients with glioblastoma multiforme: prognosis, extent of resection, and survival. J Neurosurg. 2001;95 (2):190–8.
7. Sanai NN. Glioma extent of resection and its impact on patient outcome. Neurosurgery. 2008;62(4):753–66.
8. Claus EBEB. Survival rates in patients with low-grade glioma after intraoperative magnetic resonance image guidance. Cancer. 2005;103(6):1227–33.
9. Keles GEG. Low-grade hemispheric gliomas in adults: a critical review of extent of resection as a factor influencing outcome. J Neurosurg. 2001;95 (5):735–45.
10. Kuhnt DD. Correlation of the extent of tumor volume resection and patient survival in surgery of glioblastoma multiforme with high-field intraoperative MRI guidance. Neuro-oncology (Charlottesville, Va). 2011;13(12):1339–48.
11. Omay SBSB. Surgical navigation for meningioma surgery. J Neurooncol. 2010;99(3):357–64.
12. Orringer DADA. Neuronavigation in the surgical management of brain tumors: current and future trends. Expert Rev Med Devices. 2012;9(5):491–500.
13. Barnett GHG. Intracranial meningioma resection using frameless stereotaxy. J Image Guided Surg. 1995;1(1):46–52.
14. D'Amico RSRS. Neurosurgical oncology: advances in operative technologies and adjuncts. J Neurooncol. 2014;119(3):451–63.
15. Kumar AA. The role of neuronavigation-guided functional MRI and diffusion tensor tractography along with cortical stimulation in patients with eloquent cortex lesions. Br J Neurosurg. 2014;28 (2):226–33.
16. Bello LL. Intraoperative use of diffusion tensor imaging fiber tractography and subcortical mapping for resection of gliomas: technical considerations. Neurosurg Focus. 2010;28(2):E6.
17. Bello LL. Motor and language DTI Fiber Tracking combined with intraoperative subcortical mapping for surgical removal of gliomas. NeuroImage (Orlando, Fla). 2008;39(1):369–82.

18. Mikuni NN. Clinical impact of integrated functional neuronavigation and subcortical electrical stimulation to preserve motor function during resection of brain tumors. J Neurosurg. 2007;106(4):593–8.
19. Widmann GG. Frameless stereotactic targeting devices: technical features, targeting errors and clinical results. Int J Med Robot Comp Assist Sur. 2012;8(1):1–16.
20. Mascott CRCR. In vivo accuracy of image guidance performed using optical tracking and optimized registration. J Neurosurg. 2006;105(4):561–7.
21. Spetzger UU. Error analysis in cranial neuronavigation. Minim Invasive Neurosurg. 2002;45(1):6–10.
22. Ferrant MM. Serial registration of intraoperative MR images of the brain. Med Image Anal. 2002;6 (4):337–59.
23. Ivanov MM. Intraoperative ultrasound in neurosurgery—a practical guide. Br J Neurosurg. 2010;24(5):510–7.
24. Lam AMA. Intraoperative use of transcranial Doppler ultrasonography. Neurosurg Clin N Am. 1996;7 (4):709–22.
25. Cheon J-EJE. Intraoperative neurosonography revisited: effective neuronavigation in pediatric neurosurgery. Ultrasonography (Seoul, Korea). 2015;34 (2):79–87.
26. Catalano O, Nunziata A, Siani A. Fundamentals in oncologic ultrasound: sonographic imaging and intervention in the cancer patient. Italy: Springer-Verlag; 2009.
27. Solheim OO. Ultrasound-guided operations in unselected high-grade gliomas–overall results, impact of image quality and patient selection. Acta Neurochir (Wien). 2010;152(11):1873–86.
28. El Beltagy MAMA. Role of intraoperative ultrasound in resection of pediatric brain tumors. Child's nervous system. 2010;26(9):1189–93.
29. Sæther CAC. Did survival improve after the implementation of intraoperative neuronavigation and 3D ultrasound in glioblastoma surgery? A retrospective analysis of 192 primary operations. J Neurol Sur Part A. 2012;73(2):73–8.
30. Moiyadi AVAV. Usefulness of three-dimensional navigable intraoperative ultrasound in resection of brain tumors with a special emphasis on malignant gliomas. Acta Neurochir (Wien). 2013;155 (12):2217–25.
31. Gerganov VMVM. Typical 3-D localization of tumor remnants of WHO grade II hemispheric gliomas–lessons learned from the use of intraoperative high-field MRI control. Acta Neurochir (Wien). 2011;153(3):479–87.
32. Woydt MM. Correlation of intra-operative ultrasound with histopathologic findings after tumour resection in supratentorial gliomas. A method to improve gross total tumour resection. Acta Neurochir (Wien). 1996;138(12):1391–8.
33. Selbekk TT. Ultrasound imaging in neurosurgery: approaches to minimize surgically induced image artefacts for improved resection control. Acta Neurochir (Wien). 2013;155(6):973–80.
34. Šteňo AA. Intraoperative ultrasound in low-grade glioma surgery. Clin Neurol Neurosurg. 2015;135:96–9.
35. Jakola ASAS. Quality of life in patients with intracranial gliomas: the impact of modern image-guided surgery. J Neurosurg. 2011;114 (6):1622–30.
36. Moiyadi AVAV. Direct navigated 3D ultrasound for resection of brain tumors: a useful tool for intraoperative image guidance. Neurosurg Focus. 2016;40(3):E5.
37. Unsgaard GG. Intra-operative 3D ultrasound in neurosurgery. Acta Neurochir (Wien). 2006;148 (3):235–53.
38. Engelhardt M, Hansen C, Eyding J, Wilkening W, Brenke C, Krogias C, et al. Feasibility of contrast-enhanced sonography during resection of cerebral tumours: initial results of a prospective study. Ultrasound Med Biol. 2007;33(4):571–5.
39. Nimsky CC. Intraoperative high-field-strength MR imaging: implementation and experience in 200 patients. Radiology. 2004;233(1):67–78.
40. Schwartz RBR. Intraoperative MR imaging guidance for intracranial neurosurgery: experience with the first 200 cases. Radiology. 1999;211(2):477–88.
41. Black PMP. Development and implementation of intraoperative magnetic resonance imaging and its neurosurgical applications. Neurosurgery. 1997;41 (4):831.
42. Steinmeier RR. Intraoperative magnetic resonance imaging with the magnetom open scanner: concepts, neurosurgical indications, and procedures: a preliminary report. Neurosurgery. 1998;43(4):739.
43. Hall WAW. High-field strength interventional magnetic resonance imaging for pediatric neurosurgery. Pediatr Neurosurg. 1998;29(5):253.
44. Senft CC. Intraoperative MRI guidance and extent of resection in glioma surgery: a randomised, controlled trial. Lancet Oncol. 2011;12(11):997–1003.
45. Hatiboglu MAMA. Impact of intraoperative high-field magnetic resonance imaging guidance on glioma surgery: a prospective volumetric analysis. Neurosurgery. 2009;64(6):1073–81.
46. Kuhnt DD. Quantification of glioma removal by intraoperative high-field magnetic resonance imaging: an update. Neurosurgery. 2011;69(4):852–63.
47. Livne OO. Intraoperative magnetic resonance imaging for resection of intra-axial brain lesions: a decade of experience using low-field magnetic resonance imaging, Polestar N–10, 20, 30 systems. World Neurosur. 2014;82(5):770–6.
48. Mohammadi AMAM. Use of high-field intraoperative magnetic resonance imaging to enhance the extent of resection of enhancing and nonenhancing gliomas. Neurosurgery. 2014;74(4):339–50.
49. Napolitano MM. Glioblastoma surgery with and without intraoperative MRI at 3.0T. Neurochirurgie. 2014;60(4):143–50.

50. Olubiyi OIOI. Intraoperative magnetic resonance imaging in intracranial glioma resection: a single-center, retrospective blinded volumetric study. World Neurosurg. 2015;84(2):528–36.
51. Raheja AA. Initial experience of using high field strength intraoperative MRI for neurosurgical procedures. J Clin Neurosci. 2015;22(8):1326–31.
52. Roder CC. Maximizing the extent of resection and survival benefit of patients in glioblastoma surgery: high-field iMRI versus conventional and 5-ALA-assisted surgery. Eur J Surg Oncol. 2014;40(3):297–304.
53. Sakurada KK. Usefulness of multimodal examination and intraoperative magnetic resonance imaging system in glioma surgery. Neurol Med Chir. 2012;52(8):553.
54. Senft CC. Influence of iMRI-guidance on the extent of resection and survival of patients with glioblastoma multiforme. Technol Cancer Res Treat. 2010;9(4):339.
55. Senft CC. Optimizing the extent of resection in eloquently located gliomas by combining intraoperative MRI guidance with intraoperative neurophysiological monitoring. J Neurooncol. 2012;109(1):81–90.
56. G-cGC Sun. Intraoperative high-field magnetic resonance imaging combined with fiber tract neuronavigation-guided resection of cerebral lesions involving optic radiation. Neurosurgery. 2011;69(5):1070.
57. Wu J-SJS. 3.0-T intraoperative magnetic resonance imaging-guided resection in cerebral glioma surgery: interim analysis of a prospective, randomized, triple-blind, parallel-controlled trial. Neurosurgery. 2014;61 Suppl 1:145–54.
58. Kubben PLPL. Intraoperative magnetic resonance imaging versus standard neuronavigation for the neurosurgical treatment of glioblastoma: a randomized controlled trial. Surgical Neurol Int. 2014;5:70.
59. Childs S, Bruch P. Successful management of risk in the hybrid OR. AORN J. 2015;101(2):223–34; quiz 35–7.
60. Ene CICI. Flow-related aneurysm within glioblastoma: a case report and review of literature. World neurosurgery. 2016.
61. Nguyen HSHS. Coincidence of an anterior cerebral artery aneurysm and a glioblastoma: case report and review of literature. Int Med Case Rep J. 2015;8:295–9.
62. Shah AHAH. The role of preoperative embolization for intracranial meningiomas. J Neurosurg. 2013;119(2):364–72.

Mapping the Brain for Primary Brain Tumor Surgery

5

Emmanuel Mandonnet and Hugues Duffau

Abbreviations

ACEPS	Axonal-cortical evoked potentials
CCEPs	Cortico-cortical evoked potentials
CST	Cortico-spinal tract
DES	Direct electrical stimulation
DTI	Diffusion tensor imaging
ECoG	Electrocortiograms
HGA	High-gamma activity
IFOF	Inferior fronto-occipital fasciculus
PPTT	Pyramid-palm-tree test
R-fMRI	Rest-based fMRI
rTMS	Repetitive transcranial magnetic stimulation
SLF	Superior longitudinal fasciculus
SMA	Supplementary motor area
T-fMRI	Task-based fMRI
vPMC	Ventral premotor cortex
VWFA	Visual word from area

Introduction

The goal of surgery in primary brain tumors is to optimize the extent of resection, in order to significantly increase the survival, while preserving or even improving quality of life (for example by controlling intractable epilepsy). In other words,

E. Mandonnet
Department of Neurosurgery, Lariboisière Hospital, Paris, France
e-mail: emmanuel.mandonnet@aphp.fr

H. Duffau (✉)
Department of Neurosurgery, Gui de Chauliac Hospital, Montpellier, France
e-mail: h-duffau@chu-montpellier.fr

J. Moliterno Günel et al. (eds.), *Malignant Brain Tumors*,
DOI 10.1007/978-3-319-49864-5_5

the aim is to find the best "onco-functional balance", that is, to give the opportunity to the patients to enjoy a normal life as long as possible. To this end, due to a considerable inter-individual anatomo-functional variability, structural landmarks are important but not enough. Furthermore, in essence, "tumoral limits" do not exist in diffuse gliomas, because these tumors migrate within brain parenchyma, especially along the white matter tracts. As a consequence, in the past decade, it has been proposed to switch from "image-guided surgery" to "functional mapping-guided surgery", i.e., to achieve resection up to eloquent structures, both at cortical and subcortical levels. Indeed, advances in brain mapping have deeply improved the surgical management of glioma patients, regarding functional as well as oncological outcomes. In this chapter, we summarize the preoperative and intraoperative methods that allows to map the brain and we review the cortical and axonal mapping of the main cognitive functions.

Preoperative Mapping

The preoperative planning is likely to be the most important step in functional brain tumor resection. Apart the non-invasive techniques of brain mapping that will be discussed in this section, the preoperative time is essential for selecting the intraoperative tasks.

The choice of those tasks rely on three parameters:

- location of the tumor, in relation to the knowledge we have about the functional anatomy and neural networks [1],
- the deficit evidenced on extensive neuropsychological assessment. Indeed, any slight deficit in a cognitive domain testifies that plasticity limitations of the lesioned networks have been reached, meaning that this specific domain should be tested if it should be preserved (see for e.g. Chapter 19 in [2]),
- in-depth discussion with the patient. The choice of functions to be preserved depends on the patient's way of life (profession, hobbies ...) [3].

Over the last twenty years, several methods have been developed to map preoperatively brain functions. Although none of these methods is reliable enough to get rid of awake brain mapping by direct electrical stimulation, their combined use can be of help when there is a contra-indication to awake surgery. We rapidly review these methods and refer the reader to more specific review papers on this topic.

Preoperative Cortical Methods

Task-Based fMRI (T-fMRI)

The link between non-invasive T-fMRI mapping and intraoperative DES mapping remains poorly understood. For primary motor areas, the degree of correlation is quite high [4], although not perfect (for e.g., sensitivity of 71% reported in [5]). The problem is far more complex for higher cognitive functions, like complex motor task or language. Previous studies have approached the problem through simple comparison between activated areas on task-based fMRI and DES eloquent sites. It has been concluded that sensitivity and specificity of T-fMRI (with respect to DES areas) are much too low to rely solely on T-fMRI for determining functional boundaries. Depending on the T-fMRI paradigm, some studies concluded to a high sensitivity and low specificity, and some others to the reverse [6]. Of note, the advent of 3T MRI did not improve the reliability of fMRI (for e.g., sensitivity of 37.1% and specificity of 83.4% in [7]). At least two caveats might explain the discrepancy between T-fMRI and DES. First, as mentioned in [8], the two methods are intrinsically different: DES will jam some networks preventing their functionality. But, through instantaneous dynamic reorganization of the undisturbed networks, the function can eventually still be implemented by compensatory networks. This would explain some false positive of fMRI (i.e. an activated area on T-fMRI is not found eloquent by DES). To explain false negatives of fMRI, there are two possibilities: either they correspond to "false positives of DES" (i.e. removal of an eloquent DES areas would not cause any deficit) or it is a real false negative of fMRI (the site is eloquent and not detected by fMRI). This last situation is grounded by our recent understanding of the link between neuronal activity and BOLD signal. Indeed, it has been shown that BOLD contrast indicate areas with input and local computations rather than output spiking activity [9].

In the same vein, a recent study has shown that in temporal regions, high-gamma band power (which is believed to be the best surrogate of BOLD signal) on electrocorticography during picture naming and word reading vanishes after a short duration of 10 s [10]. On the contrary, in frontal areas, this activity lasted all along the 60 s of analysis. Such dissociation in neuronal activity between frontal and temporal areas during a language task likely explains that temporal areas are more difficult to detect on T-fMRI than frontal areas (see [11] and references therein).

Rest-Based fMRI (R-fMRI)

Although the first observation of low-frequency (0.1 Hz) correlations within distinct brain networks in a resting subject dates back to 1995 [12], it is only 10 years later that a seminal paper offered to use this technique to perform a segregation of brain areas in different functional networks [13]. Among others, have been recognized motor, language, attention (dorsal and ventral), and default mode networks. According to preliminary reports, R-fMRI could be a promising tool, with better correlations with DES [14, 15]. Moreover, a very important study revealed a high degree of correlations between R-fMRI and cortico-cortical evoked potentials (CCEPs) [16]. Last but not least, positive and negative correlations exhibited by R-fMRI have been found to exist also electrophysiologically (by measuring the correlations in the high-gamma band) [17]. All these datas support the idea that the partitioning of the brain based on low-frequency correlations in R-fMRI could be a powerful method to achieve in a very short time a global brain mapping for each patient.

rTMS: Motor/Language

The interest of rTMS regarding motor function mapping has been established. The motor maps obtained through neuronavigated rTMS are highly correlated with the intraoperative maps obtained by DES [18]. Moreover, for high-grade tumors, due to edema and vascular redistribution, T-fMRI might be unable to locate primary motor areas, whereas rTMS is still effective. For that reason, rTMS appears to be the gold standard for preoperative mapping of primary motor areas. Nonetheless, as it will be discussed in the paragraph about intraoperative methods, there is currently no reports testing by rTMS higher motor functions (like grasping, fine movements, bimanual coordination …). Moreover, there are conflicting results regarding the interest of rTMS for mapping language functions [19, 20]. Its specificity for language mapping is only 23.8%, with a positive predictive value of 35.6% according to [21]. A recent study investigated the relationship between T-fMRI, rTMS and DES maps [22]. It was found that rTMS was more sensitive compared to DES. On the contrary, T-fMRI was not enough sensitive with regards to DES. More specifically, T-fMRI failed to detect temporal language areas, as previously discussed.

Preoperative Axonal Mapping

Preoperative tractography is gaining interest among neurooncological surgeons. This MRI modality enables to locate the main white matter fiber tracts of the brain. In the past few years, several new algorithmic methods have been developed to infer fibers directions from diffusion-weighted images. Diffusion tensor estimation is the most widely used. It allows to draw RGB maps superimposed on a 3D-T1 anatomy, which is the simplest way to visualize white matter anisotropy. But this diffusion tensor estimation was unable to resolve the problem of crossing fibers. Two different new categories of algorithm attempted to overcome this limitation: the constrained spherical deconvolution and q-ball. Finally, it should be reminded that there is another layer of algorithms to determine the continuous line of a pathway: tracking algorithms. These algorithm are classified in two broad categories: deterministic or probabilistic. Tractograms can then be uploaded in the neuronavigation systems, allowing to correlated images with intraoperative stimulation, both for motor functions of the pyramidal tract and language functions of the dorsal and ventral streams. However, clinical interest of tractography is quite limited for two reasons:

- First, the variability of the trackings with the different methods. CSD and q-ball are supposed to resolve the problem of crossing fibers, however, there is currently no way to validate the obtained tractograms. As a consequence, a recent study by the DTI challenge concluded that there are still limitations for clinical use of DTI in neurosurgery [23]. Moreover, the problem of kissing fibers is even more challenging.
- Second, even if tractography would be perfect, this imaging method cannot inform us about the functional deficit that would be encountered after resection of a tracked fasciculus.

All in all, preoperative mapping methods are becoming more informative about individual brain functional and structural anatomy. It can be anticipated that datas coming from all these methods (T-fMRI, R-fMRI, tractography, rTMS) could be integrated by means of biocomputationals models of the brain, allowing better correlations with DES and surgical outcome.

Intraoperative Mapping

Cortical Mapping Under General Anesthesia

Motor: DES Versus Train of Five

The primary motor areas can be identified under GA by direct electrical stimulation. This seminal technique, introduced by Penfield, consists to apply a 60 Hz current for a few seconds (what we call Ojemann stimulation, OS), until a movement is elicited. About 20 years ago, the train of five (To5) technique has been introduced [24]. Since then, very few papers have studied the pro and cons of the two techniques. In a large series of glioma patients, Bello et al. very recently compared the two techniques and concluded that whereas To5 is always applicable, OS is not recommended for cases with increased excitability [25]. This excitability can be predicted from preoperative parameters, including long seizure history, diffuse margins on FLAIR, infiltration of CST, preoperative deficits.

However, it should be kept in mind that theTo5 technique is more challenging in terms of equipments and that interpretation of motor-evoked potentials has to be made by a qualified neurophysiologist. For this reason, many teams prefer to awake the patient also for motor functions.

Non-motor Functions: Cortico-Cortical Evoked Potentials

Up to now, awake surgery was the only way to identify cortical areas eloquent for non-motor functions. However, the technique of CCEP, initiated in 2004 by Matusmoto et al. (although there are some sporadic earlier reports cited in the paper of Matsumoto et al.) shows promising results regarding the possibility to map language functions under GA. In their initial report, these authors have shown, in an extraoperative recordings of grids put all over the perisylvian language areas, that 1 Hz stimulation of anterior frontal language areas (as detected by functional disturbances at 60 Hz stimulation) generates CCEPs in a wide posterior temporal region (including the 60 Hz temporal language site). And reciprocally, the posterior temporal language site also elicited CCEPs in the frontal operculum. Importantly, it has been recently shown the shape of these CCEPs is quite similar in awake and asleep patients [26]. More studies are needed to evaluate the clinical value of this new tool.

Cortical Mapping in Awake Condition

Several techniques can be used for intraoperative mapping in an awake patient. The first kind of methods is just to record electrical activity (by electrocortiograms, ECoG) while the patient is performing a task. Although high-gamma activity (HGA) of ECoG was the focus of several previous studies [27–31], it is only recently that this activity was analyzed on-line for language mapping [10]. It was shown to be highly correlated with direct electrical stimulation. This method is appealing, because all the brain surface can be mapped in a very short period of time. However, this technique is quite sophisticated, limiting currently its spread in daily practice [32].

Moreover, it should be noted that, similarly to T-fMRI, HGA mapping is in essence inadequate for distinguishing participating areas from essential ones. Hence, only methods interfering with neuronal networks can make the distinction. There are two different ways to interfere with brain networks: cooling and electrical stimulation. Cooling as been reported once in humans, and showed somewhat different results compared to electrical stimulation [33]. For some reason, this method has not been used by any other team to our knowledge, and consequently, we will focus, in the next sections, on brain mapping by direct electrical stimulation.

Sensori-Motor Functions

In comparison to the motor mapping that can be done asleep, awake motor mapping offers the possibility to test not only the ability to move, but also to perform complex movements or motor behavior. Although there exists a variety of tasks (repetitive movement of flexion and extension of the different segments of the superior limb, grasping, using a screw-driver, in-phase and out-of-phase bimanual movements), their use remains rare during awake surgery. In fact, the first cases have been reported during extraoperative mapping for epilepsy surgery [34, 35]. A recent review [36] discussed these so called negative motor areas (negative, because they stop the on-going motor behavior). Two clusters have been found on each hemisphere: the posterior end of inferior frontal gyrus (pars opercularis) together with the lower end of precentral gyrus on the lateral surface, and the SMA on the mesial surface. In a somehow contradictory study about the exact location of these sites on the superior frontal gyrus, it has been shown recently that, in fact, 95% of sites blocking repetitive complex movements or bilateral coordination are located in the convexity of the superior frontal gyrus (see also Fig. 5.1), while only 5% are located in the mesial part of the superior frontal gyrus [37]. Last but not least, awake condition allows the patient to report about sensory functions: for example, he can warn the surgeon by telling during stimulation (usually of parietal areas) «I do not feel my leg anymore» and the preservation of these sites is crucial to keep such a fundamental function as walking.

Primary Visual Areas

The preservation of the primary visual areas on both sides of the calcarine sulcus is in some cases of utmost importance. Indeed, it should be reminded to the patient that the driving license is no more valid in case of hemianopsia. As initially reported in 1968 [38], electrical stimulation generates mainly positive visual phenomena, like phosphene, flash of light, … Of note, as for any primary motor or sensory areas, there is almost no plasticity, meaning that anatomical landmarks allow to locate primary visual areas reliably.

Language

Language is the most widely mapped function during awake surgery. Since the very first reports by Penfield, the technology did not change that much: applying electrical stimulation for a period of 3–4 s disturbs the language task. However, the

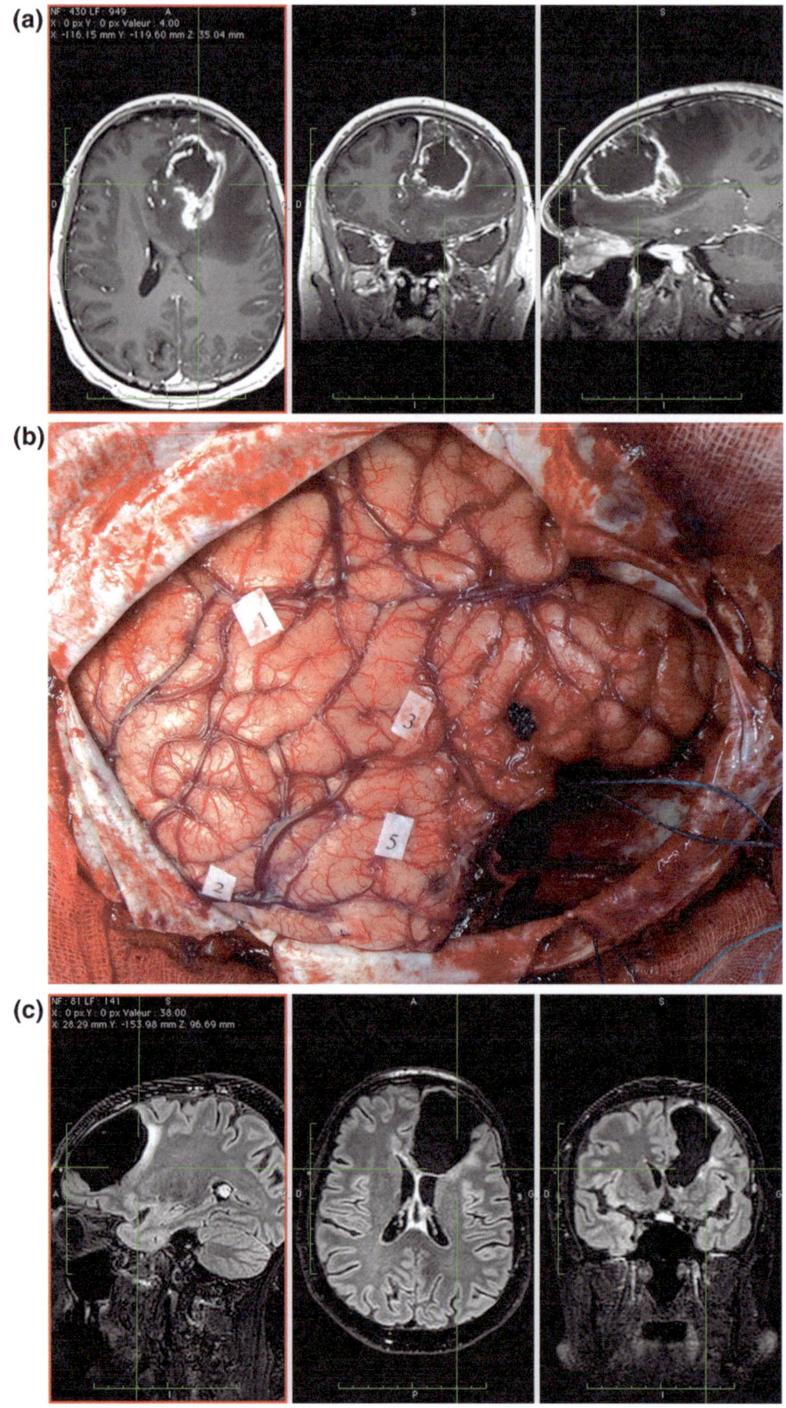
(a)
NF : 430 LF : 949
X : 0 px Y : 0 px Valeur : 4.00
X: -116.15 mm Y: -119.60 mm Z: 35.04 mm
(b)
1
3
5
2
(c)
NF : 81 LF : 141
X : 0 px Y : 0 px Valeur : 38.00
X: 28.29 mm Y: -153.98 mm Z: 96.69 mm

◀ **Fig. 5.1** Illustrative case of a 50 years-old frustrated left-handed patient diagnosed with a left frontal glioblastoma revealed by headaches and language disturbances. **a Preoperative T1-gadolinium enhanced MRI**, showing a large enhancing mass of the superior frontal gyrus, extending towards the ventricle and the head of the caudate nucleus. **b Intraoperative mapping**, cortical mapping evidenced a complete anarthria in the parietal operculum (tag 1), primary motor area of the thumb (tag 2), negative motor areas, stopping repetitive movement of upper limb (tag 3 and 4), and disturbances of PPTT with preservation of picture naming (tag 5). Axonally, resection was stopped in the lateral vicinity of the head of the caudate nucleus, where stimulation at the cross-road between aslant tract and IFOF generated perseverations and semantic paraphasias. **c Postoperative FLAIR MRI** showing a small residue in the posterior wall (the enhancement was completely removed). Patient was then treated with radiotherapy with concomitant Temozolomide, followed by 6 cycles of Temozolomide. He was able to resume his professional activity of sales representative full time. He remained recurrence-free for 18 months

classification of the different types of observed errors has been only recently clarified: it is of utmost importance to distinguish motor arrest, speech arrest, and anomia. A simple algorithm has been proposed, in order to optimize the initial testing for differentiating the areas to these different types of error [39]. Most commonly, the language assessment is performed through a picture naming task. This raises a still debated question: is it enough to assess a function as complex as language just by naming pictures? In a first response, it is important to notice that picture naming allows to investigate the two main components of language: phonology and semantics [40]. Indeed, the speech therapist can make the on-line distinction between phonological paraphasia (e.g. log instead of dog) versus semantic paraphasia (for e.g. cat instead of dog) [41]. The current anatomo-functional model maps these two components on the dorsal pathway for phonology and ventral stream for semantics [42]. However, on the cortical surface, there is no clear-cut spatial segregation between phonological and semantic sites [43]. There is for each domain, three clusters in the left hemisphere: one in the pars triangularis, one at the posterior end of the middle frontal gyrus, and one in the posterior part of the superior temporal gyrus. The great well known inter-patients variability [44] proves once again the necessity of intraoperative mapping in an awake patient. Of note, there is a striking resemblance between this map and the clusters evidenced by a meta-analysis of T-fmRI studies [45]. This overlapping suggests that the phonological and semantic systems are not anatomically separable at the 5 mm scale at the cortical level. Of note, when the patient's response is an anomia, one cannot conclude whether this is a disturbance of the phonological or semantic system, or both.

Hence, the ability to name a picture insures that both phonological and lexico-semantic abilities are preserved. However, it should be kept in mind that naming does not warrant full semantic judgment. Indeed, a dissociation has been shown between picture naming and pyramid-palm-tree test (PPTT), a supramodal semantic association task: in some fronto-opercular and superior temporal sites (see also Fig. 5.1), patients were able to name pictures, without being able to make semantic association [46, 47].

Moreover, language requires more than phonology and basic semantics: syntax, that is the ability to find the meaning of a sentence from rules and links between words, is also an essential part of language. Interestingly, although some patients exhibit difficulties to understand syntactically complex sentences in the immediate postoperative course, permanent syntactic deficit after picture-naming based awake surgery are rarely observed [48]. Similarly, there are no reported case of patients with a long lasting deficit of repetition (i.e. a language task with an auditory rather than visual input). Still, many authors have proposed numerous tasks for better evaluating language intraoperatively (see following review papers [49–51]), and some new protocols are still under investigation [52, 53].

Nevertheless, it should be mentioned that proper name deficits have been reported after left anterior temporal lobectomy [54, 55]. Whereas this deficit can be prevented by adding a task of naming famous faces, this should be balanced on a case-by-case basis with the oncological benefit:

indeed, the impact in daily life of an inability to name proper names is highly variable for each patient.

Similarly, one should not forget to test patients in mother-tongue and secondary learned languages for bilingual patients [56–60].

Last but not least, reading is an essential part of language abilities. Removal of visual word form area (VWFA) has been shown to result in long lasting reading deficit [61], while its identification by DES allows to preserve reading abilities [62, 63]. Apart in the basal temporo-occipital areas, different studies reported specific reading disturbances when stimulating posterior superior left temporal gyrus and left supramarginal gyrus [64], but also posterior part of inferior and middle left frontal gyrus [65]. These latter sites were generally superimposed or close to naming sites, meaning that they would have been preserved even if lecture would not have been tested. Finally, stimulation of FEF areas also induced reading troubles, by generating involuntary ocular movements (but this area can be detected just by looking at eyes movements [66]). On a practical point of view, these results show that reading per se needs to be tested only in (left) dominant posterior temporo-occipital regions. Of note, disturbances were very infrequently observed in the anterior temporal lobe. This is somehow in disagreement with the triangle model, in which it has been shown recently that the semantico-phonological conversion in reading is thought to be supported by the anterior temporal lobe [67]. Moreover, in this model, the role of posterior inferior and middle frontal regions was not assigned. Hence, electrostimulation datas should be better integrated in the currents neurocomputational models of reading.

Spatial Consciousness

It has been well known from stroke studies that right parietal lobe lesions can result in spatial neglect of the opposite hemi-space. Because such deficit can be as debilitating in daily life, the importance of preventing this syndrome cannot be overemphasized. In a seminal report in 2005, Thiebaut de Schotten et al. described two cases of right parietal tumor resection with spatial consciousness monitoring [68]. The bisection test is very simple: the patient is asked to draw the middle of a 20 cm line. In case of unilateral spatial neglect (transiently generated by the electrical stimulation), patient will deviate on the right of the line. Two cortical deviations sites were identified, in the caudal superior temporal gyrus and in the supramarginal gyrus. Since then, two studies reported larger series of spatial consciousness mapping [69, 70]. Roux et al. found several cortical regions with rightward but also leftward deviations. Those regions were centered around the temporo-parietal junction and deviations in the superior parietal lobule were uncommon. On the contrary, Vallar et al. observed rightward deviations mainly in Broadman's area 7b. Like for language, it is likely that spatial consciousness is supported by a distributed set of interconnected cortical areas.

Calculation

The neural correlates of mental calculation have been intensively studied by T-fMRI studies. It involves a large set of areas, grouped in three different networks [71]: the bilateral horizontal segment of intraparietal sulcus for quantity processing, the left angular gyrus for numbers manipulation in verbal modality, and the bilateral superior parietal regions for focusing attention (and this network is not specific to number manipulations). Accordingly, several authors reported disruption of calculation in various cortical areas, such as left angular gyrus [72–74], right angular gyrus [75, 76], left superior parietal lobule [77], horizontal portion of left intraparietal sulcus and left supramarginal gyrus [74]. In all these studies, some sites were specific to calculation and even to a subtype of computations (susbtraction vs. multiplication), while some others were also related to language disturbances. It should be noted that, in comparison with language mapping, there are very few reports about mental calculation mapping. This might be in relation to the relative rarity of parietal diffuse low-grade glioma. Moreover, the functional benefit of preserving mental calculation should be balanced with the oncological benefit to remove these areas: indeed, except for some very specific professions requiring mathematical abilities, patients usually do not care to keep their mental calculation abilities (probably because we are more and more relying on computers for daily arithmetic).

Double Task

The importance in efficient cognition of being able to perform simultaneously two tasks cannot be overemphasized. Fortunately, this can be easily tested intraoperatively: a motor task can be added to any other cognitive task. Hence, patients can be asked to do picture naming or PPTT or mental calculation while simultaneously performing a repetitive movement of the upper limb. This double task greatly enhances the sensitivity to electrical stimulation, that is, some sites will respond only to the double task, while each task separately would be efficiently performed [42]. Again, depending on the preoperative discussion with the patient, one can decide to preserve or not such areas requiring a high-level of cognitive functioning.

Mentalizing

Emotions have a major influence in daily life, particularly for decision making. Assessing the subjective experience of others in terms of mental states is a brain function referred to as mentalizing. Recent theories hypothesizes a two levels hierarchical network: a low-level network for emotion recognition or motor intention (theory of mind), and a higher-level network of mentalizing per se for complex inferences about other's state of mind and intentions. The low-level network is supposed to be linked to the mirror neuron system, whereas the higher-level is related to the default-mode network, in particular the ability to attribute the intentions of others [78]. Interestingly, the low-level network can be monitored intraoperatively by the Read the Mind in the Eyes test. A first study reported responses in the right superior temporal gyrus, middle temporal gyrus and supramarginal gyrus [79]. In another study, responses were found in the pars opercularis and triangularis of the right frontal operculum [80]. If it is safer to preserve these sites, it should be noted that this function is likely to be distributed over redundant areas, ensuring a high plastic potential: indeed, in a series without intraoperative testing, only two patients out of ten kept an impairment on the assessment 3 months after surgery [81]. Of note, whereas mentalizing per se can be objectively evaluated with the comic strips task, there is currently no way to test the higher-level network in an intraoperative setting. It could be anticipated that this higher-level function is even more prone to plasticity than its lower-level counterpart. This would explain the very low risk of permanent deficit (10%).

Other Self-reported Effects of Stimulations

A major advantage of on-line monitoring during awake surgery is the possibility for the patient to continuously report any inner conscious and subjective feeling induced by electrical stimulation. For example, intention to move (by stimulation in the posterior parietal cortex [82]) or out-of-body experiments (interpreted as a disruption of multisensory information by stimulating the (right) temporo-parietal junction [83]) have been described by patients.

In the same vein, disruption of consciousness of the external environment (induced by stimulating the ventral part of the posterior cingulate cortex) has been reported [84]. After recovering from the stimulation, the patients could describe their state as if «in a dream».

Axonal Mapping Under General Anesthesia

Motor: DES Versus Train of Five

The To5 technique is becoming a popular tool for axonal mapping of the cortico-spinal tract.

Continuous monitoring can be achieved by stimulating with the resective surgical tool, either the ultrasonic aspirator [85] or a suction device [86].

All in all, To5 appears to be a powerful method, for both cortical and axonal identification of cortico-spinal pathway. However, it should be kept in mind that with this technique, it is currently not possible to assess higher order motor function (like grasping, fine movements, bimanual coordination …) and the only way to monitor these functions is intraoperative electrical mapping in an awake patient.

Non-motor Functions: ACEPs

Until very recently, there was no technique to map non-motor function axonally under GA. A very recent study reported the identification of the arcuate fasciculus by axono-cortical evoked potentials [26]. The basic idea is to stimulate at 1 Hz during white matter removal and to record in anterior and posterior language areas identified by CCEPs. The reliability of this technique needs to be assessed further, but seems promising.

Axonal Mapping in Awake Patients

Motor Functions

The possibility to test repetitive movements and bimanual coordination opened new avenues in the axonal mapping of motor functions. In particular, the stimulation of the fibers located in the depth of the precentral sulcus generates impairments of repetitive movements of unilateral or bilateral limbs. It has been argued that the stimulated pathway has direct projection to the spinal cord [87]. In addition, the network for motor control might also involve the frontal aslant tract (linking the SMA to the pars opercularis/vPMC) and the fronto-striatal tract [88, 89]. This is not surprising, considering that the aslant tract makes the link between the two clusters of «negative motor areas». From past experience in surgery with motor mapping under GA, it is known that resection of these pathways will lead to the so called «SMA syndrome», with a transient akinesia (and mutism on the left dominant side). Again, the oncological benefit should be carefully balance for each patient: it is certainly important to preserve a high level of motor coordination in a tennis player or a pianist, while it might be not necessary for a sales manager.

Language Function

Since the seminal paper in 2002 [90], great advances have been made in our understanding of error patterns elicited by white matter pathways stimulation. These advances were concomitant with the development of new neuropsychological models of language (identifying phonological and semantic as the two main subsystems [40], and hypothesizing that they are sustained anatomically by two parallel pathways, the dorsal and ventral streams respectively [91]) and with the (re)-discovery of white matter anatomy by diffusion tensor imaging and cadaveric fiber dissections. For example, the inferior fronto-occipital fasciculus has been rediscovered by DTI [92] and detailed by fiber dissections [93, 94], and new pathways (aslant [95–97], middle longitudinal fasciculus [98–100]) were discovered by virtual dissections and then confirmed by fiber dissections [96, 97, 101]. On the other side, as explained above, tracking algorithms can lead to unrealistic pathways: for example, the trajectory of the SLF I as described by DTI [102] is the subject of debate among fiber dissection experts (see [103] for initial controversy, and [104] for recent discussion). In the same vein, a long standing debate about the putative existence of a superior occipital-frontal fasciculus seems to be resolved [105].

The datas gathered from axonal mapping can be summarized in two ways:

- Probabilistic maps, either of functional tumor remnants [106] or of eloquent sites [107].
- Neuropsychological models with anatomical substrate [41, 42].

In brief, phonological errors are more frequently encountered by stimulation of the arcuate fasciculus [108, 109], while perseverations and semantic errors are more frequently encountered by stimulation of IFOF (see Fig. 5.1) [110, 111]. This is in line with the dual stream model of language [91, 112]. Articulatory aspects are supported by the SLF III [113], while disturbances of speech fluency are observed in relation to the aslant and fronto-striatal tracts [114, 115], linking the SMA area to the pars opercularis/vPMC and the head of caudate nucleus respectively. The connectivity of the reading system has also been investigated [116]. The results show that: stimulation of inputs to the VWFA (i.e. the posterior part of the inferior longitudinal fasciculus) induces complete alexia; stimulation of the white matter anteriorly adjacent to the VWFA induces difficulties for irregular words reading (i.e. for the semantic/addressed pathway in the triangle model); while stimulation of the white matter located superiorly to the VWFA generates difficulties for both irregular and pseudo-words, but not for regular words. This intriguing observation suggest that the posterior part of the arcuate fasciculus is involved in the executive control that normally regulates the balance between the semantic/addressed and phonological/assembled pathways.

Visual Functions

Whenever the patients cannot accept to live with a hemianopsia, the visual pathways should be preserved by DES mapping. The anatomical complexity of the visuals pathways has recently been revisited, thanks to DTI and fiber dissection studies [117–121]. It should be mentioned that intraoperative testing of vision in a hemi-field remains a challenge, because axonal stimulation can generate visual defect rather than positive phenomena. Hence, it is necessary to use for example picture naming with images distributed in the different quadrants. However, because the patient can compensate with ocular movements, this is not a 100% reliable methodology [122] and this should be taken into account in the onco-functional balance [3].

Spatial Consciousness

In a seminal study [68], the 2nd branch of the superior longitudinal fasciculus was identified as the tract whose stimulation generated rightward deviations in line bisection test. Since this first description, two other teams reported their observations of intraoperative line bisection [69, 70]. Results are not easy to compare, as methodology were slightly different (line on paper versus tablet, use of right hand or left hand to mark the midpoint). Interestingly, leftward as well as rightward deviations were observed. Remarkably, both studies agreed that it is the stimulation of the second branch of the superior longitudinal fasciculus that generates massive deviations. How these observations (and especially the leftward deviations) could be integrated in the general model of spatial neglect as an interaction between right dominant stimulus-driven ventral attention network (sustained by SLF III) and goal-directed bilateral dorsal attention network (sustained by SLF II) [123] remains an open question.

Mentalizing

A lesion study suggested that disconnection of the right arcuate fasciculus and/or SLF III was associated with poorer low-level mentalizing, while disconnection of the right cingulum was associated with poorer high-level mentalizing [78]. Accordingly, stimulation of the white matter of the right frontal operculum generated error in the Read the Mind in the Eyes test, at a location that could correspond to the terminations of the the arcuate fasciculus/SLF III [80]. More studies are needed to make the link with the more posterior sites observed cortically, that is to stimulate the arcuate fasciculus/SLF III in the depth of a tumor located to the right supramarginal gyrus.

Mental Calculation

While a first study did not report any disturbances of mental calculation when stimulating white matter of the left angular gyrus [73], such effects were observed when stimulating the white matter in the right parietal lobe [124].

Plasticity and Remapping

Whenever the resection has been pushed until encountering functional responses in an awake patient, an immediate postoperative decline is usually observed in one or several cognitive domains. The onset of this deterioration is not always immediate, and usually takes place between postoperative day 1 and 3 [125]. The classical explanation of this delay is that deterioration is concomitant to the peak of edema. In addition, it can be hypothesized that in the first postoperative days, the brain is massively reorganizing its connection weights, resulting in a transient abnormal functioning. Recovery usually occurs in two steps: a rapid spontaneous postoperative recovery in the first week after deterioration, and a slow rehabilitation-guided long-term recovery (lasting about 3 months). The importance of intensive rehabilitation cannot be overemphasized. It should be started as soon as possible, right after the surgery [126, 127], and it should be under the supervision of a trained speech therapist or neuropsychologist. On a patho-physiological point of view, this long-term recovery is directly related to the patient's potential of plasticity, and it has been observed that it took longer time in older patients.

All in all, for low-grade glioma, postoperative plasticity is driven first by rehabilitation and then by the slow regrowth of the tumor. As a consequence, it should be kept in mind that, thanks to this plasticity, responsive sites identified during a first surgery might be unresponsive some years later. This opens the possibility to reoperate on low-grade glioma and to remove the second time some areas found eloquent at first surgery—thus to increase the extent of resection without eliciting permanent functional deficits [128, 129].

Conclusions

Advances in brain mapping techniques have allowed a better understanding of the dynamic organization of human brain, i.e. in large-scale, parallel, delocalized and interactive sub-networks. Therefore, anatomical landmarks are not enough to preserve an optimal quality of life in brain tumor patients undergoing maximal resective surgery: individual functional mapping is mandatory to tailor the resection according to cortical and subcortical eloquent structures for each patient. Because non-invasive preoperative functional neuroimaging is currently not reliable enough to identify the cortices and white matter tracts crucial for brain processing, in particular with regard to high order cognitive functions, intraoperative mapping using direct electrical stimulation is the goal standard to remove diffuse gliomas. In awake patients, it is now possible to achieve an extensive mapping, not only of sensorimotor and language functions, but also of cognitive and emotional functions. Cortical and axonal stimulation enables a precise investigation of the neural circuits of glioma patients, to detect a possible remapping elicited by the tumor itself, in addition to the interindividual variability, and to define in real-time the boundaries of surgical resection in order to improve both the oncological results (e.g. by performing a supratotal resection, extended beyond the enhancement in high-grade gliomas and beyond the FLAIR abnormalities in low-grade glioma) as well as the functional outcomes. The ultimate goal is to increase the quantity of quality of life, based upon a personalized surgical strategy taking into account the wishes of the patient. Therefore, a comprehensive explanation of the natural history of the disease, but also the determination of the individual quality of life (according notably to the job and hobby of the patient) is essential before the surgical act, with the aim to adapt the selection of cognitive tasks during resection, and then to optimize the onco-functional balance of surgery.

References

1. Fernández Coello A, Moritz-Gasser S, Martino J, Martinoni M, Matsuda R, Duffau H. Selection of intraoperative tasks for awake mapping based on relationships between tumor location and functional networks. J Neurosurg. 2013;119(6):1380–94.
2. Diffuse Low-Grade Gliomas in Adults—Natural History, Interaction with the Brain, and New Individualized [Internet]. Springer. Hugues Duffau; [cited 2013 Dec 8]. Available from: http://www.springer.com/medicine/oncology/book/978-1-4471-2212-8.
3. Duffau H, Mandonnet E. The, "onco-functional balance" in surgery for diffuse low-grade glioma: integrating the extent of resection with quality of life. Acta Neurochir (Wien). 2013;155(6):951–7.
4. Gabriel M, Brennan NP, Peck KK, Holodny AI. Blood oxygen level dependent functional magnetic resonance imaging for presurgical planning. Neuroimaging Clin N Am. 2014;24(4):557–71.
5. Bartos R, Jech R, Vymazal J, Petrovický P, Vachata P, Hejcl A, et al. Validity of primary motor area localization with fMRI versus electric cortical stimulation: a comparative study. Acta Neurochir (Wien). 2009;151(9):1071–80.
6. Giussani C, Roux F-E, Ojemann J, Sganzerla EP, Pirillo D, Papagno C. Is preoperative functional magnetic resonance imaging reliable for language

areas mapping in brain tumor surgery? Review of language functional magnetic resonance imaging and direct cortical stimulation correlation studies. Neurosurgery. 2010;66(1):113–20.
7. Kuchcinski G, Mellerio C, Pallud J, Dezamis E, Turc G, Rigaux-Viodé O, et al. Three-tesla functional MR language mapping: comparison with direct cortical stimulation in gliomas. Neurology. 2015;84(6):560–8.
8. Mandonnet E. Intraoperative electrical mapping: advances, limitations and perspectives. In: MD PHD, editor. Brain mapping [Internet]. Springer Vienna; 2011 [cited 2016 Feb 6]. p. 101–8. Available from: http://link.springer.com/chapter/10.1007/978-3-7091-0723-2_8.
9. Logothetis NK. The neural basis of the blood-oxygen-level-dependent functional magnetic resonance imaging signal. Philos Trans R Soc Lond B Biol Sci. 2002;357(1424):1003–37.
10. Ogawa H, Kamada K, Kapeller C, Hiroshima S, Prueckl R, Guger C. Rapid and minimum invasive functional brain mapping by real-time visualization of high gamma activity during awake craniotomy. World Neurosurg. 2014;82(5):912.e1–10.
11. Kunii N, Kamada K, Ota T, Kawai K, Saito N. Characteristic profiles of high gamma activity and blood oxygenation level-dependent responses in various language areas. Neuroimage. 2013;15 (65):242–9.
12. Biswal B, Yetkin FZ, Haughton VM, Hyde JS. Functional connectivity in the motor cortex of resting human brain using echo-planar MRI. Magn Reson Med. 1995;34(4):537–41.
13. Fox MD, Snyder AZ, Vincent JL, Corbetta M, Van Essen DC, Raichle ME. The human brain is intrinsically organized into dynamic, anticorrelated functional networks. Proc Natl Acad Sci USA. 2005;102(27):9673–8.
14. Mitchell TJ, Hacker CD, Breshears JD, Szrama NP, Sharma M, Bundy DT, et al. A novel data-driven approach to preoperative mapping of functional cortex using resting-state functional magnetic resonance imaging. Neurosurgery. 2013;73(6):969–982; discussion 982–983.
15. Qiu T, Yan C, Tang W, Wu J, Zhuang D, Yao C, et al. Localizing hand motor area using resting-state fMRI: validated with direct cortical stimulation. Acta Neurochir (Wien). 2014;156(12):2295–302.
16. Keller CJ, Bickel S, Entz L, Ulbert I, Milham MP, Kelly C, et al. Intrinsic functional architecture predicts electrically evoked responses in the human brain. Proc Natl Acad Sci USA. 2011;108 (25):10308–13.
17. Keller CJ, Bickel S, Honey CJ, Groppe DM, Entz L, Craddock RC, et al. Neurophysiological investigation of spontaneous correlated and anticorrelated fluctuations of the BOLD signal. J Neurosci. 2013;33(15):6333–42.
18. Picht T, Schmidt S, Brandt S, Frey D, Hannula H, Neuvonen T, et al. Preoperative functional mapping for rolandic brain tumor surgery: comparison of navigated transcranial magnetic stimulation to direct cortical stimulation. Neurosurgery. 2011;69 (3):581–588; discussion 588.
19. Krieg SM, Shiban E, Buchmann N, Gempt J, Foerschler A, Meyer B, et al. Utility of presurgical navigated transcranial magnetic brain stimulation for the resection of tumors in eloquent motor areas. J Neurosurg. 2012;116(5):994–1001.
20. Krieg SM, Tarapore PE, Picht T, Tanigawa N, Houde J, Sollmann N, et al. Optimal timing of pulse onset for language mapping with navigated repetitive transcranial magnetic stimulation. Neuroimage. 2014;15(100):219–36.
21. Picht T, Krieg SM, Sollmann N, Rösler J, Niraula B, Neuvonen T, et al. A comparison of language mapping by preoperative navigated transcranial magnetic stimulation and direct cortical stimulation during awake surgery. Neurosurgery. 2013;72(5):808–19.
22. Ille S, Sollmann N, Hauck T, Maurer S, Tanigawa N, Obermueller T, et al. Impairment of preoperative language mapping by lesion location: a functional magnetic resonance imaging, navigated transcranial magnetic stimulation, and direct cortical stimulation study. J Neurosurg. 2015;123(2): 314–24.
23. Pujol S, Wells W, Pierpaoli C, Brun C, Gee J, Cheng G, et al. The DTI challenge: toward standardized evaluation of diffusion tensor imaging tractography for neurosurgery. J Neuroimaging. 2015;25(6):875–82.
24. Taniguchi M, Cedzich C, Schramm J. Modification of cortical stimulation for motor evoked potentials under general anesthesia: technical description. Neurosurgery. 1993;32(2):219–26.
25. Bello L, Riva M, Fava E, Ferpozzi V, Castellano A, Raneri F, et al. Tailoring neurophysiological strategies with clinical context enhances resection and safety and expands indications in gliomas involving motor pathways. Neuro-oncology. 2014;16 (8):1110–28.
26. Yamao Y, Matsumoto R, Kunieda T, Arakawa Y, Kobayashi K, Usami K, et al. Intraoperative dorsal language network mapping by using single-pulse electrical stimulation. Hum Brain Mapp. 2014;35 (9):4345–61.
27. Canolty RT, Edwards E, Dalal SS, Soltani M, Nagarajan SS, Kirsch HE, et al. High gamma power is phase-locked to theta oscillations in human neocortex. Science. 2006;313(5793):1626–8.
28. Canolty RT, Soltani M, Dalal SS, Edwards E, Dronkers NF, Nagarajan SS, et al. Spatiotemporal dynamics of word processing in the human brain. Front Neurosci. 2007;1(1):185–96.
29. Edwards E, Nagarajan SS, Dalal SS, Canolty RT, Kirsch HE, Barbaro NM, et al. Spatiotemporal imaging of cortical activation during verb generation and picture naming. Neuroimage. 2010;50 (1):291–301.

30. Mainy N, Jung J, Baciu M, Kahane P, Schoendorff B, Minotti L, et al. Cortical dynamics of word recognition. Hum Brain Mapp. 2008;29(11):1215–30.
31. Pei X, Leuthardt EC, Gaona CM, Brunner P, Wolpaw JR, Schalk G. Spatiotemporal dynamics of electrocorticographic high gamma activity during overt and covert word repetition. Neuroimage. 2011;54(4):2960–72.
32. Pallud J. A concept car or an all-road car to drive all along glioma resection? World Neurosurg. 2015;84 (1):187.
33. Bakken HE, Kawasaki H, Oya H, Greenlee JDW, Howard MA. A device for cooling localized regions of human cerebral cortex. Technical note. J Neurosurg. 2003;99(3):604–8.
34. Lüders HO, Dinner DS, Morris HH, Wyllie E, Comair YG. Cortical electrical stimulation in humans. The negative motor areas. Adv Neurol. 1995;67:115–29.
35. Mikuni N, Ohara S, Ikeda A, Hayashi N, Nishida N, Taki J, et al. Evidence for a wide distribution of negative motor areas in the perirolandic cortex. Clin Neurophysiol. 2006;117(1):33–40.
36. Filevich E, Kühn S, Haggard P. Negative motor phenomena in cortical stimulation: implications for inhibitory control of human action. Cortex. 2012;48 (10):1251–61.
37. Martino J, Gabarrós A, Deus J, Juncadella M, Acebes JJ, Torres A, et al. Intrasurgical mapping of complex motor function in the superior frontal gyrus. Neuroscience. 2011;14(179):131–42.
38. Brindley GS, Lewin WS. The visual sensations produced by electrical stimulation of the medial occipital cortex. J Physiol (Lond). 1968;194(2):54–5.
39. Mandonnet E, Sarubbo S, Duffau H. Proposal of an optimized strategy for intraoperative testing of speech and language during awake mapping. Neurosurgical Review. In Press.
40. Indefrey P, Levelt WJM. The spatial and temporal signatures of word production components. Cognition. 2004;92(1–2):101–44.
41. Duffau H, Moritz-Gasser S, Mandonnet E. A re-examination of neural basis of language processing: Proposal of a dynamic hodotopical model from data provided by brain stimulation mapping during picture naming. Brain Lang. 2013.
42. Duffau H. Stimulation mapping of white matter tracts to study brain functional connectivity. Nat Rev Neurol. 2015;11(5):255–65.
43. Tate MC, Herbet G, Moritz-Gasser S, Tate JE, Duffau H. Probabilistic map of critical functional regions of the human cerebral cortex: Broca's area revisited. Brain. 2014.
44. Ojemann GA. Individual variability in cortical localization of language. J Neurosurg. 1979;50 (2):164–9.
45. Vigneau M, Beaucousin V, Hervé PY, Duffau H, Crivello F, Houdé O, et al. Meta-analyzing left hemisphere language areas: phonology, semantics, and sentence processing. Neuroimage. 2006;30 (4):1414–32.
46. Gatignol P, Capelle L, Le Bihan R, Duffau H. Double dissociation between picture naming and comprehension: an electrostimulation study. NeuroReport. 2004;15(1):191–5.
47. Bello L, Gallucci M, Fava M, Carrabba G, Giussani C, Acerbi F, et al. Intraoperative subcortical language tract mapping guides surgical removal of gliomas involving speech areas. Neurosurgery. 2007;60(1):67–80; discussion 80–82.
48. Teichmann M, Rosso C, Martini J-B, Bloch I, Brugières P, Duffau H, et al. A cortical-subcortical syntax pathway linking Broca's area and the striatum. Hum Brain Mapp. 2015;36(6):2270–83.
49. De Witte E, Mariën P. The neurolinguistic approach to awake surgery reviewed. Clin Neurol Neurosurg. 2013;115(2):127–45.
50. Rofes A, Miceli G. Language mapping with verbs and sentences in awake surgery: a review. Neuropsychol Rev. 2014;24(2):185–99.
51. Talacchi A, Santini B, Casartelli M, Monti A, Capasso R, Miceli G. Awake surgery between art and science. Part II: language and cognitive mapping. Funct Neurol. 2013;28(3):223–39.
52. De Witte E, Satoer D, Robert E, Colle H, Verheyen S, Visch-Brink E, et al. The Dutch Linguistic Intraoperative Protocol: a valid linguistic approach to awake brain surgery. Brain Lang. 2015;140:35–48.
53. Rofes A, de Aguiar V, Miceli G. A minimal standardization setting for language mapping tests: an Italian example. Neurol Sci. 2015;36(7):1113–9.
54. Papagno C, Casarotti A, Comi A, Pisoni A, Lucchelli F, Bizzi A, et al. Long-term proper name anomia after removal of the uncinate fasciculus. Brain Struct Funct. 2014.
55. Papagno C, Miracapillo C, Casarotti A, Romero Lauro LJ, Castellano A, Falini A, et al. What is the role of the uncinate fasciculus? Surgical removal and proper name retrieval. Brain. 2011;134(Pt 2):405–14.
56. Roux F-E, Trémoulet M. Organization of language areas in bilingual patients: a cortical stimulation study. J Neurosurg. 2002;97(4):857–64.
57. Giussani C, Roux F-E, Lubrano V, Gaini SM, Bello L. Review of language organisation in bilingual patients: what can we learn from direct brain mapping? Acta Neurochir (Wien). 2007;149 (11):1109–1116; discussion 1116.
58. Lucas TH, McKhann GM, Ojemann GA. Functional separation of languages in the bilingual brain: a comparison of electrical stimulation language mapping in 25 bilingual patients and 117 monolingual control patients. J Neurosurg. 2004;101 (3):449–57.
59. Walker JA, Quiñones-Hinojosa A, Berger MS. Intraoperative speech mapping in 17 bilingual patients undergoing resection of a mass lesion.

Neurosurgery. 2004;54(1):113–117; discussion 118.
60. Bello L, Acerbi F, Giussani C, Baratta P, Taccone P, Songa V, et al. Intraoperative language localization in multilingual patients with gliomas. Neurosurgery. 2006;59(1):115–125; discussion 115–125.
61. Gaillard R, Naccache L, Pinel P, Clémenceau S, Volle E, Hasboun D, et al. Direct intracranial, FMRI, and lesion evidence for the causal role of left inferotemporal cortex in reading. Neuron. 2006;50 (2):191–204.
62. Gil-Robles S, Carvallo A, Jimenez MDM, Gomez Caicoya A, Martinez R, Ruiz-Ocaña C, et al. Double dissociation between visual recognition and picture naming: a study of the visual language connectivity using tractography and brain stimulation. Neurosurgery. 2013;72(4):678–86.
63. Mandonnet E, Gatignol P, Duffau H. Evidence for an occipito-temporal tract underlying visual recognition in picture naming. Clin Neurol Neurosurg. 2009;111(7):601–5.
64. Roux F-E, Durand J-B, Jucla M, Réhault E, Reddy M, Démonet J-F. Segregation of lexical and sub-lexical reading processes in the left perisylvian cortex. PLoS ONE. 2012;7(11):e50665.
65. Roux F-E, Lubrano V, Lauwers-Cances V, Trémoulet M, Mascott CR, Démonet J-F. Intra-operative mapping of cortical areas involved in reading in mono- and bilingual patients. Brain. 2004;127(Pt 8):1796–810.
66. Milea D, Lobel E, Lehéricy S, Duffau H, Rivaud-Péchoux S, Berthoz A, et al. Intraoperative frontal eye field stimulation elicits ocular deviation and saccade suppression. NeuroReport. 2002;13 (10):1359–64.
67. Hoffman P, Lambon Ralph MA, Woollams AM. Triangulation of the neurocomputational architecture underpinning reading aloud. Proc Natl Acad Sci USA. 2015;112(28):E3719–28.
68. Thiebaut de Schotten M, Urbanski M, Duffau H, Volle E, Lévy R, Dubois B, et al. Direct evidence for a parietal-frontal pathway subserving spatial awareness in humans. Science. 2005;309 (5744):2226–8.
69. Roux F-E, Dufor O, Lauwers-Cances V, Boukhatem L, Brauge D, Draper L, et al. Electrostimulation mapping of spatial neglect. Neurosurgery. 2011;69(6):1218–31.
70. Vallar G, Bello L, Bricolo E, Castellano A, Casarotti A, Falini A, et al. Cerebral correlates of visuospatial neglect: a direct cerebral stimulation study. Hum Brain Mapp. 2014;35(4):1334–50.
71. Dehaene S, Piazza M, Pinel P, Cohen L. Three parietal circuits for number processing. Cogn Neuropsychol. 2003;20(3):487–506.
72. Whalen J, McCloskey M, Lesser RP, Gordon B. Localizing arithmetic processes in the brain: evidence from a transient deficit during cortical stimulation. J Cogn Neurosci. 1997;9(3):409–17.
73. Duffau H, Denvil D, Lopes M, Gasparini F, Cohen L, Capelle L, et al. Intraoperative mapping of the cortical areas involved in multiplication and subtraction: an electrostimulation study in a patient with a left parietal glioma. J Neurol Neurosurg Psychiatr. 2002;73(6):733–8.
74. Pu S, Li Y, Wu C, Wang Y, Zhou X, Jiang T. Cortical areas involved in numerical processing: an intraoperative electrostimulation study. Stereotact Funct Neurosurg. 2011;89(1):42–7.
75. Yu X, Chen C, Pu S, Wu C, Li Y, Jiang T, et al. Dissociation of subtraction and multiplication in the right parietal cortex: evidence from intraoperative cortical electrostimulation. Neuropsychologia. 2011;49(10):2889–95.
76. Roux F-E, Boetto S, Sacko O, Chollet F, Trémoulet M. Writing, calculating, and finger recognition in the region of the angular gyrus: a cortical stimulation study of Gerstmann syndrome. J Neurosurg. 2003;99(4):716–27.
77. Roux F-E, Boukhatem L, Draper L, Sacko O, Démonet J-F. Cortical calculation localization using electrostimulation. J Neurosurg. 2009;110 (6):1291–9.
78. Herbet G, Lafargue G, Bonnetblanc F, Moritz-Gasser S. Menjot de Champfleur N, Duffau H. Inferring a dual-stream model of mentalizing from associative white matter fibres disconnection. Brain. 2014;137(Pt 3):944–59.
79. Giussani C, Pirillo D, Roux F-E. Mirror of the soul: a cortical stimulation study on recognition of facial emotions. J Neurosurg. 2010;112(3):520–7.
80. Herbet G, Lafargue G, Moritz-Gasser S, Bonnetblanc F, Duffau H. Interfering with the neural activity of mirror-related frontal areas impairs mentalistic inferences. Brain Struct Funct. 2015;220(4):2159–69.
81. Herbet G, Lafargue G, Bonnetblanc F, Moritz-Gasser S, Duffau H. Is the right frontal cortex really crucial in the mentalizing network? A longitudinal study in patients with a slow-growing lesion. Cortex. 2013;49(10):2711–27.
82. Desmurget M, Reilly KT, Richard N, Szathmari A, Mottolese C, Sirigu A. Movement intention after parietal cortex stimulation in humans. Science. 2009;324(5928):811–3.
83. Knight J. An out of body experience. Nature. 2002;419(6903):106–7.
84. Herbet G, Lafargue G, de Champfleur NM, Moritz-Gasser S, le Bars E, Bonnetblanc F, et al. Disrupting posterior cingulate connectivity disconnects consciousness from the external environment. Neuropsychologia. 2014;56:239–44.
85. Shiban E, Krieg SM, Obermueller T, Wostrack M, Meyer B, Ringel F. Continuous subcortical motor

evoked potential stimulation using the tip of an ultrasonic aspirator for the resection of motor eloquent lesions. J Neurosurg. 2015;123(2):301–6.
86. Raabe A, Beck J, Schucht P, Seidel K. Continuous dynamic mapping of the corticospinal tract during surgery of motor eloquent brain tumors: evaluation of a new method. J Neurosurg. 2014;120(5):1015–24.
87. Schucht P, Moritz-Gasser S, Herbet G, Raabe A, Duffau H. Subcortical electrostimulation to identify network subserving motor control. Hum Brain Mapp. 2013;34(11):3023–30.
88. Rech F, Herbet G, Moritz-Gasser S, Duffau H. Disruption of bimanual movement by unilateral subcortical electrostimulation. Hum Brain Mapp. 2013.
89. Rech F, Herbet G, Moritz-Gasser S, Duffau H. Somatotopic organization of the white matter tracts underpinning motor control in humans: an electrical stimulation study. Brain Struct Funct. 2015.
90. Duffau H, Capelle L, Sichez N, Denvil D, Lopes M, Sichez J-P, et al. Intraoperative mapping of the subcortical language pathways using direct stimulations. An anatomo-functional study. Brain. 2002;125(Pt 1):199–214.
91. Hickok G, Poeppel D. Dorsal and ventral streams: a framework for understanding aspects of the functional anatomy of language. Cognition. 2004;92(1–2):67–99.
92. Catani M, Howard RJ, Pajevic S, Jones DK. Virtual in vivo interactive dissection of white matter fasciculi in the human brain. Neuroimage. 2002;17(1):77–94.
93. Martino J, Brogna C, Robles SG, Vergani F, Duffau H. Anatomic dissection of the inferior fronto-occipital fasciculus revisited in the lights of brain stimulation data. Cortex. 2010;46(5):691–9.
94. Sarubbo S, De Benedictis A, Maldonado IL, Basso G, Duffau H. Frontal terminations for the inferior fronto-occipital fascicle: anatomical dissection, DTI study and functional considerations on a multi-component bundle. Brain Struct Funct. 2013;218(1):21–37.
95. Catani M, Dell'acqua F, Vergani F, Malik F, Hodge H, Roy P, et al. Short frontal lobe connections of the human brain. Cortex. 2012;48(2):273–91.
96. Ford A, McGregor KM, Case K, Crosson B, White KD. Structural connectivity of Broca's area and medial frontal cortex. Neuroimage. 2010;52(4):1230–7.
97. Kinoshita M, Shinohara H, Hori O, Ozaki N, Ueda F, Nakada M, et al. Association fibers connecting the Broca center and the lateral superior frontal gyrus: a microsurgical and tractographic anatomy. J Neurosurg. 2012;116(2):323–30.
98. Makris N, Preti MG, Asami T, Pelavin P, Campbell B, Papadimitriou GM, et al. Human middle longitudinal fascicle: variations in patterns of anatomical connections. Brain Struct Funct. 2013;218(4):951–68.
99. Makris N, Preti MG, Wassermann D, Rathi Y, Papadimitriou GM, Yergatian C, et al. Human middle longitudinal fascicle: segregation and behavioral-clinical implications of two distinct fiber connections linking temporal pole and superior temporal gyrus with the angular gyrus or superior parietal lobule using multi-tensor tractography. Brain Imaging Behav. 2013;7(3):335–52.
100. Makris N, Papadimitriou GM, Kaiser JR, Sorg S, Kennedy DN, Pandya DN. Delineation of the middle longitudinal fascicle in humans: a quantitative, in vivo, DT-MRI study. Cereb Cortex. 2009;19(4):777–85.
101. Maldonado IL, de Champfleur NM, Velut S, Destrieux C, Zemmoura I, Duffau H. Evidence of a middle longitudinal fasciculus in the human brain from fiber dissection. J Anat. 2013;223(1):38–45.
102. Makris N, Kennedy DN, McInerney S, Sorensen AG, Wang R, Caviness VS, et al. Segmentation of subcomponents within the superior longitudinal fascicle in humans: a quantitative, in vivo, DT-MRI study. Cereb Cortex. 2005;15(6):854–69.
103. Maldonado IL, Mandonnet E, Duffau H. Dorsal fronto-parietal connections of the human brain: a fiber dissection study of their composition and anatomical relationships. Anat Rec (Hoboken). 2012;295(2):187–95.
104. Yagmurlu K, Middlebrooks EH, Tanriover N, Rhoton AL. Fiber tracts of the dorsal language stream in the human brain. J Neurosurg. 2015;20:1–10.
105. Forkel SJ, Thiebaut de Schotten M, Kawadler JM, Dell'Acqua F, Danek A, Catani M. The anatomy of fronto-occipital connections from early blunt dissections to contemporary tractography. Cortex. 2014;56:73–84.
106. Ius T, Angelini E. Thiebaut de Schotten M, Mandonnet E, Duffau H. Evidence for potentials and limitations of brain plasticity using an atlas of functional resectability of WHO grade II gliomas: towards a "minimal common brain". Neuroimage. 2011;56(3):992–1000.
107. Sarubbo S, De Benedictis A, Merler S, Mandonnet E, Balbi S, Granieri E, et al. Towards a functional atlas of human white matter. Hum Brain Mapp. 2015;36(8):3117–36.
108. Maldonado IL, Moritz-Gasser S, Duffau H. Does the left superior longitudinal fascicle subserve language semantics? A brain electrostimulation study. Brain Struct Funct. 2011;216(3):263–74.
109. Maldonado IL, Moritz-Gasser S, de Champfleur NM, Bertram L, Moulinié G, Duffau H. Surgery for gliomas involving the left inferior parietal lobule: new insights into the functional anatomy provided by stimulation mapping in awake patients. J Neurosurg. 2011;115(4):770–9.

110. Duffau H, Gatignol P, Mandonnet E, Peruzzi P, Tzourio-Mazoyer N, Capelle L. New insights into the anatomo-functional connectivity of the semantic system: a study using cortico-subcortical electrostimulations. Brain. 2005;128(Pt 4):797–810.
111. Khan OH, Herbet G, Moritz-Gasser S, Duffau H. The role of left inferior fronto-occipital fascicle in verbal perseveration: a brain electrostimulation mapping study. Brain Topogr. 2013.
112. Hickok G, Poeppel D. The cortical organization of speech processing. Nat Rev Neurosci. 2007;8(5):393–402.
113. Duffau H, Gatignol P, Denvil D, Lopes M, Capelle L. The articulatory loop: study of the subcortical connectivity by electrostimulation. NeuroReport. 2003;14(15):2005–8.
114. Kemerdere R, de Champfleur NM, Deverdun J, Cochereau J, Moritz-Gasser S, Herbet G, et al. Role of the left frontal aslant tract in stuttering: a brain stimulation and tractographic study. J Neurol. 2015.
115. Kinoshita M, de Champfleur NM, Deverdun J, Moritz-Gasser S, Herbet G, Duffau H. Role of fronto-striatal tract and frontal aslant tract in movement and speech: an axonal mapping study. Brain Struct Funct. 2014.
116. Zemmoura I, Herbet G, Moritz-Gasser S, Duffau H. New insights into the neural network mediating reading processes provided by cortico-subcortical electrical mapping. Hum Brain Mapp. 2015;36(6):2215–30.
117. Goga C, Türe U. The anatomy of Meyer's loop revisited: changing the anatomical paradigm of the temporal loop based on evidence from fiber microdissection. J Neurosurg. 2015;122(6):1253–62.
118. Sarubbo S, De Benedictis A, Milani P, Paradiso B, Barbareschi M, Rozzanigo U, et al. The course and the anatomo-functional relationships of the optic radiation: a combined study with "post mortem" dissections and "in vivo" direct electrical mapping. J Anat. 2015;226(1):47–59.
119. Sincoff EH, Tan Y, Abdulrauf SI. White matter fiber dissection of the optic radiations of the temporal lobe and implications for surgical approaches to the temporal horn. J Neurosurg. 2004;101(5):739–46.
120. Rubino PA, Rhoton AL, Tong X, Oliveira E de. Three-dimensional relationships of the optic radiation. Neurosurgery. 2005;57(4 Suppl.):219–27; discussion 219–227.
121. Ebeling U, Reulen HJ. Neurosurgical topography of the optic radiation in the temporal lobe. Acta Neurochir (Wien). 1988;92(1–4):29–36.
122. Gras-Combe G, Moritz-Gasser S, Herbet G, Duffau H. Intraoperative subcortical electrical mapping of optic radiations in awake surgery for glioma involving visual pathways. J Neurosurg. 2012;117(3):466–73.
123. Corbetta M, Kincade MJ, Lewis C, Snyder AZ, Sapir A. Neural basis and recovery of spatial attention deficits in spatial neglect. Nat Neurosci. 2005;8(11):1603–10.
124. Della Puppa A, De Pellegrin S, Lazzarini A, Gioffrè G, Rustemi O, Cagnin A, et al. Subcortical mapping of calculation processing in the right parietal lobe. J Neurosurg. 2015;122(5):1038–41.
125. Wilson SM, Lam D, Babiak MC, Perry DW, Shih T, Hess CP, et al. Transient aphasias after left hemisphere resective surgery. J Neurosurg. 2015;123(3):581–93.
126. Bartolo M, Zucchella C, Pace A, Lanzetta G, Vecchione C, Bartolo M, et al. Early rehabilitation after surgery improves functional outcome in inpatients with brain tumours. J Neurooncol. 2012;107(3):537–44.
127. Zucchella C, Capone A, Codella V, De Nunzio AM, Vecchione C, Sandrini G, et al. Cognitive rehabilitation for early post-surgery inpatients affected by primary brain tumor: a randomized, controlled trial. J Neurooncol. 2013;114(1):93–100.
128. Martino J, Taillandier L, Moritz-Gasser S, Gatignol P, Duffau H. Re-operation is a safe and effective therapeutic strategy in recurrent WHO grade II gliomas within eloquent areas. Acta Neurochir (Wien). 2009;151(5):427–36; discussion 436.
129. Southwell DG, Hervey-Jumper SL, Perry DW, Berger MS. Intraoperative mapping during repeat awake craniotomy reveals the functional plasticity of adult cortex. J Neurosurg. 2015;6:1–10.

Fluorescence-Guided Resection of Malignant Gliomas

6

Walter Stummer

Introduction

During surgery for malignant gliomas, it is sometimes excruciatingly difficult to distinguish gross tumor and a more or less broad region of infiltrated and functionally intact tissue from surrounding "healthy" brain. Tactile or optical information, the latter obtained with the operating microscope, is not sufficient for reliable differentiation and neurosurgeons strongly tend to overestimate resection based on their subjective impression, as first demonstrated by Albert et al. [1]. Neuronavigation has been investigated as a tool for overcoming these difficulties but suffers from brain shift [2, 3]. Re-referencing with the intra-operative MRI helps resolve this problem, but the MRI is itself expensive and incontrovertibly prolongs surgery. Further, MRI provides images, which rely on contrast-enhancement for identifying malignant gliomas tissue. Tissue damage during surgery might lead to unspecific extravasation of Gd-containing contrast agents, a phenomenon that has to be taken into account during resection. Further, even though enhancing tissue is the accepted aim of resection in malignant glioma surgery [4–9], enhancing regions mark only a core region of the angiogenic tumor with a high cell density, which is surrounded by a broad rim of infiltrated tissue.

Obvious limitations of traditional methods for adequately identifying tumor tissue intra-operatively have spawned novel concepts, among which fluorescence, based on active or passive accumulation of so-called fluorophores in tumor tissue, is receiving increasing attention.

Utilizing special wavelengths of light for excitation (usually of a short wavelength) and filter combinations for fluorescence detection, these fluorophores can be selectively visualized, because fluorophores emit light at a wavelength differing and exceeding the excitation wavelength (Fig. 6.1). The obvious practical advantage for surgeons, given selectivity of accumulation, is real-time detection of tumor during surgery based on the contrast of tissues containing the fluorophore as opposed to tissues without the fluorophore. With fluorescence information available using modified surgical microscopes, and light conditions allowing, the surgeon can resect using the fluorescence mode. Tumor detection by this method is independent of neuronavigation and brain shift.

A Brief History

Historically, the use of a fluorophore for highlighting malignant glioma tissue was first described by Moore et al. [10] as a means of localizing brain tumors. Equipped only with topographical information from neurological examinations and vague morphological–anatomical data from

W. Stummer (✉)
Department of Neurosurgery, University of Münster, Albert-Schweitzer-Campus 1, Geb. A1, 48146 Münster, Germany
e-mail: walter.stummer@ukmuenster.de

J. Moliterno Günel et al. (eds.), *Malignant Brain Tumors*, DOI 10.1007/978-3-319-49864-5_6

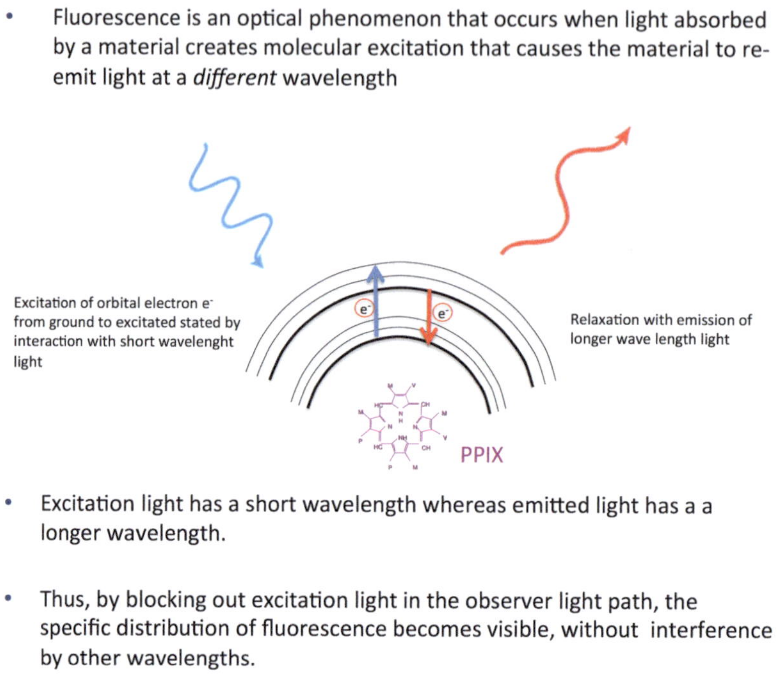

Fig. 6.1 Scheme illustrating the nature of fluorescence and how it is visualized

ventriculographic studies, and intra-operatively with a brain needle for finding tumor-afflicted brain and biopsies of tissue, these authors employed a mercury vapor lamp and a Wood's filter together with intravenous fluorescein to locate and resect tumors. They noted that in some cases, they were able to identify additional small regions of tumor, which escaped notice when viewed with ordinary illumination, thus first defining the two key elements of the use of fluorescence for surgery of brain tumors:

- initial detection of the tumor in the brain
- optimizing resection based on tissue fluorescence

Regarding fluorescein, they acknowledged, however, that "the brain tissue immediately surrounding the tumor is edematous and edematous brain tissue is shown to retain a greater amount of dye than otherwise normal brain" and "edematous tissue surrounding the tumor does fluoresce, but to a lesser degree…" thus already pointing out possible limitations of dyes which reach the brain tumor via a breached blood–brain barrier in the tumor, i.e., of passive permeability markers. At that point of time, the concept of a blood–brain barrier was long accepted, but the lack of such in tumor was still in the realm of theory and put forward by Moore et al. [10] as a possible explanation for the differential uptake of dye when comparing tumor, edematous tissue, and normal brain. In summary however, the authors felt fluorescence to have "definitive clinical value." On a by note, this paper already envisages a coupling of 131-iodine to fluorescein dyes for better diagnosis of malignant brain tumors.

After this first report little was heard about fluorescence in neurosurgery until the late 1990s when Kuoriwa and co-workers from Japan presented three publications on fluorescein for glioma surgery the last in 1999 [11–13].

In 1998, we published our first reports [14–16] on 5-aminolevulinic acid (5-ALA) for fluorescence-guided resections providing data on both experimental data and data on the first use of this compound in humans in a small phase I/II patient cohort. In contradistinction to fluorescein, 5-ALA is a prodrug, which is converted into a fluorescing fluorophore within tumor cells [17, 18] and thus is unique so far, compared to other fluorophores that have been investigated. 5-ALA has been studied extensively for fluorescence-guided resections since then.

Recently, with new filters integrated into operating microscopes, fluorescein is again receiving some, albeit controversial, interest [19–22].

Both fluorochromes will be discussed in detail in the course of this paper. Currently, new approaches with fluorophores targeted to surface markers of tumors cells are being investigated and are on the verge of clinical translation.

ALA for Fluorescence-Guided Resections

5-Aminolevulinic acid (ALA) is a natural metabolite, which is involved in heme-biosynthesis. When given in excess, this compound results in the accumulation and/or selective retention of fluorescing porphyrins, particularly protoporphyrin IX (PPIX) in epithelia and more predominantly in cancers arising from such epithelia and in many brain tumors [17, 18, 23]. Under physiological circumstances, PPIX is converted into non-fluorescent proto-heme by iron chelation and from there into hemoglobin. In experiments utilizing the C6 glioma cell line in vitro and in vitro we were able to first demonstrate selective retention in malignant glioma cells [15], an observation, which was safely extended to human malignant gliomas [16]. The reasons for this selectivity are not completely understood. Relationships have been postulated to decreased expression of ferrochelatase in tumors [24], an enzyme which converts PPIX to proto-heme by chelating iron into the porphyrin ring. Other possible explanations have been put forward, such as a decreased activity of the ATP-binding cassette transporter (ABCB6) [25] which eliminates porphyrins from cells, as well as tumor cell density, tumor cell proliferative activity and a disturbed blood–brain barrier permeability in the region of the tumor [26, 27].

PPIX is strongly fluorescent with an excitation maximum at approximately 405 nm (the so-called Soret band) with two emission peaks at 635 and 704 nm (Fig. 6.2) [28]. In vivo, the spectrum detected from tissue has an additional peak at between 450 and 500 nm, i.e., in the green range, resulting from underlying brain tissue autofluorescence from NADH, riboflavins and carotenoids and other autofluorophores in normal tissue. This autofluorescence is equally stimulated by blue excitation light [29]. Surgical microscopes adapted for protoporphyrin IX detection currently use xenon excitation light filtered for violet-blue with a wavelength peak at 375–440 nm. For observing fluorescence they do not simply use a long-pass or barrier filter for visualizing the 635 nm peak of protoporphyrin IX, that is, cutting away all wavelengths below for instance 600 nm. This would result in PPIX being visible on a black background, without allowing any background discrimination. We considered the possibility of background discrimination to be important for enabling resection and tissue manipulation by the surgeon using the fluorescence mode. Rather, microscopes by the major manufactures use barrier filters for fluorescence detection, which open at slightly below 440 nm. This allows a small fraction of the excitation light to be included in the observation pathway of the microscopes. In addition, tissue autofluorescence, which is located in the blue-green range, is also visualized. Remitted excitation light and tissue autofluorescence together enable background brain tissue to become visible with a green-blue tone [14].

5-ALA is currently approved for resections of malignant gliomas in many countries of the world after initial approval by the European Medicines Agency (EMA). Approval was granted based on a study [30], which randomized patients with malignant gliomas to be operated on either with or without 5-ALA for fluorescence-guided resections. Groups were compared for extent of resection and safety as well as for progression-free survival. Extents of resection were greater in the 5-ALA group,

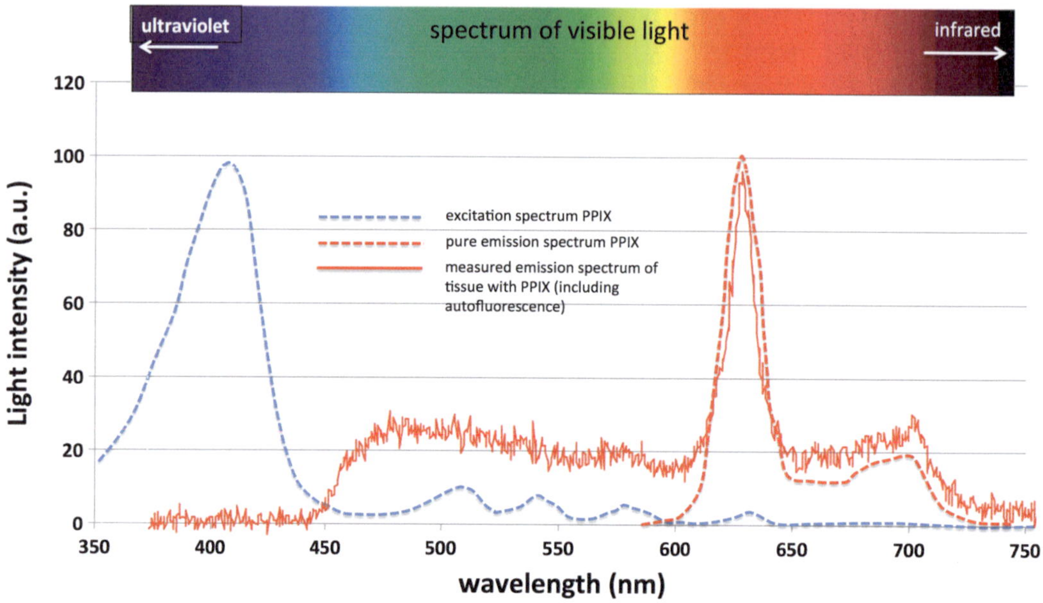

Fig. 6.2 Fluorescence excitation and emission in tissues containing PPIX, compared to the visible light spectrum. PPIX has an absorption maximum at 405 nm, the so-called Soret band, which is located in the *blue* range. Excitation light sources typically used for microscopes feature a wavelength range of 375 to about 440 nm. PPIX emission peaks are at 635 and 705 nm, both in the *red* range. Brain tissue additionally contains autofluorophores (carotenoids, riboflavin, NADH). In vivo, autofluorescence is superimposed over the pure PPIX signal. By choosing a barrier filter, which allows the passage of light of longer wavelengths than about 440 nm, a small part of the excitation light and autofluorescence together provide background "illumination" with superimposed red tumor fluorescence

resulting in a prolongation of progression-free survival without significantly more frequent neurological deficits. Rates of complete resection of contrast-enhancing tumor were 65% for the 5-ALA versus 35% for the control arm with conventional white light illumination.

On a by note, the rate of 65% is frequently cited as the limit to what can be achieved using 5-ALA. This may not be the case however, since patients operated on using 5-ALA in the context of the study were the first dozen or so patients ever to be operated on by surgeons with relatively little experience with the novel technology. Newer studies put forward by experienced surgeons indicate a much higher potential of 5-ALA for facilitating gross total resections of enhancing tumors in up to 96% of cases (Table 6.1), when used in conjunction with neurophysiological mapping and monitoring [31–35]. In one recent study, intra-operative MRI in combination with neurophysiological methods resulted in 82% "complete" resections [35]. When augmented with 5-ALA-induced fluorescence, gross total tumor resection rates were stated to have been reached in 100%. Overall, a meta-analysis by Eljamel [36] indicated a rate of gross total resection, i.e., resection of more than 98% of enhancing tumor in over 75% of a total of 565 patients.

In retrospect, utilizing resection rates as a primary study aim for a randomized study may not have been a well-chosen endpoint for testing the usefulness of 5-ALA. Resection depends on many factors other than visualizing the tumor, foremost the worry about maintaining function, which depends strongly on the surgeon, the surgeon's convictions regarding the value of resection and the use of mapping/monitoring for safely extending resections. Particularly, the concepts and views regarding these factors have changed over time. Today the value of safe resection is more generally accepted in the

Table 6.1 Resection rates using 5-ALA as reported in the literature

Publication	*n*	Location	ioMR	Monitoring mapping	Study type	Resection rate (%)	Comment
Stummer et al. [37]	50	Eloquent and non-eloquent	No	No	Prospective monocentric cohort	65	
Stummer et al. [30]	135	Eloquent and non-eloquent	No	No	Prospective multicentric two-arm randomized	65	
De la Puppa et al. [34]	25	Eloquent only (motor, language)	No	Yes	Prospective monocentric cohort	80	
Diez Valle et al. [33]	36	Eloquent and non-eloquent	No	Yes	Prospective monocentric cohort	83.3	
Coburger et al. [35]	33	Eloquent and non-eloquent	Yes	Yes	Prospective Monocentric cohort, historical matched pair	100	ioMR alone 82%
Schucht et al. [32]	67	Eloquent only (motor)	No	Yes	Prospective monocentric cohort	76	
Schucht et al. [31]	103	Eloquent and non-eloquent	No	Yes	Prospective Monocentric cohort	96	

neurosurgical community and mapping/monitoring has become a common adjunct for surgery of malignant gliomas. Thus, it may have been more appropriate to test 5-ALA as an intra-operative diagnostic agent or contrast medium. This would have involved testing the compound for toxicological safety as well as for measures of diagnostic accuracy only, e.g., looking at the positive predictive value of fluorescence for demonstrating tumor rather than attempting to prove a *therapeutic* value of the use of 5-ALA. This potential therapeutic value is the sum of patient selection and intra-operative tumor detection *but mostly of the surgeon performing the surgery and utilizing any available technology*, the surgeon's role being highly uncontrollable and variable.

5-ALA is presently being marketed as "Gliolan®" in the EU and other parts of the world, and surgical microscopes modified for fluorescence-guided resections are available from the leading microscope manufacturers, for which fluorescence modules can be purchased as accessories. These microscopes uniformly feature xenon light sources generating conventional white light and are switchable to blue light illumination and the appropriate observation filters, usually by operating a switch or foot pedal, thus enabling free shuttling between both illumination modes.

What Does Visible PPIX Fluorescence Signify in the Context of Glioma Surgery?

Selectivity

Relying on 5-ALA-induced PPIX for fluorescence-guided resection requires knowing how accurately fluorescence indicates bulk tumor or infiltrated brain. The authors have almost unanimously determined a high positive predictive value (PPV, the probability that fluorescence indicates tumor) of over 95% [33, 35–42]. The values for specificity and sensitivity are more varied in the literature, the reason being that both these traditional measures *depend on tissue sampling in non-fluorescing, normally appearing tissue* (Fig. 6.3, adapted from Stummer et al. [43]).

Importantly, the results of such sampling strongly depend on the distance from the tumor the samples are collected because in malignant gliomas cell density rapidly decreases with distance from the tumor mass along with likelihood for finding tumor-infiltrated biopsies. Therefore, determining specificity and sensitivity depends critically on the distance at which samples from non-fluorescent marginal tissue are taken. Since authors of different studies employ different sampling algorithms, they will understandably determine different values for these traditional measures of diagnostic accuracy.

The PPV, on the other hand, is the only measure of diagnostic accuracy that does not require biopsies from non-fluorescing, normally appearing tissue (Fig. 6.3). The negative predictive value (NPV, the probability that non-fluorescing tissue shows tumor cells) similarly depends on the location in non-fluorescing tissue from which samples are taken. If investigators collect samples close to macroscopically fluorescing tissue, the NPV will be lower compared to the NPV determined by investigators who collect samples at a larger distance from macroscopically fluorescing tissue. The varying values calculated by different authors are reflected in Table 6.2.

According to our recent experience [42], fluorescence can be visualized using the microscope down to a cell density of 10% in malignant

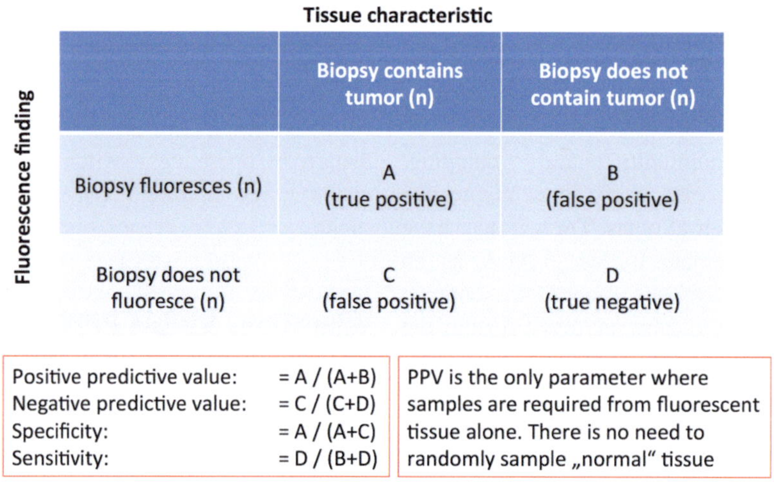

Fig. 6.3 Scheme for illustrating the calculation of measures of diagnostic accuracy, which are frequently used for determining the value of a diagnostic method. In studies on fluorescence-guided resection, "specificity" and "sensitivity" are highly variable when comparing the results of different investigators, since these measures require random biopsies from "normal" appearing brain. The distance to the main tumor mass at which these biopsies are obtained is crucial, because with increasing distance from the tumor cell density rapidly drops. This distance is rarely defined in various studies (adapted from [43])

Table 6.2 Accuracy of intra-operative fluorescence for predicting tumor

Publication	PPV	NPV	Sensitivity	Specificity
Stummer et al. [37]	99	50	89	96
Coburger et al. [35]	99	22	91	80
Yamada et al. [41]	92	69	95	53
Diez Valle et al. [33]	100 (strong) 97 (weak)	66	N.g.	N.g.
Idoate et al. [38]	100 (solid tumor) 97 (infiltrating tumor)	67	N.g.	N.g.
Stummer et al. [42]	96	40	N.g.	N.g.

gliomas. Using more sensitive spectrometry, more infiltrating cells can be detected [42, 44], which are not visible through the microscope due the low intensity of fluorescence.

Although we were able to establish a relationship between WHO grade and fluorescence as well as the MIB (Ki-67) index and fluorescence in gliomas, we were unable to detect a relationship to other molecular markers, which are currently being determined on a routine basis for gliomas, e.g., 1p19q co-deletions, MGMT promoter methylation, or IDH1 mutations [45].

False Positive Fluorescence Induced by 5-ALA

False positive fluorescence, when described, was usually related to tissue areas in close proximity to the resection cavity [37, 39, 46, 47] or on a microscopic basis [48] but was never observed at a meaningful distance from the tumor cavity. Such fluorescence has been attributed to reactive astrocytes or inflammation, especially in patients with recurrent malignant gliomas, but not to normal brain tissue [46–49]. In 313 patients with imaging suggestive of recurrence of glioblastomas after multimodal therapy, 3% of patients showed fluorescence in tissue where pathological examination revealed radiation necrosis [49]. This fluorescence was described as weak. Fluorescence in normal brain was not described in that report.

Relationship Between 5-ALA-Induced Fluorescence and Enhancement on the MRI

Fluorescence has been related to contrast-enhancement of malignant gliomas on the MRI [39]. However, a number of investigators have provided data demonstrating fluorescence to extend beyond contrast-enhancement [35, 37, 42, 50–52] (Fig. 6.4). Resection of this area of fluorescence tissue, which extends beyond contrast-enhancing tumor, has been associated with extended survival [51]. A number of groups have provided evidence that fluorescence even in non-enhancing tumors can be predicted by amino acid positron emission tomography (PET) with ^{18}F-fluoroethyl-tyrosine (FET) or ^{11}C-methionine [45, 52–55].

In Which Tumors Is 5-ALA of Value?

Use in Gliomas Apart from Gbm

The use of 5-ALA for fluorescence-guided resections of brain tumors was first described for malignant gliomas [16], and the use in glioblastoma is the most common use described so far. Other gliomas may be amenable to fluorescence-guided resections as well, as is the case for approximately 16–20% of grade II gliomas [45, 53, 56, 57], despite the accepted lack of significant blood–brain perturbations in such tumors. In gliomas, which do not show typical imaging characteristics of glioblastoma, tumor size and patient age were predictive of finding useful fluorescence intra-operatively, either for fluorescence-guided resections or for finding an anaplastic focus [45]. In the case of gliomas without imaging features suggestive of glioblastoma (i.e., necrosis marginal enhancement and perifocal edema), any enhancement on the MRI resulted in the likelihood of useful fluorescence of 78%; if patients were older than 44 years and tumors were larger than 7 cm^3, this likelihood was 97%. In non-enhancing tumors, tumor size and the FET-PET ratio were predictive of fluorescence. Patients with non-enhancing tumors and a FET-PET uptake ratio of at least 1.85 demonstrated a likelihood of 23% for showing fluorescence. If tumors were additionally larger than 11 cm^3, this probability was increased to 46% [45].

Thus, in our practice all patients with non-enhancing tumors are subjected to FET-PET for assessing whether 5-ALA would be of value for surgery. FET-PET is also helpful for determining the location of anaplastic foci in otherwise apparently low-grade gliomas [53–55], which would be identified during surgery based on fluorescence and be specifically biopsied for

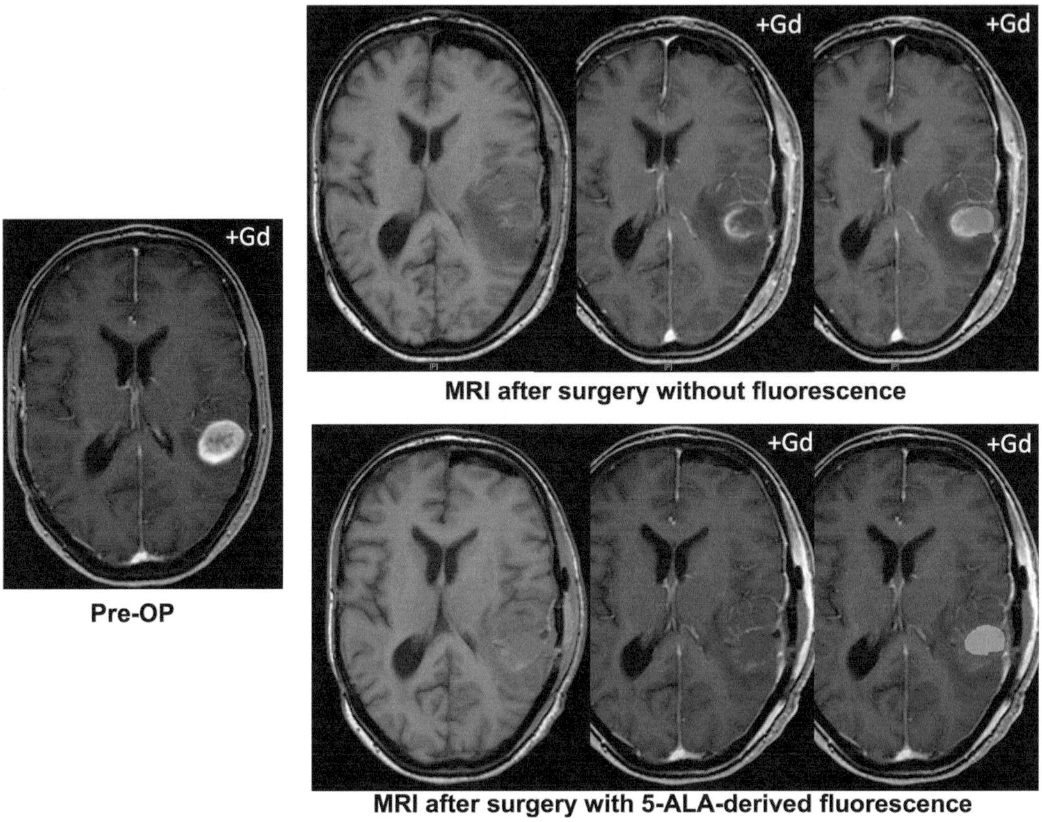

Fig. 6.4 5-ALA-induced tumor fluorescence extends beyond enhancing tumor. This patient with a left angular gyrus glioblastoma was operated on first without fluorescence. Residual enhancing tumor is visible and the resection cavity is slightly smaller than the original tumor (*yellow insert*), due to decompression. *Bottom row* surgery was repeated using 5-ALA and mapping/monitoring. All fluorescing tissue was removed safely. The final resection cavity (*red insert*) extends considerably further than the enhancing tumor regions

targeted histological interrogation. Such hot spots, if macroscopically fluorescent, were found to indicate high-grade areas in otherwise low-grade tumors [54], thus avoiding undergrading of these tumors.

It is, however, important to understand that the fluorescence visible to the surgeon through the microscope is actually quite strong, and too strong to be absorbed by the microscope lenses and filters. Thus, the observation of fluorescence in 16–20% of LGG gliomas alludes to macroscopic fluorescence, i.e., the fluorescence visible to the surgeon through the microscope. In addition, light from the tumor cavity is divided between surgeon, observer, and camera system.

Using spectrometry or confocal microscopy [42, 58, 59], porphyrins can be detected even when no macroscopic fluorescence can be observed. These findings indicate that low-grade gliomas commonly accumulate porphyrins which are difficult to perceive using the surgical microscope, based in part on the comparative amount of accumulation per cell but also on the low cell density observed in low-grade gliomas.

Tumors Other Than Gliomas that Accumulate Useful Fluorescence

Multiple groups have investigated brain tumors apart from gliomas regarding their capability of accumulating visible porphyrin fluorescence (e.g., Marbacher et al. [60]). Also, several reports provide data on children [61–64] regarding the specific pathologies in this patient population. In children with high-grade gliomas, similar usefulness of 5-ALA-induced porphyrins has been reported as with adults. Grade II and III ependymomas seem to avidly accumulate porphyrins. Medulloblastomas, pilocytic astrocytomas, and PNETs were found to display fluorescence in up to 50% of cases, which was found useful by surgeons in about 20% of patients (Table 6.3).

As is our own experience and from the literature available so far, meningiomas have a strong propensity for accumulating protoporphyrin IX (Table 6.3). This characteristic may not be of much practical value in the typical low-grade convexity meningioma that is easily identified and resected using conventional illumination. On the other hand, porphyrins have been observed in zones of bony invasion as well as in the dural infiltration zone [65–73]. In recurrent atypical or anaplastic meningiomas, especially after surgery and radiotherapy with inherent scarring, 5-ALA-induced porphyrins help identify residual tumor cells [70]. The use of ALA has been reported for pituitary adenoma, hemangioblastoma, ependymomas, metastasis, and gangliogliomas (Table 6.3). Schwannomas have been found not to accumulate significant fluorescence [60].

It is of interest to note that all investigators of tumors apart from malignant gliomas use the same dose and timing of application for 5-ALA as initially published by our group in 1998, i.e., 20 mg/kg orally 3 h prior to induction of anesthesia. Particularly in low-grade gliomas or other benign cerebral tumors, metabolism of 5-ALA to porphyrins may well differ from its metabolism in highly proliferative malignant gliomas. The question of using different doses or timelines of application of 5-ALA has not been addressed so far for these tumors. Even in high-grade gliomas, we are now giving 5-ALA earlier, 4–5 h prior to induction of anesthesia. Our recent data (manuscript in preparation) suggest that porphyrin accumulation peaks at 7–8 h rather than 6 h after ingestion. Thus, assuming a time period of 3 h from induction of anesthesia to surgically approaching the marginal tumor after positioning, draping, craniotomy, and debulking,

Table 6.3 Non-glioma brain tumors and ALA versatility

Tumor type	Visible fluorescence	Useful?	Reference examples
Meningioma Low-grade High-grade Dural infiltration Bony infiltration	+++ +++ ++ ++	−+[a] +++ ++ ++	Coluccia et al. [73], Valdes et al. [72], Motekallemi et al. [68], Cornelius et al. [69], Della Puppa et al. [65]
Ependymoma Grade I Grade II Grade III	+++ +++ +++	++ ++ ++	Inoue et al. [91], Arai et al. [92], Stummer et al. [64], Bernal Garcia et al. [93]
Hemangioblastoma	+++	+	Utsuki et al. [94]
PNET	+, 40%	−+, 20%	Stummer et al. [64]
Ganglioglioma	+, 40%	+, 40%	Stummer et al. [64]
Medulloblastoma	+, 50%	+−, 20%	Stummer et al. [64], Eicker et al. [95]
Pilocytic astrocytoma	+, 22%	[a]−, 18%	Stummer et al. [64]
Pituitary	+	+	Eljamel et al. [79]
Metastasis	++, 70%	+	Kamp et al. [77]
Stereotactic biopsy (lymphoma, inflammation, HGG, metastasis)	+++	+++	Moriuchi et al. [74], Widhalm et al. [75], von Campe [76]

[a]Not considered necessary

administration 4–5 h prior to surgery appears recommendable.

5-ALA has been suggested to be useful in the context of stereotactic biopsies [74–76]. Investigators argue that detecting fluorescence in a stereotactic biopsy will prove that the target has been correctly located, thus reducing the need for intra-operative pathology or serial sampling. While this may be true for malignant gliomas and lymphomas, lesions such as abscesses or metastasis may show unspecific fluorescence in perifocal tissue [77].

Practical Implementation of 5-ALA

Patient Selection

If a patient presents with imaging suggestive of a malignant glioma (contrast-enhancement, necrosis, edema) and a metastasis is unlikely, these patients will be given 5-ALA 4–5 h prior to induction of anesthesia. In suspected gliomas without contrast-enhancement, we will base our decision to give 5-ALA on FET-PET. If the uptake ratio in the lesion exceeds 1.85, such patients will also be treated with 5-ALA. We do not restrict ourselves to tumors where gross total resections can be expected. Investigators currently assume that resection rates beyond 70% will improve outcome in patients with glioblastomas [6] and that above this threshold, survival will depend on the amount of tumor additional resected, optimally all of contrast-enhancing tumor. Thus, whenever we perform resections for malignant gliomas, we utilize 5-ALA for maximizing resection even if we are at times forced to leave infiltrating or gross tumor behind, the latter if there is a risk that perforators are involved in the tumor or due to the proximity to important tracts or areas of cortex.

Phototoxicity

5-ALA-induced porphyrins also accumulate in the skin, sensitizing skin up to a period of 24 h. If skin is exposed to sufficient light, patients might develop rubor of the skin or sunburn. The risk of skin phototoxicity is highest between 6 and 8 h after administration. During this time, patients are draped during surgery and are in the operating room. Up to the time point of surgery, we do not implement particular measures for light protection. After surgery, patients are transferred to a recovery ward and from there to the intensive care ward for postoperative surveillance. During this time until the next morning, we close window shades and avoid direct light reaching the patient. Ambient light, to our knowledge, has not resulted in phototoxic reactions. Care must be taken in patients whose surgery is postponed unexpectedly, e.g., due to an intervening emergency. If such patients are unintentionally exposed to sunlight, they will develop rubor of the skin or sunburn.

If surgery has to be postponed, we still try to perform surgery on the same day. Re-dosing 5-ALA in case same-day surgery is canceled has not been related to adverse events [78], but systematic and prospective data are not available. This also alludes to early redo surgery if unexpectedly resectable tumor is detected during early postoperative MRI.

All patients are given a dose of approximately 20 mg/kg dissolved in 50 ml of tap water. Pharmacological data (unpublished data) show that orally ingested 5-ALA at a dose of 30 mg/kg body weight will result in a peak plasma concentration at 0.94 h after ingestions and is cleared from plasma rapidly thereafter. Concerns by anesthesiologists regarding the volume of water with which 5-ALA is ingested can be mitigated by this observation, since at the time of induction of anesthesia almost all of the drug will have passed from the digestive tract into the plasma and from there into cells.

We do not recommend 5-ALA to be dissolved in other liquids apart from clear water (e.g., orange juice) [79] to improve taste. The 5-ALA solution tastes slightly acidic, the taste not being complained about by patients. Dissolving 5-ALA in other liquids might change pharmacokinetics.

Surgery is planned using technical adjuncts as necessary. Neuronavigation is standard at our institution, supplemented by ultrasound.

Electrophysiological monitoring and mapping, including "awake" craniotomies, will be implemented depending on the location of tumors. After craniotomy and cortical mapping, we resect the tumor usually in critical regions first, especially when patients are awake, to ensure compliance during this time. Resection will include subcortical mapping, either with the "train-of-five" technique for eliciting motor evoked potentials or with the 60-Hz method for ablating function, as in language mapping.

The information derived from tissue fluorescence can be utilized immediately at the beginning after exposing the cortex for locating the tumor. If the tumor reaches or almost reaches the cortical surface, the exact location of fluorescence will demonstrate where initial corticotomy might best be planned. When approaching a subcortical tumor based on navigation or ultrasound, the fluorescent margins will become visible at an early stage, confirming the correct trajectory of approach.

As part of our standard, we always obtain a frozen section to rule out metastasis, lymphoma, or abscess. These lesions might mimic high-grade glioma on the MRI but require different therapies (lymphoma or abscess) or harbor the danger of unspecific fluorescence (e.g., in metastasis [77]).

In case intra-operative imaging (MRI, CT) is not available, care must be taken not to lose the fluorescing margin because this margin might later be hidden by overhanging edges, may collapse, and may not be visible on the surface or be covered by necrosis (Fig. 6.5). Several groups have pointed out synergies between intra-operative MRI and 5-ALA. Resection is performed using fluorescence and shuttling back and

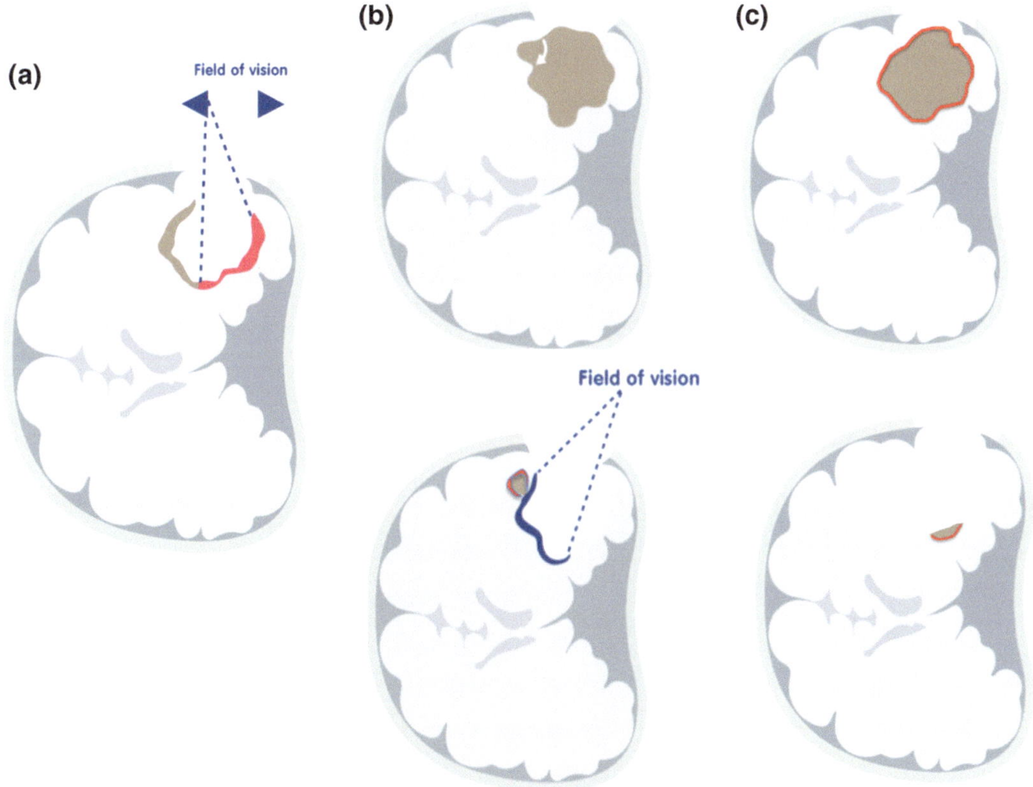

Fig. 6.5 Possible pitfalls in fluorescence-guided resections potentially resulting in inadvertent residual tumor on post-op MRI. *A* Residual tumor is hidden under overhanging edges and is outside the direct field of vision; *B* cystic regions that collapse. Fluorescing tumor is not visible on the surface; *C* non-fluorescent necrotic tumor obscures residual enhancing tumor. Surgeons should take to resect following the margin of fluorescence

forth between the fluorescence-mode and conventional white light illumination until fluorescing tissue is no longer visible. If subsequent MRI demonstrates regions of residual tumor, surgeons can return to these areas and will usually find these areas to fluoresce, but to have been outside the initial field of vision or covered by blood or debris [80].

Using mapping and monitoring, we extend resections to encompass all fluorescing tissue if in any way possible without jeopardizing function. We do not uncritically resect all tissues that fluoresce, also if we are concerned about perforators traversing the tumor that, if damaged, will result in a significant remote ischemic deficit.

Tissue Fluorescence Qualities

Usually two types of fluorescence can be distinguished during resection, a more central strong ("lava," "red," "solid") and a marginal weaker ("pink," "salmon," as previously termed by surgeons; Figs. 6.6 and 6.7). We have established that these fluorescence qualities can reproducibly be found in malignant glioma surgery [42]. Strong red fluorescence is associated with solidly proliferating tumor with a high cell density and neovascularization, whereas weaker pink fluorescence is associated with infiltrating tumor down to a tumor cell density of 10%. This phenomenon can be used for guiding resections, since functional tissue cannot be located in the region of strong fluorescence, which can be safely removed, provided this region is not transversed by perforators supplying remote and functionally important brain. With pink fluorescence (highlighting infiltrating tumor), surgeons will approach such functionally intact brain, i.e., deep white matter tracts. In this situation, it is necessary to have information whether adjacent tissue carries critical function, e.g., by mapping. Complete resection of fluorescence even outside of the enhancing tumor has been associated with extended survival [37, 51].

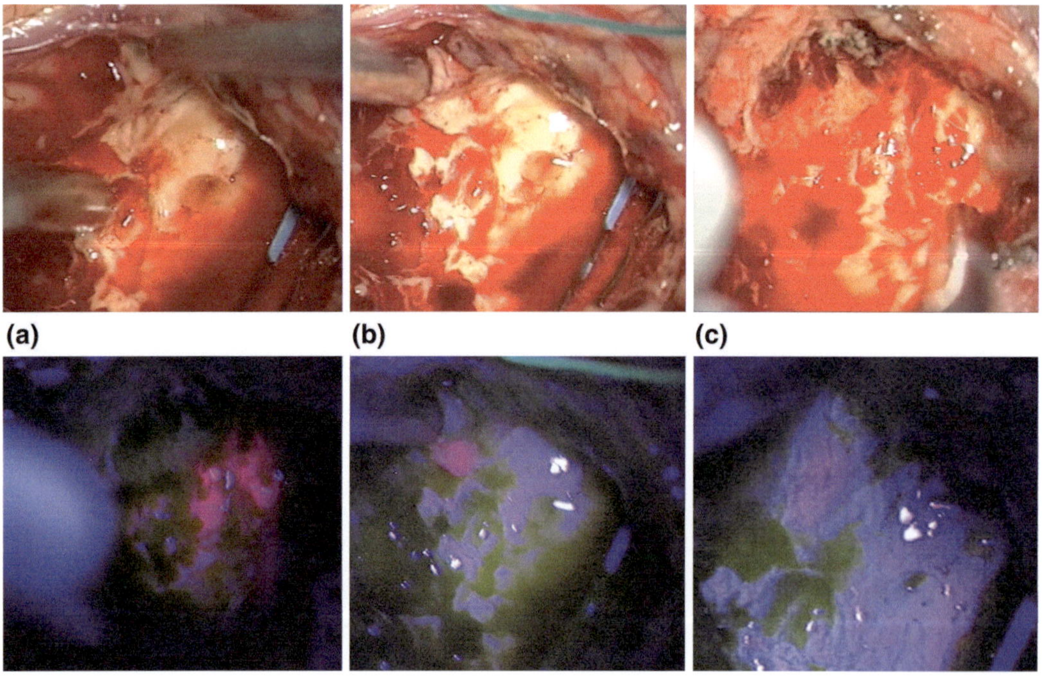

Fig. 6.6 Different fluorescence qualities. After debulking, *dark red* fluorescence becomes visible, signifying solidly proliferating, angiogenic tumor (*A*); after removal of tissue with "*red*" fluorescence, areas of *pink* fluorescence become visible (*B*). Residual "*pink*" fluorescence at the margins, signifying residual infiltrating tumor (*C*)

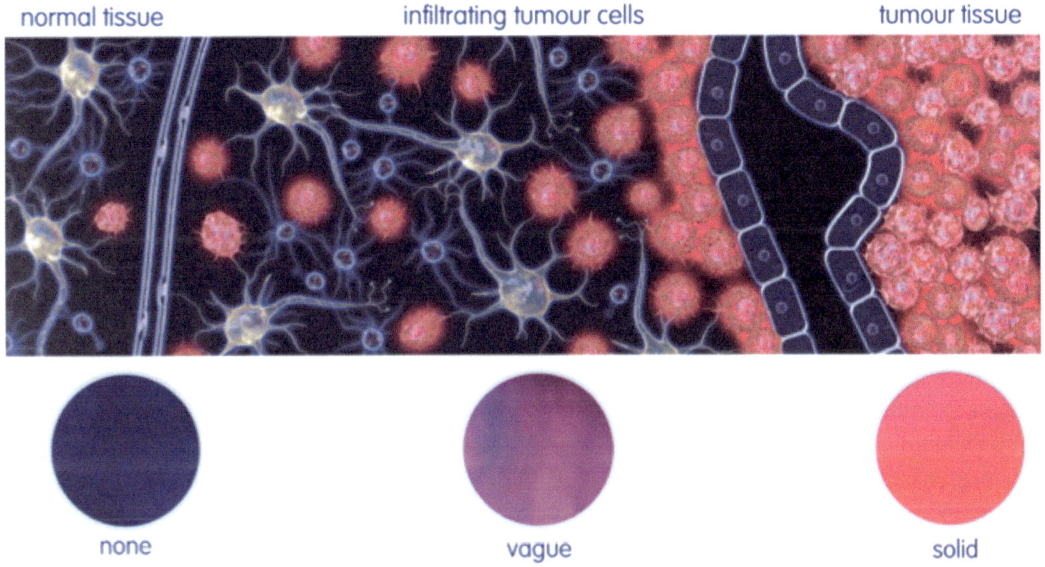

Fig. 6.7 Scheme illustrating the relationship between fluorescence qualities and tissue morphology. "*Red*" fluorescence signifies solidly proliferating tumor with neovasculature, "*pink*" infiltrating tumor to a density of about 10%, which borders on functionally intact brain tissue [42]

Necrotic tissue, on the other hand, does not fluoresce as this part of the tumor upholds no metabolism.

> ***Remember:*** 5-ALA-induced fluorescence is a technique for identifying tumor. Giving 5-ALA for resection of malignant gliomas does not alleviate the necessity for immaculate surgical technique, intra-operative mapping and monitoring in eloquently located tumors, profound knowledge of anatomy and a judicious approach to resection, being aware of pitfalls such as overhanging edges or fluorescence being hidden by blood, cotton patties, or necrotic tumor. Hardware needs to be tested for correct function prior to surgery.

In principle, resections can be performed using fluorescence alone over large parts of surgery. Blood slowly oozing into the resection cavity will hide fluorescence, because hemoglobin is a very strong absorber of light. The low light intensity under blue-violet illumination does not allow accurate hemostasis. In case oozing needs to be controlled, surgeons will switch back to conventional illumination. Due to the additional information derived from fluorescence at all stages of surgery (finding the tumor, resecting along its margins), we liberally shuttle to the fluorescence mode from the beginning of surgery. We take care to not have the illumination intensity under white light at too strong a level because switching to subdued blue-violet light will otherwise be harder to adapt to. Modern microscopes have excess light, the full magnitude of which is not necessary for surgery of a malignant glioma. We do not recommend changing to the fluorescence mode only when the surgeon feels the gross tumor has been resected completely under white light illumination. The surgeon misses important information during the course of surgery, which guides his resection strategy and renders resections as efficient as possible. Also, there is a worry about photobleaching of PPIX during the course of surgery. As with any dye, PPIX degrades under the influence of strong light. This process is not immediate but takes a matter of many minutes. Nevertheless, under adverse circumstances marginal pink fluorescence might be bleached away [16].

For resections of gliomas using 5-ALA-induced fluorescence, we traditionally use the ultrasound aspirator at the margins of the tumor. We do try to avoid coagulation in critical subcortical areas to reduce the risk of perilesional ischemic brain damage. If we do use coagulation, we note superficial PPIX fluorescence also to be destroyed, which can be replenished by sucking away the superficial level of tissue debris.

Usually we rely on the optical impression under the microscope for distinguishing fluorescent from non-fluorescing tissue. The camera image has a much lower resolution compared to eye. In addition, the camera gain can be changed and images integrated over different periods of time by varying the shutter speed. However, while longer integration times will increase contrast, they will cause the images to blur and to stutter, whereas increasing the gain and amplifying image pixels will distort colors away from the natural tone visible to the eye through the microscope.

Fluorescein for Fluorescence-Guided Resections

After its introduction by Moore et al. [10], fluorescein has recently enjoyed a renaissance for fluorescence-guided resections of malignant gliomas [19–22]. This renaissance was based on the popularity of older intra-operative fluorescence techniques (ICG, 5-ALA) as well as the introduction of new filter combinations (Yellow 560; Carl Zeiss, Oberkochen) incorporated into surgical microscopes for visualizing fluorescein. Fluorescein sodium is approved in ophthalmology for retinal angiography but is not approved for intra-operative fluorescence-guided resections in the brain and should only be used in the context of clinical studies. Fluorescein appears toxicologically safe apart from rare instances of anaphylaxis, which have been described during resection of a brain tumor [81].

Fluorescein is injected intravenously and gives a strong yellow fluorescence and, in conjunction with special microscope filters, provides vivid background information.

Fluorescein enters the malignant glioma through the breached blood–brain barrier. There is no specific affinity to tumor cells [21]. Extravasation results in co-location of fluorescence and regions of blood–brain barrier disruption. This phenomenon is used for locating tumor tissue. In practice, the fluorescent image appears brighter than what is observed using 5-ALA and the filters are constructed to allow more light reflected from normal tissue to pass, giving greater background detail.

However, there are a number of pitfalls and challenges involved in using fluorescein or other fluorophores entering the tumor based on increased blood–brain barrier permeability within malignant gliomas, as illustrated in Fig. 6.8.

1. After i.v. injection, concentrations of the fluorophores will be highest in vessels and will highlight all perfused tissues and not necessarily the tumor. The contrast from tumor to normal tissue will be weak.
2. The fluorophore will be extravasated within areas of blood–brain disruption in the brain tumor, while concentrations in plasma and in perfused tissues will slowly subside.
3. Extravasated fluorophore will flow into peritumoral tissue with edema. Tumor-related edema has been shown to traverse tissue at a rate of more than 2 mm/h [82]. Depending on the duration between administration and tumor resection, the distance of unspecific spread of fluorescein will be significant.

Thus, even without surgical manipulation the pharmacokinetics of i.v. fluorophores such as fluorescein in plasma, tumor tissue, and perifocal edema are complex. Further complexity is introduced into the equation by surgical manipulation of tissue, resulting in blood–brain barrier breakdown in regions of surgical tissue injury and unspecific extravasation at resection margins. Furthermore, blood or plasma containing the fluorophore and oozing into the resection cavity will unselectively stain tissue.

Together, intravenously administered, unselective fluorophores are wrought with many

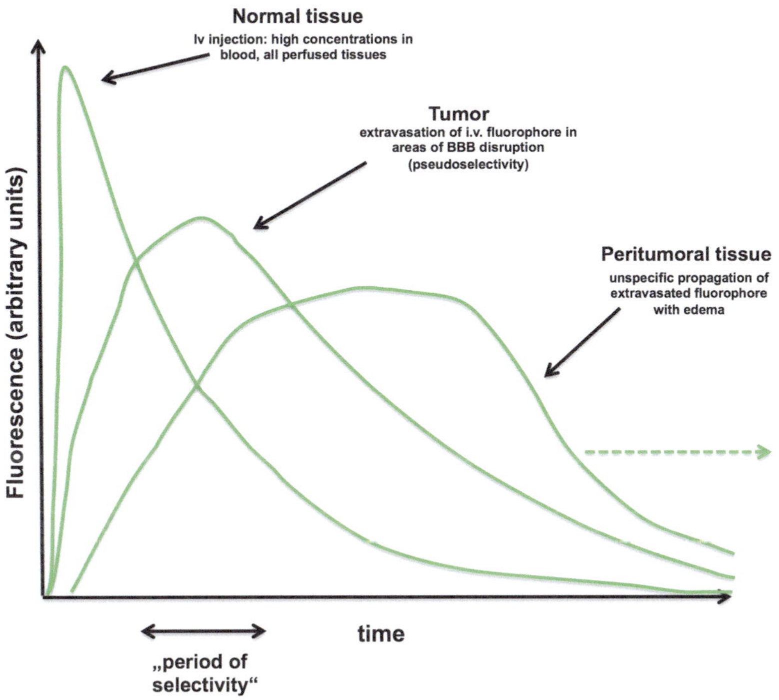

Fig. 6.8 Scheme illustrating the pharmacokinetics of intravenously applied fluorophores, which reach the tumor via the broken down blood–brain barrier. After injection, concentrations of fluorophores in vessels and therefore in all perfused tissues are high. Extravasation within the tumor leads to co-location of fluorophore in the tumor resulting in a period of pseudo selectivity, which can be used for fluorescence-guided detection. Fluorophore extravasated in the tumor spreads with edema into perilesional tissue at a speed of approximately 2 mm/h [82]. These physiological phenomena need to be considered when using such fluorophores for fluorescence-guided resections

Table 6.4 Time points and doses used for fluorescein in glioma surgery (publications after 2010)

Publication	Fluorescein dose (mg/kg)	Timing of injection
Rey-Dios et al. [88]	4	Fifteen minutes before dural opening, 4 mg/kg fluorescein
Schebesch et al. [22]	3–4	After bone flap removal prior to durotomy
Acerbi et al. [19, 20]	5–10	After intubation and before skin incision
Chen et al. [89]	15–20	After the dura at the craniotomy site was opened
Diaz et al. [21]	3	At the time of anesthesia induction
Okuda [90]	20	After induction of anesthesia and opening of the dura

pitfalls, and timing and dose of administration are crucial. Currently, fluorescein is being used at multiple doses and times of administration (Table 6.4) and not according to a uniform protocol. We have investigated various time points of application [83], ranging from acute injections to injections after induction of anesthesia. With acute injections, the amount of fluorescein in vessels was high, resulting in strong staining of all perfused tissues but also in extravasation with blood and strong unspecific contamination of tissue. With early injections after induction of anesthesia, we still faced the problem of unspecific oozing from resection margins.

Clearly, further research is necessary if fluorescein and similar substances should be used for fluorescence-guided resection. Ultimately, randomized studies will be necessary.

Dual-Labeling Approach

In a novel approach, we now attempt to combine unspecific fluorescein tissue fluorescence for contrasting normal brain with selective PPIX fluorescence. For simultaneously visualizing red PPIX fluorescence and yellow fluorescein fluorescence, we exploit the fact that both fluorochromes can be visualized using a single barrier filter that opens at about 500 nm, since fluorescein has a fluorescence maximum at 525 nm and PPIX at 635 nm. For excitation, we combine the excitation light optimized for PPIX (375–440 nm) together with light optimized for exciting fluorescein (370–510 nm). The combination highlights perfused tissue background while allowing visualization of red porphyrin fluorescence. In case of co-location of fluorescein and 5-ALA-induced porphyrins, tissues appear a vivid orange (Fig. 6.9, manuscript in preparation).

Future Developments in Fluorescence-Guided Resection

A number of newer agents for fluorescence-guided resections are in the pipeline and are being translated into clinical use. For the future, more selective agents are being sought with selective binding to malignant glioma cells. One approach is to use the tumor ligand chlorotoxin, a scorpion venom with established affinity to malignant tumor cells [84]. CTX is non-toxic to humans and is conjugated to indocyanine green (ICG). "Tumor Paint BLZ-100" is presently being tested in phase I clinical studies.

Huang et al. [85] have constructed a near-infrared dye targeted to integrin $\alpha_v\beta_3$. Integrins play an important role in tumor angiogenesis, growth, and metastasis. So far, in vivo data are available showing utility of the probe for detecting malignant gliomas with high integrin expression.

In the same year, Wang et al. [86] evaluated the use of monoclonal antibodies targeting vascular endothelial growth factor receptor 1 (VEGF-1) conjugated to fluorophores in a transgenic mouse model of medulloblastoma. Since the antibodies do not cross the blood–brain barrier, antibodies were topically applied, demonstrating preferential binding to tumor cells, and thus suggesting utility for intra-operative detection of tumor.

Recently, cancer-selective alkylphosphocholine (APC) analogs were used experimentally for intra-operative tumor detection [87]. Coupled to infrared fluorophores, these analogs appear to be incorporated and selectively retained in tumor cell membranes. Early-phase clinical trials are underway for exploring this possibility of intra-operative tissue diagnosis.

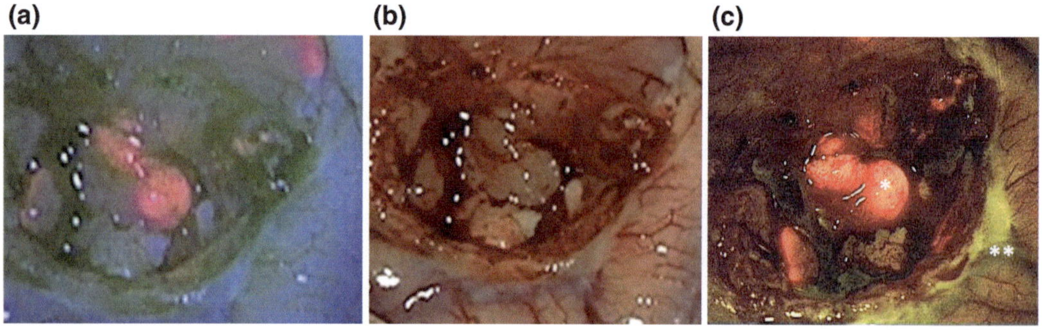

Fig. 6.9 Dual-labeling approach. This is an experimental approach in which fluorescein (4 mg/kg, administered immediately after induction of anesthesia, as previously described [19, 20]) and 5-ALA (20 mg/kg, administered 4 h prior to induction of anesthesia) are simultaneously visualized using a suitable combination of excitation light and emission filters. Fluorescein in vessels highlights perfused tissues, giving enhanced background information to the surgeon, whereas 5-ALA-induced porphyrins selectively highlight tumor. Regions with both fluorophores appear *orange* (*single asterisk*). *Note* Extravasation of fluorescein at resection margins (*double asterisk*)

Conclusions

Tissue fluorescence has become a helpful adjunct for malignant glioma surgery. In this context, 5-ALA is unique because it elicits synthesis and accumulation of the fluorochrome PPX within the tumor cell. Its full potential for other brain tumors has not been determined completely.

Fluorescein is being investigated in depth as an agent with stronger fluorescence but, based on the passive nature of its accumulation in tumors via the leaky blood–brain barrier, low selectivity based on the theoretical basis of its accumulation. Further research with this compound, possibly in conjunction with 5-ALA, is being performed.

Several other targeted and fluorescing compounds are slowly translating into clinical use.

References

1. Albert FK, Forsting M, Sartor K, Adams HP, Kunze S. Early ostoperative magnetic resonance imaging after resection of malignant glioma: objective evaluation of residual tumor and its influence on regrowth and prognosis. Neurosurgery. 1994;34 (1):45–60.
2. Willems PW, van der Sprenkel JW, Tulleken CA, Viergever MA, Taphoorn MJ. Neuronavigation and surgery of intracerebral tumours. J Neurol. 2006;253 (9):1123–36 (Epub 2006 Sep 20. Review).
3. Nimsky C, Ganslandt O, Cerny S, Hastreiter P, Greiner G, Fahlbusch R. Quantification of, visualization of, and compensation for brain shift using intraoperative magnetic resonance imaging. Neurosurgery. 2000;47(5):1070–9 (Discussion 1079–1080).
4. Kreth FW, Thon N, Simon M, et al. Gross total but not incomplete resection of glioblastoma prolongs survival in the era of radiochemotherapy. Ann Oncol. 2013;24(12):3117–23.
5. Lacroix M, Abi-Said D, Fourney DR, et al. A multivariate analysis of 416 patients with glioblastoma multiforme: prognosis, extent of resection, and survival. J Neurosurg. 2001;95(2):190–8.
6. Sanai N, Polley MY, McDermott MW, Parsa AT, Berger MS. An extent of resection threshold for newly diagnosed glioblastomas. J Neurosurg. 2011;115(1):3–8.
7. Stummer W, Meinel T, Ewelt C, Martus P, Jakobs O, Felsberg J, Reifenberger G. Prospective cohort study of radiotherapy with concomitant and adjuvant temozolomide chemotherapy for glioblastoma patients with no or minimal residual enhancing tumor load after surgery. J Neurooncol. 2012;108 (1):89–97.
8. Stummer W, Tonn JC, Mehdorn HM, Nestler U, Franz K, Goetz C, Bink A, Pichlmeier U. Counterbalancing risks and gains from extended resections in malignant glioma surgery: a supplemental analysis from the randomized 5-aminolevulinic acid glioma resection study. Clinical article. J Neurosurg. 2011;114(3):613–23.
9. Pichlmeier U, Bink A, Schackert G, Stummer W. ALA Glioma Study Group resection and survival in glioblastoma multiforme: an RTOG recursive partitioning analysis of ALA study patients. Neuro Oncol. 2008;10(6):1025–34.
10. Moore GE, Peyton WT, French LA, Walker WW. The clinical use of fluorescein in neurosurgery; the localization of brain tumors. J Neurosurg. 1948;5 (4):392–8.
11. Kuroiwa T, Kajimoto Y, Ohta T. Comparison between operative findings on malignant glioma by a fluorescein surgical microscopy and histological findings. Neurol Res. 1999;21(1):130–4.
12. Kuroiwa T, Kajimoto Y, Ohta T. Development of a fluorescein operative microscope for use during malignant glioma surgery: a technical note and preliminary report. Surg Neurol. 1998;50(1):41–8 (discussion 48-9).
13. Kuroiwa T, Kajimoto Y, Ohta T. Surgical management for supratentorial astrocytic tumors. Minim Invasive Neurosurg. 1999;42(4):182–6.
14. Stummer W, Stepp H, Möller G, Ehrhardt A, Leonhard M, Reulen HJ. Technical principles for protoporphyrin-IX-fluorescence guided microsurgical resection of malignant glioma tissue. Acta Neurochir (Wien). 1998;140(10):995–1000.
15. Stummer W, Stocker S, Novotny A, Heimann A, Sauer O, Kempski O, Plesnila N, Wietzorrek J, Reulen HJ. In vitro and in vivo porphyrin accumulation by C6 glioma cells after exposure to 5-aminolevulinic acid. J Photochem Photobiol. 1998;B 45(2–3):160–9.
16. Stummer W, Stocker S, Wagner S, Stepp H, Fritsch C, Goetz C, Goetz AE, Kiefmann R, Reulen HJ. Intraoperative detection of malignant gliomas by 5-aminolevulinic acid-induced porphyrin fluorescence. Neurosurgery. 1998;42(3):518–25.
17. Bottomley SS, Muller-Eberhard U. Pathophysiology of heme synthesis. Semin Hematol. 1988;25(4):282–302.
18. Colditz MJ, Leyen KV, Jeffree RL. Aminolevulinic acid (ALA)-protoporphyrin IX fluorescence guided tumour resection. Part 2: theoretical, biochemical and practical aspects. J Clin Neurosci. 2012;19 (12):1611–6.
19. Acerbi F, Broggi M, Eoli M, Anghileri E, Cavallo C, Boffano C, Cordella R, Cuppini L, Pollo B, Schiariti M, Visintini S, Orsi C, La Corte E, Broggi G, Ferroli P. Is fluorescein-guided technique able to help

in resection of high-grade gliomas? Neurosurg Focus. 2014;2014(36):E5.
20. Acerbi F, Broggi M, Eoli M, Anghileri E, Cuppini L, Pollo B, Schiariti M, Visintini S, Ori C, Franzini A, Broggi G, Ferroli P. Fluorescein-guided surgery for grade IV gliomas with a dedicated filter on the surgical microscope: preliminary results in 12 cases. Acta Neurochir (Wien). 2013;155:1277–86.
21. Diaz RJ, Dios RR, Hattab EM, Burrell K, Rakopoulos P, Sabha N, Hawkins C, Zadeh G, Rutka JT, Cohen-Gadol AA. Study of the biodistribution of fluorescein in glioma-infiltrated mouse brain and histopathological correlation of intraoperative findings in high-grade gliomas resected under fluorescein fluorescence guidance. J Neurosurg. 2015;3:1–10.
22. Schebesch KM, Proescholdt M, Höhne J, et al. Sodium fluorescein-guided resection under the YELLOW 560 nm surgical microscope filter in malignant brain tumor surgery—a feasibility study. Acta Neurochir (Wien). 2013;155(4):693–9.
23. Van Hillegersberg R, Van den Berg JW, Kort WJ, Terpstra OT, Wilson JH. Selective accumulation of endogenously produced porphyrins in a liver metastasis model in rats. Gastroenterology. 1992;103 (2):647–51.
24. Teng L, Nakada M, Zhao SG, Endo Y, Furuyama N, Nambu E, Pyko IV, Hayashi Y, Hamada JI. Silencing of ferrochelatase enhances 5-aminolevulinic acid-based fluorescence and photodynamic therapy efficacy. Br J Cancer. 2011;104(5):798–807.
25. Zhao SG, Chen XF, Wang LG, Yang G, Han DY, Teng L, Yang MC, Wang DY, Shi C, Liu YH, Zheng BJ, Shi CB, Gao X, Rainov NG. Increased expression of ABCB6 enhances protoporphyrin IX accumulation and photodynamic effect in human glioma. Ann Surg Oncol. 2013;20(13):4379–88.
26. Ennis SR, Novotny A, Xiang J, et al. Transport of 5-aminolevulinic acid between blood and brain. Brain Res. 2003;959(2):226–34.
27. Stummer W, Reulen HJ, Novotny A, Stepp H, Tonn JC. Fluorescence-guided resections of malignant gliomas—an overview. Acta Neurochir Suppl. 2003;88:9–12.
28. Valentine RM, Ibbotson SH, Wood K, Brown CT, Moseley H. Modelling fluorescence in clinical photodynamic therapy. Photochem Photobiol Sci. 2013;12(1):203–13.
29. Pascu A, Romanitan MO, Delgado JM, Danaila L, Pascu ML. Laser-induced autofluorescence measurements on brain tissues. Anat Rec (Hoboken). 2009;292(12):2013–22.
30. Stummer W, Pichlmeier U, Meinel T, Wiestler OD, Zanella F, Reulen HJ. Fluorescence-guided surgery with 5-aminolevulinic acid for resection of malignant glioma: a randomised controlled multicentre phase III trial. Lancet Oncol. 2006;7(5):392–401.
31. Schucht P, Beck J, Abu-Isa J, et al. Gross total resection rates in contemporary glioblastoma surgery: results of an institutional protocol combining 5-aminolevulinic acid intraoperative fluorescence imaging and brain mapping. Neurosurgery. 2012;71 (5):927–35 (discussion 935–936).
32. Schucht P, Seidel K, Beck J, et al. Intraoperative monopolar mapping during 5-ALA-guided resections of glioblastomas adjacent to motor eloquent areas: evaluation of resection rates and neurological outcome. Neurosurg Focus. 2014;37(6):E16.
33. Diez Valle R, Tejada Solis S, Idoate Gastearena MA, García de Eulate R, Dominguez Echávarri P, Aristu Mendiroz J. Surgery guided by 5-aminolevulinic fluorescence in glioblastoma: volumetric analysis of extent of resection in single-center experience. J Neurooncol. 2011;102(1):105–13.
34. Della Puppa A, De Pellegrin S, d'Avella E, et al. 5-aminolevulinic acid (5-ALA) fluorescence guided surgery of high-grade gliomas in eloquent areas assisted by functional mapping. Our experience and review of the literature. Acta Neurochir (Wien). 2013;155(6):965–72 (discussion 972).
35. Coburger J, Engelke J, Scheuerle A, et al. Tumor detection with 5-aminolevulinic acid fluorescence and Gd-DTPA-enhanced intraoperative MRI at the border of contrast-enhancing lesions: a prospective study based on histopathological assessment. Neurosurg Focus. 2014;36(2):E3.
36. Eljamel S. 5-ALA fluorescence image guided resection of glioblastoma multiforme: a meta-analysis of the literature. Int J Mol Sci. 2015;16(5):10443–56.
37. Stummer W, Novotny A, Stepp H, Goetz C, Bise K, Reulen HJ. Fluorescence-guided resection of glioblastoma multiforme by using 5-aminolevulinic acid-induced porphyrins: a prospective study in 52 consecutive patients. J Neurosurg. 2000;93(6): 1003–13.
38. Idoate MA, Diez Valle R, Echeveste J, Tejada S. Pathological characterization of the glioblastoma border as shown during surgery using 5-aminolevulinic acid-induced fluorescence. Neuropathology. 2011;31(6):575–82 (18).
39. Roberts DW, Valdés PA, Harris BT, et al. Coregistered fluorescence-enhanced tumor resection of malignant glioma: relationships between d-aminolevulinic acid-induced protoporphyrin IX fluorescence, magnetic resonance imaging enhancement, and neuropathological parameters. Clinical article. J Neurosurg. 2011;114(3):595–603.
40. Hefti M, von Campe G, Moschopulos M, Siegner A, Looser H, Landolt H. 5-Aminolevulinic acid induced protoporphyrin IX fluorescence in high-grade glioma surgery: a one-year experience at a single institution. Swiss Med Wkly. 2008;138(11–12):180–5.
41. Yamada S, Muragaki Y, Maruyama T, Komori T, Okada Y. Role of neurochemical navigation with 5-aminolevulinic acid during intraoperative MRI-guided resection of intracranial malignant gliomas. Clin Neurol Neurosurg. 2015;130:134–9.
42. Stummer W, Tonn JC, Goetz C, et al. 5-Aminolevulinic acid-derived tumor fluorescence: the diagnostic accuracy of visible fluorescence

qualities as corroborated by spectrometry and histology and postoperative imaging. Neurosurgery. 2014;74(3):310–9 (discussion 319–320).
43. Stummer W. Response to journal club: 5-aminolevulinic acid-derived tumor fluorescence: the diagnostic accuracy of visible fluorescence qualities as corroborated by spectrometry and histology and postoperative imaging. Neurosurgery. 2015;76 (2):230–1.
44. Valdés PA, Moses ZB, Kim A, Belden CJ, Wilson BC, Paulsen KD, Roberts DW, Harris BT. Gadolinium- and 5-aminolevulinic acid-induced protoporphyrin IX levels in human gliomas: an ex vivo quantitative study to correlate protoporphyrin IX levels and blood-brain barrier breakdown. J Neuropathol Exp Neurol. 2012;71(9):806–13.
45. Jaber M, Wölfer J, Ewelt C, Holling M, Hasselblatt M, Niederstadt T, Zoubi T, Weckesser M, Stummer W. The value of 5-Aminolevulinic acid in low-grade gliomas and high-grade gliomas lacking glioblastoma imaging features: an analysis based on fluorescence, magnetic resonance imaging, 18F-fluoroethyl tyrosine positron emission tomography, and tumor molecular factors. Neurosurgery. 2016;78(3):401–11.
46. Nabavi A, Thurm H, Zountsas B, et al. Five-aminolevulinic acid for fluorescence-guided resection of recurrent malignant gliomas: a phase II study. Neurosurgery. 2009;65(6):1070–6 (discussion 1076–1077).
47. Utsuki S, Oka H, Sato S, et al. Histological examination of false positive tissue resection using 5-aminolevulinic acid-induced fluorescence guidance. Neurol Med Chir (Tokyo). 2007;47(5):210–3 (discussion 213–214).
48. Ando T, Kobayashi E, Liao H, et al. Precise comparison of protoporphyrin IX fluorescence spectra with pathological results for brain tumor tissue identification. Brain Tumor Pathol. 2011;28(1): 43–51.
49. Kamp MA, Felsberg J, Sadat H, Kuzibaev J, Steiger HJ, Rapp M, Reifenberger G, Dibué M, Sabel M. 5-ALA-induced fluorescence behavior of reactive tissue changes following glioblastoma treatment with radiation and chemotherapy. Acta Neurochir (Wien). 2015;157(2):207–13 (discussion 213–4).
50. Schucht P, Knittel S, Slotboom J, et al. 5-ALA complete resections go beyond MR contrast enhancement: shift corrected volumetric analysis of the extent of resection in surgery for glioblastoma. Acta Neurochir (Wien). 2014;156(2):305–12 (discussion 312).
51. Aldave G, Tejada S, Pay E, Marigil M, Bejarano B, Idoate MA, Díez-Valle R. Prognostic value of residual fluorescent tissue in glioblastoma patients after gross total resection in 5-aminolevulinic acid-guided surgery. Neurosurgery. 2013;72 (6):915–20 (discussion 920-1).
52. Roessler K, Becherer A, Donat M, Cejna M, Zachenhofer I. Intraoperative tissue fluorescence using 5-aminolevolinic acid (5-ALA) is more sensitive than contrast MRI or amino acid positron emission tomography ((18)F-FET PET) in glioblastoma surgery. Neurol Res. 2012;34(3):314–7.
53. Widhalm G, Wolfsberger S, Minchev G, et al. 5-Aminolevulinic acid is a promising marker for detection of anaplastic foci in diffusely infiltrating gliomas with nonsignificant contrast enhancement. Cancer. 2010;116(6):1545–52.
54. Ewelt C, Floeth FW, Felsberg J, Steiger HJ, Sabel M, Langen KJ, Stoffels G, Stummer W. Finding the anaplastic focus in diffuse gliomas: the value of Gd-DTPA enhanced MRI, FET-PET, and intraoperative, ALA-derived tissue fluorescence. Clin Neurol Neurosurg. 2011;113(7):541–7.
55. Stockhammer F, Misch M, Horn P, Koch A, Fonyuy N, Plotkin M. Association of F18-fluoro-ethyl-tyrosin uptake and 5-aminolevulinic acid-induced fluorescence in gliomas. Acta Neurochir (Wien). 2009;151(11):1377–83.
56. Widhalm G, Kiesel B, Woehrer A, Traub-Weidinger T, Preusser M, Marosi C, Prayer D, Hainfellner JA, Knosp E, Wolfsberger S. 5-Aminolevulinic acid induced fluorescence is a powerful intraoperative marker for precise histopathological grading of gliomas with non-significant contrast-enhancement. PLoS ONE. 2013;8(10):e76988.
57. Nishikawa R. Fluorescence illuminates the way .... Neuro Oncol. 2011;13(8):805.
58. Valdés PA, Jacobs V, Harris BT, Wilson BC, Leblond F, Paulsen KD, Roberts DW. Quantitative fluorescence using 5-aminolevulinic acid-induced protoporphyrin IX biomarker as a surgical adjunct in low-grade glioma surgery. J Neurosurg. 2015;123 (3):771–80.
59. Sanai N, Snyder LA, Honea NJ, et al. Intraoperative confocal microscopy in the visualization of 5-aminolevulinic acid fluorescence in low-grade gliomas. J Neurosurg. 2011;115(4):740–8.
60. Marbacher S, Klinger E, Schwyzer L, Fischer I, Nevzati E, Diepers M, Roelcke U, Fathi AR, Coluccia D, Fandino J. Use of fluorescence to guide resection or biopsy of primary brain tumors and brain metastases. Neurosurg Focus. 2014;36(2):E10.
61. Beez T, Sarikaya-Seiwert S, Steiger HJ, Hänggi D. Fluorescence-guided surgery with 5-aminolevulinic acid for resection of brain tumors in children—a technical report. Acta Neurochir (Wien). 2014;156 (3):597–604.
62. Preuß M, Renner C, Krupp W, Christiansen H, Fischer L, Merkenschlager A, Kieß W, Müller W, Manzo N, Meixensberger J, Nestler U. The use of 5-aminolevulinic acid fluorescence guidance in resection of pediatric brain tumors. Childs Nerv Syst. 2013;29(8):1263–7.
63. Skjøth-Rasmussen J, Bøgeskov L, Sehested A, Klausen C, Broholm H, Nysom K. The use of

5-ALA to assist complete removal of residual non-enhancing part of childhood medulloblastoma: a case report. Childs Nerv Syst. 2015;31(11):2173–7.
64. Stummer W, Rodrigues F, Schucht P, Preuss M, Wiewrodt D, Nestler U, Stein M, Artero JM, Platania N, Skjøth-Rasmussen J, Della Puppa A, Caird J, Cortnum S, Eljamel S, Ewald C, González-García L, Martin AJ, Melada A, Peraud A, Brentrup A, Santarius T, Steiner HH, European ALA Pediatric Brain Tumor Study Group. Predicting the "usefulness" of 5-ALA-derived tumor fluorescence for fluorescence-guided resections in pediatric brain tumors: a European survey. Acta Neurochir (Wien). 2014;156(12):2315–24.
65. Della Puppa A, Rustemi O, Gioffrè G, Troncon I, Lombardi G, Rolma G, Sergi M, Munari M, Cecchin D, Gardiman MP, Scienza R. Predictive value of intraoperative 5-aminolevulinic acid-induced fluorescence for detecting bone invasion in meningioma surgery. J Neurosurg. 2014;120 (4):840–5.
66. Potapov AA, Goryaynov SA, Okhlopkov VA, Shishkina LV, Loschenov VB, Savelieva TA, Golbin DA, Chumakova AP, Goldberg MF, Varyukhina MD, Spallone A. Laser biospectroscopy and 5-ALA fluorescence navigation as a helpful tool in the meningioma resection. Neurosurg Rev. 2016 Feb 18 [Epub ahead of print] PubMed PMID: 26887580.
67. El-Khatib M, Tepe C, Senger B, Dibué-Adjei M, Riemenschneider MJ, Stummer W, Steiger HJ, Cornelius JF. Aminolevulinic acid-mediated photodynamic therapy of human meningioma: an in vitro study on primary cell lines. Int J Mol Sci. 2015;16 (5):9936–48.
68. Motekallemi A, Jeltema HR, Metzemaekers JD, van Dam GM, Crane LM, Groen RJ. The current status of 5-ALA fluorescence-guided resection of intracranial meningiomas-a critical review. Neurosurg Rev. 2015;38(4):619–28.
69. Cornelius JF, Slotty PJ, Kamp MA, Schneiderhan TM, Steiger HJ, El-Khatib M. Impact of 5-aminolevulinic acid fluorescence-guided surgery on the extent of resection of meningiomas—with special regard to high-grade tumors. Photodiagnosis Photodyn Ther. 2014;11(4):481–90.
70. Wilbers E, Hargus G, Wölfer J, Stummer W. Usefulness of 5-ALA (Gliolan®)-derived PPX fluorescence for demonstrating the extent of infiltration in atypical meningiomas. Acta Neurochir (Wien). 2014;156(10):1853–4.
71. Cornelius JF, Slotty PJ, Stoffels G, Galldiks N, Langen KJ, Steiger HJ. 5-Aminolevulinic acid and (18)F-FET-PET as metabolic imaging tools for surgery of a recurrent skull base meningioma. J Neurol Surg B Skull Base. 2013;74(4):211–6.
72. Valdes PA, Bekelis K, Harris BT, Wilson BC, Leblond F, Kim A, Simmons NE, Erkmen K, Paulsen KD, Roberts DW. 5-Aminolevulinic acid-induced protoporphyrin IX fluorescence in meningioma: qualitative and quantitative measurements in vivo. Neurosurgery. 2014;10(Suppl 1):74–82 (discussion 82-3).
73. Coluccia D, Fandino J, Fujioka M, Cordovi S, Muroi C, Landolt H. Intraoperative 5-aminolevulinic-acid-induced fluorescence in meningiomas. Acta Neurochir (Wien). 2010;152 (10):1711–9. doi:10.1007/s00701-010-0708-4 (Epub 2010 Jun 10).
74. Moriuchi S, Yamada K, Dehara M, Teramoto Y, Soda T, Imakita M, Taneda M. Use of 5-aminolevulinic acid for the confirmation of deep-seated brain tumors during stereotactic biopsy. Report of 2 cases. J Neurosurg. 2011;115(2):278–80.
75. Widhalm G, Minchev G, Woehrer A, Preusser M, Kiesel B, Furtner J, Mert A, Di Ieva A, Tomanek B, Prayer D, Marosi C, Hainfellner JA, Knosp E, Wolfsberger S. Strong 5-aminolevulinic acid-induced fluorescence is a novel intraoperative marker for representative tissue samples in stereotactic brain tumor biopsies. Neurosurg Rev. 2012;35(3):381–91.
76. von Campe G, Moschopulos M, Hefti M. 5-Aminolevulinic acid-induced protoporphyrin IX fluorescence as immediate intraoperative indicator to improve the safety of malignant or high-grade brain tumor diagnosis in frameless stereotactic biopsies. Acta Neurochir (Wien). 2012;154(4):585–8.
77. Kamp MA, Grosser P, Felsberg J, Slotty PJ, Steiger HJ, Reifenberger G, Sabel M. 5-aminolevulinic acid (5-ALA)-induced fluorescence in intracerebral metastases: a retrospective study. Acta Neurochir (Wien). 2012;154(2):223–8.
78. Schucht P, Murek M, Jilch A, Seidel K, Hewer E, Wiest R, Raabe A, Beck J. Early re-do surgery for glioblastoma is a feasible and safe strategy to achieve complete resection of enhancing tumor. PLoS ONE. 2013;8(11):e79846.
79. Eljamel MS, Leese G, Moseley H. Intraoperative optical identification of pituitary adenomas. J Neurooncol. 2009;92(3):417–21.
80. Eyüpoglu IY, Hore N, Savaskan NE, Grummich P, Roessler K, Buchfelder M, Ganslandt O. Improving the extent of malignant glioma resection by dual intraoperative visualization approach. PLoS ONE. 2012;7(9):e44885. doi:10.1371/journal.pone.0044885.
81. Dilek O, Ihsan A, Tulay H. Anaphylactic reaction after fluorescein sodium administration during intracranial surgery. J Clin Neurosci. 2011;18 (3):430–1.
82. Gröger U, Huber P, Reulen HJ. Formation and resolution of human peritumoral brain edema. Acta Neurochir Suppl (Wien). 1994;60:373–4.
83. Schwake M, Stummer W, Suero Molina EJ, Wölfer J. Simultaneous fluorescein sodium and 5-ALA in fluorescence-guided glioma surgery. Acta Neurochir (Wien). 2015;157(5):877–9. doi:10.1007/s00701-015-2401-0.
84. Butte PV, Mamelak A, Parrish-Novak J, Drazin D, Shweikeh F, Gangalum PR, Chesnokova A,

Ljubimova JY, Black K. Near-infrared imaging of brain tumors using the tumor paint BLZ-100 to achieve near-complete resection of brain tumors. Neurosurg Focus. 2014;36(2):E1.
85. Huang R, Vider J, Kovar JL, Olive DM, Mellinghoff IK, Mayer-Kuckuk P, Kircher MF, Blasberg RG. Integrin αvβ3-targeted IRDye 800CW near-infrared imaging of glioblastoma. Clin Cancer Res. 2012;18(20):5731–40.
86. Wang D, Chen Y, Leigh SY, Haeberle H, Contag CH, Liu JT. Microscopic delineation of medulloblastoma margins in a transgenic mouse model using a topically applied VEGFR-1 Probe. Transl Oncol. 2012;5(6):408–14.
87. Swanson KI, Clark PA, Zhang RR, Kandela IK, Farhoud M, Weichert JP, Kuo JS. Fluorescent cancer-selective alkylphosphocholine analogs for intraoperative glioma detection. Neurosurgery. 2015;76(2):115–23.
88. Rey-Dios R, Cohen-Gadol AA. Technical principles and neurosurgical applications of fluorescein fluorescence using a microscope-integrated fluorescence module. Acta Neurochir (Wien). 2013;155:701–6.
89. Chen B, Wang H, Ge P, Zhao J, Li W, Gu H, Wang G, Luo Y, Chen D. Gross total resection of glioma with the intraoperative fluorescence-guidance of fluorescein sodium. Int J Med Sci. 2012;9:708–14.
90. Okuda T, Yoshioka H, Kato A. Fluorescence-guided surgery for glioblastoma multiforme using high-dose fluorescein sodium with excitation and barrier filters. J Clin Neurosci. 2012;19:1719–22.
91. Inoue T, Endo T, Nagamatsu K, Watanabe M, Tominaga T. 5-aminolevulinic acid fluorescence-guided resection of intramedullary ependymoma: report of 9 cases. Neurosurgery. 2013;72(2 Suppl Operative):ons159–68 (discussion ons168).
92. Arai T, Tani S, Isoshima A, Nagashima H, Joki T, Takahashi-Fujigasaki J, Abe T. (Intraoperative photodynamic diagnosis for spinal ependymoma using 5-aminolevulinic acid: technical note). No Shinkei Geka. 2006;34(8):811–7 (Japanese).
93. Bernal García LM, Cabezudo Artero JM, Marcelo Zamorano MB, Gilete Tejero I. Fluorescence-guided resection with 5-aminolevulinic Acid of subependymomas of the fourth ventricle: report of 2 cases: technical case report. Neurosurgery. 2015;11(Suppl 2):E364–71; discussion E371.
94. Utsuki S, Oka H, Sato K, Shimizu S, Suzuki S, Fujii K. Fluorescence diagnosis of tumor cells in hemangioblastoma cysts with 5-aminolevulinic acid. J Neurosurg. 2010;112(1):130–2.
95. Eicker S, Sarikaya-Seiwert S, Borkhardt A, Gierga K, Turowski B, Heiroth HJ, Steiger HJ, Stummer W. ALA-induced porphyrin accumulation in medulloblastoma and its use for fluorescence-guided surgery. Cent Eur Neurosurg. 2011;72(2):101–3.

7 The Role of Laser-Induced Thermal Therapy in the Management of Malignant Gliomas

Elena Fomchenko and Veronica L.S. Chiang

Introduction

Current standard-of-care treatment for patients with newly diagnosed HGGs includes maximally cytoreductive tumor resection followed by a combination of radiation and concomitant or subsequent alkylating agent temozolomide, based on the protocol described by Stupp et al. [1–5]. Unfortunately, regardless of the success of the initial treatment, these tumors often recur both locally and at distant sites in the brain. No standard protocols currently exist for management of non-resectable HGGs or salvage management of HGGs, and treatment options are often limited by their cumulative toxicities. Novel systemic agents including targeted therapies and immunotherapies are being actively developed but have not been shown as yet to be successful without surgical cytoreduction.

Rationale for Use of LITT for HGGs

Typically, the role of surgical resection is to assist in making the diagnosis of HGG and facilitate rapid reduction of intracranial hypertension to maximize recovery of mass-related neurological dysfunction. Multiple retrospective studies suggest significant improvement in progression-free survival (PFS) and overall survival (OS) with gross total resection (GTR) [6–22]. The average survival in patients with untreated *glioblastoma multiforme* is merely 9 weeks [23] but can be significantly improved to an average of 6.6 months with biopsy only versus 10.4 months with partial resection versus 14.6 months with gross total resection followed by chemotherapy and radiation, with a quarter of patients surviving for up to 2 years and around 10% surviving for up to 5 years [3].

Other studies, however, call aggressive resection into question. A recent study of 306 patients with newly diagnosed GBMs by McGirt et al. [7] showed a 6% incidence of surgically acquired motor deficits and a 5% incidence of surgically acquired language deficits, resulting in the lower OS times of 9.6 and 9 months, respectively, as compared to 12.8 months OS in patients without surgically acquired deficits [7]. This translated into a significant reduction in two-year survival from 23 to 8% with newly acquired motor deficits and 0% with newly acquired language deficits [7]. Gulate et al. [25] likewise reported that 15.3% of their patients developed surgically related new neurological deficits resulting in a significantly decreased Karnofsky performance score (KPS) in 39% of patients, which in addition to age was a significant predictor of worse functional outcome [25]. Further, patients with surgically acquired neurological deficits were less likely to receive

E. Fomchenko (✉) · V.L.S. Chiang
Department of Neurosurgery, Yale University School of Medicine, 15 York Street LLCI 810, P.O. Box 208082, New Haven, CT 06510, USA
e-mail: elena.fomchenko@yale.edu

V.L.S. Chiang
e-mail: veronica.chiang@yale.edu

J. Moliterno Günel et al. (eds.), *Malignant Brain Tumors*,
DOI 10.1007/978-3-319-49864-5_7

adjuvant radiation therapy or chemotherapy, which has been shown to worsen survival [25].

Because of the potential risk of additional neurological injury, the surgical management of deep lesions requiring an approach through eloquent brain, such as the left insula or subcortical motor regions, basal ganglia and the thalamus, and tumors that cross the midline, such as those involving the corpus callosum, may include only a diagnostic biopsy. To improve surgical cytoreduction of these surgically difficult-to-access tumors, several novel methods have been developed including radiosurgery, laser interstitial thermal therapy (LITT), photodynamic therapy, and most recently, high-intensity-focused ultrasound. LITT, which is the focus of this chapter, is a minimally invasive technique involving stereotactic placement of a single or multiple high-energy laser fibers into the substance of the tumor in order to deliver thermal therapy for tumor ablation. Delivery of heat is performed under the guidance of MRI with intra-procedural monitoring and verification of successful energy delivery (Fig. 7.1).

Lasers in History

The most common use of lasers in the nervous system includes the use of argon, ruby, and CO_2 lasers to perform cutting and vaporization, and to achieve tissue hemostasis [26, 27]. The first use of interstitial laser photochemotherapy to nervous tissue, however, traces back to 1987, when Powers et al. [28] described the use of mitochondria-specific rhodamine-123 dye and a 150 mW blue-green argon light for treatment of flank and intracerebral rat gliomas, resulting in progressive central tumor shrinkage and necrosis over time, but eventual tumor recurrence at its periphery, where light penetration was limited by distance [28]. Further studies investigated effects of variations in wavelength and types of thermal energy emitting tips, including the end emitting bare tip versus diffusion emitting sapphire tip optical fiber probes [29] (Fig. 7.2), showing that elevations in tissue temperature are related to surface area of the probe, which directly affects rate of energy delivery, and rate of temperature change near the light source affected distance of

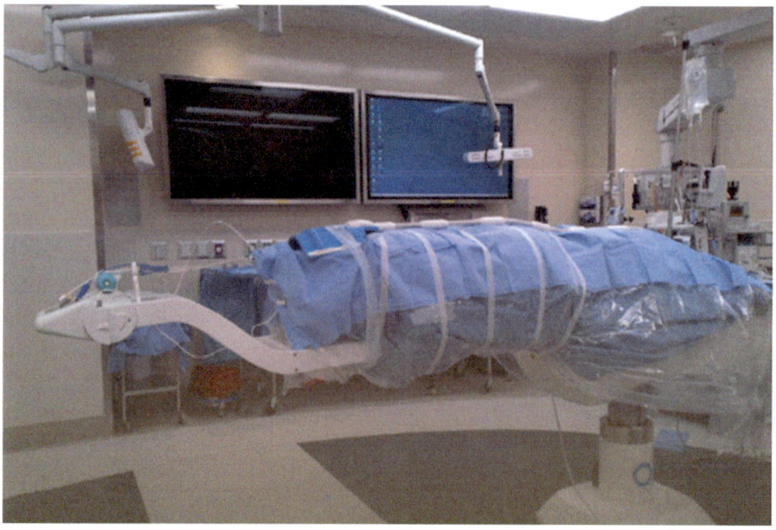

Fig. 7.1 MRI-compatible surgical suite at Yale New Haven Hospital. Patient positioning and preparation prior to obtaining pre-LITT MRI. Heat delivery is performed under MRI guidance for intra-procedural monitoring and confirmation of successful energy delivery

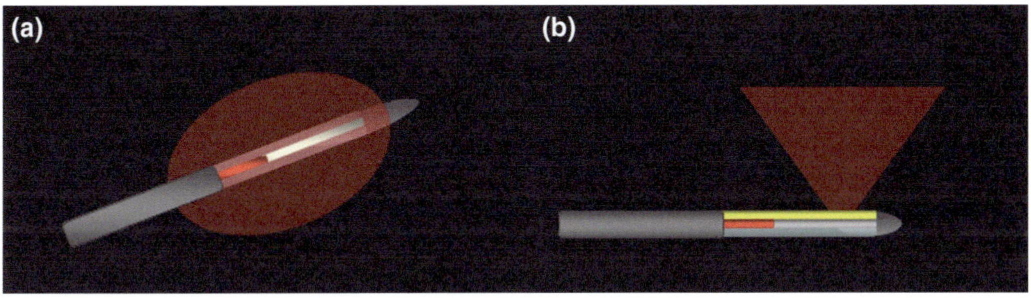

Fig. 7.2 Types of probe tips commonly used to target intracranial lesions with laser interstitial thermal therapy. Diffusion-tip probe creates an ellipse-shaped LITT lesion **a** and directional tip creates a wedge-shaped LITT lesion **b**

heat penetration independent of light wavelength [29]. Laser effect on tissues is also known to be dependent on tissue thermal and optical properties, including thermal conductivity, hemoglobin and fluid content, tissue density, and specific heat, in addition to laser wavelength, mode, and fluence [30].

Despite significant knowledge regarding the factors that influence laser effect on the in vitro tissues, the most significant barrier to the use of laser thermocoagulation remained the inability to predict the size of thermal lesioning in vivo. Its re-invigoration in clinical practice in the past decade is due solely to the development of MR thermometry by Frank Jolesz in 1981 [31–34]. MR thermometry is the ability to interpret MR gradient echo image changes in order to follow thermal tissue changes (Fig. 7.3). Initial feasibility work was performed in cat, dog, rabbit, and pig brains, showing good correlation between changes in gradient echo image information and histological evidence of cell death [21–25]. Further, three histologically distinct zones of post-laser regions of injury, including (a) peri-laser vaporization zone, (b) zone of coagulation necrosis, and (c) zone of peri-lesional edema, can be clearly depicted using gadolinium enhanced T1-weighted spin-echo MR images [35–39] (Fig. 7.4).

Current Indications for Use in LITT in Neurosurgical Patients

Over the past decade, the indications for the use of MR-guided LITT have significantly expanded. Treatment of glial tumors and brain metastases failing radiation and surgery remain the major indications for the use of LITT [40–42] (Fig. 7.5). Within this group also fall the cases of radiation necrosis, with which our center has had significant treatment success [43–45]. Increasingly, however, as the technology advances, LITT has expanded its use into the areas of epilepsy, particularly in patients with mesial temporal sclerosis, or lesion-based seizures [46–48], the area of neurovascular neurosurgery such as LITT use for treatment of cavernous malformations [49, 50], and for the treatment of benign tumors such as meningiomas [51, 52]. The largest advantage of LITT over the more traditional approaches is its ability to minimize the intracranial approach through the normal brain parenchyma in order to access the lesion. In addition, with a stab incision in the skin and a small drill hole in the skull, intra-operative blood loss and postoperative pain associated with the surgery are also significantly minimized. Lastly, the ability to visualize heat delivery based on real-time MRI allows the

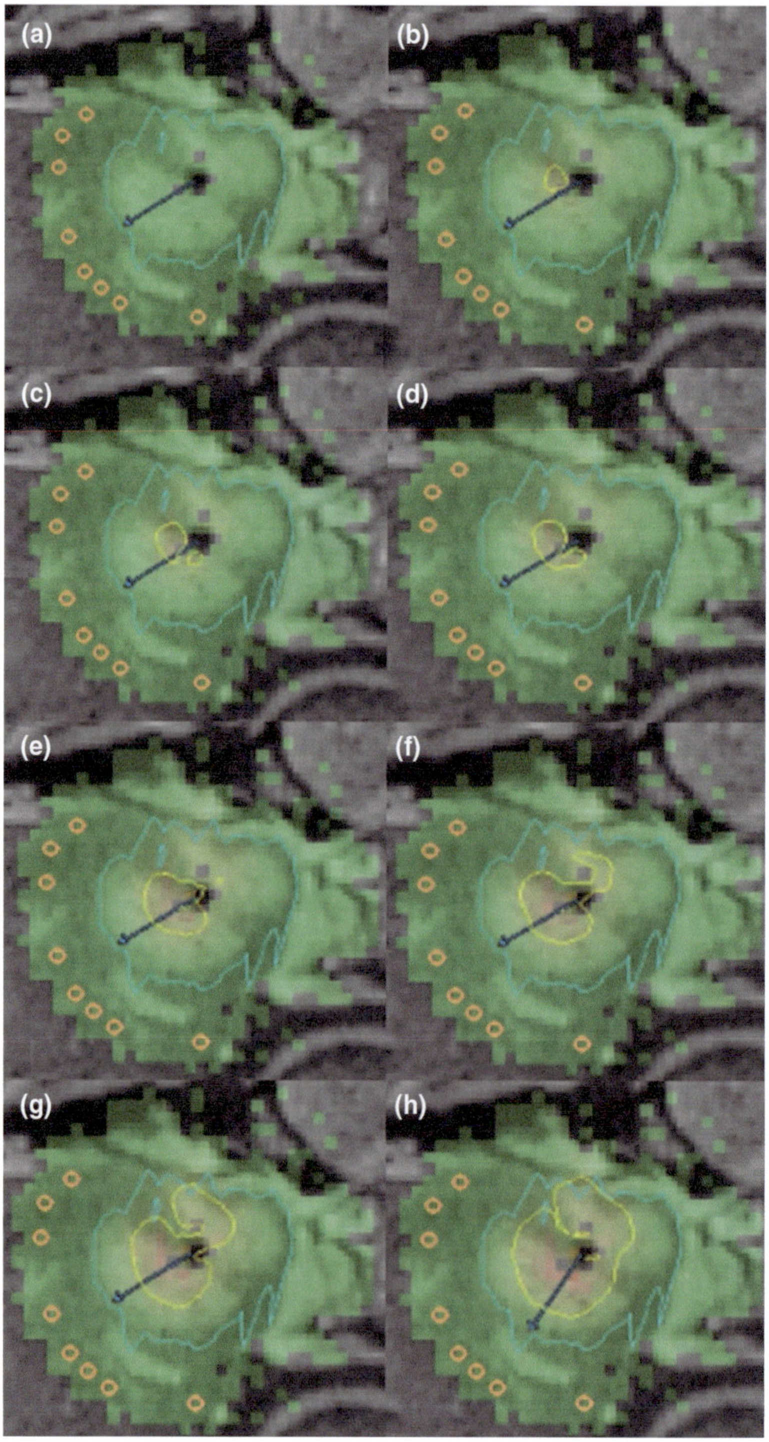

Fig. 7.3 Intra-operative LITT imaging showing heat delivery (*yellow line*) and lesion outline (*light blue*). Serial images (**a**–**h**) show radial growth of area of tissue destruction (*shaded green*)

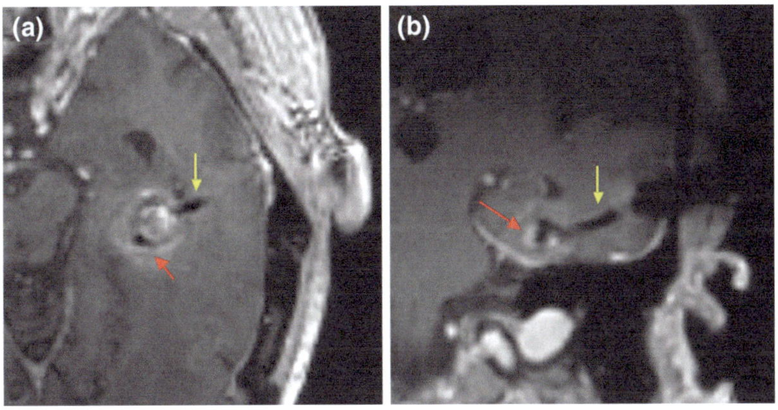

Fig. 7.4 Immediate post-LITT imaging showing laser trajectory (*yellow arrow*) in axial (**a**) and coronal (**b**) planes. Post-LITT MRI shows a hyperdense center with a dark rim consistent with coagulation products, surrounded by a thin rim of contrast enhancement (*red arrow*) that shows the extent of laser-treated tissue at the edge of ablation zone

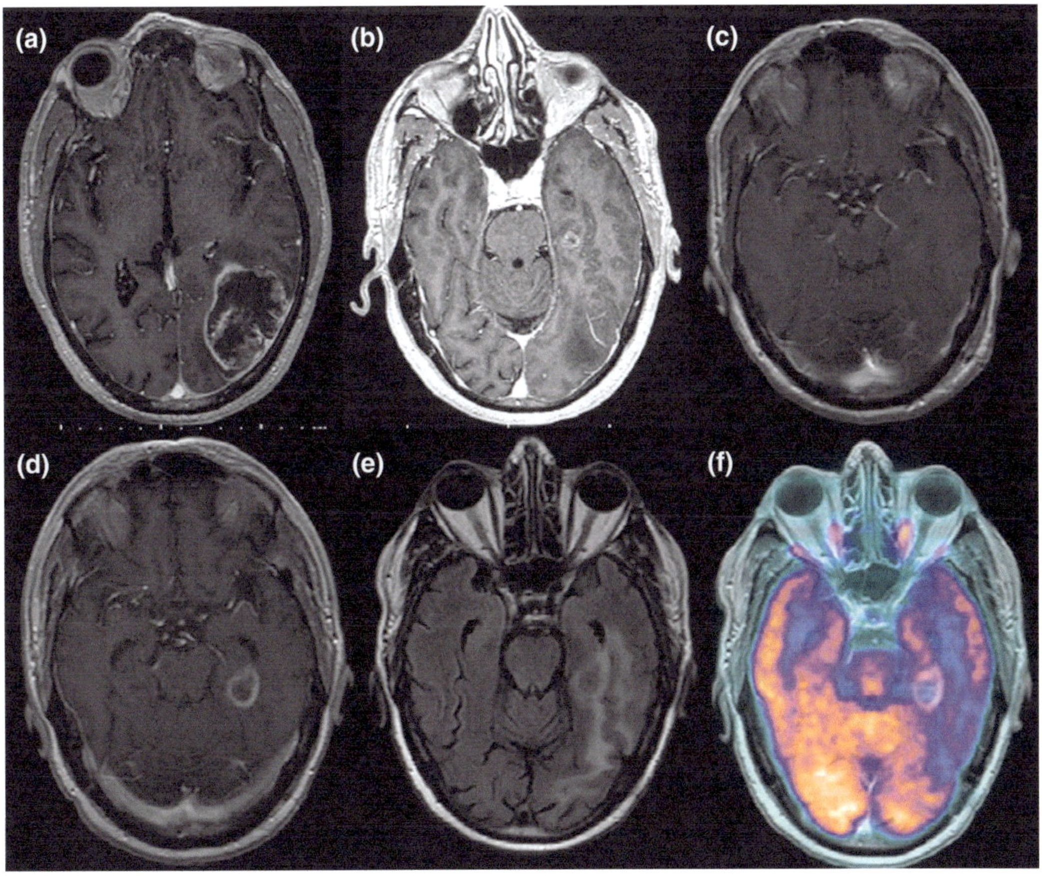

Fig. 7.5 Response to LITT in a 50-year-old male patient diagnosed with a multifocal GBM and treated with partial surgical resection of a larger GBM focus, followed by laser ablation of all GBM foci. **a** T1-weighted Gadolinium sequence showing a large left occipital GBM focus that was resected and treated by 54 Gy of fractionated radiation; **b** second left temporal GBM focus treated by 54 Gy of fractionated radiation alone without resection; **c** left temporal GBM focus showed good initial response; (**d** and **e**) follow-up T1-weighted gadolinium and FLAIR sequences showing recurrence of the left temporal GBM focus; (**f**) follow-up PET scan confirming tumor recurrence

surgeon to determine adequacy of treatment in real time [35–39] (Fig. 7.3).

The LITT Procedure

LITT procedures can be performed both in the operating room, if an intra-operative MRI is available, and in a diagnostic MRI suite (Fig. 7.1). Prior to starting surgery, at our facility, we spend a significant amount of time planning the laser trajectory (Fig. 7.6). Using our neuro-navigation planning software, we estimate that each laser pass will allow us to cover a cylinder of tissue of up to 25–30 mm in diameter. By overlaying each trajectory onto the lesion, one can plan the number of trajectories required to cover the lesion and the direction from which the laser is best introduced. While there is no current data to support trajectory recommendations, we have found that treatment is usually most easily achieved if the laser is brought along the long axis of the lesion with the structures most at risk at the tip of the fiber.

LITT can be performed under general anesthesia or conscious sedation along with local anesthetics. In our facility, we have access to an intra-operative MRI, and the ability to perform LITT under general anesthesia has allowed us to perform complex multiple trajectory treatments more easily. Prior to starting the procedure, the patient is medicated with 10 mg dexamethasone and antibiotics. Mannitol is not administered in order to minimize brain shift during surgery. Following the administration of general anesthesia, the patient is placed in pins so that when the head is secured to the operating table, the head holder is in neutral position. In addition, the trajectory of the laser needs to be taken into account so that as it protrudes from the head, it is directed as much as possible directly out the bore of the magnet. If this is not possible, in general, it is better for the laser fiber to be pointing off to the side than straight up in the bore. At this time, we obtain a preoperative MRI, since in our experience best results are obtained if the imaging for the procedure is performed the day of surgery. A T2-weighted MRI sequence is usually obtained first, and if the target can be well defined on this sequence, then gadolinium is not administered. If, however, the T2 sequence is insufficient, then a half dose of gadolinium is

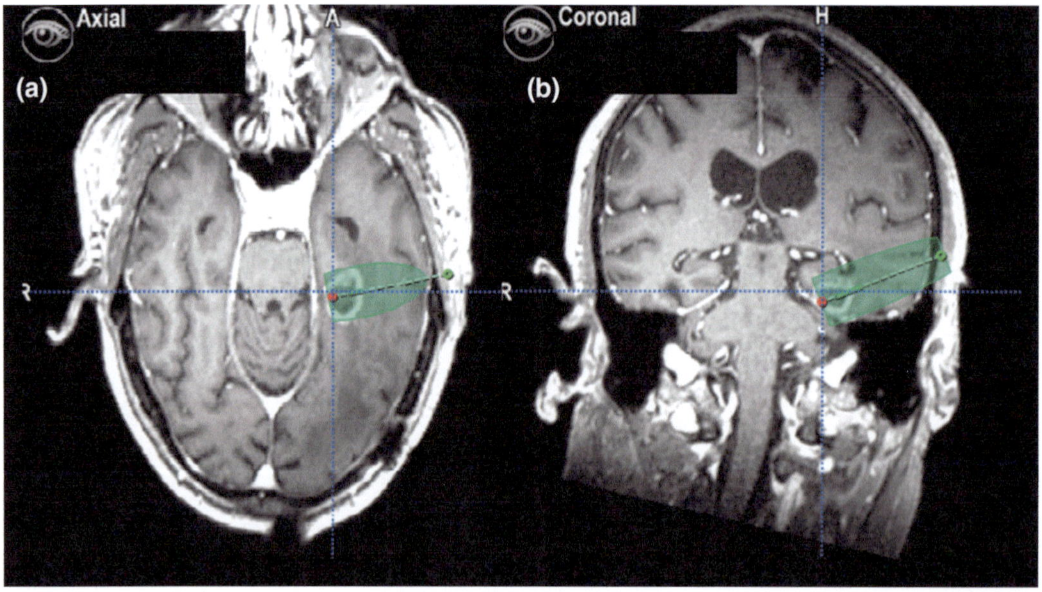

Fig. 7.6 Pre-LITT trajectory planning using BrainLab. Coronal and axial images depicting direction of the laser placement are projected using BrainLab software based on the intra-operative MRI, with an intent to cover the lesion being treated with an estimated cylinder of heat 20 mm in diameter (**a** and **b**)

administered only. Throughout the course of treatment, repeat doses of gadolinium are required and minimizing the amount of gadolinium used initially can decrease potential overall toxicity.

Placement of the laser fiber is then guided by neuro-navigation based on this preoperative MRI scan. For most cases, a stab incision is first made in the scalp and then a twist-drill hole is made in the direction of laser fiber placement. In our experience, not only is it essential to use neuro-navigation to guide the drilling of this hole, but if the hole is not directly perpendicular to the skull, then it is important to ensure that skiving of the drill bit does not occur. In rare cases, if the laser needs to be placed through a burr hole instead of a twist-drill hole, we still recommend drilling the burr hole in the direction of laser placement; otherwise, significant difficulty can occur with having to remove extra bone around the edges of the burr hole. Once the dura is opened, it has been our practice at this time to obtain tissue biopsy, both to confirm the diagnosis and the tumor grade, as well as to obtain tissue in some cases to determine subsequent clinical trial eligibility. Following biopsy, an MR-compatible anchor bolt used for laser probe insertion is placed. The laser is then inserted to a depth determined using the preoperative MRI planning (Fig. 7.6).

At this time, a T1-weighted MPRAGE sequence is obtained with full-dose gadolinium, and in our system, drawing of the target is then performed and the location of the laser within the target is confirmed (Fig. 7.3). Laser heating is then initiated and stopped when adequate heat has been delivered to the margins of the target (Fig. 7.4). Additional ablation can be achieved by retraction, advancement, or rotation of the laser fiber. Once it is felt that lesion ablation is sufficient, T1-weighted MPRAGE images with gadolinium are obtained again to assess thermal injury margin (Fig. 7.4). If thermal injury margin is satisfactory, then the bolt is removed, and the surgical site is closed. All our patients have been admitted to the ICU for overnight observation. In addition to continuing steroids and antibiotics, patients with lesion diameters greater than 4 cm are sometimes administered mannitol overnight. Most patients can be discharged home the following day with a dexamethasone taper over the subsequent 2–3 weeks. Post-ablation MRI imaging is then obtained at 2 weeks postoperatively to help guide postoperative dexamethasone taper and then repeated at 1.5, 3, 6, and 12 months post-LITT (Fig. 7.7).

LITT Systems

Two FDA-approved LITT systems are commercially available today in the USA. These are as follows:

(1) NeuroBlate—Monteris Medical, Inc; Minnesota.
(2) Visualase—Medtronic, Inc; Minnesota.

The NeuroBlate system uses a 1064 nm neodymium:yttrium aluminum garnet (Nd:YAG) laser that is cooled using CO2 [53]. The system offers two probe types: a diffuse firing tip and a directional firing tip, both of which create a disk-shaped lesion circular around the probe but flat proximally and distally. The directional tip can potentially provide a larger radius of treatment with better conformity to the actual tumor shape but requires a larger cooling catheter. Directional firing seems to be more successful at lower power settings which therefore will make treatment time longer. The laser power settings range between 12 and 16 Watts, and the rapidity of lesional heating is controlled by the ratio of pulsed “time on”: “time off”; less “time off” results in faster heating. Maximum temperatures reached during LITT range from 45 to 70°. It has also been suggested that use of less power may be beneficial for lesions located in the eloquent brain and for post-LITT edema reduction [54, 55]. In addition to options for laser firing direction and power settings, the NeuroBlate system also offers flexibility in laser mounting to the skull. In addition to the anchor bolt, the laser can be held in place using a tripod in the case of salvage surgical situations, where bone may not be present at the site where the laser needs to be introduced.

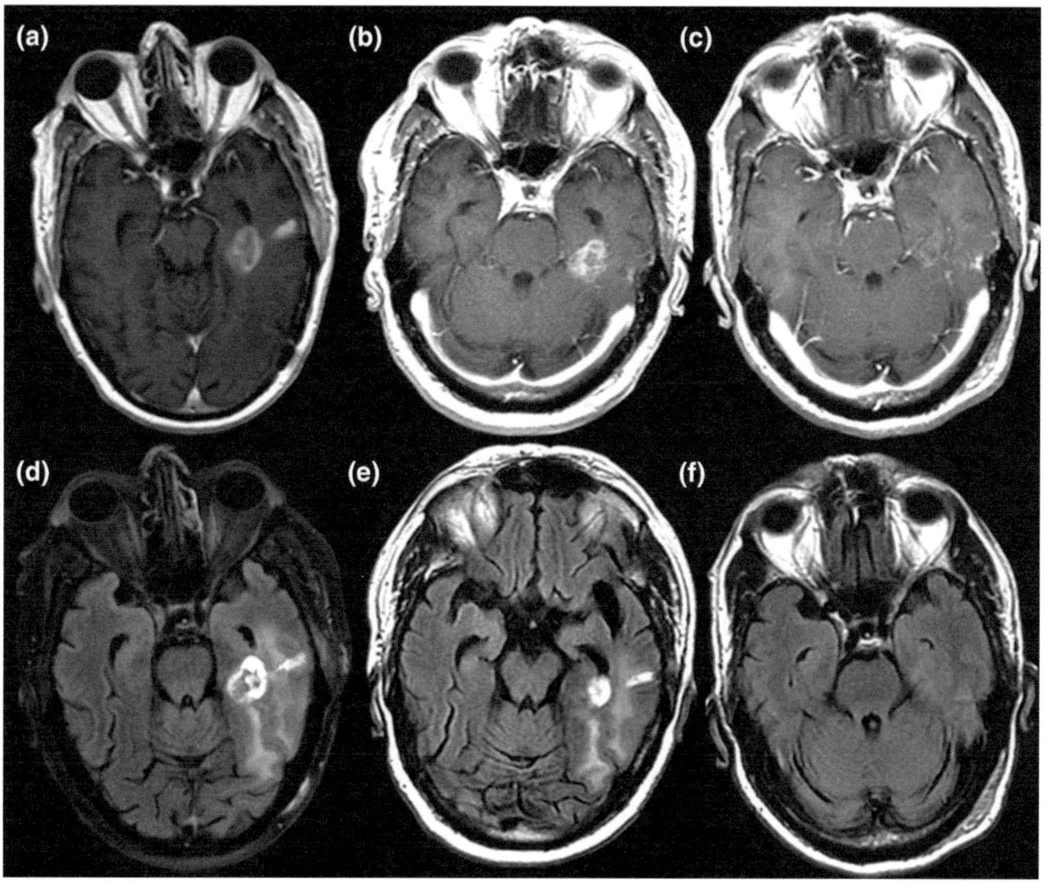

Fig. 7.7 Postoperative imaging of LITT-treated lesion at 2, 6 weeks and 3 months after laser thermal coagulation. T1-weighted gadolinium sequences (**a**, **c**, **e**) show stable or marginally increased in size lesion over the first 6 weeks after treatment, followed by a decrease in size by 3 months after treatment. FLAIR abnormalities (**b**, **d**, **f**) resolve earlier if the lesion is controlled by the LITT treatment and disappear by 3 months post-LITT (**e** and **f**)

The Visualase system uses a 15 W 980-nm diode laser and a diffusion-tip probe with a silicone fiberoptic core surrounded by a cooling sheath, and creates an ellipse-shaped LITT lesion centered at the probe tip (Fig. 7.2). Lesion size is time-sensitive due to its ability for rapid tissue heating [48, 56, 57]. Maximum LITT temperatures reach into the 80–90° range. Only the zone of irreversible damage as calculated by the Arrhenius equation is used with this system [39, 58]. Given the hotter temperatures, the laser "on time" tends to be shorter with this system. In our experience, while this system lacks directional control, the heat does tend to conform to the shape of the lesion well in most cases due to the difference in composition of tumor versus surrounding edematous brain.

The innovation that is unique to the NeuroBlate system, however, is an MR-compatible robotic driver that is attached to the laser and allows control of depth and rotational movement of the laser from the control room, thus minimizing the need for the surgeon to manually manipulate the laser fiber and to be able to accurately move the laser to the needed depth and direction without the surgeon having to put their head into the magnet bore and move the fiber an estimated amount, or withdraw the magnet each time a change in laser position is needed.

With the laser turned on, both systems designated planes of imaging. For NeuroBlate, monitoring is performed in 3 parallel planes whereas with the Visualase system, monitoring is performed in 2 orthogonal planes. Both then use the Arrhenius equation [39, 58] to calculate the effect of the heat on the cells surrounding the laser over time. The Visualase system only calculates a single cell kill line compared with the NeuroBlate system that allows calculation of zones of potentially reversible (protein denaturation) versus irreversible (cell kill) injury. In our experience, while the initial heating pattern of both the diffuse tip and the directional firing tip can start off equivalent, we have clearly seen an advantage in using the directional tip in pushing heat out beyond a 15 mm radius in a single direction. Given that many high-grade gliomas lesions are not round but rather quite irregular, this system's versatility seems advantageous in treating these lesions. What is much needed is a planning prediction model that helps the surgeon decide where best to place the laser fiber based on predicted heat diffusion patterns. With the current imaging versatility and robotic driving system within the magnet bore, development of this technology should hopefully ultimately allow for automation of LITT treatment delivery in the future.

Reported Results of LITT Use for HGG

A comprehensive review of the literature describing the results of LITT use for HGGs can be found in the article by Hawasli et al. [59]. The number of studies that describe the risks and benefits of potential LITT use in treatment of patients with HGGs published since the 1990s is less than 20 (Table 7.1 [60–73]). Most of these

Table 7.1 Articles of LITT use in newly diagnosed and recurrent HGG

Citation	Type	#Patients	WHO III	WHO IV	New	Recurrent	Location	Size
Mohammadi et al. [42]	CS	34	10	24	16	19	15f, 5p, 5t, 2i, 1cc, 7thal	V: 0.7–49.9
Sloan et al. [60]	CS	10	0	10	0	10	3f, 3p, 2t, 1to, 1tp	V: 2.6–19
Hawasli et al. [41]	CS	17	1	10	7	4	3f, 2p, 1cc, 4thal, 1bg	V: 14.1 SD:10.7
Carpentier et al. [61]	CS	4	0	4	0	4	1f, 2t, 1f/cc	V: 3.8–8.9
Jethwa et al. [55]	CS	20	1	6	3	4	5f, 1t, 1mb	V: 0.4–68.9
Schwarzmaier et al. [62]	CS	16	0	16	0	16	4f, 2p, 1o, 2t, 3po, 2tp, 1cc, 1ft	V: 21.6 SD: 18.6
Schwarzmaier et al. [63]	CS	2	0	2	0	2	1t, 1po	V: 20
Schulze et al. [64]	CS	8	3	5	?	?	?	?
Leonardi and Lumenta [65]	CS	24	11	6		~17	?	D: 2.1–2.6
Lumenta et al. [66]	CS	24	11	7	13	5	?	D: 2.8
Leonardi et al. [38]	CS	24	12	9	0	21	?	D: 2.2
Reimer et al. [67]	CS	4	3	1	0	4	3f, 1t	D: 1–3.5
Schwabe et al. [68]	CS	18	1	3	?	?	2f, 1tp, 1fp	D: 2–3.5
Kahn et al. [69]	CS	8	2	1	?	?	1p, 1tp, 1cc	D: 1.8–2.7
Bettag et al. [70]	CS	5	?	?	?	?	?	D: 2–3.5
Sakai et al. [71]	CS	5	0	2	1	1	2p	?
Bettag et al. [72]	CS	5	?	?	?	?	2f, 2t, 1thal	?
Sugiyama et al. [73]	CS	3	?	?	?	?	?	D: 1.2–3

studies are case series, and there are no large randomized controlled trials available to date.

In summary, a total of 230 patients with 161 high-grade LITT-treated lesions have been described; 55 (34.2%) of these lesions were diagnosed as grade III gliomas and 106 (65.8%) as GBMs, with 40 (24.8%) being newly diagnosed and 107 (66.5%) being recurrent lesions. A wide variation of tumor sizes treated is reported, with diameters of up to 5.5 cm in a few studies, but mostly ranging from 0.4 to 68.9 cm^3 [41, 42, 60–73]. Only 21 (13%) of these lesions were in locations where LITT would be considered a first-line approach for treatment, including the insula, corpus callosum, basal ganglia, or the thalamus. What makes it difficult to interpret outcome following LITT is a similarly large range of percentages of lesion heat coverage by LITT. Cell kill coverage with LITT can range from 100% of lesions usually in those less than 3.5 cm in diameter, to frequently quoted ranges of 78–98% (but as low as 28%) in studies that include larger and more complex lesions using a variety (high versus low) of LITT energies [38, 41, 42, 55, 60–69]. This analysis is further complicated by the use of multiple trajectories for lesioning, which in some studies amounted to nearly half of all treated patients [42]. Reported procedural length times can therefore also range significantly from 2 to 16 h.

In studies comparing LITT-treated grade III tumors with LITT-treated GBMs, progression-free survival (PFS) in patients with LITT-treated GBMs was reported as 3–4 months, while PFS in patients with LITT-treated grade III tumors was 10–17 months, with corresponding OS of 7–9 months in patients with LITT-treated GBMs and 30 months in patients with LITT-treated grade III tumors [38, 65, 66] (Table 7.2). Review of other studies that predominantly included patients with GBMs similarly showed average PFS of 4 months and OS of 8.7 months after LITT treatment [41, 60–63]. When looking specifically at LITT use in newly diagnosed HGGs, results are limited with regard to number of patients included across these studies (24.8%, or 40/161), lack of subgroup analysis, inconsistent use of surgical interventions in addition to LITT, and relatively short follow-up times [41, 42, 66]. Studies that predominantly included patients with LITT-treated recurrent GBMs contain significantly larger numbers of patients and reported OS of 6.9–15 months post-LITT [60, 62].

In a recent multicentered study by Mohammadi et al. [42], 19 new and 16 salvage HGG patients were treated with LITT. Median PFS was again 5.1 months, and 71% of cases progressed during follow-up. Multivariate analysis of factors that may affect outcome showed that patient gender, age, tumor recurrence, use of prior chemotherapy or radiation therapy, or tumor grade were not factors that determined the OS. PFS, however, was doubled (from 4.6 to >9.7 months) if only <0.05 cm^3 of tumor volume was missed by the protein denaturation line and <1.5 cm^3 of tumor volume was uncovered by the cell kill line. In addition, the only significant prognostic factor in the study was preoperative KPS which has also been demonstrated in the previous studies [41, 42, 66].

Complications associated with LITT are described in Table 7.3 and are associated with roughly a third of LITT procedures (53 of 161 LITT treatments). Of these, 15.5% (25/161) represented neuro-deficits including aphasia or paresis, around half of which were transient; 4% (7/161) involved an infection; 2.5% (4/161) involved transient cerebral edema; 1.9% (3/161) were associated with seizures or an intracerebral hemorrhage post-LITT. KPSs for LITT-treated patients ranged from 70–100 pre-LITT and 40–90 post-LITT, with most studies reporting same or worse average KPS in treated patients as compared to pre-LITT, and only a single study quoting an improved KPS post-LITT [60].

Imaging Changes Following LITT

At our institution, a postoperative CT scan is often obtained within 24 h of LITT completion. This scan frequently shows centrally located hyperdense blood breakdown products correlating with ground glass appearing T1 hyperintensities seen on MRI consistent with coagulation necrosis in the center of targeted lesions

Table 7.2 Outcomes of LITT in new and recurrent HGG

Citation	#HGG	KPS pre	KPS post	Follow-up time	Radiologic response	Clinical response
Mohammadi et al. [42]	34	50–90 (80)	–	7.2 mth	5 w/central, 12 w/peripheral, 6 distant progression	PFS ave 5.1 mth (4.6–>9.7 mth); 1 year survival 68 ± 9%
Sloan et al. [60]	10	70–90 (80)	10–20 better	3.6–39 mth (15)	57–90% (78% ave) targeted	OS 10.4 (7.4, 6.5, 14.3 mth vs. dosing)
Hawasli et al. [41]	11	74.1	40–90	0.1–11.2 mth (5.8)	Decrease to 91.4 ± 17.1% at 5 mth, 67.4 ± 8.4% at 10 mth	PFS: 2.6, 3.2, 7.6, 8.4, 9.2 mths OS: 0.1, 1.7, 4.1 mh
Carpentier et al. [61]	4	50, 70, 90, 90	–	Till expired	Peripheral enhancement, partial; decrease at 0.5, 1, 1.5, and 2 mth	PFS: 1 mth OS: 10 mth
Jethwa et al. [55]	7	–	–	–	–	–
Schwarzmaier et al. [62]	16	70	–	9.1 ± 6.3 mth	Decreased	OS: 6.9 mth (5.2–11.2)
Schwarzmaier et al. [63]	2	60, 70	50, 70	15, 30 mth	Decrease at 12 mth	PFS: 5 mth OS: 13, 15 mth
Schulze et al. [64]	8	–	–	–	Decrease at 2 mth	PFS 2 mth in 1/8
Leonardi and Lumenta [65]	17	78 (III) 69 (IV)	Same to worse	–	–	PFS: 10 (III), 4 (IV) mth OS: 30 (III), 9 (IV) mth
Lumenta et al. [66]	18	–	–	3.5–4.2 mth	Necrosis, peripheral enhancement; partial	PFS: 17 (III), 3 mth; OS: 7 (IV) mth
Leonardi et al. [38]	21	–	–	–	Necrosis, peripheral enhancement	–
Reimer et al. [67]	4	–	–	–	Decreased at 6 mth	PFS: 6, 6, 8, 12 mth
Schwabe et al. [68]	4	–	–	–	Immediate necrosis and edema, all decreased	–
Kahn et al. [69]	3	–	–	6, 9, 13 mth	15–87% decrease at 1 mth	–
Bettag et al. [70]	?5	–	–	–	Necrosis, decrease in size at 1 mth	–
Sakai et al. [71]	2	0, 90	–	12, 23 mth	Response at 15 mth, 12 mth	PFS: 12, 15 mth; OS: 23 mth
Bettag et al. [72]	?5	–	–	–	Necrosis, edema in all	–
Sugiyama et al. [73]	?3	0, 80, 100	–	9, 23, 31 mth	All resolved	OS: 12, 23a, 31a mth

(Fig. 7.4a). Uniformity in timing of post-LITT MR imaging is also lacking. Most studies quote radiographic response based on T1-weighted or T2-weighted MRI sequences ranging from 7 days to 3 months after surgery [41, 60, 61, 64, 66, 67, 69]. The most commonly reported radiographic response following LITT has been a transient increase in the size of the rim-enhancing lesion with central necrosis seen on T1-weighted imaging representing the ablation lesion—which

Table 7.3 Complications and adjuvants, LITT-treated patients with new and recurrent HGGs

Citation	#HGG	Complications	Adjuvants
Mohammadi et al. [42]	34	5 transient 2 permanent deficits; 1 seizure, 1 hypoNa, 1 DVT, 2 infection, 3 ICH	New: temozolamide + XRT; recurrent: temozolomide, bevacizumab, procarbazine, lomustine, cytoxan
Sloan et al. [60]	10	1 pseudoaneurysm, 1 paresis, 1 transient hemianopia, 1 transient dysphasia	–
Hawasli et al. [41]	11	3 transient aphasia, 2 transient paresis, 2 hypoNa, 1 DVT, 1 infection	New: temozolamide + XRT; recurrent: bevacizumab
Carpentier et al. [61]	4	1 aphasia, 1 seizure, 1 CSF leak	Irinotecan, bevacizumab, BCNU, temozolomide
Jethwa et al. [55]	7	1 cerebral edema	–
Schwarzmaier et al. [62]	16	1 paresis, 3 neutropenia, 1 thrombocytopenia, 1 transaminitis	Temozolomide, doxorubicin, nimustine, teniposide, thalidomide
Schwarzmaier et al. [63]	2	–	Temozolomide
Schulze et al. [64]	8	–	–
Leonardi and Lumenta [65]	17	2 neuro-deficit, 1 infection	–
Lumenta et al. [66]	18	1 neuro-deficit, 1 seizure, 1 apraxia, 3 infection/abscess	–
Leonardi et al. [38]	21	2 neuro-deficits	–
Reimer et al. [67]	4	1 transient aphasia	–
Schwabe et al. [68]	4	3 transient edema	–
Kahn et al. [69]	3	–	XRT
Bettag et al. [70]	?5	–	–
Sakai et al. [71]	2	–	Nimustine
Bettag et al. [72]	?5	–	–
Sugiyama et al. [73]	?3	–	–

should be larger than the original tumor (Fig. 7.7a, b, d, and e). LITT-treated lesions can additionally develop a rim of restricted diffusion in the area of pretreatment enhancement, with concomitant development of peripheral enhancement at the margin of the heat ablation consistent with breakdown of blood-brain barrier [47, 64, 68, 71, 74, 75] (Fig. 7.4b). Central necrosis without peripheral enhancement, however, was noted in at least 57 (35.4%) patients. 38.5% of patients then showed a decrease in radiographic size of enhancement at various time-points ranging from 0.5–10 months. This can be associated with a variable decrease in amount of associated T2-weighted signal although the timing of this is also not well documented. In our experience, best imaging results are seen around 3 months post-LITT although lesions can take up to 6 months to regress fully to their new baseline (Figs. 7.5 and 7.7).

Radiographic recurrence has also not been carefully addressed in most of these studies; however, several studies report radiographic recurrence in as many as 67% of patients, with most recurrences observed at the periphery of the treated lesion as would be expected based on laser physics [41, 42, 67, 71]. There is a lack of literature discussing which MR series would be best for detecting recurrence although Tiwari et al. [47] suggested that the standard T1-weighted MRI in conjunction with a T2 GRE sequences may be useful in detecting recurrence. In our experience, it is possible to see areas of nodularity develop and then regress making evidence of progression on T1-weighted MRI difficult to interpret. Clinical tumor progression has been reported at any time between 1 and 17 months. Given that sometimes it is unclear whether or not there is evidence of tumor recurrence after LITT, the optimal time-points to restart bevacizumab or other chemotherapy agents for patients that underwent LITT are also unknown. Anecdotally, most patients were restarted on systemic agents when cleared postoperatively as would be used after standard surgical resection.

Conclusions

MR-guided LITT is a rapidly developing, minimally invasive, and promising surgical technique. In theory, the ability to induce rapid cytoreduction in tumors that are otherwise not surgically accessible without significant morbidity remains attractive. While in some patients LITT can result in meaningful PFS and OS, a neurological deterioration rate that can be as high as one in every three patients makes the role of its use in HGGs unclear. Which patients would benefit most from the use of LITT, whether LITT in fact improves outcomes, at what time point LITT fits into the overall treatment algorithm and how LITT treatment should be delivered to achieve best outcomes also remain unclear. Ideally multicentered studies comparing LITT to best alternative management should be performed to determine its true efficacy.

Currently, LITT is only being used for its cytoreductive capacity. However, there are animal studies that suggest LITT causes blood-brain barrier disruption and the induction of neovascularization [75]. In addition, coagulated tumor tissue would likely generate a robust immune response lasting days to weeks. Both of these properties raise the possibility for its role in enhancing the efficacy of immunotherapy or the local delivery of chemotherapies or adjuvant radiation.

Lastly, the development of LITT technology is intimately intertwined with the understanding of both laser science and application of MRI. Currently, the ability to ablate the entire lesion is not guaranteed and often cannot be predicted preoperatively. Several research groups have focused on development of processing algorithms for desired lesioning, including deformable registration scheme Thirion's Demons algorithm corrected by Gaussian smoothing (GaSR) of the deformation field, or the Anisotropic smoothing regularizer [76]. Improvement of LITT therefore requires ongoing cooperative developments in the area of preoperative planning based on an analysis of prior treatments to determine heat diffusion prediction algorithms, as well as better imaging techniques to assist with intra- and postoperative understanding of the effect of LITT on the tumor tissue and the surrounding brain parenchyma.

References

1. CBTRUS. Ostrom QT, Gittleman H, et al. CBTRUS statistical report: primary brain and central nervous system tumor diagnosed in the united states in 2007–2011. Neuro-Oncology. 2014;16:iv1–63.
2. Stupp R, Dietrich PY, Ostermann Kraljevic S, Pica A, Maillard I, Maeder P, Meuli R, Janzer R, Pizzolato G, Miralbell R, Porchet F, Regli L, de Tribolet N, Mirimanoff RO, Leyvraz S. Promising survival for patients with newly diagnosed glioblastoma multiforme treated with concomitant radiation plus temozolomide followed by adjuvant temozolomide. J Clin Oncol. 2002;20(5):1375–82.
3. Stupp R, Mason WP, van den Bent MJ, Weller M, Fisher B, Taphoorn MJ, Belanger K, Brandes AA, Marosi C, Bogdahn U, Curschmann J, Janzer RC, Ludwin SK, Gorlia T, Allgeier A, Lacombe D, Cairncross JG, Eisenhauer E, Mirimanoff RO; European Organisation for Research and Treatment of Cancer Brain Tumor and Radiotherapy GROUPS; National Cancer Institute of Canada Clinical Trials Group. Radiotherapy plus concomitant and adjuvant temozolomide for glioblastoma. N Engl J Med. 2005;352(10):987–96.
4. Stupp R, Hegi ME, Mason WP, van den Bent MJ, Taphoorn MJ, Janzer RC, Ludwin SK, Allgeier A, Fisher B, Belanger K, Hau

P, Brandes AA, Gijtenbeek J,Marosi C, Vecht CJ, Mokhtari K, Wesseling P, Villa S, Eisenhauer E, Gorlia T, Weller M, Lacombe D, Cairncross JG, Mirimanoff RO; European Organisation for Research and Treatment of Cancer Brain Tumour and Radiation Oncology Groups; National Cancer Institute of Canada Clinical Trials Group. Effects of radiotherapy with concomitant and adjuvant temozolomide versus radiotherapy alone on survival inglioblastoma in a randomised phase III study: 5-year analysis of the EORTC-NCIC trial. Lancet Oncol. 2009;10(5):459–66. Doi:10.1016/S1470-2045(09)70025-7. Epub 2009 Mar 9.

5. Hegi ME, Diserens AC, Godard S, Dietrich PY, Regli L, Ostermann S, Otten P, Van Melle G, de Tribolet N, Stupp R. Clinical trial substantiates the predictive value of O-6-methylguanine-DNA methyltransferase promoter methylation in glioblastoma patients treated with temozolomide. Clin Cancer Res. 2004;10(6):1871–4.
6. Oszvald A, Güresir E, Setzer M, Vatter H, Senft C, Seifert V, Franz K. Glioblastoma therapy in the elderly and the importance of the extent of resection regardless of age. J Neurosurg. 2012;116(2):357–64. Doi:10.3171/2011.8.JNS102114. Epub 2011 Sep 23.
7. McGirt MJ, Mukherjee D, Chaichana KL, Than KD, Weingart JD, Quinones-Hinojosa A. Association of surgically acquired motor and language deficits on overall survival after resection of glioblastoma multiforme. Neurosurgery. 2009;65 (463–470):44.
8. Stummer W, Reulen HJ, Meinel T, Pichlmeier U, Schumacher W, Tonn JC, Rohde V, Oppel F, Turowski B, Woiciechowsky C, Franz K, Pietsch T; ALA-Glioma Study Group. Extent of resection and survival in glioblastoma multiforme: identification of and adjustment for bias. Neurosurgery. 2008;62(3):564–76; discussion 564–76. Doi:10.1227/01.neu.0000317304.31579.17.
9. Nomiya T, Nemoto K, Kumabe T, Takai Y, Yamada S. Prognostic significance of surgery and radiation therapy in cases of anaplastic astrocytoma: retrospective analysis of 170 cases. J Neurosurg. 2007;106(4):575–81.
10. Stark AM, Nabavi A, Mehdorn HM, Blömer U. Glioblastoma multiforme-report of 267 cases treated at a single institution. Surg Neurol. 2005;63(2):162–9; discussion 169.
11. Ushio Y, Kochi M, Hamada J, Kai Y, Nakamura H. Effect of surgical removal on survival and quality of life in patients with supratentorial glioblastoma. Neurol Med Chir (Tokyo). 2005;45(9):454–60; discussion 460–1.
12. Brown PD, Maurer MJ, Rummans TA, Pollock BE, Ballman KV, Sloan JA, Boeve BF, Arusell RM, Clark MM, Buckner JC. A prospective study of quality of life in adults with newly diagnosed high-grade gliomas: the impact of the extent of resection on quality of life and survival. Neurosurgery. 2005;57(3):495–504; discussion 495–504.
13. Lamborn KR, Chang SM, Prados MD. Prognostic factors for survival of patients with glioblastoma: recursive partitioning analysis. Neuro Oncol. 2004;6 (3):227–35.
14. Tortosa A, Viñolas N, Villà S, Verger E, Gil JM, Brell M, Caral L, Pujol T, Acebes JJ, Ribalta T, Ferrer I, Graus F. Prognostic implication of clinical, radiologic, and pathologic features in patients with anaplastic gliomas. Cancer. 2003;97(4):1063–71.
15. Puduvalli VK, Hashmi M, McAllister LD, Levin VA, Hess KR, Prados M, Jaeckle KA, Yung WK, Buys SS, Bruner JM, Townsend JJ, Davis R, Sawaya R, Kyritsis AP. Anaplastic oligodendrogliomas: prognostic factors for tumor recurrence and survival. Oncology. 2003;65(3):259–66.
16. Levin VA, Yung WK, Bruner J, Kyritsis A, Leeds N, Gleason MJ, Hess KR, Meyers CA, Ictech SA, Chang E, Maor MH. Phase II study of accelerated fractionation radiation therapy with carboplatin followed by PCV chemotherapy for the treatment of anaplastic gliomas. Int J Radiat Oncol Biol Phys. 2002;53(1):58–66.
17. Buckner JC, Schomberg PJ, McGinnis WL, Cascino TL, Scheithauer BW, O'Fallon JR, Morton RF, Kuross SA, Mailliard JA, Hatfield AK, Cole JT, Steen PD, Bernath AM. A phase III study of radiation therapy plus carmustine with or without recombinant interferon-alpha in the treatment of patients with newly diagnosed high-grade glioma. Cancer. 2001;92(2):420–33.
18. Sanai N, Polley MY, McDermott MW, Parsa AT, Berger MS. An extent of resection threshold for newly diagnosed glioblastomas. J Neurosurg. 2011;115(1):3–8. Doi:10.3171/2011.2.JNS10998. Epub 2011 Mar 18.
19. Keles GE, Chang EF, Lamborn KR, Tihan T, Chang CJ, Chang SM, et al. Volumetric extent of resection and residual contrast enhancement on initial surgery as predictors of outcome in adult patients with hemispheric anaplastic astrocytoma. J Neurosurg. 2006;105:34–40. Doi:10.3171/jns.2006.105.1.34.
20. Lacroix M, Abi-Said D, Fourney DR, Gokaslan ZL, Shi W, DeMonte F, Lang FF, McCutcheon IE, Hassenbusch SJ, Holland E, Hess K, Michael C, Miller D, Sawaya R. A multivariate analysis of 416 patients with glioblastoma multiforme: prognosis, extent of resection, and survival. J Neurosurg. 2001;95(2):190–8.
21. Pope WB, Sayre J, Perlina A, Villablanca JP, Mischel PS, Cloughesy TF. MR imaging correlates of survival in patients with high-grade gliomas. AJNR Am J Neuroradiol. 2005;26(10):2466–74.
22. Keles GE, Anderson B, Berger MS. The effect of extent of resection on time to tumor progression and survival in patients with glioblastoma multiforme of the cerebral hemisphere. Surg Neurol. 1999;52 (4):371–9.
23. Fazeny-Dörner B, Wenzel C, Veitl M, Piribauer M, Rössler K, Dieckmann K, et al. Survival and

prognostic factors of patients with unresectable glioblastoma multiforme. Anticancer Drugs. 2003;14:305–12.
24. Keles GE, Lamborn KR, Chang SM, Prados MD, Berger MS. Volume of residual disease as a predictor of outcome in adult patients with recurrent supratentorial glioblastomas multiforme who are undergoing chemotherapy. J Neurosurg. 2004;100(1):41–6.
25. Gulati S, Jakola AS, Nerland US, Weber C, Solheim O. The risk of getting worse: surgically acquired deficits, perioperative complications, and functional outcomes after primary resection of glioblastoma. World Neurosurg. 2011;76:572–9.
26. Skinner MG, Iizuka MN, Kolios MC, Sherar MD. A theoretical comparison of energy sources–microwave, ultrasound and laser–for interstitial thermal therapy. Phys Med Biol. 1998;43(12):3535–47.
27. Seegenschmiedt MH, Sauer R. The current role of interstitial thermo-radiotherapy. Strahlenther Onkol. 1992;168(3):119–40.
28. Powers SK, Beckman WC Jr, Brown JT, Kolpack LC. Interstitial laser photochemotherapy of rhodamine-123-sensitized rat glioma. J Neurosurg. 1987;67(6):889–94.
29. Elias Z, Powers SK, Atstupenas E, Brown JT. Hyperthermia from interstitial laser irradiation in normal rat brain. Lasers Surg Med. 1987;7(4):370–5.
30. Devaux BC, Roux FX. Experimental and clinical standards, and evolution of lasers in neurosurgery. Acta Neurochir (Wien). 1996;138(10):1135–47.
31. Jolesz FA. Functional imaging of the brain. 1983;17(1):59–62.
32. Sapareto SA, Dewey WC. Thermal dose determination in cancer therapy. Int J Radiat Oncol Biol Phys. 1984;10:787–800.
33. Sapareto SA. Thermal isoeffect dose: addressing the problem of thermotolerance. Int J Hyperthermia. 1987;3:297–305.
34. Cline HE, Schenck JF, Hynynen K, Watkins RD, Souza SP, Jolesz FA. MR-guided focused ultrasound surgery. J Comput Assist Tomogr. 1992;16:956–65.
35. Tracz RA, Wyman DR, Little PB, Towner RA, Stewart WA, Schatz SW, Pennock PW, Wilson BC. Magnetic resonance imaging of interstitial laser photocoagulation in brain. Lasers Surg Med. 1992;12(2):165–73.
36. Tracz RA, Wyman DR, Little PB, Towner RA, Stewart WA, Schatz SW, Wilson BC, Pennock PW, Janzen EG. Comparison of magnetic resonance images and the histopathological findings of lesions induced by interstitial laser photocoagulation in the brain. Lasers Surg Med. 1993;13(1):45–54.
37. Menovsky T, Beek JF, Phoa SS, Brouwer PA, Klein MG, Verlaan CW, van Acker RE, van Gemert MJ. Ultrasonography in acute interstitial laser irradiation of the pig brain: preliminary results. J Image Guid Surg. 1995;1(4):237–41.
38. Leonardi MA, Lumenta CB, Gumprecht HK, von Einsiedel GH, Wilhelm T. Stereotactic guided laser-induced interstitial thermotherapy (SLITT) in gliomas with intraoperative morphologic monitoring in an open MR-unit. Minim Invasive Neurosurg. 2001;44(1):37–42.
39. McNichols RJ, Gowda A, Kangasniemi M, Bankson JA, Price RE, Hazle JD. MR thermometry-based feedback control of laser interstitial thermal therapy at 980 nm. Lasers Surg Med. 2004;34(1):48–55.
40. Hawasli AH, Ray WZ, Murphy RK, Dacey RG Jr, Leuthardt EC. Magnetic resonance imaging-guided focused laser interstitial thermal therapy for subinsular metastatic adenocarcinoma: technical case report. Neurosurgery. 2012;70(2 Suppl. Operative):332–7; discussion 338. Doi:10.1227/NEU.0b013e318232fc90.
41. Hawasli AH, Bagade S, Shimony JS, Miller-Thomas M, Leuthardt EC. Magnetic resonance imaging-guided focused laser interstitial thermal therapy for intracranial lesions: single-institution series. Neurosurgery. 2013;73(6):1007–17. Doi:10.1227/NEU.0000000000000144.
42. Mohammadi AM, Hawasli AH, Rodriguez A, Schroeder JL, Laxton AW, Elson P, Tatter SB, Barnett GH, Leuthardt EC. The role of laser interstitial thermal therapy in enhancing progression-free survival of difficult-to-access high-grade gliomas: a multicenter study. Cancer Med. 2014;3(4):971–9. Doi:10.1002/cam4.266. Epub 2014 May 9.
43. Torres-Reveron J, Tomasiewicz HC, Shetty A, Amankulor NM, Chiang VL. Stereotactic laser induced thermotherapy (LITT): a novel treatment for brain lesions regrowing after radiosurgery. J Neurooncol. 2013;113(3):495–503. Doi:10.1007/s11060-013-1142-2. Epub 2013 May 16.
44. Rahmathulla G, Recinos PF, Valerio JE, Chao S, Barnett GH. Laser interstitial thermal therapy for focal cerebral radiation necrosis: a case report and literature review. Stereotact Funct Neurosurg. 2012;90(3):192–200. Doi:10.1159/000338251. Epub 2012 Jun 5.
45. Chao ST, Ahluwalia MS, Barnett GH, Stevens GH, Murphy ES, Stockham AL, Shiue K, Suh JH. Challenges with the diagnosis and treatment of cerebral radiation necrosis. Int J Radiat Oncol Biol Phys. 2013;87(3):449–57. Doi:10.1016/j.ijrobp.2013.05.015. Epub 2013 Jun 19.
46. Kang JY, Wu C, Tracy J, Lorenzo M, Evans J, Nei M, Skidmore C, Mintzer S, Sharan AD, Sperling MR. Laser interstitial thermal therapy for medically intractable mesial temporal lobe epilepsy. Epilepsia. 2016;57(2):325–34. Doi:10.1111/epi.13284. Epub 2015 Dec 24.
47. Tiwari P, Danish S, Madabhushi A. Identifying MRI markers associated with early response following laser ablation for neurological disorders: preliminary findings. PLoS One. 2014;9(12):e114293. Doi:10.1371/journal.pone.0114293. eCollection 2014.
48. Curry DJ, Gowda A, McNichols RJ, Wilfong AA. MR-guided stereotactic laser ablation of epileptogenic

foci in children. Epilepsy Behav. 2012;24(4):408–14. Doi:10.1016/j.yebeh.2012.04.135. Epub 2012 Jun 9.
49. Consiglieri GD, Killory BD, Germain RS, Spetzler RF. Utility of the CO_2 laser in the microsurgical resection of cavernous malformations. World Neurosurg. 2013;79(5–6):714–8. Doi:10.1016/j.wneu.2011.12.088. Epub 2011 Dec 28.
50. Wang NK, Hung KL, Liao HC, Lin YM. A patient with PHACE syndrome with marked ipsilateral cerebral atrophy. Pediatr Neonatol. 2010;51(2):130–4. Doi:10.1016/S1875-9572(10)60023-X.
51. Passacantilli E, Antonelli M, D'Amico A, Delfinis CP, Anichini G, Lenzi J, Santoro A. Neurosurgical applications of the 2-µm thulium laser: histological evaluation of meningiomas in comparison to bipolar forceps and an ultrasonic aspirator. Photomed Laser Surg. 2012;30(5):286–92. Doi:10.1089/pho.2011.3137. Epub 2012 Mar 9.
52. Passacantilli E, Anichini G, Delfinis CP, Lenzi J, Santoro A. Use of 2-µm continuous-wave thulium laser for surgical removal of a tentorial meningioma: case report. Photomed Laser Surg. 2011;29(6):437–40. Doi:10.1089/pho.2010.2809. Epub 2010 Dec 23.
53. Feyh J, Gutmann R, Leunig A, Jäger L, Reiser M, Saxton RE, Castro DJ, Kastenbauer E. MRI-guided laser interstitial thermal therapy (LITT) of head and neck tumors: progress with a new method. J Clin Laser Med Surg. 1996;14(6):361–6.
54. Riordan M, Tovar-Spinoza Z. Laser induced thermal therapy (LITT) for pediatric brain tumors: case-based review. Trans Pediatr. 2014;3(3):229–35. Doi:10.3978/j.issn.2224-4336.2014.07.07.
55. Jethwa PR, Barrese JC, Gowda A, Shetty A, Danish SF. Magnetic resonance thermometry-guided laser-induced thermal therapy for intracranial neoplasms: initial experience. Neurosurgery. 2012;71(1 Suppl. Operative):133–44; 144–5.
56. Carpentier A, McNichols RJ, Stafford RJ, Itzcovitz J, Guichard JP, Reizine D, Delaloge S, Vicaut E, Payen D, Gowda A, George B. Real-time magnetic resonance-guided laser thermal therapy for focal metastatic brain tumors. Neurosurgery. 2008;63(1 Suppl. 1):ONS21–8; discussion ONS28-9. Doi:10.1227/01.neu.0000335007.07381.df.
57. Tovar-Spinoza Z, Carter D, Ferrone D, et al. The use of MRI-guided laser-induced thermal ablation for epilepsy. Childs Nerv Syst. 2013;29:2089–94.
58. Welch AJ, Cain CP. Combination sensor for measurement of light and temperature. Lasers Surg Med. 1995;16(4):397–400.
59. Hawasli AH, Kim AH, Dunn GP, Tran DD, Leuthardt EC. Stereotactic laser ablation of high-grade gliomas. Neurosurg Focus. 2014;37(6):E1. Doi:10.3171/2014.9.FOCUS14471.
60. Sloan AE, Ahluwalia MS, Valerio-Pascua J, Manjila S, Torchia MG, Jones SE, Sunshine JL, Phillips M, Griswold MA, Clampitt M, Brewer C, Jochum J, McGraw MV, Diorio D, Ditz G, Barnett GH. Results of the NeuroBlate System first-in-humans Phase I clinical trial for recurrent glioblastoma: clinical article. J Neurosurg. 2013;118(6):1202–19. Doi:10.3171/2013.1.JNS1291. Epub 2013 Apr 5.
61. Carpentier A, Chauvet D, Reina V, Beccaria K, Leclerq D, McNichols RJ, Gowda A, Cornu P, Delattre JY. MR-guided laser-induced thermal therapy (LITT) for recurrent glioblastomas. Lasers Surg Med. 2012;44(5):361–8. Doi:10.1002/lsm.22025. Epub 2012 Apr 5.
62. Schwarzmaier HJ, Eickmeyer F, von Tempelhoff W, Fiedler VU, Niehoff H, Ulrich SD, Yang Q, Ulrich F. MR-guided laser-induced interstitial thermotherapy of recurrent glioblastoma multiforme: preliminary results in 16 patients. Eur J Radiol. 2006;59(2):208–15. Epub 2006 Jul 18.
63. Schwarzmaier HJ, Eickmeyer F, von Tempelhoff W, Fiedler VU, Niehoff H, Ulrich SD, Ulrich F. MR-guided laser irradiation of recurrent glioblastomas. J Magn Reson Imaging. 2005;22(6):799–803.
64. Schulze PC, Vitzthum HE, Goldammer A, Schneider JP, Schober R. Laser-induced thermotherapy of neoplastic lesions in the brain—underlying tissue alterations, MRI-monitoring and clinical applicability. Acta Neurochir (Wien). 2004;146:803–12.
65. Leonardi MA, Lumenta CB. Stereotactic guided laser-induced interstitial thermotherapy (SLITT) in gliomas with intraoperative morphologic monitoring in an open MR: clinical expierence. Minim Invasive Neurosurg. 2002;45(4):201–7.
66. Lumenta CB, Leonardi MA, von Einsiedel H. Stereotactic guided laser-induced interstitial thermotherapy (SLITT) in gliomas with intraoperative morphologic monitoring in open MR. 2001. SPIE (Abstract).
67. Reimer P, Bremer C, Horch C, Morgenroth C, Allkemper T, Schuierer G. MR-monitored LITT as a palliative concept in patients with high grade gliomas: preliminary clinical experience. J Magn Reson Imaging. 1998;8(1):240–4.
68. Schwabe B, Kahn T, Harth T, Ulrich F, Schwarzmaier HJ. Laser-induced thermal lesions in the human brain: short- and long-term appearance on MRI. J Comput Assist Tomogr. 1997;21(5):818–25.
69. Kahn D, Follett KA, Bushnell DL, Nathan MA, Piper JG, Madsen M, Kirchner PT. Diagnosis of recurrent brain tumor: value of 201Tl SPECT vs 18F-fluorodeoxyglucose PET. AJR Am J Roentgenol. 1994;163(6):1459–65.
70. Bettag M, Ulrich F, Schober R, Hessel S, Sabel M: Experimental and first clinical results of Nd:YAG laser-induced hyperthermia in brain tumours. In: Waidelich W, Waidelich R, Hofstetter A, editors. Laser in medicine. Berlin: Springer-Verlag; 1992. pp. 210–213.
71. Sakai T, Fujishima I, Sugiyama K, Ryu H, Uemura K. Interstitial laserthermia in neurosurgery. J Clin Laser Med Surg. 1992;10(1):37–40.

72. Bettag M, Ulrich F, Schober R, Fürst G, Langen KJ, Sabel M, Kiwit JC. Stereotactic laser therapy in cerebral gliomas. Acta Neurochir Suppl (Wien). 1991;52:81–3.
73. Sugiyama K, Sakai T, Fujishima I, Ryu H, Uemura K, Yokoyama T. Stereotactic interstitial laser-hyperthermia using Nd-YAG laser. Stereotact Funct Neurosurg. 1990;54–55:501–5.
74. Sabel M, Rommel F, Kondakci M, Gorol M, Willers R, Bilzer T. Locoregional opening of the rodent blood-brain barrier for paclitaxel using Nd:YAG laser-induced thermo therapy: a new concept of adjuvant glioma therapy? Lasers Surg Med. 2003;33:75–80.
75. Nakagawa M, Matsumoto K, Higashi H, Furuta T, Ohmoto T. Acute effects of interstitial hyperthermia on normal monkey brain—magnetic resonance imaging appearance and effects on blood-brain barrier. Neurol Meg Chir (Tokyo). 1994;34:668–75.
76. Hwuang E, Danish S, Rusu M, Sparks R, Toth R, Madabhushi A. Anisotropic smoothing regularization (AnSR) in Thirion's Demons registration evaluates brain MRI tissue changes post-laser ablation. Conf Proc IEEE Eng Med Biol Soc. 2013;2013:4006–9. Doi:10.1109/EMBC.2013.6610423.

Part III

Adjuvant Therapies

Current Standard Treatment Options for Malignant Glioma

8

Kevin P. Becker and Joachim M. Baehring

Introduction

The Central Brain Tumor Registry estimates that there will be more than 24,000 new cases of primary malignant brain and central nervous system (CNS) tumors diagnosed in the United States in the year 2016. Eighty percent or more than 19,000 of these cases will be malignant gliomas consisting of World Health Organization (WHO) grade 3 anaplastic tumors and grade 4 glioblastoma. WHO grade 3 tumors can be further broken down into threes anaplastic subtypes: astrocytoma, oligodendroglioma, and oligoastrocytoma based upon morphologic and molecular features.

Glioblastoma is the most common (46%) and aggressive primary malignant brain tumor (Fig. 8.1a). WHO grade 4 tumors are distinguished from grade 3 tumors by the presence of pseudopalisading necrosis and vascular proliferation which are morphologic hallmarks of their aggressive nature. Except in rare circumstances, glioblastoma is a fatal diagnosis with current median overall survival of 15–23 months and a five-year survival of less than 5% [1].

Anaplastic gliomas (Fig. 8.1b) can be defined based upon morphologic features of increased hypercellularity, nuclear atypia with alteration of the nuclear–cytoplasmic ratio, and increased mitotic activity. Although early studies often did not distinguish among the various subtypes (or even WHO grade 3 from grade 4 tumors), we now know that the oligodendroglioma feature is often associated with 1p/19q co-deletion and a favorable prognosis. The current median life expectancy after diagnosis of a WHO grade 3 tumor is 2–3 years [2] for the general patient population; however, this can be further broken down when taking into account IDH1 mutation status and 1p/19 co-deletion [3].

Chemotherapy

Nitrosoureas

Nitrosoureas such as carmustine (BCNU) and lomustine (CCNU) are highly lipophilic compounds that exhibit excellent blood–brain barrier penetration with lomustine reaching brain concentrations nearly equal to serum levels. Nitrosoureas are spontaneously broken down into two active metabolites; chloroethyldiazohydroxide and an isocyanate group. The chloroethyldiazohydroxide moiety mediates DNA–DNA and DNA–protein cross-linking and the isocyanate group carbamoylates amino acids which leads to disruption of RNA synthesis and DNA repair.

K.P. Becker (✉)
Department of Neurology, Yale School of Medicine, 15 York Street, LCI-9, RM 920, New Haven, CT 06520, USA
e-mail: kevin.becker@yale.edu

J. M. Baehring
Department of Neurology,
Department of Neurosurgery,
Yale School of Medicine, New Haven, USA

J. Moliterno Günel et al. (eds.), *Malignant Brain Tumors*,
DOI 10.1007/978-3-319-49864-5_8

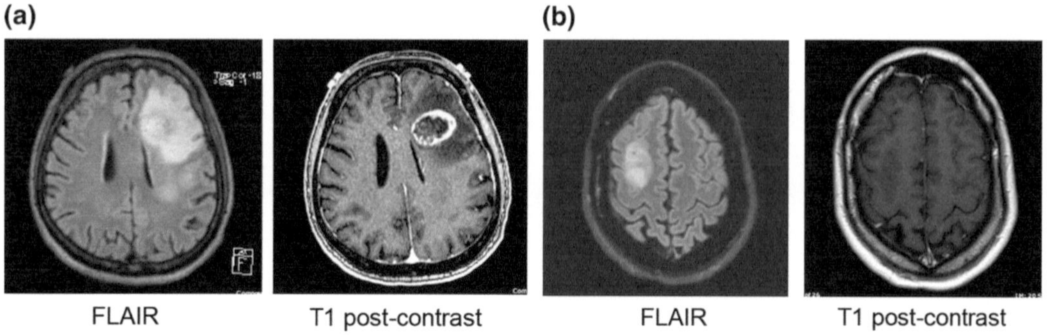

Fig. 8.1 **a** Magnetic resonance imaging of brain—glioblastoma magnetic resonance imaging reveals the aggressive nature of glioblastoma with the typical ring enhancement, central necrosis, and significant mass effect. **b** Magnetic resonance imaging of brain—anaplastic astrocytoma. Magnetic resonance imaging demonstrates the radiographic features of a WHO grade III anaplastic astrocytoma with bulky FLAIR signal suggestive of mass and absence of contrast enhancement

The use of these agents is dose-limited by cumulative myelosuppression and potential pulmonary toxicity.

Nitrosoureas—Newly Diagnosed Anaplastic Gliomas

Historically, nitrosoureas have been the most common chemotherapy class used in the management of malignant gliomas with widespread use since the 1970s. The approval of temozolomide in March 2005, with its improved adverse effect profile and efficacy, largely relegated these agents to the treatment of recurrent disease with several notable exceptions. In the RTOG 9402 clinical trial, lomustine combined with vincristine and procarbazine as part of the "PCV protocol" was evaluated for newly diagnosed malignant gliomas [4]. In this study, 291 patients with either anaplastic oligodendroglioma or anaplastic oligoastrocytoma were randomized to receive radiation therapy alone or up to 4 cycles of PCV chemotherapy followed by radiation therapy. In the end, there was no difference in median survival between the PCV-radiation group versus the radiation therapy-alone group (4.6 vs. 4.7 years; hazard ratio [HR] = 0.79; 95% CI, 0.60–1.04); however, subgroup analysis demonstrated that patients with 1p/19q co-deletions had a significant survival advantage when treated with PCV radiation compared to patients treated with radiation therapy alone (14.7 vs. 7.3 years; HR = 0.59; 95% CI, 0.37–0.95; $p = 0.03$). These findings suggested that 1p/19q co-deletion was predictive for chemotherapy response.

A role for the use of PCV chemotherapy for patients with 1p/19 co-deleted tumors was further defined by the findings of EORTC 26951 clinical trial which randomized 368 patients with anaplastic oligodendroglioma or anaplastic oligoastrocytoma to receive either radiation therapy or radiation followed by up to six cycles of PCV [5]. Unlike the RTOG trial, survival in the radiation group combined with chemotherapy was prolonged versus the radiation therapy-alone group (42.3 vs. 30.6 months, hazard ratio [HR], 0.75; 95% CI, 0.60–0.95); however, in the 80 patients identified with 1p/19q co-deletion survival was further augmented by addition of PCV following radiation (OS not reached in the RT/PCV group versus 112 months; HR, 0.56; 95% CI, 0.31–1.03). These findings support the use of chemotherapy for malignant tumors with 1p/19q co-deletion, i.e., oligodendrogliomas and mixed gliomas.

Several questions arose out of these findings including whether temozolomide could be substituted for the PCV regimen and whether it is important to start with radiation followed by chemotherapy or chemotherapy followed by radiation. An attempt to address both these questions was undertaken with the NOA-04 clinical trial [6]. In this phase III clinical trial, patients with newly diagnosed anaplastic glioma were randomly assigned to receive either 60 Gy fractionated radiation, 4 cycles of PCV, or 8 cycles of temozolomide. At the time of disease progression or with the development of unacceptable toxicity, patients were then allowed to cross-over to receive either radiation (PCV and temozolomide arms) or PCV or temozolomide (radiation arm, randomized 1:1). Initial analysis revealed there were no differences between progression-free survival between the radiation versus chemotherapy group (30.6 months vs. 31.9 months, HR 1.0; $p = 0.87$) or median overall survival (72 months vs. 82 months, HR 1.2). This was further confirmed with long-term analysis after following patients for 11.8 years which showed there were no differences among the treatment groups [7]. Several conclusions arose out of this study. It appeared that PCV and temozolomide had equivalent efficacy at least for all gliomas and that there was no difference in survival whether patients were treated with radiation or chemotherapy upfront or at recurrence; however, the mature data from this trial have yet to be published in a peer-reviewed journal. Molecular analysis also revealed that isocitrate dehydrogenase 1 mutations were stronger positive prognostic factors than either MGMT methylation status or 1p/19 co-deletion.

There are ongoing studies including the Alliance trial—CODEL clinical trial which is currently recruiting patients with 1p/19q co-deleted anaplastic gliomas (astrocytoma, oligoastrocytoma, and oligodendroglioma) and WHO grade II low-grade gliomas. This study is evaluating temozolomide and PCV chemotherapy head to head following fractionated radiation therapy. Another trial, the EORTC 26053/RTOG 0834 CATNON phase III clinical trial is an ongoing study evaluating the timing of temozolomide and whether adding temozolomide to fractionated radiation is beneficial compared to radiation treatment alone for patients with 1p/19q intact anaplastic gliomas. Given the nature of clinical trials and the involvement of both low-grade and anaplastic tumors, it will likely be many years before we have definitive data regarding this important question; however, a general trend at least in the USA is to treat patients with oligodendrogliomas with PCV and other tumors with temozolomide.

Nitrosoureas—Recurrent Glioblastoma

The phase II "BELOB" clinical trial investigated the role of lomustine alone and combined with bevacizumab versus monotherapy bevacizumab for recurrent glioblastoma. This study enrolled 153 patients with recurrent glioblastoma who were randomized to receive either lomustine 110 mg/m^2 every 6 weeks, lomustine at either 90 or 110 mg/m^2 along with bevacizumab 10 mg/kg given every 2 weeks, or bevacizumab alone. The investigators found that the nine-month overall survival was 43% in the lomustine arm, 38% in the bevacizumab arm, and 63% in the bevacizumab and lomustine (combined 90 and 110 mg/m^2) arm and progression-free survival at 6 months was 13% for lomustine, 16% for bevacizumab, and 42% for combined bevacizumab and lomustine. Although these results appear to be an improvement over the results of bevacizumab and irinotecan studied in the BRAIN trial [8], a more definitive answer awaits the conclusions of the EORTC 26101 phase III clinical trial which has recently completed enrollment of patients with progressive glioblastoma to either lomustine 90 mg/m^2 every six weeks along with bevacizumab 10 mg/kg every two weeks versus monotherapy lomustine 110 mg/m^2 every six weeks.

The first clinical trial to prospectively evaluate nitrosoureas and temozolomide head to head for recurrent glioblastoma (and a small subset of anaplastic gliomas—26% of enrollees) was undertaken by Brada et al. [9]. In this study, 447 chemotherapy-naïve patients at first relapse following radiotherapy were randomized to receive either 6 cycles of PCV every six weeks or temozolomide at 150–200 mg/m^2/day on a 5 of 28-day schedule or 100 mg/m^2/day on a 21 of 28-day schedule. After a median follow-up time of 10.4 months for the PCV and 14 months for the temozolomide arm, there was no survival benefit seen when comparing PCV to the combined arms of temozolomide (6.7 months for

PCV and 7.2 months for combined temozolomide, HR 0.91; 95% CI 0.74–1.11, $p = 0.36$); however, the 5 of 28-day schedule of temozolomide did modestly improve survival compared to PCV (5 months for temozolomide and 3.6 months for PCV; HR 0.8; 95% CI, 0.63–1.03, $p = 0.038$). The conclusion of this trial was that PCV and temozolomide on a 5 of 28-day schedule were similar in efficacy but given an observed improvement in quality of life and ease of administration, temozolomide should be favored over PCV.

Temozolomide

Temozolomide is an oral alkylating chemotherapy agent whose drug development arose out of the clinical trial failure of dacarbazine and mitozolomide for patients with melanoma. At physiologic pH, temozolomide undergoes base catalyzation to monomethyl-triazeno-imidazole-carboxamide (MTIC) which spontaneously converts to the bio-reactive methyldiazonium cation. Methyldiazonium goes on to alkylate the N^7 and O^6 positions of guanine and N^3 position of O^6 alkylation of guanine is thought to mediate the predominant anti-tumor effect. Although early studies demonstrated a variety of adverse effects including fatigue, nausea/vomiting, and myelosuppression, these have proven to be relatively mild in clinical practice and predictable compared to previously used cytotoxic agents.

The first clinical trial evaluating temozolomide solely for malignant glioma was conducted by O'Reilly et al. [10] who enrolled 28 patients with 18 of the patients having a high-grade glioma. Of the 10 evaluable patients who received adjuvant temozolomide, 5 patients (4 had WHO grade IV tumors) experienced significant clinical and radiographic improvement. These findings led Roger Stupp and colleagues to design a phase II study and ultimately the seminal EORTC-NCIC phase III study which established temozolomide along with fractionated radiation followed by adjuvant temozolomide administered at 150–200 mg/m^2/day on a 5 of 28-day schedule as the standard of care for patients with newly diagnosed glioblastoma. This combination led to median survival ranges of 15–23 months or a 3- to 11-month median survival improvement beyond surgery followed by radiation therapy alone [11, 12].

An additional important finding that arose from the EORTC-NCIC trial was that patients with methyl-guanine-methyltransferase (MGMT) methylation were more responsive to temozolomide and had prolonged survival compared to patients with hypomethylated MGMT [13]. This led to the hypothesis that temozolomide given over a prolonged period could possibly lead to MGMT depletion and improved chemoresponsiveness. This theory was tested in a randomized phase II study which enrolled 85 patients with newly diagnosed glioblastoma treated with six weeks of concurrent radiation and temozolomide to receive adjuvant treatment with either dose-dense temozolomide (150 mg/m^2/day—7 days on, 7 days off) or metronomic (daily) temozolomide (50 mg/m^2/day) [14]. One-year survival for patients treated with the dose-dense regimen was 80% which was superior to metronomic dosing (69% survival at one year) and also an improvement from the 61% one-year survival observed with the EORTC-NCIC clinical trial [11]. This was further studied in the randomized phase III RTOG 0525 clinical trial which compared adjuvant temozolomide given on a 5 of 28-day schedule at 150–200 mg/m^2/day versus temozolomide at 75 mg/m^2/day on a 21 of 28-day schedule [15]. Both dosing schedules were given up to 12 cycles. No survival benefit was seen for dose-dense temozolomide (median overall survival 14.9 months, 95%, CI 13.7–16.5 months) versus standard dosing (16.6 months, 95% CI, 14.9–31.5 months, HR, 1.03, $p = 0.63$). On the basis of these studies and others [9], there is currently no role for dose-dense temozolomide for newly diagnosed glioblastoma.

Gliadel Wafers

Gliadel wafers are biodegradable wafers consisting of a poly (carboxyphenoxy-propane sebacic acid) matrix embedded with the nitrosourea, carmustine (BCNU). The wafers were developed by Henry Brem and colleagues in an attempt to avoid the hematologic and pulmonary toxicity associated with the systemic administration of BCNU [16].

In 1993, Tamargo et al. were the first to demonstrate that the interstitial release of BCNU through BCNU-embedded polymer wafers was superior to systemic administration in a gliosarcoma animal model [17]. This ultimately led to a series of clinical trials for patients with malignant gliomas. Gliadel was approved by the Federal Drug Administration (FDA) in 1996 for the treatment of recurrent glioma on the basis of the findings of a phase III clinical trial. In this randomized, placebo-controlled trial, 222 patients with recurrent malignant glioma were randomized to receive either surgically implanted wafers embedded with 3.85% BCNU or placebo. The median overall survival for patients on the experimental arm was 31 weeks versus 23 weeks for patients receiving placebo wafers (HR = 0.67, $p = 0.06$). Subanalysis of glioblastoma patients demonstrated a survival advantage of 50 % at six months (44% vs. 64%, $p = 0.02$), and there were no significant adverse events observed [18].

A large, international, randomized phase III clinical trial [19] for patients with newly diagnosed malignant glioma was initiated after the encouraging results of a small randomized, placebo-controlled trial [20]. In this trial, 240 patients with newly diagnosed glioma were randomized to receive either BCNU wafer or placebo at the time of the initial surgical resection followed by fractionated radiation therapy. At the time of early follow-up (12–30 months), a survival benefit was observed for patients treated with BCNU wafers (13.9 vs. 11.6 months, $p = 0.03$). These findings were confirmed in a long-term (59 months) follow-up report [21]. A meta-analysis of these two trials by Meldorf et al. [22] further demonstrated a reduction in the risk of death of 29% with the implantation of BCNU wafers. On the basis of these findings, FDA approved Gliadel for patients with newly diagnosed glioma in 2003.

Although the development of Gliadel represented a significant advance for the treatment of newly diagnosed and recurrent glioma, their widespread use and acceptance has subsequently been limited due to a high rate of postoperative infections, problems with wound healing, chemical meningitis, cerebral edema, obstructive hydrocephalus, cyst formation, and pseudoprogression [23, 24].

Bevacizumab

Almost 50 years ago, Judah Folkman and colleagues hypothesized that targeting the tumor vasculature of solid tumors would represent an effective treatment strategy [25]. Ultimately, it was discovered that the family of soluble ligand vascular endothelial growth factor (VEGF) mediates tumor neovascularization in a wide range of tumors. VEGF was subsequently shown to be an important mediator of angiogenesis in malignant gliomas with 30-fold higher concentrations in glioblastoma when compared to low-grade gliomas [26]. Bevacizumab is a humanized monoclonal antibody that binds vascular endothelial growth factor with high affinity ($K_d \sim 0.5$ nM) and has been approved for a variety of tumors including relapsed glioblastoma [27]. Despite initial concerns about intra-cranial hemorrhage and stroke, bevacizumab has been shown to be well-tolerated agent and exhibits an extended half-life of approximately 21 days.

Bevacizumab—Recurrent Glioblastoma

The first clinical trial evaluating bevacizumab for malignant glioma was undertaken in 2004 with 21 patients (11 glioblastoma and 10 anaplastic astrocytoma) who were treated with bevacizumab 5 mg/kg and irinotecan 125 mg/m^2 every two weeks [28]. This was a seminal study as it demonstrated not only the safety of bevacizumab but also a response rate of 43% which was a significant improvement from historic controls. This led to several pivotal phase II studies in which bevacizumab was used as monotherapy or in combination with irinotecan for patients with recurrent glioblastoma [29–32].

These studies demonstrated dramatically improved imaging response rates of 28–35% with bevacizumab and progression-free survival at 6 months of 29–43%. On the basis of these phase II clinical trials, on May 5, 2009, the FDA approved bevacizumab monotherapy in the United States for recurrent glioblastoma.

Bevacizumab—Newly Diagnosed Glioblastoma

Two phase III clinical trials have been undertaken to address the role of bevacizumab in the upfront setting for newly diagnosed glioblastoma. The "Avaglio" or Avastin in glioblastoma trial was a double-blind, placebo-controlled trial that randomized 921 patients with newly diagnosed glioblastoma to receive the standard of care consisting of fractionated radiation and daily temozolomide at 75 mg/m^2/day followed by six cycles adjuvant temozolomide 150–200 mg/m^2/day on a 5 of 28-day schedule along with either q2weekly bevacizumab 10 mg/kg or placebo [33]. In the end, there was no improvement in overall survival between the groups (median overall survival of 16.8 months for bevacizumab-treated patients and 16.7 months for placebo control); however, there was an improvement in progression-free survival with the addition of bevacizumab (10.6 vs. 6.2 months, HR, 0.64, $p < 0.001$). In the RTOG 0825 clinical trial, Gilbert and colleagues randomized 637 patients with newly diagnosed glioblastoma to receive the standard of care consisting of concurrent fractionated radiation and temozolomide followed by up to 12 cycles of adjuvant temozolomide with either bevacizumab 10 m/kg or placebo administered two weeks [34]. Similar to the Avaglio trial, there was no improvement in the median overall survival with the addition of bevacizumab (15.7 months vs. 16.1 months for placebo arm), but there was a modest increase in progression-free survival (10.7 months vs. 7.3 months for placebo arm). Importantly, it is unknown what effect the high level of cross-over associated with this trial had on survival. As such, at this time there is no role for the regular use of bevacizumab upfront; however, it may be beneficial in defined subgroups (patients with large volume residual disease; molecularly identifiable subgroups).

NovoTTF

In 2004, Kirson and colleagues reported that the application of very low-intensity, intermediate-frequency (100–300 kHz), alternating electrical fields ("tumor treating fields or TTFields") could disrupt the normal formation of the mitotic spindle and cause growth inhibitory effects in both cell culture lines and animal models [35]. They went on to show that this occurred in a non-thermal manner and exposure to the alternating electrical field had no deleterious effect on non-dividing cells. The mechanism of action was thought to be related to the disruption of the normal polymerization–depolymerization process that is required for cell mitosis.

These findings led to the testing of alternating electrical fields in the Fischer rat glioma model where it was observed that increasing the number of TTField directions led to significant tumor growth inhibition. This inspired the development of a single-arm pilot study with 10 patients with relapsed glioblastoma. Progression-free survival at 6 months was 50% (23–77%; 85% confidence interval) and the median overall survival was 62 weeks (20–124 weeks) with two patients alive more than two years from the start of TTField [36]. There were no serious adverse events, and the only significant toxicity was mild to moderate dermatitis at the site of electrode contact. Further studies demonstrated that the TTFields were safe and additive when administered in conjunction with chemotherapy in cell lines and animal model. As part of this publication, additional pilot studies were conducted with 10 patients with relapsed glioblastoma (failed first line) and 10 patients with newly diagnosed glioblastoma who received the TTFields along with adjuvant temozolomide [37].

NovoTTF—Newly Diagnosed Glioblastoma

A randomized, non-blinded clinical trial was initiated in July 2009 evaluating the application of TTFields in patients with newly diagnosed glioblastoma [38]. In total, 695 patients with histologically confirmed glioblastoma were randomized 2:1 to receive either adjuvant temozolomide 150–200 mg/m^2/day on a 5 of 28-day schedule along with NovoTTF delivered continuously >18 h per day or temozolomide alone. This trial was terminated prematurely after an interim analysis revealed a survival benefit. The interim analysis included 210 patients randomized to receive TTFields and temozolomide and 105 patients randomized to temozolomide alone. The median progression-free survival was 7.5 months (95% CI, 5.9–8.2 months) versus 4.0 months (95% CI, 3.3–5.2 months) in the temozolomide arm. Median overall survival was 20.5 months (95% CI, 16.7–25.0 month) in the TTFiels and temozolomide and 15.6 months (95% CI, 13.3–19.1 months) in the temozolomide arm with HR 0.64 (99.4% CI, 0.42–0.98, $p = 0.04$). There were similar adverse events between the two arms with the exception of localized skin toxicity with 45% of patients experiencing mild to moderate skin toxicity and 2% grade 3 toxicity. TTField compliance was estimated at 75% of patients enrolled on the TTField arm for more than 75% of the time in the first three months. In October 2015, NovoTTF was approved for patients with newly diagnosed glioblastoma along with temozolomide.

NovoTTF—Relapsed Glioblastoma

Stupp et al. conducted the first randomized clinical trial with NovoTTFields in patients with relapsed glioblastoma. Patients were randomized 1:1 to receive either TTFields or salvage chemotherapy of physician choice. 120 patients were randomized to receive TTFields, but only 93 patients (78%) completed >4 weeks of treatment. Median compliance in the TTF group was approximately 86% and the average daily use of TTF was 20.6 h. 117 patients were enrolled and 113 patients received salvage chemotherapy as determined by a local oncologist. In the end, there was no improvement in survival seen; however, TTfields did not appear to be inferior to the chemotherapy arm. The results of this trial led to the approval of NovoTTFields for patients with relapsed glioblastoma in March 2011 [39].

Conclusions

Despite significant advances over the last two decades, a comprehensive understanding of the molecular underpinnings of malignant glioma and the impact on clinical management is still a long way off. Increasingly, the predictive power of mgmt methylation, 1p/19q deletion, and IDH1 mutational status are being incorporated into day-to-day treatment decision making for patients with malignant glioma; however, as yet undiscovered molecular features and the implication of these findings will likely lead to more effective treatment in the future. Although as this review has illustrated there are some reasonable treatment options for patients with malignant glioma, the hope is that one day we will employ an understanding of the complex genetics of these tumors to define diagnosis, treatment, and clinical trial design.

References

1. Ostrom QT, Gittleman H, Fulop J, Liu M, Blanda R, Kromer C, et al. CBTRUS statistical report: primary brain and central nervous system tumors diagnosed in the United States in 2008–2012. Neuro Oncol. 2015;17(suppl 4):iv1–62.
2. CBTRUS. 2009–2010 CBTRUS statistical report: primary brain and central nervous system tumors diagnosed in eighteen states in 2002–2006. IL: Central Brain Tumor Registry of the United States; 2009–2010. Website: www.cbtrus.org; Available from: www.cbtrus.org.
3. Eckel-Passow JE, Lachance DH, Molinaro AM, Walsh KM, Decker PA, Sicotte H, et al. Glioma Groups based on 1p/19q, IDH, and TERT promoter mutations in tumors. N Engl J Med. 2015;372(26):2499–508.
4. Cairncross G, Wang M, Shaw E, Jenkins R, Brachman D, Buckner J, et al. Phase III trial of chemoradiotherapy for anaplastic oligodendroglioma:

long-term results of RTOG 9402. J Clin Oncol. 2013;31(3):337–43.
5. van den Bent MJ, Brandes AA, Taphoorn MJ, Kros JM, Kouwenhoven MC, Delattre JY, et al. Adjuvant procarbazine, lomustine, and vincristine chemotherapy in newly diagnosed anaplastic oligodendroglioma: long-term follow-up of EORTC brain tumor group study 26951. J Clin Oncol. 2013;31 (3):344–50.
6. Wick W, Hartmann C, Engel C, Stoffels M, Felsberg J, Stockhammer F, et al. NOA-04 randomized phase III trial of sequential radiochemotherapy of anaplastic glioma with procarbazine, lomustine, and vincristine or temozolomide. J Clin Oncol. 2009;27 (35):5874–80.
7. Wick W. Long-term analysis of the NOA-4 randomized phase III trial of sequential radiochemotherapy of anaplastic glioma with PCV or Temozolomide. J Clin Oncol. 2015;33(suppl, abstract 2001).
8. Vredenburgh JJ, Desjardins A, Herndon JE, Marcello J, Reardon DA, Quinn JA, et al. Bevacizumab plus irinotecan in recurrent glioblastoma multiforme. J Clin Oncol. 2007;25(30):4722–9.
9. Brada M, Stenning S, Gabe R, Thompson LC, Levy D, Rampling R, et al. Temozolomide versus procarbazine, lomustine, and vincristine in recurrent high-grade glioma. J Clin Oncol. 2010;28(30):4601–8.
10. O'Reilly SM, Newlands ES, Glaser MG, Brampton M, Rice-Edwards JM, Illingworth RD, et al. Temozolomide: a new oral cytotoxic chemotherapeutic agent with promising activity against primary brain tumours. Eur J Cancer (Oxford, England: 1990). 1993;29A(7):940–2.
11. Stupp R, Mason WP, van den Bent MJ, Weller M, Fisher B, Taphoorn MJ, et al. Radiotherapy plus concomitant and adjuvant temozolomide for glioblastoma. N Engl J Med. 2005;352(10):987–96.
12. Stupp R, Dietrich PY, Ostermann Kraljevic S, Pica A, Maillard I, Maeder P, et al. Promising survival for patients with newly diagnosed glioblastoma multiforme treated with concomitant radiation plus temozolomide followed by adjuvant temozolomide. J Clin Oncol. 2002;20(5):1375–82.
13. Hegi ME, Diserens AC, Gorlia T, Hamou MF, de Tribolet N, Weller M, et al. MGMT gene silencing and benefit from temozolomide in glioblastoma. N Engl J Med. 2005;352:997–1003 (United States: Massachusetts Medical Society).
14. Clarke JL, Iwamoto FM, Sul J, Panageas K, Lassman AB, DeAngelis LM, et al. Randomized phase II trial of chemoradiotherapy followed by either dose-dense or metronomic temozolomide for newly diagnosed glioblastoma. J Clin Oncol. 2009;27 (23):3861–7.
15. Gilbert MR, Wang M, Aldape KD, Stupp R, Hegi ME, Jaeckle KA, et al. Dose-dense temozolomide for newly diagnosed glioblastoma: a randomized phase III clinical trial. J Clin Oncol. 2013;31 (32):4085–91.
16. Brem H, Mahaley MS Jr, Vick NA, Black KL, Schold SC Jr, Burger PC, et al. Interstitial chemotherapy with drug polymer implants for the treatment of recurrent gliomas. J Neurosurg. 1991;74 (3):441–6.
17. Tamargo RJ, Myseros JS, Epstein JI, Yang MB, Chasin M, Brem H. Interstitial chemotherapy of the 9L gliosarcoma: controlled release polymers for drug delivery in the brain. Cancer Res. 1993;53(2):329–33.
18. Brem H, Piantadosi S, Burger PC, Walker M, Selker R, Vick NA, et al. Placebo-controlled trial of safety and efficacy of intraoperative controlled delivery by biodegradable polymers of chemotherapy for recurrent gliomas. The polymer-brain tumor treatment group. Lancet. 1995;345(8956):1008–12.
19. Westphal M, Hilt DC, Bortey E, Delavault P, Olivares R, Warnke PC, et al. A phase 3 trial of local chemotherapy with biodegradable carmustine (BCNU) wafers (Gliadel wafers) in patients with primary malignant glioma. Neuro Oncol. 2003;5 (2):79–88.
20. Valtonen S, Timonen U, Toivanen P, Kalimo H, Kivipelto L, Heiskanen O, et al. Interstitial chemotherapy with carmustine-loaded polymers for high-grade gliomas: a randomized double-blind study. Neurosurgery. 1997;41(1):44–8 (discussion 8–9).
21. Westphal M, Ram Z, Riddle V, Hilt D, Bortey E. Gliadel wafer in initial surgery for malignant glioma: long-term follow-up of a multicenter controlled trial. Acta Neurochirurgica. 2006;148(3):269–75 (discussion 75).
22. Meldorf MGRV, Agarwal S, et al. Long-term efficacy of the Gliadel wafer in patients with glioblastoma multiforme. San Diego: Annual Meeting of American Association of Neurological Surgeons; 2003.
23. Chowdhary SA, Ryken T, Newton HB. Survival outcomes and safety of carmustine wafers in the treatment of high-grade gliomas: a meta-analysis. J Neurooncol. 2015;122(2):367–82.
24. Kleinberg LR, Weingart J, Burger P, Carson K, Grossman SA, Li K, et al. Clinical course and pathologic findings after Gliadel and radiotherapy for newly diagnosed malignant glioma: implications for patient management. Cancer Invest. 2004;22(1):1–9.
25. Folkman J. Tumor angiogenesis: therapeutic implications. N Engl J Med. 1971;285(21):1182–6.
26. Cheng SY, Huang HJ, Nagane M, Ji XD, Wang D, Shih CC, et al. Suppression of glioblastoma angiogenicity and tumorigenicity by inhibition of endogenous expression of vascular endothelial growth factor. Proc Natl Acad Sci USA. 1996;93 (16):8502–7.
27. Presta LG, Chen H, O'Connor SJ, Chisholm V, Meng YG, Krummen L, et al. Humanization of an anti-vascular endothelial growth factor monoclonal antibody for the therapy of solid tumors and other disorders. Cancer Res. 1997;57(20):4593–9.

28. Stark-Vance V. Bevacizumab and CPT-11 in the treatment of relapsed malignant glioma. 2005;7 (7):7:369.
29. Friedman HS, Prados MD, Wen PY, Mikkelsen T, Schiff D, Abrey LE, et al. Bevacizumab alone and in combination with irinotecan in recurrent glioblastoma. J Clin Oncol. 2009;27:4733–40 (United States).
30. Vredenburgh JJ, Desjardins A, Herndon JE 2nd, Dowell JM, Reardon DA, Quinn JA, et al. Phase II trial of bevacizumab and irinotecan in recurrent malignant glioma. Clin Cancer Res. 2007;13 (4):1253–9.
31. Vredenburgh JJ, Desjardins A, Herndon JE, Marcello J, Reardon DA, Quinn JA, et al. Bevacizumab plus irinotecan in recurrent glioblastoma multiforme. J Clin Oncol. 2007;25:4722–9 (United States).
32. Kreisl TN, Kim L, Moore K, Duic P, Royce C, Stroud I, et al. Phase II trial of single-agent bevacizumab followed by bevacizumab plus irinotecan at tumor progression in recurrent glioblastoma. J Clin Oncol. 2009;27:P740–5 (United States).
33. Chinot OL, Wick W, Mason W, Henriksson R, Saran F, Nishikawa R, et al. Bevacizumab plus radiotherapy-temozolomide for newly diagnosed glioblastoma. N Engl J Med. 2014;370(8):709–22.
34. Gilbert MR, Dignam JJ, Armstrong TS, Wefel JS, Blumenthal DT, Vogelbaum MA, et al. A randomized trial of bevacizumab for newly diagnosed glioblastoma. N Engl J Med. 2014;370(8):699–708.
35. Kirson ED, Gurvich Z, Schneiderman R, Dekel E, Itzhaki A, Wasserman Y, et al. Disruption of cancer cell replication by alternating electric fields. Cancer Res. 2004;64(9):3288–95.
36. Kirson ED, Dbaly V, Tovarys F, Vymazal J, Soustiel JF, Itzhaki A, et al. Alternating electric fields arrest cell proliferation in animal tumor models and human brain tumors. Proc Natl Acad Sci USA. 2007;104(24):10152–7.
37. Kirson ED, Schneiderman RS, Dbaly V, Tovarys F, Vymazal J, Itzhaki A, et al. Chemotherapeutic treatment efficacy and sensitivity are increased by adjuvant alternating electric fields (TTFields). BMC Med Phys. 2009;9:1.
38. Stupp R, Taillibert S, Kanner AA, Kesari S, Steinberg DM, Toms SA, et al. Maintenance therapy with tumor-treating fields plus temozolomide vs temozolomide alone for glioblastoma: a randomized clinical trial. JAMA, J Am Med Assoc. 2015;314 (23):2535–43.
39. Stupp R, Wong ET, Kanner AA, Steinberg D, Engelhard H, Heidecke V, et al. NovoTTF-100A versus physician's choice chemotherapy in recurrent glioblastoma: a randomised phase III trial of a novel treatment modality. Eur J Cancer. 2012;48(14):2192–202 (Oxford, England: 1990).

Targeting Aberrant Signaling Pathways

9

Jacob Mandel and Santosh Kesari

Targeting Aberrant Signaling Pathways

Malignant gliomas are the most common primary brain tumor found in adults [1]. Regretfully, prognosis for these tumors remains dismal despite aggressive treatment with surgical resection, radiation, and chemotherapy. Treatment of glioblastoma patients with the current standard of care consisting of maximal resection, 6 weeks of concurrent chemoradiation with daily temozolomide followed by 6–12 cycles of adjuvant temozolomide, results in a median overall survival of only approximately 16 months [2]. Malignant gliomas have proven to be among the most difficult cancers to treat due to their genetic heterogeneity, elaborate overlapping signaling pathways, and difficulties in delivering drugs across the blood–brain barrier [3]. Recent in-depth description of the distinct molecular and genetic alterations in glioblastomas, using advanced sequencing technologies and large-scale gene expression studies, has inspired interest in the development of targeted therapies. Targeted therapies work by the inhibition of the deregulated cell signaling pathways in cancer cells by small molecules or antibodies, whereas traditional cytotoxic chemotherapies operate by impeding DNA synthesis or cell metabolism. This chapter will explore these aberrant signaling pathways in malignant gliomas and the results of the clinical trials of therapeutics targeting them.

The Cancer Genome Atlas

The Cancer Genome Atlas (TCGA), a collaboration between the National Cancer Institute (NCI) and National Human Genome Research Institute (NHGRI), was undertaken to generate comprehensive, multidimensional maps of the major genomic changes in several types of cancer. One of the first cancers studied by the TCGA was glioblastoma, and the analysis characterized a decidedly interrelated network of aberrations. It identified three key pathways: the retinoblastoma (RB) and p53 tumor suppressor pathways, and the receptor tyrosine kinases (RTKs) signaling pathway [4]. For glioblastoma patients with sequencing data, the frequencies of somatic alterations were 78, 87, and 88%, respectively, in each of these pathways (Fig. 9.1). Of further note, 74% of glioblastoma samples contained abnormalities in all three pathways [4].

J. Mandel
Baylor College of Medicine, 7200 Cambridge Ave, Suite 9A, Houston, TX 77030, USA
e-mail: Jacob.mandel@bcm.edu

S. Kesari (✉)
Department of Translational Neuro-Oncology and Neurotherapeutics, John Wayne Cancer Institute, 2200 Santa Monica Blvd, Santa Monica, CA 90404, USA
e-mail: kesaris@jwci.org

J. Moliterno Günel et al. (eds.), *Malignant Brain Tumors*,
DOI 10.1007/978-3-319-49864-5_9

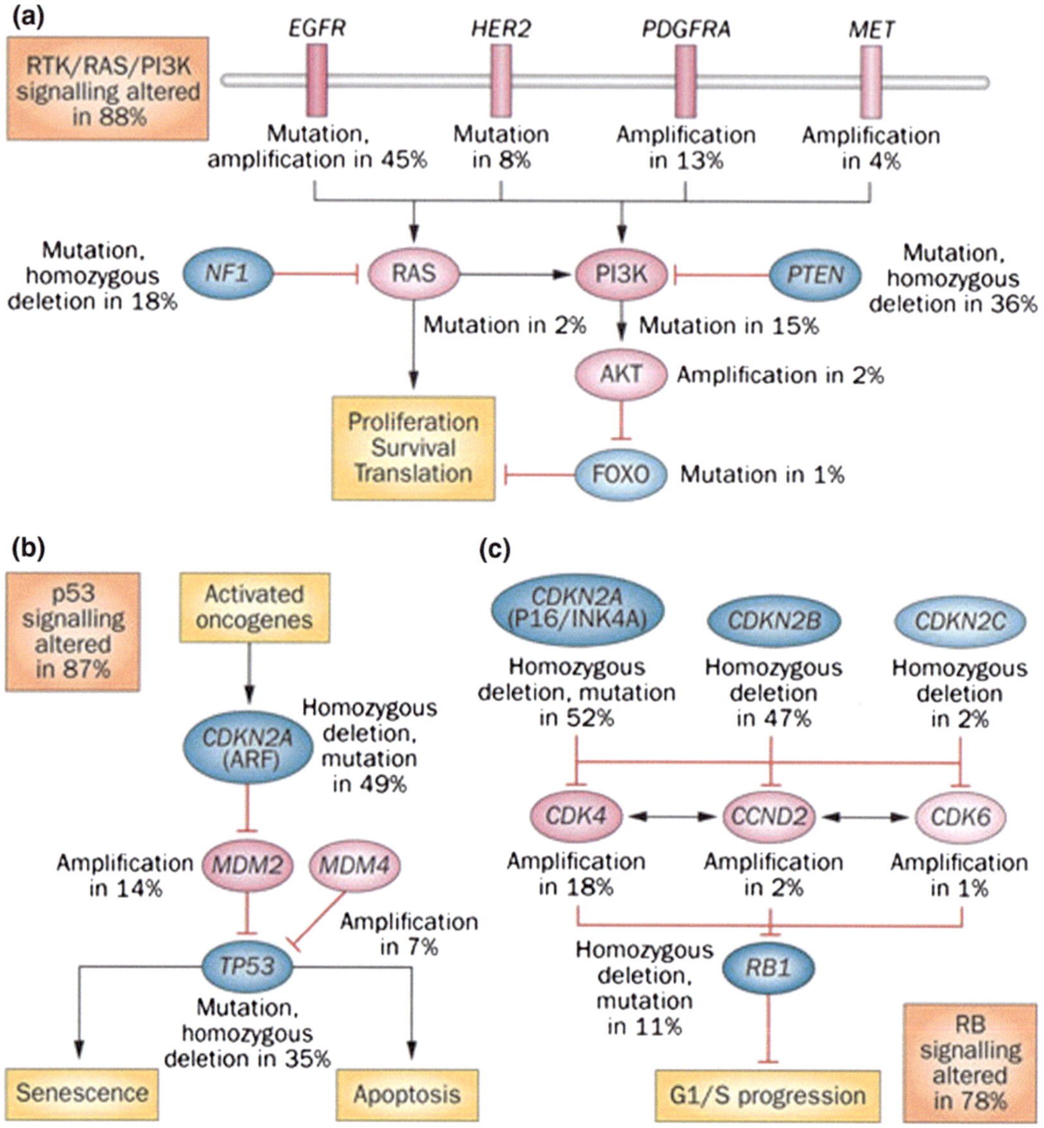

Fig. 9.1 Critical signaling pathways altered in malignant gliomas. Primary sequence alterations and significant copy number changes for the components of the **a** | RTK/RAS/PI3K, **b** | p53, and **c** | Rb signaling pathways are shown. *Red* indicates activating genetic alterations. Conversely, *blue* indicates inactivating alterations. For each altered component of a particular pathway, the nature of the alteration and the percentage of tumors affected are indicated. *Boxes* contain the final percentages of glioblastomas with alterations in at least one known component gene of the designated pathway. Abbreviation: *RTK* receptor tyrosine kinase

Retinoblastoma Tumor Suppressor Pathway

The RB protein is a tumor suppressor protein that is dysfunctional in several cancer types [5]. It is encoded by the RB gene, which is located at chromosome 13q14.1-q14.2. Normally, the RB protein prevents unwarranted cell growth by inhibiting cell cycle progression until a cell is set to undergo mitosis. When ready for cell division, the RB protein is then phosphorylated by cyclin D, cyclin-dependent kinase 4 (CDK4), and cyclin-dependent kinase 6 (CDK6) inactivating the protein and allowing for cell cycle progression [5]. Most commonly, homozygous deletion of cyclin-dependent kinase inhibitor 2A (CDKN2A) can produce loss of p16INK4a and a suppressor of CDK4, leading to dysregulation of RB signaling [5–7]. Mutations in retinoblastoma protein 1 (RB1) and CDK4 amplification can also trigger dysfunction of the RB signaling pathway. A CDK4 inhibitor, PD-0332991 (palbociclib isethionate), has been examined in two phase I trials leading to a phase II trial in recurrent RB-positive glioblastoma with results not yet reported [8–10].

p53 Tumor Suppressor Pathway

The tumor protein p53 (p53) gene is the most frequently mutated gene in human cancer and performs a critical function in preventing cancer formation [11]. It is located at chromosome 17p13.1 and reacts to DNA injury and toxic pressures by producing cell cycle arrest and apoptosis [12, 13]. Loss of p53 pathway function can be due to p53 mutation/deletion itself or by interferences in other genes that regulate p53 function such as murine double minute (MDM2/4) and the tumor suppressor protein alternate reading frame (ARF) [14–16].

The use of an intratumoral injection of a p53-containing adenovirus vector to increase wild-type p53 expression in tumor cells has been attempted in a phase 1 study in recurrent glioma, but it did not appear to achieve systemic viral dissemination [17]. Phase I trials of wild-type Ad5CMV-p53 gene therapy and recombinant adenovirus p53 (SCH-58500) in combination with surgery in recurrent malignant gliomas have been completed, but the results have yet to be published [18, 19].

SGT-53 is a nanocomplex of cationic liposome encapsulating a normal human wild-type p53 DNA sequence in a plasmid backbone exhibited to supply the p53 cDNA to the tumor cells with the goal of the p53 cDNA sequence to restore wild-type p53 function in the apoptotic pathway [20]. SGT-53 has shown to prolong survival in a mouse model and is currently undergoing investigation in a phase II trial in recurrent glioblastoma [20, 21]. An MDM2 inhibitor, JNJ-26854165, was examined in a phase I study in refractory solid tumors but has yet to be examined in brain tumor patients exclusively [22, 23]. MK-1775, a Weel kinase inhibitor, has been shown to radiosensitize p53-defective human tumor cells and is currently under investigation in a multicenter phase I trial in newly diagnosed or recurrent glioblastoma [24, 25].

Receptor Tyrosine Kinase Signaling Pathway

Receptor tyrosine kinases (RTKs) are high-affinity cell surface receptors and primary mediators of signal transduction events shown to have an essential function in the growth and progression of many cancers [26]. Twenty different RTK classes have been identified, and members of this family include the vascular endothelial growth factor receptor (VEGFR), epidermal growth factor receptor (EGFR), platelet-derived growth factor receptor (PDGFR), and hepatocyte growth factor receptor (MET). The receptor tyrosine kinase signaling pathway has been the most extensively studied pathway in malignant gliomas to date (Table 9.1).

Vascular Endothelial Growth Factor Receptor (VEGFR)

Vascular endothelial growth factor (VEGF) is a significant component implicated in the formation of new blood vessels which is a distinguishing feature of glioblastoma [27]. VEGF binding to its receptors VEGFR-1 and VEGFR-2 leads to phosphorylation of tyrosine kinase and initiation of downstream signaling pathways including phosphatidylinositol-4,5-bisphosphate 3-kinase (PI3K)/protein kinase B (Akt/PBK) and Ras/mitogen-activated protein kinases (MAPK) [28].

Bevacizumab, a monoclonal antibody that targets the VEGF-A ligand, was granted

Table 9.1 Targeted therapies for malignant gliomas in published clinical trials

Therapy	Pathway	Target/s
Bevacizumab	RTK	VEGF-A [30–37]
Cediranib	RTK	VEGFR-1, VEGFR-2, VEGFR-3, PDGFR-α/β, FGFR-1, c-Kit [38, 39]
Pazopanib	RTK	VEGFR, c-Kit, FGFR, and PDGFR [40, 41]
Sorafenib	RTK	VEGFR-2, Raf, PDGFR, c-Kit, Flt-3 [42–46]
Nintedanib	RTK	VEGFR 1-3, FGFR 1-3, PDGFR-α/β [47]
Vandetanib	RTK	VEFGR-2, EGFR [48, 49]
Sunitinib	RTK	VEGFR2, PDGFR-α, and c-Kit [50–53]
Aflibercept	RTK	VEGF and PlGF [54]
Vatalanib	RTK	VEGFR, PDGFR, and c-Kit [55–57]
Cabozantinib	RTK	VEGFR-2, MET, and RET [58]
Gefitinib	RTK	EGFR [64–69]
Erlotinib	RTK	EGFR [45, 70–80]
Cetuximab	RTK	EGFR [81, 82]
Lapatinib	RTK	EGFR and HER2 [83–85]
AEE-788	RTK	EGFR, HER2, and VEGFR2 [86]
Nimotuzumab	RTK	EGFR [92]
Imatinib	RTK	PDGFR, Bcr-Abl, and c-Kit [56, 100–105]
Dasatinib	RTK	PDGFR, Src, Bcr-Abl, c-Kit, and EphA2 [106]
PX-866	RTK	PI3K [118]
Enzastaurin	RTK	protein kinase C, PI3K, and Akt [125–128]
Everolimus	RTK	mTOR [135–137]
Temsirolimus	RTK	mTOR [46, 138–140]
Sirolimus	RTK	mTOR [49, 68, 79, 80]
Tipifarnib	RTK	Ras [151, 152]
Lonafarnib	RTK	Ras [155, 156]

Abbreviations: *RTK* receptor tyrosine kinase, *VEGF* vascular endothelial growth factor, *VEGFR* vascular endothelial growth factor receptor, *PDGFR* platelet-derived growth factor receptor, *FGFR* fibroblast growth factor receptor, *FLT3* Fms-like tyrosine kinase-3, *EGFR* epidermal growth factor receptor, *PlGF* placental growth factor receptor, *MET* hepatocyte growth factor receptor, *HER2* human epidermal growth factor receptor 2, *EphA2* ephrin type-A receptor 2, *PI3K* phosphatidylinositide 3-kinases, *mTOR* mammalian target of rapamycin

accelerated approval by the Food and Drug Administration for use as a single agent in recurrent glioblastoma in 2009 [29]. Approval was granted based on the results of two phase II clinical trials that demonstrated durable objective imaging responses based on independent radiologic review with stable or decreasing corticosteroid use [29–31]. Subsequently, two phase III clinical trials (RTOG 0825 and AVAglio) were performed examining the addition of bevacizumab or placebo to the current standard of care regimen of concurrent chemoradiation with temozolomide followed by adjuvant temozolomide in newly diagnosed glioblastoma [32, 33]. Both studies found that the addition of bevacizumab improved progression-free but not overall survival [32, 33]. While the addition of irinotecan to bevacizumab was not beneficial in the early studies of bevacizumab, a subsequent phase II study appeared to suggest that the combination of lomustine and bevacizumab may prolong overall survival compared to either treatment administered alone [30, 31, 34]. Disappointingly, the preliminary report of the results of an EORTC phase III study comparing lomustine alone versus lomustine and bevacizumab in reccurent glioblastoma failed to demonstrate an improvement in overall survival with the combination treatment [35]. Phase II trials of recurrent glioblastoma examining the addition of fotemustine or carboplatin to bevacizumab also did not demonstrate any increased survival benefit with the addition of these cytotoxic therapies [36, 37]. Despite the improvement in progression-free survival and increased imaging response rate, bevacizumab has yet to improve overall survival in either the upfront or recurrent setting.

Other VEGF inhibitors have failed to even match the limited success of bevacizumab. Cediranib, an oral pan-VEGF receptor tyrosine kinase inhibitor, demonstrated a 6-month progression-free survival of 25.8% and partial radiographic responses in 56.7% of patients in a phase II study of patients with recurrent glioblastoma [38]. However, a phase III randomized trial in recurrent glioblastoma comparing the efficacy of cediranib as monotherapy, and in combination with lomustine, versus lomustine alone failed to show any improvement with cediranib either as monotherapy or in combination with lomustine versus lomustine alone [39]. Pazopanib, a multikinase inhibitor of c-Kit, FGFR, PDGFR, and VEGFR, also did not show any prolongation of progression-free survival in a phase II study in recurrent glioblastoma [40]. A subsequent phase I/II examining pazopanib in combination with lapatinib (an EGFR inhibitor) in relapsed malignant glioma patients had limited antitumor activity leading to early termination of the study [41]. Sorafenib, an oral VEGFR-2, Raf, PDGFR, c-Kit, and Flt-3 inhibitor, was used in combination with temozolomide for initial adjuvant therapy in a phase II study for patients with glioblastoma but failed to improve the efficacy when compared to historical controls [42]. Additionally, sorafenib has been examined in several other phase II studies in recurrent glioblastoma in combination with temozolomide, bevacizumab, erlotinib, and temsirolimus of which no combination resulted in a prolongation of survival [43–46]. Nintedanib, an inhibitor that targets VEGFR 1-3, FGFR 1-3, and PDGFR-α/β, was studied in a phase II study that was terminated early following a preplanned futility analysis [47]. Vandetanib, an inhibitor of VEFGR-2 and EGFR, failed to display any significant activity in a phase I/II trial of patients with recurrent malignant glioma [48]. In addition, a phase I/II study of vandetanib plus sirolimus (an mTor inhibitor) in adults with recurrent glioblastoma failed to display benefit when compared to historical controls [49]. Sunitinib, an inhibitor of VEGFR-2, PDGFR-α, and KIT, similarly did not show any improvement in survival either as a monotherapy or in combination with irinotecan in phase I or phase II studies in recurrent glioma [50–53]. An inhibitor of VEGF and placental growth factor, aflibercept, also had minimal evidence of single-agent activity in unselected patients with recurrent malignant glioma [54]. Vatalanib, an inhibitor of VEGFR, PDGFR, and c-Kit, was examined alone in newly diagnosed glioblastoma patients and with imatinib and hydroxyurea at time of tumor recurrence in two phase I studies [55, 56]. However, a planned randomized phase II trial was terminated at its initiation (after completion of its phase I component) because of industry decision [57]. Cabozantinib, an inhibitor of VEGFR-2, MET, and RET, was used in a phase II study whose final results are yet to be published [58].

Epidermal Growth Factor Receptor (EGFR)

The epidermal growth factor receptor is located on chromosome 7p12 and is a member of the ErbB family of receptor tyrosine kinases [59]. Overexpression of EGFR is one of the most common signaling mutations in GBM and is thought to occur in around 50% of glioblastomas [60]. Glioblastomas with EGFR overexpression have been demonstrated to potentially be more radioresistant [61]. Additionally, EGFR amplification is often associated with the expression of a constitutively active, ligand-independent mutant form of the receptor called EGFRvIII generated by an in-frame deletion of exons 2–7 [61, 62].

EGFRvIII expression may be an independent prognostic factor for poor survival [63].

Unfortunately, EGFR inhibitors in malignant glioma trials have likewise been disappointing. Gefitinib, an EGFR inhibitor approved to treat non-small-cell lung cancer in 2003, failed to show any benefit when added to the treatment in newly diagnosed glioblastoma patients [64, 65]. Additionally, gefitinib in the treatment of recurrent disease has shown minimal activity alone or in combination with mammalian target of rapamycin (mTOR) inhibitors such as sirolimus or everolimus [66–69]. Another EGFR inhibitor, Erlotinib, also has shown minimal efficacy against newly diagnosed or recurrent glioblastoma [70–76]. Furthermore, several phase II studies in recurrent glioblastoma examining the combination of erlotinib with carboplatin, sorafenib, bevacizumab, or sirolimus have failed to demonstrate significant antitumor activity [45, 77–80]. Cetuximab, another EGFR inhibitor used for the treatment of metastatic colorectal cancer, metastatic non-small-cell lung cancer, and head and neck cancer, regrettably has failed to show benefit in recurrent glioblastoma when used alone or in combination with bevacizumab and irinotecan [81, 82]. Lapatinib, the first dual inhibitor of EGFR and human epidermal growth factor receptor 2 (HER2) tyrosine kinases, also did not show significant activity in recurrent glioblastoma patients [83]. Additionally, lapatinib was studied in a phase I study with temodar and a phase I/II study with pazopanib in recurrent malignant gliomas [84, 85]. The phase II study of lapatinib and pazopanib revealed limited antitumor activity of this combination leading to early study termination [84]. AEE788, another inhibitor of EGFR, HER2, and VEGFR2, was associated with unacceptable toxicity and minimal activity for the treatment of recurrent glioblastoma in a phase I trial [86].

Afatinib, an irreversible covalent inhibitor of the EGFR and HER2, is approved for first-line treatment of patients with EGFR mutation-positive non-small-cell lung carcinoma [87]. Afatinib is currently under investigation in a phase I/II trial in recurrent malignant glioma. Additionally, a phase I trial of afatinib in newly diagnosed glioblastoma patients with radiotherapy alone in patients with an unmethylated MGMT promotor or radiotherapy and temozolomide in patients with a methylated MGMT promotor is ongoing [88, 89]. Dacomitinib is another selective and irreversible inhibitor of EGFR studied in two phase II trials in recurrent glioblastoma with one of the trials limited to only patients with EGFR gene amplification and/or EGFRvIII mutation [90, 91]. Another EGFR inhibitor, nimotuzumab, has received orphan drug status in the USA and EU for glioma. A phase I/II trial in high-grade glioma with nimotuzumab showed an excellent safety profile and significant survival benefit in combination with irradiation, but unfortunately, a subsequent phase III trial of nimotuzumab in newly diagnosed glioblastoma was negative [92, 93].

Platelet-Derived Growth Factor Receptor (PDGFR)

Platelet-derived growth factor receptors (PDGFRs) are cell surface receptors for members of the PDGF family and signal through the alpha and beta PDGF receptor tyrosine kinases [94]. The PDGFR alpha (PDGFRA) gene is located on chromosome *7p22* and amplified in approximately 13% of glioblastomas [4, 95]. PDGFRA can be overexpressed, amplified, mutated, or truncated in gliomas, with *PDGFRA* point mutations being observed exclusively in glioblastomas [96].

Imatinib mesylate is an inhibitor of the PDGFR, Bcr-Abl, and c-Kit tyrosine kinases that have been found to beneficial in the treatment of chronic myelogenous leukemia b and in gastrointestinal stromal tumors [97–99]. However, imatinib alone displayed only minimal activity in recurrent malignant gliomas and in newly diagnosed glioblastoma [100, 101]. Subsequent studies looking at imatinib with the addition of hydroxyurea in recurrent malignant gliomas also failed to show clinically meaningful antitumor activity [102–105]. As discussed previously, imatinib with hydroxyurea was also examined in combination with vatalanib [56].

Dasatinib, an inhibitor of PDGFR, Src, Bcr-Abl, c-Kit, and EphA2 receptors, was studied in a phase 2 trial in target-selected patients (activation or overexpression of ≥2 putative dasatinib targets) with recurrent glioblastoma and was found ineffective with no radiographic responses [106]. Additional, phase II studies with dasatinib in combination with bevacizumab in recurrent glioblastoma and in newly diagnosed glioblastoma with chemoradiation have not yet reported results [107, 108]. A phase I multicenter trial of dasatinib in combination with CCNU was found to have substantial hematological toxicities leading to suboptimal exposure to both agents [109]. Another phase I study of dasatinib in combination with erlotinib was better tolerated [110].

Furthermore, Tandutinib, a small molecule inhibitor of PDGFR, fms-like tyrosine kinase receptor-3 (FLT3), and c-Kit, has been examined alone or with bevacizumab in recurrent glioblastoma with results awaiting publication [111, 112].

PI3K/AKT/mTOR Pathway

Along with targeting cell surface receptors, there has been a significant effort undertaken on inhibiting downstream survival signaling pathways stimulated by these receptors. The PI3K/Akt/mTOR pathway can be crucial in controlling cellular functions regulating cellular proliferation, apoptosis, cell invasion, and mobility. Activation of phosphatidylinositide 3-kinase (PI3K) complex is regulated by several growth factors in conjunction with their receptors, the most frequent of which is the amplification of EGFR [113, 114]. PI3K activation phosphorylates and activates Akt (protein kinase B) a serine/threonine-specific protein kinase [115]. Akt next activates mTOR (mammalian target of rapamycin), another serine/threonine protein kinase that controls cell growth and proliferation via the regulation of protein synthesis and transcription [116]. It is comprised of two parts, mTOR complex 1 (mTORC1) and mTOR complex 2 (mTORC2), operating as both a downstream effector and upstream regulator of PI3K [117].

PX-866, an oral PI3K inhibitor, in a recent phase II study had a low overall response rate and failed to improve progression-free survival in patients with recurrent glioblastoma [118]. BKM-120, another oral inhibitor of PI3 kinase, is currently under investigation in combination with standard of care for newly diagnosed glioblastoma and as monotherapy in recurrent glioblastoma [119, 120]. Additionally, a phase II study in recurrent glioblastoma examining the combination of BKM-120 and bevacizumab is underway [121]. XL-147 (a potent inhibitor of PI3K) and XL-765 (a dual PI3K and mTOR inhibitor) are currently being investigated as monotherapy in recurrent glioblastoma [122]. XL-765 has also been studied in combination with temozolomide in malignant glioma patients with no results published yet [123]. Pictilisib (a potent inhibitor of PI3K) and BEZ235 (a dual ATP-competitive PI3K and mTOR inhibitor) are also currently undergoing investigation in a phase II study of recurrent glioblastoma [124].

Enzastaurin is a protein kinase C and phosphoinositide-3 kinase/Akt inhibitor that failed to improve survival in newly diagnosed patients with and without O(6)-methylguanine-DNA-methyltransferase (MGMT) promotor methylation in combination with standard of care and as a monotherapy in recurrent glioblastoma [125–128]. Perifosine, an Akt inhibitor and a PI3K inhibitor, is currently being examined in recurrent malignant gliomas alone or in combination with temsirolimus [129, 130]. Ipatasertib, a highly selective pan-Akt inhibitor targeting Akt1/2/3, is also present in a phase II study of recurrent glioblastoma [131]. Nelfinavir, a protease inhibitor interfering with Akt activity, has been given neo-adjuvantly and concomitant to chemoradiotherapy with temozolomide in a phase I/II study of patients with newly diagnosed glioblastoma [132].

Several mTOR inhibitors have been developed over the past few years. mTOR is inhibited by these agents forming a complex with FK-binding protein-12 (FKBP-12) which joins to mTOR, blocking its stimulation and constraining tumor cell proliferation [133]. Everolimus, an mTOR inhibitor, has been shown to cause a marked reduction in the volume of subependymal giant cell astrocytomas and seizure frequency in patients with tuberous sclerosis [134]. Unfortunately, everolimus has not displayed durable responses as a monotherapy or when combined with gefitinib in patients with recurrent glioblastoma [69, 135]. Moreover, the addition of everolimus to standard of care in newly diagnosed glioblastoma patients did not translate into an appreciable survival benefit [136]. Furthermore, a phase II study in newly diagnosed glioblastoma patient of concurrent radiation therapy, temozolomide, and bevacizumab followed by bevacizumab/everolimus as first-line treatment failed to improve survival compared to historical controls [137].

Temsirolimus, an mTOR inhibitor approved for the treatment of renal cell carcinoma, likewise has shown limited benefit in recurrent glioblastoma as a monotherapy or in combination with sorafenib [46, 138, 139]. When temsirolimus was used in a phase I study in addition to standard of care in newly diagnosed glioblastoma, an increased risk of infection was noted [140].

Rapamycin (sirolimus), another mTOR inhibitor, has also failed to show benefit in recurrent glioblastoma when used in combination with vandetanib, erlotinib, or gefitinib as discussed earlier [49, 68, 79, 80]. Additionally, a phase II trial of rapamycin in combination with bevacizumab in recurrent glioblastoma patients was stopped early due to lack of response [141].

New mTOR-specific inhibitors are in development which can block activity of both mTOR complexes. AZD8055, one of these dual mTORC1/mTORC2 inhibitors, is currently in a phase I trial in adults with recurrent gliomas [142].

The PTEN (phosphatase and tensin homologue) gene, located on chromosome 10, is a tumor suppressor gene that negatively controls the PI3K/AKT/PKB pathway by preventing Akt signaling via the reduction of intracellular levels of phosphatidylinositol-3,4,5-triphosphate [143]. PTEN mutations have been reported in up to 40% of glioblastoma [4, 144]. In addition to inhibiting the Akt pathway, PTEN has also demonstrated the ability to enable the degradation of activated EGFR leading to the extinction of EGFR signaling [145]. Instigating expression of functional PTEN has been suggested as a potential future therapeutic approach in glioblastoma.

RAS/MAPK Pathway

The RAS/MAPK is another downstream survival signaling pathway stimulated by RTKs such as EGFR and PDGFR. Ras (rat sarcoma) gene mutations are present in a diverse group of tumor types with varying incidence [146]. Mutations in one of the three Ras genes (H-Ras, N-Ras, or K-Ras) in humans transform these genes to operating oncogenes [147]. Ras proteins have critical functions in regulating the activity of vital signaling pathways that control normal cellular proliferation. Activation and deactivation of Ras are regulated by cycling between its binding with the active guanosine triphosphate (GTP) and inactive guanosine diphosphate (GDP) forms [148]. Activated Ras results in activation of a serine/threonine kinase named Raf (rapidly accelerated fibrosarcoma). Raf subsequently phosphorylates and activates a kinase enzyme MEK (mitogen/extracellular signal-regulated Kinase) which in turn then phosphorylates and activates MAPK (mitogen-activated protein kinases).

Ras gene mutations have been found to only rarely occur in glioblastoma [4]. However, activation of Ras can occur by mechanisms that do not involve mutations in Ras. The neurofibromin 1 (NF-1) gene located on chromosomal segment 17q11.2 is a negative regulator of Ras, and loss of NF-1 may activate Ras [149]. NF-1 mutations have been reported in up to 18% of patients with glioblastoma [4].

Ras is posttranscriptionally modified by farnesyltransferase, and in vitro studies of glioblastoma with farnesyltransferase inhibitors have shown reduced cellular proliferation as well as the ability to trigger cell cycle arrest and induce apoptosis [150]. Tipifarnib is a potent and selective inhibitor of farnesyltransferase that has been examined in a phase I trial in newly diagnosed glioblastoma plus radiation therapy with and without temozolomide [151]. Unfortunately, a phase II trial of tipifarnib as a treatment for recurrent malignant glioma did not show benefit in 6-month progression-free survival compared to historical controls [152]. Lonafarnib, another farnesyltransferase inhibitor, has shown the ability to inhibit cell growth in preclinical studies [153, 154]. Two phase I studies have examined lonafarnib in combination with temozolomide, with one study in patients with malignant glioma after radiation and the other in patients with recurrent glioblastoma [155, 156].

Gene Expression-Based Molecular Classification of GBM into Subtypes

Following The Cancer Genome Atlas Network cataloging recurrent genomic abnormalities in glioblastoma, they subsequently defined four subtypes of glioblastoma (proneural, neural, classical, and mesenchymal) based on gene expression-based molecular classification [157]. Additionally, alterations and gene expression of *EGFR*, *NF1*, and *PDGFRA/IDH1* were found to distinctly delineate the classical, mesenchymal, and proneural subtypes, respectively [157]. These discoveries support the supposition that certain molecular-targeted therapies may potentially be most effective against a segment of glioblastomas. Results from a retrospective analysis of AVAglio (a randomized, placebo-controlled phase III trial examining the addition of bevacizumab to radiotherapy plus temozolomide in newly diagnosed glioblastoma) suggest that patients with IDH1 wild-type proneural glioblastoma may derive an overall survival benefit from first-line bevacizumab treatment [158]. This finding, however, still remains to be independently validated in future studies.

Furthermore, the classification of glioblastoma into unique subtypes based on genomic expression implies that there is a propensity for particular aberrations to group together. This theoretically could enable particular combinations of molecularly targeted agents to be more successful in certain subtypes.

Discussion

Large-scale gene expression studies have recently provided an in-depth description of the distinct molecular and genetic alterations in glioblastomas. This scientific progress has spurred an interest in the development of targeted therapies for these signaling pathways. Unfortunately, despite trying several agents and different pathways, targeted therapies have currently failed to improve the overall survival of glioblastoma patients. New therapies examining novel targets and innovative combinations are presently under investigation (Table 9.2).

Several possible explanations have been proposed on why early clinical results of molecularly targeted agents in malignant glioma have been so disappointing. These include the significant intratumoral heterogeneity, overlapping/redundant signaling pathways, use of molecular data from initial tumor resection as entry criteria in trials of recurrent disease, poor drug delivery to the brain, and unclear pharmacodynamic effects of drugs on tumor tissue.

Tumor heterogeneity poses a significant challenge with glioblastoma being renowned for its intratumoral heterogeneity. Due to the heterogenous nature of these tumors, it is possible that we may be inhibiting a distinct group of cells susceptible to that specific targeted pathway yet still permitting the proliferation of another group of cells whose development is independent of that pathway. A recent study has demonstrated that glioblastoma subtype classifiers can variably be expressed even across individual cells within a tumor [159].

Additionally, these tumors appear to have the intrinsic ability to respond to the inhibition of one pathway by upregulating another different pathway making a single agent unsuccessful in stopping tumor progression. For example, the use of EGFR inhibitors has demonstrated the lack of ability to change downstream targets like Akt and may even upregulate the activity of the

Table 9.2 Targeted therapy for malignant gliomas in ongoing clinical trials or trails with results not yet published

Therapy	Pathway	Target/s
PD-0332991	RB	CDK4 [10]
Ad5CMV-p53	P53	p53 [18]
Adenovirus p53 (SCH-58500)	P53	p53 [19]
SGT-53	P53	p53 [21]
MK-1775	P53	Weel [25]
Afatanib	RTK	EGFR and HER2 [88, 89]
Dacomitinib	RTK	EGFR [90, 91]
Dasatinib	RTK	PDGFR, Src, Bcr-Abl, c-Kit, and EphA2 [107, 108]
Tandutinib	RTK	PDGFR, FLT3, and c-Kit [111, 112]
BKM-120	RTK	PI3K [119–121]
XL-147	RTK	PI3K [122]
XL-765	RTK	PI3K and mTOR [122, 124]
Pictilisib	RTK	PI3K [124]
BEZ235	RTK	PI3K and mTOR [122, 124]
Perifosine	RTK	Akt and PI3K [129, 130]
Ipatasertib	RTK	Akt [124]
Nelfinavir	RTK	Akt [132]
AZD8055	RTK	mTORC1/mTORC2 [142]

Abbreviations: *RB* retinoblastoma, *P53* tumor protein p53, *RTK* receptor tyrosine kinase, *CDK4* cyclin-dependent kinase 4, *EGFR* epidermal growth factor receptor, *HER2* human epidermal growth factor receptor 2, *PDGFR* platelet-derived growth factor receptor, *EphA2* ephrin type-A receptor 2, *FLT3* Fms-like tyrosine kinase-3, *PI3K* phosphatidylinositide 3-kinases, *mTOR* mammalian target of rapamycin

PI3K/Akt pathway [160, 161]. Moreover, many of the mutations that we are currently targeting may be essential only for the early development of the tumor and subsequently are superseded by secondary pathways of tumor growth.

Another potential reason for the lack of success with these agents may be that entry into targeted therapy trials for recurrent disease is often based upon molecular characteristics from initial resection due to surgical resections at tumor recurrence not being routinely performed. However, it is possible that these targeted mutations may be altered at time of recurrence compared to initial diagnosis. A recent study in glioblastoma found that of the tumors expressing EGFRvIII at initial diagnosis, approximately one-half loses their EGFRvIII expression at tumor recurrence [162].

Additionally, with surgery at tumor recurrence being difficult, it is often challenging to determine how well the drugs are crossing the blood–brain barrier. Furthermore, even if the agent crosses into the brain, it is often uncertain whether the drug is inhibiting its intended target and having its envisioned effect without pathological confirmation.

Numerous ways to improve the success of targeted therapies in malignant glioma have been propositioned and are currently underway. These include the creation of more advanced preclinical animal models, development of more potent inhibitors that can affect multiple pathways, trials with a combination of drugs designed uniquely for each individual, identification of predictive molecular biomarkers, and novel adaptive trial designs.

Despite the discouraging results to date and the above challenges, the use of targeted therapies remains a promising approach that continues to be explored in malignant glioma and will hopefully someday prove more beneficial for this patient population in desperate need of more effective treatments.

References

1. Wen PY, Kesari S. Malignant gliomas in adults. N Engl J Med. 2008;359(5):492–507.
2. Stupp R, Mason WP, van den Bent MJ, et al. Radiotherapy plus concomitant and adjuvant temozolomide for glioblastoma. N Engl J Med. 2005;352 (10):987–96.
3. Tanaka S, Louis DN, Curry WT, Batchelor TT, Dietrich J. Diagnostic and therapeutic avenues for glioblastoma: no longer a dead end? Nature Rev Clin Oncol. 2013 Jan;10:14–26. Doi:10.1038/nrclinonc.2012.20.
4. Cancer Genomc Atlas Research Network. Comprehensive genomic characterization defines human glioblastoma genes and core pathways. Nature. 2008;455(7216):1061–8. Doi:10.1038/nature07385.
5. Murphree AL, Benedict WF. Retinoblastoma: clues to human oncogenesis. Science. 1984;223 (4640):1028–33. Doi:10.1126/science.6320372.
6. Ohgaki H, Kleihues P. Genetic alterations and signaling pathways in the evolution of gliomas. Cancer Sci. 2009;100:2235–41.
7. Lin F, de Gooijer MC, Hanekamp D, Brandsma D, Beijnen JH, van Tellingen O. Targeting core (mutated) pathways of high-grade gliomas: challenges of intrinsic resistance and drug efflux. CNS Oncol. 2013;2(3):271–88. Doi:10.2217/cns.13.15.
8. Schwartz GK, LoRusso PM, Dickson MA, et al. Phase I study of PD 0332991, a cyclin-dependent kinase inhibitor, administered in 3-week cycles (schedule 2/1). Br J Cancer. 2011;104(12):1862–8.
9. Flaherty KT, LoRusso PM, Demichele A, et al. Phase I, dose-escalation trial of the oral cyclin-dependent kinase 4/6 inhibitor PD 0332991, administered using a 21-day schedule in patients with advanced cancer. Clin Cancer Res. 2012;18(2):568–76.
10. ClinicalTrials.gov. A Study of PD 0332991 in Patients With Recurrent Rb Positive Glioblastoma (PD0332991). Identifier: NCT01227434. http://clinicaltrials.gov/show/NCT01227434.
11. Surget S, Khoury MP, Bourdon JC. Uncovering the role of p53 splice variants in human malignancy: a clinical perspective. Onco Targets Ther. 2013;7:57–68. Doi:10.2147/OTT.S53876.
12. McBride OW, Merry D, Givol D. The gene for human p53 cellular tumor antigen is located on chromosome 17 short arm (17p13). Proc Natl Acad Sci USA. 1986;83(1):130–4. Doi:10.1073/pnas.83.1.130.
13. Vousden KH, Lane DP. p53 in health and disease. Nat Rev Mol Cell Biol. 2007;8:275–83.
14. Reifenberger G, Liu L, Ichimura K, Schmidt EE, Collins VP. Amplification and overexpression of the MDM2 gene in a subset of human malignant gliomas without p53 mutations. Cancer Res. 1993;53:2736–9.
15. Riemenschneider MJ, Buschges R, Wolter M, et al. Amplification and overexpression of the MDM4 (MDMX) gene from 1q32 in a subset of malignant gliomas without TP53 mutation or MDM2 amplification. Cancer Res. 1999;59:6091–6.
16. Kamijo T, Weber JD, Zambetti G, Zindy F, Roussel MF, Sherr CJ. Functional and physical interactions of the ARF tumor suppressor with p53 and Mdm2. Proc Natl Acad Sci USA. 1998;95:8292–7.
17. Lang FF, Bruner JM, Fuller GN, Aldape K, Prados MD, Chang S, Berger MS, McDermott MW, Kunwar SM, Junck LR, Chandler W, Zwiebel JA, Kaplan RS, Yung WK. Phase I trial of adenovirus-mediated p53 gene therapy for recurrent glioma: biological and clinical results. J Clin Oncol. 2003;21:2508–18.
18. ClinicalTrials.gov. Gene Therapy in Treating Patients With Recurrent Malignant Gliomas Identifier: NCT00004041. https://clinicaltrials.gov/ct2/show/NCT00004041?term=NCT00004041&rank=1.
19. ClinicalTrials.gov. Gene Therapy in Treating Patients With Recurrent or Progressive Brain Tumors Identifier: NCT00004080. https://clinicaltrials.gov/ct2/show/NCT00004080?term=NCT00004080&rank=1.
20. Kim SS, Rait A, Kim E, Pirollo KF, Chang EH. A tumor-targeting p53 nanodelivery system limits chemoresistance to temozolomide prolonging survival in a mouse model of glioblastoma multiforme. Nanomedicine. 2015;11(2):301–11. Doi:10.1016/j.nano.2014.09.005 Epub 2014 Sep 18.
21. ClinicalTrials.gov. Phase II Study of Combined Temozolomide and SGT-53 for Treatment of Recurrent Glioblastoma Identifier: NCT02340156. https://clinicaltrials.gov/ct2/show/NCT02340156?term=sgt-53&rank=1.
22. Yuan Y, Liao YM, Hsueh CT, Mirshahidi HR. Novel targeted therapeutics: inhibitors of MDM2, ALK and PARP. J Hematol Oncol. 2011;4:16. Doi:10.1186/1756-8722-4-16.
23. Tabernero J, et al. Phase I pharmacokinetic (PK) and pharmacodynamic (PD) study of HDM-2 antagonist JNJ-26854165 in patients with advanced refractory solid tumors. J Clin Oncol (Meet Abs). 2009;27(15S):3514.
24. Bridges KA, Hirai H, Buser CA, Brooks C, Liu H, Buchholz TA, Molkentine JM, Mason KA, Meyn RE. MK-1775, a novel Wee1 kinase inhibitor, radiosensitizes p53-defective human tumor cells. Clin Cancer Res. 2011;17(17):5638–48. Doi:10.1158/1078-0432.CCR-11-0650 Epub 2011 Jul 28.
25. ClinicalTrials.gov. WEE1 Inhibitor MK-1775, Radiation Therapy, and Temozolomide in Treating Patients With Newly Diagnosed or Recurrent Glioblastoma Multiforme. Identifier: NCT01849146. https://

clinicaltrials.gov/ct2/show/study/NCT01849146?term=wee1+glioblastoma&rank=1&show_desc=Y#desc.

26. Zwick E, Bange J, Ullrich A. Receptor tyrosine kinase signalling as a target for cancer intervention strategies. Endocr. Relat Cancer. 2001;8(3):161–73. Doi:10.1677/erc.0.0080161.
27. Plate KH, Breier G, Weich HA, et al. Vascular endothelial growth factor is a potential tumour angiogenesis factor in human gliomas in vivo. Nature. 1992;359:845–8.
28. Rini BI, Small EJ. Biology and clinical development of vascular endothelial growth factor-targeted therapy in renal cell carcinoma. J Clin Oncol. 2005;23(5):1028–43.
29. Cohen MH, Shen YL, Keegan P, Pazdur R. FDA drug approval summary: bevacizumab (Avastin) as treatment of recurrent glioblastoma multiforme. Oncologist. 2009;14:1131–8.
30. Friedman HS, Prados MD, Wen PY, Mikkelsen T, Schiff D, Abrey LE, Yung WK, Paleologos N, Nicholas MK, Jensen R, Vredenburgh J, Huang J, Zheng M, Cloughesy T. Bevacizumab alone and in combination with irinotecan in recurrent glioblastoma. J Clin Oncol. 2009;27(28):4733–40. Doi:10.1200/JCO.2008.19.8721 Epub 2009 Aug 31.
31. Kreisl TN, Kim L, Moore K, et al. Phase II trial of single-agent bevacizumab followed by bevacizumab plus irinotecan at tumor progression in recurrent glioblastoma. J Clin Oncol. 2009;27:740–5.
32. Gilbert MR, Dignam JJ, Armstrong TS, Wefel JS, Blumenthal DT, Vogelbaum MA, Colman H, Chakravarti A, Pugh S, Won M, Jeraj R, Brown PD, Jaeckle KA, Schiff D, Stieber VW, Brachman DG, Werner-Wasik M, Tremont-Lukats IW, Sulman EP, Aldape KD, Curran WJ Jr, Mehta MP. A randomized trial of bevacizumab for newly diagnosed glioblastoma. N Engl J Med. 2014;370(8):699–708. Doi:10.1056/NEJMoa1308573.
33. Chinot OL, Wick W, Mason W, Henriksson R, Saran F, Nishikawa R, Carpentier AF, Hoang-Xuan K, Kavan P, Cernea D, Brandes AA, Hilton M, Abrey L, Cloughesy T. Bevacizumab plus radiotherapy-temozolomide for newly diagnosed glioblastoma. N Engl J Med. 2014;370(8):709–22. Doi:10.1056/NEJMoa1308345.
34. Taal W, Oosterkamp HM, Walenkamp AM, Dubbink HJ, Beerepoot LV, Hanse MC, Buter J, Honkoop AH, Boerman D, de Vos FY, Dinjens WN, Enting RH, Taphoorn MJ, van den Berkmortel FW, Jansen RL, Brandsma D, Bromberg JE, van Heuvel I, Vernhout RM, van der Holt B, van den Bent MJ. Single agent bevacizumab or lomustine versus a combination of bevacizumab plus lomustine in patients with recurrent glioblastoma (BELOB trial): a randomised controlled phase 2 trial. Lancet Oncol. 2014;15(9):943–53. Doi:10.1016/S1470-2045(14)70314-6 Epub 2014 Jul 15.
35. ClinicalTrials.gov. Bevacizumab and Lomustine for Recurrent GBM. Identifier: NCT01290939. https://clinicaltrials.gov/ct2/show/NCT01290939?term=ccnu+and+bevacizumab+and+ccnu&rank=4.
36. Soffietti R1, Trevisan E, Bertero L, Cassoni P, Morra I, Fabrini MG, Pasqualetti F, Lolli I, Castiglione A, Ciccone G, Rudà R. Bevacizumab and fotemustine for recurrent glioblastoma: a phase II study of AINO (Italian Association of Neuro-Oncology). J Neurooncol. 2014 Feb;116(3):533–41. Doi:10.1007/s11060-013-1317-x Epub 2013 Dec 1.
37. Field KM, Simes J, Nowak AK, Cher L, Wheeler H, Hovey EJ, Brown CS, Barnes EH, Sawkins K, Livingstone A, Freilich R, Phal PM, Fitt G, CABARET/COGNO investigators, Rosenthal MA. Randomized phase 2 study of carboplatin and bevacizumab in recurrent glioblastoma. Neuro Oncol 2015 Nov;17(11):1504–13. Doi:10.1093/neuonc/nov104. Epub 2015 Jun 30.
38. Batchelor TT, Duda DG, di Tomaso E, Ancukiewicz M, Plotkin SR, Gerstner E, Eichler AF, Drappatz J, Hochberg FH, Benner T, Louis DN, Cohen KS, Chea H, Exarhopoulos A, Loeffler JS, Moses MA, Ivy P, Sorensen AG, Wen PY, Jain RK. Phase II study of cediranib, an oral pan-vascular endothelial growth factor receptor tyrosine kinase inhibitor, in patients with recurrent glioblastoma. J Clin Oncol. 2010;28(17):2817–23. Doi:10.1200/JCO.2009.26.3988 Epub 2010 May 10.
39. Batchelor TT, Mulholland P, Neyns B, Nabors LB, Campone M, Wick A, Mason W, Mikkelsen T, Phuphanich S, Ashby LS, Degroot J, Gattamaneni R, Cher L, Rosenthal M, Payer F, Jürgensmeier JM, Jain RK, Sorensen AG, Xu J, Liu Q, van den Bent M. Phase III randomized trial comparing the efficacy of cediranib as monotherapy, and in combination with lomustine, versus lomustine alone in patients with recurrent glioblastoma. J Clin Oncol. 2013;31(26):3212–8. Doi:10.1200/JCO.2012.47.2464 Epub 2013 Aug 12.
40. Iwamoto FM, Lamborn KR, Robins HI, Mehta MP, Chang SM, Butowski NA, Deangelis LM, Abrey LE, Zhang WT, Prados MD, Fine HA. Phase II trial of pazopanib (GW786034), an oral multi-targeted angiogenesis inhibitor, for adults with recurrent glioblastoma (North American Brain Tumor Consortium Study 06-02). Neuro Oncol. 2010;12(8):855–61. Doi:10.1093/neuonc/noq025 Epub 2010 Mar 3.
41. Reardon DA, Groves MD, Wen PY, Nabors L, Mikkelsen T, Rosenfeld S, Raizer J, Barriuso J, McLendon RE, Suttle AB, Ma B, Curtis CM, Dar MM, de Bono J. A phase I/II trial of pazopanib in combination with lapatinib in adult patients with relapsed malignant glioma. Clin Cancer Res. 2013;19(4):900–8. Doi:10.1158/1078-0432.CCR-12-1707 Epub 2013 Jan 30.
42. Hainsworth JD, Ervin T, Friedman E, Priego V, Murphy PB, Clark BL, Lamar RE. Concurrent radiotherapy and temozolomide followed by

temozolomide and sorafenib in the first-line treatment of patients with glioblastoma multiforme. Cancer. 2010;116(15):3663–9. Doi:10.1002/cncr.25275.

43. Reardon DA, Vredenburgh JJ, Desjardins A, Peters K, Gururangan S, Sampson JH, Marcello J, Herndon JE 2nd, McLendon RE, Janney D, Friedman AH, Bigner DD, Friedman HS. Effect of CYP3A-inducing anti-epileptics on sorafenib exposure: results of a phase II study of sorafenib plus daily temozolomide in adults with recurrent glioblastoma. J Neurooncol. 2011;101(1):57–66. Doi:10.1007/s11060-010-0217-6 Epub 2010 May 5.
44. Galanis E, Anderson SK, Lafky JM, Uhm JH, Giannini C, Kumar SK, Kimlinger TK, Northfelt DW, Flynn PJ, Jaeckle KA, Kaufmann TJ, Buckner JC. Phase II study of bevacizumab in combination with sorafenib in recurrent glioblastoma (N0776): a north central cancer treatment group trial. Clin Cancer Res. 2013;19(17):4816–23. Doi:10.1158/1078-0432.CCR-13-0708 Epub 2013 Jul 5.
45. Peereboom DM, Ahluwalia MS, Ye X, Supko JG, Hilderbrand SL, Phuphanich S, Nabors LB, Rosenfeld MR, Mikkelsen T, Grossman SA. New Approaches to Brain Tumor Therapy Consortium. NABTT 0502: a phase II and pharmacokinetic study of erlotinib and sorafenib for patients with progressive or recurrent glioblastoma multiforme. Neuro Oncol. 2013;15(4):490–6. Doi:10.1093/neuonc/nos322 Epub 2013 Jan 17.
46. Lee EQ, Kuhn J, Lamborn KR, Abrey L, DeAngelis LM, Lieberman F, Robins HI, Chang SM, Yung WK, Drappatz J, Mehta MP, Levin VA, Aldape K, Dancey JE, Wright JJ, Prados MD, Cloughesy TF, Gilbert MR, Wen PY. Phase I/II study of sorafenib in combination with temsirolimus for recurrent glioblastoma or gliosarcoma: North American Brain Tumor Consortium study 05-02. Neuro Oncol. 2012;14(12):1511–8. Doi:10.1093/neuonc/nos264 Epub 2012 Oct 24.
47. Muhic A, Poulsen HS, Sorensen M, Grunnet K, Lassen U. Phase II open-label study of nintedanib in patients with recurrent glioblastoma multiforme. J Neurooncol. 2013;111(2):205–12. Doi:10.1007/s11060-012-1009-y Epub 2012 Nov 27.
48. Kreisl TN, McNeill KA, Sul J, Iwamoto FM, Shih J, Fine HA. A phase I/II trial of vandetanib for patients with recurrent malignant glioma. Neuro Oncol. 2012;14(12):1519–26. Doi:10.1093/neuonc/nos265 Epub 2012 Oct 25.
49. Chheda MG, Wen PY, Hochberg FH, Chi AS, Drappatz J, Eichler AF, Yang D, Beroukhim R, Norden AD, Gerstner ER, Betensky RA, Batchelor TT. Vandetanib plus sirolimus in adults with recurrent glioblastoma: results of a phase I and dose expansion cohort study. J Neurooncol. 2015 Feb;121(3):627–34. Doi:10.1007/s11060-014-1680-2 Epub 2014 Dec 13.
50. Neyns B, Sadones J, Chaskis C, Dujardin M, Everaert H, Lv S, Duerinck J, Tynninen O, Nupponen N, Michotte A, De Greve J. Phase II study of sunitinib malate in patients with recurrent high-grade glioma. J Neurooncol. 2011;103(3):491–501. Doi:10.1007/s11060-010-0402-7 Epub 2010 Sep 25.
51. Pan E, Yu D, Yue B, Potthast L, Chowdhary S, Smith P, Chamberlain M. A prospective phase II single-institution trial of sunitinib for recurrent malignant glioma. J Neurooncol. 2012;110(1):111–8. Doi:10.1007/s11060-012-0943-z Epub 2012 Jul 26.
52. Kreisl TN, Smith P, Sul J, Salgado C, Iwamoto FM, Shih JH, Fine HA. Continuous daily sunitinib for recurrent glioblastoma. J Neurooncol. 2013;111(1):41–8. Doi:10.1007/s11060-012-0988-z Epub 2012 Oct 20.
53. Reardon DA, Vredenburgh JJ, Coan A, Desjardins A, Peters KB, Gururangan S, Sathornsumetee S, Rich JN, Herndon JE, Friedman HS. Phase I study of sunitinib and irinotecan for patients with recurrent malignant glioma. J Neurooncol. 2011;105(3):621–7. Doi:10.1007/s11060-011-0631-4 Epub 2011 Jul 9.
54. de Groot JF1, Lamborn KR, Chang SM, Gilbert MR, Cloughesy TF, Aldape K, Yao J, Jackson EF, Lieberman F, Robins HI, Mehta MP, Lassman AB, Deangelis LM, Yung WK, Chen A, Prados MD, Wen PY. Phase II study of aflibercept in recurrent malignant glioma: a North American Brain Tumor Consortium study. J Clin Oncol. 2011 Jul 1;29(19):2689–95. Doi:10.1200/JCO.2010.34.1636 Epub 2011 May 23.
55. Gerstner ER, Eichler AF, Plotkin SR, Drappatz J, Doyle CL, Xu L, Duda DG, Wen PY, Jain RK, Batchelor TT. Phase I trial with biomarker studies of vatalanib (PTK787) in patients with newly diagnosed glioblastoma treated with enzyme inducing anti-epileptic drugs and standard radiation and temozolomide. J Neurooncol. 2011;103(2):325–32. Doi:10.1007/s11060-010-0390-7 Epub 2010 Sep 7.
56. Reardon DA, Egorin MJ, Desjardins A, Vredenburgh JJ, Beumer JH, Lagattuta TF, Gururangan S, Herndon JE 2nd, Salvado AJ, Friedman HS. Phase I pharmacokinetic study of the vascular endothelial growth factor receptor tyrosine kinase inhibitor vatalanib (PTK787) plus imatinib and hydroxyurea for malignant glioma. Cancer. 2009;115(10):2188–98. Doi:10.1002/cncr.24213.
57. Brandes AA, Stupp R, Hau P, Lacombe D, Gorlia T, Tosoni A, Mirimanoff RO, Kros JM, van den Bent MJ. EORTC study 26041-22041: phase I/II study on concomitant and adjuvant temozolomide (TMZ) and radiotherapy (RT) with PTK787/ZK222584 (PTK/ZK) in newly diagnosed glioblastoma. Eur J Cancer. 2010;46(2):348–54. Doi:10.1016/j.ejca.2009.10.029 Epub 2009 Nov 27.
58. Wen PY, Prados M, Schiff D, Reardon DA, Cloughesy T, Mikkelsen T, Batchelor T, Drappatz J, Chamberlain MC, De Groot JF. Phase II study of XL184 (BMS 907351), an inhibitor of MET,

VEGFR2, and RET, in patients (pts) with progressive glioblastoma (GB) [abstract]. J Clin Oncol. 2010;28(15 suppl):181s.
59. Normanno N, De Luca A, Bianco C, et al. Epidermal growth factor receptor (EGFR) signaling in cancer. Gene. 2006;366:2–16.
60. Ekstrand AJ, James CD, Cavenee WK, et al. Genes for epidermal growth factor receptor, transforming growth factor alpha, and epidermal growth factor and their expression in human gliomas in vivo. Cancer Res. 1991;51:2164–72.
61. Barker FG 2nd, SimmonsML Chang SM, et al. EGFR overexpression and radiation response in glioblastoma multiforme. Int J Radiat Oncol Biol Phys. 2001;51:410–8.
62. Pelloski CE, Ballman KV, Furth AF, et al. Epidermal growth factor receptor variant III status defines clinically distinct subtypes of glioblastoma. J Clin Oncol. 2007;25:2288–94.
63. Shinojima N, Tada K, Shiraishi S, Kamiryo T, Kochi M, Nakamura H, Makino K, Saya H, Hirano H, Kuratsu J, Oka K, Ishimaru Y, Ushio Y. Prognostic value of epidermal growth factor receptor in patients with glioblastoma multiforme. Cancer Res. 2003;63:6962–70.
64. Uhm JH, Ballman KV, Wu W, et al. Phase II evaluation of gefitinib in patients with newly diagnosed grade 4 astrocytoma: Mayo/North Central Cancer Treatment Group Study N0074. Int J Radiat Oncol Biol Phys. 2011;80(2):347–53.
65. Chakravarti A, Wang M, Robins HI, et al. RTOG 0211: a phase ½ study of radiation therapy with concurrent gefitinib for newly diagnosed glioblastoma patients. Int J Radiat Oncol Biol Phys. 2013;85(5):1206–11.
66. Rich JN, Reardon DA, Peery T, et al. Phase II trial of gefitinib in recurrent glioblastoma. J Clin Oncol. 2004;22(1):133–42.
67. Franceschi E, Cavallo G, Lonardi S, et al. Gefitinib in patients with progressive high-grade gliomas: a multicenter phase II study by Gruppo Italiano Cooperativo di Neuro-Oncologia (GICNO). Br J Cancer. 2007;96:1047–51.
68. Reardon DA, Quinn JA, Vredenburgh JJ, et al. Phase I trial of gefitinib plus sirolimus in adults with recurrent malignant glioma. Clin Cancer Res. 2006;12(3 Pt 1):860–8.
69. Kreisl TN, Lassman AB, Mischel PS, et al. A pilot study of everolimus and gefitinib in the treatment of recurrent glioblastoma (GBM). J Neurooncol. 2009;92(1):99–105.
70. YungWK, Vredenburgh JJ, Cloughesy TF, et al. Safety and efficacy of erlotinib in first-relapse glioblastoma: a phase II open-label study. Neuro Oncol. 2010;12(10):1061–70.
71. Raizer JJ, Abrey LE, Lassman AB, et al. A phase II trial of erlotinib in patients with recurrent malignant gliomas and nonprogressive glioblastoma multiforme postradiation therapy. Neuro Oncol. 2010;12 (1):95–103.
72. Peereboom DM, Shepard DR, Ahluwalia MS, et al. Phase II trial of erlotinib with temozolomide and radiation in patients with newly diagnosed glioblastoma multiforme. J Neurooncol. 2010;98(1):93–9.
73. Prados MD, Chang SM, Butowski N, et al. Phase II study of erlotinib plus temozolomide during and after radiation therapy in patients with newly diagnosed glioblastoma multiforme and gliosarcoma. J Clin Oncol. 2009;27(4):579–84.
74. Brown PD, Krishnan S, Sarkaria JN, et al. Phase I/II trial of erlotinib and temozolomide with radiation therapy in the treatment of newly diagnosed glioblastoma multiforme: North Central Cancer Treatment Group Study N0177. J Clin Oncol. 2008;26(34):5603–9.
75. Krishnan S, Brown PD, Ballman KV, et al. Phase I trial of erlotinib with radiation therapy in patients with glioblastoma multiforme: results of North Central Cancer Treatment Group protocol N0177. Int J Radiat Oncol Biol Phys. 2006;65(4):1192–9.
76. Prados MD, Lamborn KR, Chang S, et al. Phase 1 study of erlotinib HCl alone and combined with temozolomide in patients with stable or recurrent malignant glioma. Neuro Oncol. 2006;8(1):67–78.
77. De Groot JF, Gilbert MR, Aldape K, et al. Phase II study of carboplatin and erlotinib (Tarceva, OSI-774) in patients with recurrent glioblastoma. J Neurooncol. 2008;90(1):89–97.
78. Sathornsumetee S, Dejardins A, Vredenburgh JJ, et al. Phase II trial of bevacizumab and erlotinib in patients with recurrent malignant glioma. Neuro Oncol. 2010;12(12):1300–10.
79. Nghiemphu PL, Lai A, Green RM, et al. A dose escalation trial for the combination of erlotinib and sirolimus for recurrent malignant gliomas. J Neurooncol. 2012;110(2):245–50.
80. Reardon DA, Desjardin A, Vredenburgh JJ, et al. Phase 2 trial of erlotinib plus sirolimus in adults with recurrent glioblastoma. J Neurooncol. 2010;96 (2):219–30.
81. Neyns B, Sadones J, Joosens E, et al. Stratified phase II trial of cetuximab in patients with recurrent high-grade glioma. Ann Oncol. 2009;20:1596–603.
82. Hasselbalch B, Lassen U, Hansen S, Holmberg M, Sørensen M, Kosteljanetz M, Broholm H, Stockhausen MT, Poulsen HS. Cetuximab, bevacizumab, and irinotecan for patients with primary glioblastoma and progression after radiation therapy and temozolomide: a phase II trial. Neuro Oncol. 2010;12(5):508–16. Doi:10.1093/neuonc/nop063 Epub 2010 Feb 5.
83. Thiessen B, Stewart C, Tsao M, Kamel-Reid S, Schaiquevich P, Mason W, Easaw J, Belanger K, Forsyth P, McIntosh L, Eisenhauer E. A phase I/II trial of GW572016 (lapatinib) in recurrent glioblastoma multiforme: clinical outcomes, pharmacokinetics and molecular correlation. Cancer Chemother Pharmacol. 2010;65(2):353–61. Doi:10.1007/s00280-009-1041-6.
84. Reardon DA, Groves MD, Wen PY, Nabors L, Mikkelsen T, Rosenfeld S, Raizer J, Barriuso J,

McLendon RE, Suttle AB, Ma B, Curtis CM, Dar MM, de Bono J. A phase I/II trial of pazopanib in combination with lapatinib in adult patients with relapsed malignant glioma. Clin Cancer Res. 2013;19(4):900–8. Doi:10.1158/1078-0432.CCR-12-1707 Epub 2013 Jan 30.
85. Karavasilis V, Kotoula V, Pentheroudakis G, Televantou D, Lambaki S, Chrisafi S, Bobos M, Fountzilas G. A phase I study of temozolomide and lapatinib combination in patients with recurrent high-grade gliomas. J Neurol. 2013;260(6):1469–80. Doi:10.1007/s00415-012-6812-z Epub 2013 Jan 5.
86. Reardon DA, Conrad CA, Cloughesy T, et al. Phase I study of AEE788, a novel multitarget inhibitor of ErbB and VEGF receptor-family tyrosine kinases, in recurrent glioblastoma patients. Cancer Chemother Pharmacol. 2012;69(6):1507–18.
87. Minkovsky N, Berezov A. BIBW-2992, a dual receptor tyrosine kinase inhibitor for the treatment of solid tumors. Curr Opin Investig Drugs. 2008 Dec;9(12): 1336–46. PMID 19037840.
88. ClinicalTrials.gov. BIBW 2992 (Afatinib) With or Without Daily Temozolomide in the Treatment of Patients With Recurrent Malignant Glioma. Identifier: NCT00727506. https://clinicaltrials.gov/ct2/show/NCT00727506?term=Afatinib+glioma&rank=1.
89. ClinicalTrials.gov. Open Label Trial to Explore Safety of Combining Afatinib (BIBW 2992) and Radiotherapy With or Without Temozolomide in Newly Diagnosed Glioblastoma Multiform. Identifier: NCT00977431. https://clinicaltrials.gov/ct2/show/NCT00977431?term=Afatinib+glioma&rank=3.
90. ClinicalTrials.gov. PF-00299804 in Adult Patients With Relapsed/Recurrent Glioblastoma. Identifier: NCT01112527 https://clinicaltrials.gov/ct2/show/NCT01112527?term=Dacomitinib+GLIOMA&rank=.
91. ClinicalTrials.gov. Safety and Efficacy of PF-299804 (Dacomitinib), a Pan-HER Irreversible Inhibitor, in Patients With Recurrent Glioblastoma With EGFR Amplification or Presence of EGFRvIII Mutation. A Phase II CT. Identifier: NCT01520870. https://clinicaltrials.gov/ct2/show/NCT01520870?term=Dacomitinib+GLIOMA&rank=1.
92. Solomón MT, Selva JC, Figueredo J, Vaquer J, Toledo C, Quintanal N, Salva S, Domíngez R, Alert J, Marinello JJ, Catalá M, Griego MG, Martell JA, Luaces PL, Ballesteros J, de-Castro N, Bach F, Crombet T. Radiotherapy plus nimotuzumab or placebo in the treatment of high grade glioma patients: results from a randomized, double blind trial. BMC Cancer. 2013 Jun 19;13:299. Doi:10.1186/1471-2407-13-299.
93. Westphal M, Heese O, Steinbach JP, Schnell O, Schackert G, Mehdorn M, Schulz D, Simon M, Schlegel U, Senft C, Geletneky K, Braun C, Hartung JG, Reuter D, Metz MW, Bach F, Pietsch T. A randomised, open label phase III trial with nimotuzumab, an anti-epidermal growth factor receptor monoclonal antibody in the treatment of newly diagnosed adult glioblastoma. Eur J Cancer. 2015;51(4):522–32. Doi:10.1016/j.ejca.2014.12.019 Epub 2015 Jan 20.
94. Matsui T, Heidaran M, Miki T, Popescu N, La Rochelle W, Kraus M, Pierce J, Aaronson S. Isolation of a novel receptor cDNA establishes the existence of two PDGF receptor genes. Science. 1989;243(4892):800–4. Doi:10.1126/science.2536956.
95. Stenman G, Rorsman F, Huebner K, Betsholtz C. The human platelet-derived growth factor alpha chain (PDGFA) gene maps to chromosome 7p22. Cytogenet Cell Genet. 1992;60(3–4):206–7. Doi:10.1159/000133337.
96. Alentorn A, Marie Y, Carpentier C, et al. Prevalence, clinicopathological value, and co-occurrence of PDGFRA abnormalities in diffuse gliomas. Neuro Oncol. 2012;14:1393-140.
97. Buchdunger E, Cioffi CL, Law N, et al. Abl protein-tyrosine kinase inhibitor STI571 inhibits in vitro signal transduction mediated by c-Kit and platelet-derived growth factor receptors. J Pharmacol Exp Ther. 2000;295:139–45.
98. Druker BJ, Talpaz M, Resta DJ, et al. Efficacy and safety of a specific inhibitor of the BCR-ABL tyrosine kinase in chronic myeloid leukemia. N Engl J Med. 2001;344:1031–7.
99. Demetri GD, von Mehren M, Blanke CD, et al. Efficacy and safety of imatinib mesylate in advanced gastrointestinal stromal tumors. N Engl J Med. 2002;347:472–80.
100. Wen PY, Yung WK, Lamborn KR, et al. Phase I/II study of imatinib mesylate for recurrent malignant gliomas: North American Brain Tumor Consortium Study 99-08. Clin Cancer Res. 2006;12(16):4899–907.
101. Razis E, Selviaridis P, Labropoulos S, et al. Phase II study of neoadjuvant imatinib in glioblastoma: evaluation of clinical and molecular effects of the treatment. Clin Cancer Res. 2009;15(19):6258–66.
102. Reardon DA, Dresemann G, Taillibert S, et al. Multicentre phase II studies evaluating imatinib plus hydroxyurea in patients with progressive glioblastoma. Br J Cancer. 2009;101(12):1995–2004.
103. Dresemann G, Weller M, Rosenthal MA, et al. Imatinib in combination with hydroxyurea versus hydroxyurea alone as oral therapy in patients with progressive pretreated glioblastoma resistant to standard dose temozolomide. J Neurooncol. 2010;96(3):393–402.
104. Desjardins A, Quinn JA, Vredenburgh JJ, Sathornsumetee S, Friedman AH, Herndon JE, McLendon RE, Provenzale JM, Rich JN, Sampson JH, Gururangan S, Dowell JM, Salvado A, Friedman HS, Reardon DA. Phase II study of imatinib mesylate and hydroxyurea for recurrent grade III malignant gliomas. J Neurooncol. 2007;83(1):53–60 Epub 2007 Jan 24.

105. Reardon DA, Egorin MJ, Quinn JA, et al. Phase II study of imatinib mesylate plus hydroxyurea in adults with recurrent glioblastoma multiforme. J Clin Oncol. 2005;23(36):9359–68.
106. Lassman AB, Pugh SL, Gilbert MR, Aldape KD, Geinoz S, Beumer JH, Christner SM, Komaki R, DeAngelis LM, Gaur R, Youssef E, Wagner H, Won M, Mehta MP. Phase 2 trial of dasatinib in target-selected patients with recurrent glioblastoma (RTOG 0627). Neuro Oncol. 2015;17(7):992–8. Doi:10.1093/neuonc/nov011 Epub 2015 Mar 10.
107. ClinicalTrials.gov. Dasatinib and Bevacizumab in Treating Patients With Recurrent or Progressive High-Grade Glioma or Glioblastoma Multiforme. Identifier: NCT00892177. https://clinicaltrials.gov/ct2/show/NCT00892177?term=Dasatinib+glioma&rank=5.
108. ClinicalTrials.gov. Dasatinib or Placebo, Radiation Therapy, and Temozolomide in Treating Patients With Newly Diagnosed Glioblastoma Multiforme Identifier: NCT00869401. https://clinicaltrials.gov/ct2/show/NCT00869401?term=Dasatinib+glioma&rank=11.
109. Franceschi E, Stupp R, van den Bent MJ, et al. EORTC 26083 phase I/II trial of dasatinib in combination with CCNU in patients with recurrent glioblastoma. Neuro Oncol. 2012;12(12):1503–10.
110. Reardon DA, Vredenburgh JJ, Desjardins A, Peters KB, Sathornsumetee S, Threatt S, Sampson JH, Herndon JE 2nd, Coan A, McSherry F, Rich JN, McLendon RE, Zhang S. Friedman HS. Phase 1 trial of dasatinib plus erlotinib in adults with recurrent malignant glioma. J Neurooncol. 2012;108(3):499–506. Doi:10.1007/s11060-012-0848-x Epub 2012 Mar 10.
111. ClinicalTrials.gov. Tandutinib in Treating Patients With Recurrent or Progressive Glioblastoma. Identifier: NCT00379080. https://clinicaltrials.gov/ct2/show/NCT00379080?term=Tandutinib+glioma&rank=31.
112. ClinicalTrials.gov. Tandutinib Plus Bevacizumab to Treat Recurrent Brain Tumors. Identifier: NCT00667394. https://clinicaltrials.gov/ct2/show/NCT00667394?term=Tandutinib+glioma&rank=1.
113. Watanabe K, Tachibana O, Sata K, Yonekawa Y, Kleihues P, Ohgaki H. Overexpression of the EGF receptor and p53 mutations are mutually exclusive in the evolution of primary and secondary glioblastomas. Brain Pathol. 1996;6:217–23.
114. Wong AJ, Ruppert JM, Bigner SH, et al. Structural alterations of the epidermal growth factor receptor gene in human gliomas. Proc Natl Acad Sci USA. 1992;89:2965–9.
115. Manning BD, Cantley LC. AKT/PKB Signaling: Navigating Downstream. Cell. 2007;129(7):1261–74. Doi:10.1016/j.cell.2007.06.009.
116. Hay N, Sonenberg N. Upstream and downstream of mTOR. Genes Dev. 2004;18(16):1926–45. Doi:10.1101/gad.1212704. PMID 15314020.
117. Akhavan D, Cloughesy TF, Mischel PS. mTOR signaling in glioblastoma: lessons learned from bench to bedside. Neuro Oncol. 2010;12:882–9.
118. Pitz MW, Eisenhauer EA, MacNeil MV, Thiessen B, Easaw JC, Macdonald DR, Eisenstat DD, Kakumanu AS, Salim M, Chalchal H, Squire J, Tsao MS, Kamel-Reid S, Banerji S, Tu D, Powers J, Hausman DF, Mason WP. Phase II study of PX-866 in recurrent glioblastoma. Neuro Oncol. 2015 Sep;17(9):1270–4. Doi:10.1093/neuonc/nou365 Epub 2015 Jan 20.
119. ClinicalTrials.gov. A Phase I Dose Escalation Study of BKM120 With Radiation Therapy and Temozolomide in Patients With Newly Diagnosed Glioblastoma. Identifier: NCT01473901. https://clinicaltrials.gov/ct2/show/NCT01473901?term=NCT01473901&rank=1.
120. ClinicalTrials.gov. Phase II Study of BKM120 for Subjects With Recurrent Glioblastoma. Identifier: NCT01339052. https://clinicaltrials.gov/ct2/show/NCT01339052?term=NCT01339052&rank=1.
121. ClinicalTrials.gov. Combination of BKM120 and Bevacizumab in Refractory Solid Tumors and Relapsed/Refractory Glioblastoma Multiforme. Identifier: NCT01349660. https://clinicaltrials.gov/ct2/show/NCT01349660?term=pi3k+glioma&rank=6.
122. ClinicalTrials.gov. Exploratory Study of XL765 (SAR245409) or XL147 (SAR245408) in Subjects With Recurrent Glioblastoma Who Are Candidates for Surgical Resection. Identifier: NCT01240460. https://clinicaltrials.gov/ct2/show/NCT01240460?term=pi3k+glioma&rank=5.
123. ClinicalTrials.gov. A Study of XL765 (SAR245409) in combination with temozolomide with and without radiation in adults with malignant gliomas. Identifier: NCT00704080. https://clinicaltrials.gov/ct2/show/NCT00704080?term=pi3k+glioma&rank=2.
124. ClinicalTrials.gov. Evaluation of the treatment effectiveness of glioblastoma/ gliosarcoma through the suppression of the PI3K/Akt pathway in compared with MK-3475. Identifier: NCT02430363. https://clinicaltrials.gov/ct2/show/NCT02430363?term=pi3k+glioma&rank=4.
125. Butowski N, Chang SM, Lamborn KR, Polley MY, Pieper R, Costello JF, Vandenberg S, Parvataneni R, Nicole A, Sneed PK, Clarke J, Hsieh E, Costa BM, Reis RM, Hristova-Kazmierski M, Nicol SJ, Thornton DE, Prados MD. Phase II and pharmacogenomics study of enzastaurin plus temozolomide during and following radiation therapy in patients with newly diagnosed glioblastoma multiforme and gliosarcoma. Neuro Oncol. 2011;13(12):1331–8. Doi:10.1093/neuonc/nor130 Epub 2011 Sep 6.
126. Wick W, Steinbach JP, Platten M, Hartmann C, Wenz F, von Deimling A, Shei P, Moreau-Donnet V, Stoffregen C, Combs SE. Enzastaurin before and concomitant with radiation therapy, followed by

enzastaurin maintenance therapy, in patients with newly diagnosed glioblastoma without MGMT promoter hypermethylation. Neuro Oncol. 2013;15 (10):1405–12. Doi:10.1093/neuonc/not100 Epub 2013 Aug 1.
127. Wick W, Puduvalli VK, Chamberlain MC, van den Bent MJ, Carpentier AF, Cher LM, Mason W, Weller M, Hong S, Musib L, Liepa AM, Thornton DE, Fine HA. Phase III study of enzastaurin compared with lomustine in the treatment of recurrent intracranial glioblastoma. J Clin Oncol. 2010;28(7):1168–74. Doi:10.1200/JCO.2009.23.2595 Epub 2010 Feb 1.
128. Kreisl TN, Kotliarova S, Butman JA, Albert PS, Kim L, Musib L, Thornton D, Fine HA. A phase I/II trial of enzastaurin in patients with recurrent high-grade gliomas. Neuro Oncol. 2010;12 (2):181–9. Doi:10.1093/neuonc/nop042 Epub 2010 Jan 22.
129. ClinicalTrials.gov. Clinical and Molecular-Metabolic Phase II trial of perifosine for recurrent/progressive malignant gliomas. Identifier: NCT00590954. https://clinicaltrials.gov/ct2/show/NCT00590954?term=akt+glioma&rank=5.
130. ClinicalTrials.gov. Perifosine and Torisel (Temsirolimus) for recurrent/progressive malignant gliomas. Identifier: NCT02238496. https://clinicaltrials.gov/ct2/show/NCT02238496?term=akt+glioma&rank=4.
131. ClinicalTrials.gov. Evaluation of the treatment effectiveness of glioblastoma/gliosarcoma through the suppression of the PI3K/Akt pathway in compared with MK-3475. Identifier: NCT02430363. https://clinicaltrials.gov/ct2/show/NCT00694837?term=akt+glioma&rank=9.
132. ClinicalTrials.gov. Study with Nelfinavir and combined radiochemotherapy for glioblastoma identifier: NCT00694837. https://clinicaltrials.gov/ct2/show/NCT00694837?term=akt+glioma&rank=9.
133. Faivre S, Kroemer G, Raymond E. Current development of mTOR inhibitors as anticancer agents. Nat Rev Drug Discov. 2006;5:671–88.
134. Krueger DA, Care MM, Holland K, et al. Everolimus for subependymal giant-cell astrocytomas in tuberous sclerosis. N Engl J Med. 2010;363: 1801–11.
135. Cloughesy T, Raizer J, Drappatz J, et al. A phase II trial of everolimus in patients with recurrent glioblastoma multiforme. Neuro Oncol. 2011;13 (suppl 3):42–3.
136. Ma DJ, Galanis E, Anderson SK, Schiff D, Kaufmann TJ, Peller PJ, Giannini C, Brown PD, Uhm JH, McGraw S, Jaeckle KA, Flynn PJ, Ligon KL, Buckner JC, Sarkaria JN. A phase II trial of everolimus, temozolomide, and radiotherapy in patients with newly diagnosed glioblastoma: NCCTG N057K. Neuro Oncol. 2015;17(9):1261–9. Doi:10.1093/neuonc/nou328 Epub 2014 Dec 18.
137. Hainsworth JD, Shih KC, Shepard GC, Tillinghast GW, Brinker BT, Spigel DR. Phase II study of concurrent radiation therapy, temozolomide, and bevacizumab followed by bevacizumab/everolimus as first-line treatment for patients with glioblastoma. Clin Adv Hematol Oncol. 2012;10(4):240–6.
138. Chang SM, Wen P, Cloughesy T, Greenberg H, Schiff D, Conrad C, et al. Phase II study of CCI-779 in patients with recurrent glioblastoma multiforme. Invest New Drugs. 2005;23:357–61.
139. Galanis E, Buckner JC, Maurer MJ, Kreisberg JI, Ballman K, Boni J, et al. Phase II trial of temsirolimus (CCI-779) in recurrent glioblastoma multiforme: a North Central Cancer Treatment Group Study. J Clin Oncol. 2005;23:5294–304.
140. Sarkaria JN1, Galanis E, Wu W, Dietz AB, Kaufmann TJ, Gustafson MP, Brown PD, Uhm JH, Rao RD, Doyle L, Giannini C, Jaeckle KA, Buckner JC. Combination of temsirolimus (CCI-779) with chemoradiation in newly diagnosed glioblastoma multiforme (GBM) (NCCTG trial N027D) is associated with increased infectious risks. Clin Cancer Res. 2010 Nov 15;16(22):5573–80. Doi:10.1158/1078-0432.CCR-10-1453 Epub 2010 Oct 4.
141. Lassen U, Sorensen M, Gaziel TB, Hasselbalch B, Poulsen HS. Phase II study of bevacizumab and temsirolimus combination therapy for recurrent glioblastoma multiforme. Anticancer Res. 2013;33 (4):1657–60.
142. ClinicalTrials.gov. AZD8055 for adults with recurrent gliomas. Identifier: NCT01316809. https://clinicaltrials.gov/ct2/show/NCT01316809?term=AZD8055&rank=2.
143. Stambolic V, Suzuki A, de la Pompa JL, Brothers GM, Mirtsos C, Sasaki T, Ruland J, Penninger JM, Siderovski DP, Mak TW. Negative regulation of PKB/Akt-dependent cell survival by the tumor suppressor PTEN. Cell. 1998;95(1):29–39.
144. Schmidt EE, Ichimura K, Goike HM, Moshref A, Liu L, Collins VP. Mutational profile of the PTEN gene in primary human astrocytic tumors and cultivated xenografts. J Neuropathol Exp Neurol. 1999;58(11):1170–83.
145. Vivanco I, Rohle D, Versele M, et al. The phosphatase and tensin homolog regulates epidermal growth factor receptor (EGFR) inhibitor response by targeting EGFR for degradation. Proc Natl Acad Sci USA. 2010;107:6459–64.
146. Bos J. ras oncogenes in human cancer: a review. Cancer Res. 1989;49(17):4682–9.
147. Downward J. Targeting RAS signalling pathways in cancer therapy. Nat. Rev. Cancer. 2003 Jan;3 (1):11–22.
148. Hurley JB, Simon MI, Teplow DB, Robishaw JD, Gilman AG. Homologies between signal transducing G proteins and ras gene products. Science. 1984;226(4676):860–2.
149. Dasgupta B, Li W, Perry A, Gutmann DH. Glioma formation in neurofibromatosis 1 reflects preferential activation of K-RAS in astrocytes. Cancer Res. 2005;65:236–45.

150. Feldkamp MM, Lau N, Guha A. Growth inhibition of astrocytoma cells by farnesyl transferase inhibitors is mediated by a combination of anti-proliferative, pro-apoptotic and antiangiogenic effects. Oncogene. 1999;18:7514–26.
151. Nghiemphu PL1, Wen PY, Lamborn KR, Drappatz J, Robins HI, Fink K, Malkin MG, Lieberman FS, DeAngelis LM, Torres-Trejo A, Chang SM, Abrey L, Fine HA, Demopoulos A, Lassman AB, Kesari S, Mehta MP, Prados MD, Cloughesy TF, North American Brain Tumor Consortium. A phase I trial of tipifarnib with radiation therapy, with and without temozolomide, for patients with newly diagnosed glioblastoma. Int J Radiat Oncol Biol Phys. 2011 Dec 1;81 (5):1422–7. Doi:10.1016/j.ijrobp.2010.07.1997 Epub 2010 Oct 8.
152. Cloughesy TF, Wen PY, Robins HI, Chang SM, Groves MD, Fink KL, et al. Phase II trial of tipifarnib in patients with recurrent malignant glioma either receiving or not receiving enzyme-inducing antiepileptic drugs: a North American Brain Tumor Consortium Study. J Clin Oncol. 2006;24:3651–6.
153. Glass TL, Liu TJ, Yung WK. Inhibition of cell growth in human glioblastoma cell lines by farnesyltransferase inhibitor SCH66336. Neuro Oncol. 2000;2(3):151–8.
154. Chaponis D, Barnes JW, Dellagatta JL, Kesari S, Fast E, Sauvageot C, Panagrahy D, Greene ER, Ramakrishna N, Wen PY, Kung AL, Stiles C, Kieran MW. Lonafarnib (SCH66336) improves the activity of temozolomide and radiation for orthotopic malignant gliomas. J Neurooncol. 2011;104 (1):179–89. Doi:10.1007/s11060-010-0502-4 Epub 2011 Jan 19.
155. Desjardins A, Reardon DA, Peters KB, Threatt S, Coan AD, Herndon JE 2nd, Friedman AH, Friedman HS, Vredenburgh JJ. A phase I trial of the farnesyl transferase inhibitor, SCH 66336, with temozolomide for patients with malignant glioma. J Neurooncol. 2011;105(3):601–6. Doi:10.1007/s11060-011-0627-0 Epub 2011 Jul 7.
156. Yust-Katz S, Liu D, Yuan Y, Liu V, Kang S, Groves M, et al. Phase 1/1b study of lonafarnib and temozolomide in patients with recurrent or temozolomide refractory glioblastoma. Cancer. 2013;119:2747–53.
157. Verhaak RG, Hoadley KA, Purdom E, Wang V, Qi Y, Wilkerson MD, et al. Integrated genomic analysis identifies clinically relevant subtypes of glioblastoma characterized by abnormalities in PDGFRA, IDH1, EGFR, and NF1. Cancer Cell. 2010;17:98–110.
158. Sandmann T, Bourgon R, Garcia J, Li C, Cloughesy T, Chinot OL, Wick W, Nishikawa R, Mason W, Henriksson R, Saran F, Lai A, Moore N, Kharbanda S, Peale F, Hegde P, Abrey LE, Phillips HS, Bais C. Patients With Proneural Glioblastoma May Derive Overall Survival Benefit From the Addition of Bevacizumab to First-Line Radiotherapy and Temozolomide: Retrospective Analysis of the AVAglio Trial. J Clin Oncol. 2015;33(25):2735–44. Doi:10.1200/JCO.2015.61.5005 Epub 2015 Jun 29.
159. Patel AP, Tirosh I, Trombetta JJ, Shalek AK, Gillespie SM, Wakimoto H, Cahill DP, Nahed BV, Curry WT, Martuza RL, Louis DN, Rozenblatt-Rosen O, Suvà ML, Regev A, Bernstein BE. Single-cell RNA-seq highlights intratumoral heterogeneity in primary glioblastoma. Science. 2014;344(6190):1396–401. Doi:10.1126/science.1254257 Epub 2014 Jun 12.
160. Hegi ME, Diserens AC, Bady P, Kamoshima Y, Kouwenhoven MC, Delorenzi M, et al. Pathway analysis of glioblastoma tissue after preoperative treatment with the EGFR tyrosine kinase inhibitor gefitinib—a phase II trial. Mol Cancer Ther. 2011;10:1102–12.
161. Chakravarti A, Loeffler JS, Dyson NJ. Insulin-like growth factor receptor I mediates resistance to anti-epidermal growth factor receptor therapy in primary human glioblastoma cells through continued activation of phosphoinositide 3-kinase signaling. Cancer Res. 2002;62(1):200–7.
162. van den Bent MJ, Gao Y, Kerkhof M, Kros JM, Gorlia T, van Zwieten K, Prince J, van Duinen S, Sillevis Smitt PA, Taphoorn M, French PJ. Changes in the EGFR amplification and EGFRvIII expression between paired primary and recurrent glioblastomas. Neuro Oncol. 2015 Jul;17(7):935–41. Doi:10.1093/neuonc/nov013 Epub 2015 Feb 16.

Targeted Therapy of IDH1-Mutated Tumors

10

Owen Clark and Christian Grommes

Introduction

Almost a hundred years have passed since Otto Warburg's seminal hypothesis that cancer ultimately stems from deregulated metabolism [1]. Indeed, since this time, it has been well established that increased energetic and anabolic demands of tumor cells result in numerous metabolic alterations [2, 3]. However, skepticism still remains as to whether such metabolic reprogramming is a cause or consequence of tumorigenesis. The first evidence that genetic alterations in metabolic genes are directly involved in tumorigenesis came early in this century, with the discovery of loss of function mutations in the mitochondrial enzymes *succinate dehydrogenase* and *fumarate hydratase* in renal cell carcinoma and paragangliomas [4, 5]. However, the observation that an enzyme involved in the TCA cycle, *isocitrate dehydrogenase* (*IDH*), is mutated at high frequency in a wide array of cancers represented a pivotal point in the field of cancer metabolism. Here, we aim to summarize such findings in the context of how the relatively nascent IDH field has progressed, and shed light on exciting potential future directions.

O. Clark (✉)
Human Oncology and Pathogenesis Program (HOPP), Memorial Sloan Kettering Cancer Center, 1275 York Avenue, New York, NY 10065, USA
e-mail: clarko@mskcc.org

C. Grommes
Department of Neurology, Memorial Sloan Kettering Cancer Center, 1275 York Avenue, New York, NY 10065, USA
e-mail: grommesc@mskcc.org

Background

The first discovery of an *IDH* mutation appeared in one of the earliest comprehensive analyses of mutations in protein-coding genes in cancer, representing an infrequent event in colorectal cancer [6]. Two years later, the same group applied genome wide, next-generation sequencing to 22 WHO Grade IV glioblastoma multiforme (GBM) tumors, identifying highly recurrent mutations in the *IDH1* isoform of *IDH* in 12% of sequenced tumors [7]. Here, the majority of *IDH*-mutant GBMs (5/6) were found in tumors that had progressed overtime from lower grade (WHO grade II/III) gliomas. This seminal finding was confirmed in a follow-up study with a much larger sample of tumors, reporting that *IDH* mutations were remarkably frequent (>70%) in low-grade gliomas [8]. Since these initial studies, *IDH* mutations have been observed in a number of hematopoietic neoplasms, most notably cytogenetically normal-acute myelocytic leukemia (AML; ~10–15%) [9, 10]; blast-phase myeloproliferative neoplasms (20%) [11]; and angioimmunoblastic T-cell lymphoma (20%) [12]. Mutations also occur in chondrosarcoma (56%) [13]; and less frequently (<5%) in other solid tumors [14].

The vast majority of *IDH* mutations arise in the catalytic pocket of the enzyme. Mutations in

J. Moliterno Günel et al. (eds.), *Malignant Brain Tumors*, DOI 10.1007/978-3-319-49864-5_10 the cytoplasmic and peroxisome-localized IDH isoform *IDH1* predominantly occur at arginine 132, resulting in substitutions including R132H, R132C, R132L, R132S, and R132G, with the former representing the most common alteration. The mitochondrial counterpart *IDH2* is also mutated at low frequency in glioma, at either the analogous residue R140, or R172. Mutations in *IDH1* and *IDH2* are mutually exclusive, suggesting redundancy between the two isoforms.

Molecular Alterations: Basic Biochemistry

IDH functions in the TCA cycle where it catalyzes the NADP$^+$-dependent oxidative decarboxylation of isocitrate to alpha ketoglutarate (α-KG), producing CO_2 and NADPH in the process [15]. IDH1 and IDH2 share 69% structural similarity, the main difference being the presence of a C-terminal peroxisomal targeting sequence in the cytosolic IDH1 [16]. Loss of function of the wild-type protein was put forward as an early explanation for the prevalence of *IDH* mutations. However, this contrasts with the highly recurrent and monoallelic nature of such mutations. In 2009, a landmark study conducted a large-scale metabolomics screen in *IDH*-mutant glioblastoma cells, finding that $IDH1^{R132H}$ conferred a gain of function or 'neomorphic' ability to produce the R(−) enantiomer of the metabolite 2-hydroxyglutarate (R-2-HG), resulting in millimolar cytoplasmic levels [17]. R-2-HG was shown to accumulate in glioma samples at up to 100-fold (5–35 μmol/g) higher levels versus *IDH* wild-type gliomas, as well as leukemias [10], and was subsequently shown to underlie all *IDH* mutations [18]. Production of the R-2-HG 'oncometabolite' involves direct conversion from α-KG and relies on the presence of a wild-type allele [19], likely explaining the rareness of loss of heterozygosity.

Current data suggests that the R-2-HG oncometabolite is responsible for many, if not all, biologic effects of *IDH* mutations (Fig. 10.1). Cell permeable esters of R-2-HG phenocopy the effects of mutant *IDH* in experimental models [20, 21], and ectopic expression of the dehydrogenase [22] that converts R-2-HG into α-KG, and thus counteracts the activity of mutant IDH, is sufficient to reverse the cellular effects of cancer-associated IDH mutations [23]. Due to their utilization of α-KG as a cofactor, R-2-HG competitively inhibits 2-oxoglutarate (2-OG)-dependent dioxygenases [24], a diverse family of ~80 enzymes that maintain a number of different cellular functions, many of which are still currently unknown [25].

Molecular Alterations: Epigenetic Modifications

Numerous lines of evidence suggest that *IDH* mutations contribute to widescale epigenetic modifications. One subgroup of the 2-OG dioxygenase family that is potently inhibited by R-2-HG is the jumonji domain containing (Jmjc) family of histone lysine demethylases [26], responsible for the removal of methyl groups from lysine (K) residues of histone tails [27, 28]. Methylation of K residues on the tail of histone 3 (H3) is generally associated with either transcriptionally silenced (H3K9, H3K27, H3K20) or active (H3K4, H3K36, H3K79) regions of chromatin and thus repressed or activated gene expression, respectively [29]. These enzymes are particularly sensitive to inhibition by R-2-HG [26], and knockdown of *Jmjd2c* (also known as *Kdm4c*) is sufficient to phenocopy the effects of mutant *Idh* on adipocyte differentiation in 3T3-L1 cells [20].

R-2-HG also inhibits ten-eleven translocation 2 (TET2) [24]—a 2-OG-dependent dioxygenase that catalyzes the conversion of 5-methylcytosine (5mC) to 5-hydroxy-methylcytosine (5-hmC)—thus effectively reversing gene silencing by DNA methylation [30]. *TET2* is itself mutated in myeloid malignancies [31], with mutations occurring in a mutually exclusive fashion to those of *IDH* [32]. This along with the observation of decreased 5-hmC levels in *IDH*-mutant AML [32], and the identification of TET2 as a candidate effector of mutant IDH in a short hairpin RNA library screen of 2-OG dioxygenases [21], suggests that this

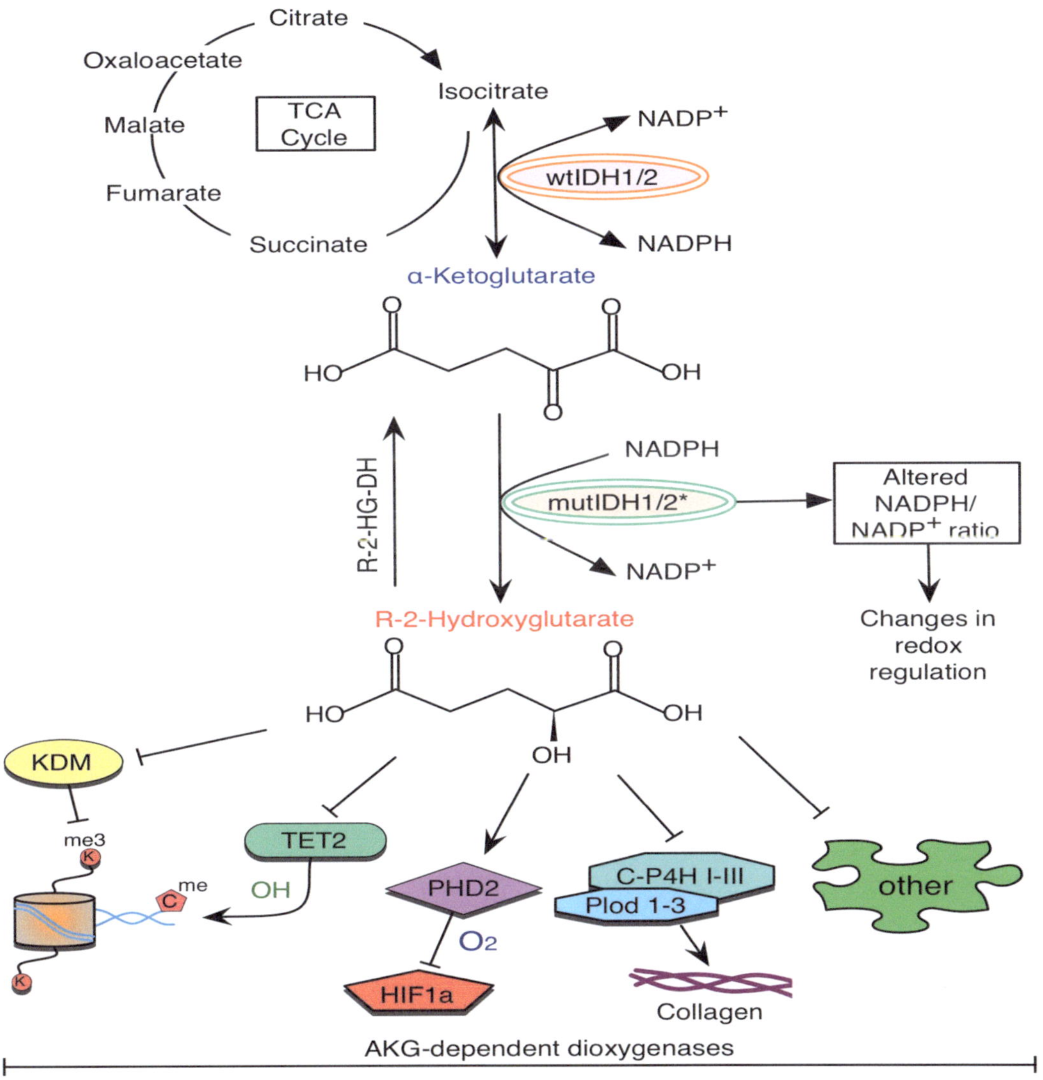

Fig. 10.1 Molecular mechanisms of *IDH*-associated tumorigenesis. Wild-type IDH1/2 (wtIDH1/2) converts isocitrate (generated through the citric acid (TCA) cycle) into α-KG, producing NADPH in the process. Mutant IDH1/2 (mutIDH1/2) converts isocitrate (generated through the citric acid (TCA) cycle) into α-KG, producing NADPH in the process. Epigenetic modifications result from inhibition of histone lysine demethylases (KDMs) and the 5-methyl cytosine hydroxylase TET2. Inhibition of prolyl-hydroxylation impairs collagen maturation. R-2-HG has been reported to activate the enzyme prolyl-hydroxylase 2 (PHD2) that inhibits hypoxia-inducible factor 1-alpha (HIF-1α) [37], although other studies suggest that it may be inhibited [24]. Mutant IDH may also change the cellular redox environment by altering the ratio of NADPH to $NADP^+$. IDH3 has been omitted from this figure for simplicity

enzyme is an important mediator of the effects of *IDH* mutation, at least in myeloid malignancies. Indeed, *IDH* mutations in AML are associated with a hypermethylation phenotype, resulting from increases in global methylcytosine, where widespread DNA methylation results in epigenetic silencing of gene expression [33].

In glioma, mutant IDH establishes a widescale DNA methylation signature [34] known as glioma CpG island methylator phenotype

(G-CIMP), observed in the majority of *IDH*-mutant tumors [20, 35]. In this study, ectopic expression of mutant IDH1 in human astrocytes led to a time-dependent build up of histone methylation at H3K9, H3K27, and H3K36, in addition to increases in global methylcytosine. Treatment of IDH1-mutant glioma cells with a mutant-specific IDH inhibitor decreases histone methylation both in vitro and in vivo, although this is not clearly linked to growth inhibition [36].

Molecular Alterations: Hypoxia and Metabolism

Despite its status as a 2-OG-dependent dioxygenase, prolyl-hydroxylase 2 (PHD2—also referred to as EGLN1) has been reported to be stimulated by mutant IDH [37]. This enzyme is responsible for regulating the expression of hypoxia-inducible factor (HIF)-1α through a post-translational modification involving hydroxylation of a proline residue in HIF's alpha subunit, leading to targeting by the Von Hippel–Lindau (VHL) ubiquitin ligase complex under normoxic conditions [38, 39]. R-2-HG stimulates the activity of both PHD2 and the functionally similar PHD1 at tumor-relevant concentrations, resulting in a decrease in HIF1α and its target genes [37]. Notably, knockdown of *HIF1α* and overexpression of PHD2 in $IDH1^{R132H}$-expressing astrocytes, both had transforming effects in soft agar colony formation assays. The same group noted that knockdown of *PHD2* abrogated growth factor independence, and restored differentiation ability in $IDH1^{R132H}$ leukemia cells [21]. However, other reports have suggested that R-2-HG inhibits PHD2-mediated HIF1α modification [24], which has been suggested as an explanation for the observed stabilization of *Hif1a*, and increased transcription of downstream target genes, reported in an $Idh1^{R132H}$ knock-in mouse [40].

Alterations in the TCA cycle resulting from *IDH* mutations would be expected to disrupt the balance of intracellular redox signaling. Due to impaired oxidative decarboxylation of isocitrate, *IDH*-mutant tumors exhibit alterations in the NADPH/$NADP^+$ ratio [15, 41]. In addition to scavenging mitochondrial free radicals itself, NADPH is required as a hydrogen anion donor in the generation of the reduced form of glutathione (GSH), which constitutes the cells' major defense mechanism against reactive oxygen species (ROS) [42]. *IDH*-mutant cells exhibit both reduced levels of NADPH and a corresponding reduction in GSH [43]. It has also been noted that glioblastoma cells ectopically expressing mutant IDH exhibit elevated levels of ROS, rendering them more sensitive to radiation [44, 45], which has been put forward as an explanation for the favorable therapeutic response [46, 47] and prognosis [48] of mutant *IDH* [49]. However, elevation of ROS levels has not been observed in transgenic models of mutant *Idh* [40, 50].

Recent reports suggest that alterations in metabolism and mitochondrial bioenergetics may render *IDH*-mutant cancer cells more sensitive to cell death. For instance, Tateishi et al. [51] found that mutant IDH1 lowers NAD+ levels, sensitizing cells to further NAD+ depletion that resulted in autophagy and cytotoxicity. While Chan et al. [52] found that R-2-HG-mediated inhibition of the mitochondrial enzyme COX rendered *IDH*-mutant AML cells sensitive to inhibition of the anti-apoptotic protein BCL-2. These studies raise the interesting notion that *IDH* mutations might endow tumor cells with an Achille's heal that could form the basis of targeted therapy, rather than drugging the mutant protein itself.

The Contribution of Mutant IDH to Tumor Formation

Large-scale analyses of clinical data suggest that *IDH* mutations are an important event in tumorigenesis. Analyzing over 300 gliomas, Watanabe et al. [53] found that in the 51 cases with multiple biopsies, neither acquisition of a mutation in *TP*53 nor loss of 1p/19q occurred prior to a mutation in *IDH1*, highlighting its early occurrence. Whole-exome sequencing of matched biopsy pairs from glioma samples taken at initial diagnosis and at the time of recurrence showed that *IDH1*^{R132H} was the only mutation that was consistently present in both the initial and recurrent biopsy specimen [54]. In leukemia patients, *IDH2* mutations were observed to occur in the absence of *NPM1c* mutations in both mature and progenitor cell populations, suggesting that *IDH2* mutation might occur as a pre-leukemic event [55].

Numerous studies have explored whether *IDH* mutations can transform nonmalignant cells of various lineages. Expression of mutant *Idh* in mouse myeloid progenitor 32D cells and primary mouse bone marrow cells impaired hematopoietic differentiation and increased stem/progenitor cell marker expression, suggesting a pro-leukemogenic effect [56]. A more recent study suggested that retrovirally mediated expression of mutant *Idh2*^{R140Q} in murine primary hematopoietic bone marrow stem and progenitor cell populations was sufficient to induce myeloproliferative-like neoplasms, T-cell lymphoma, or B-cell lymphoma, when transplanted into irradiated mice [57]. However, these hematological malignancies occurred at low penetrance and with long latency, suggesting that they did not arise solely due to mutant *Idh2* expression. Expression of mutant *Idh2* in a non-transformed mesenchymal multipotent mouse cell line (C3H10T) impaired their differentiation into adipocytic and chondrocytic lineages and resulted in loss of contact inhibition and tumor formation in vivo [58]. In immortalized human astrocytes, expression of mutant *IDH*, but not wild-type *IDH* or a catalytically inactive *IDH* mutant, resulted in anchorage-independent growth [37].

Further insights into the role of mutant *IDH* in tumor initiation have emerged from experiments with genetically engineered mice (Fig. 10.2). Tamoxifen-induced global expression of *Idh2*^{R140Q} or ^{R172K} resulted in cardiomyopathy, white matter abnormalities throughout the central nervous system, and muscular dystrophy, while mice engineered to express mutant *Idh2* in specific tissues developed carcinomas, albeit with very long latencies [59]. In a hematopoietic tissue-specific model, mice that expressed a doxycycline-inducible *Idh2*^{R140Q} allele did not develop leukemia after 1 year of continuous doxycycline treatment [60]. The most common cancer-associated *IDH* mutation, *IDH1*^{R132H}, has also been inserted into the endogenous murine *Idh1* locus, and expression of the mutant enzyme subsequently targeted to specific cell populations. Expression of *Idh1*^{R132H} in hematopoietic cells resulted in increased numbers of hematopoietic progenitors, but no overt leukemia [61]. Expression of *Idh1*^{R132H} in nestin-expressing neural stem cells resulted in perinatal lethality due to cerebral hemorrhage [40]. Expression of *Idh1*^{R132H} in GFAP-expressing astrocytes resulted in more subtle defects, including impaired collagen maturation and basement membrane function, likely due to R-2-HG-mediated inhibition of prolyl-/lysyl-hydroxylation of collagen proteins, but did not result in glioma formation. Tamoxifen-inducible expression of mutant *Idh1* in chondrocytes resulted in the development of enchondromas—benign cartilage tumors that are precursors to malignant chondrosarcomas [62]. Doxycycline-induced expression of mutant *Idh2* (*Idh2*^{R140Q} or *Idh2*^{R172K}) increased hepatocyte proliferation in a liver injury model, but was not sufficient to induce tumors [63].

The current data from knock-in mice suggest that mutant *Idh* likely cooperates with other genetic or epigenetic events to initiate cancer. Using a mouse transplantation assay, Chaturvedi et al. [64] found that mutant *IDH1* alone did not transform hematopoietic cells but greatly accelerated the onset of leukemia in cooperation with *HoxA9*. Chen et al. [65] applied a mosaic mouse modeling approach in which hematopoietic stem and progenitor cells (HPSC) from *Flt3-ITD* or *Nras*^{G12D} mice were transduced with a retroviral vector expressing mutant *Idh2* and then assessed for tumorigenic potential following transplantation into syngeneic recipient mice. *Idh2* mutants were found to cooperate with *Flt3* or *Nras* alleles to drive leukemia formation. This cooperativity between mutant *Idh2*^{R140Q} and other leukemia-relevant pathway alterations (e.g., Flt3-ITD or homeobox proteins HoxA9 and Meis1a) was confirmed in the aforementioned

Cancer Type	Promoter	Tumor Formation	Phenotype
Acute Myeloid Leukemia (AML)	Lysozyme 2; Vav 1	None	Splenomegaly; Anaemia
Acute Myeloid Leukemia (AML)	Collagen A1	Leukemia In combination with *Flt3*^{ITD}	Splenomegaly
Chondrosarcoma	Collagen, type 2, A1	Enchondroma	None

Cancer Type	Promoter	Tumor Formation	Phenotype
Glioma	Nestin; GFAP	No gliomas	Brain hemorrhage

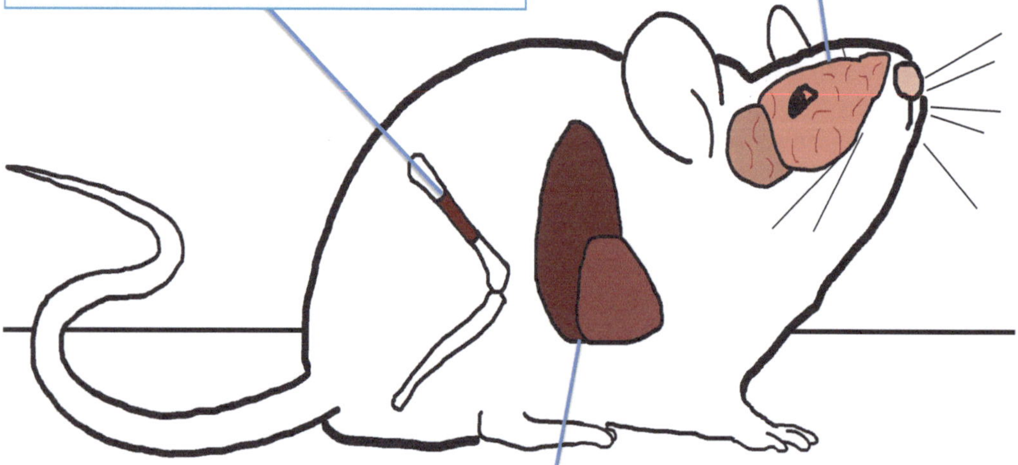

Cancer Type	Promoter	Tumor Formation	Phenotype
Intrahepatic Cholangiocarcinoma (IHCC)	Albumin	IHCC In combination with Kras^{G12D}	None

Fig. 10.2 Transgenic models of mutant *IDH*. Transgenic knock-in systems have been used in an attempt to model *Idh*-mutant AML, glioma, chondrosarcoma, and IHCC, both alone and in combination of other genetic lesions

doxycycline-inducible transgenic model [60] and another mosaic mouse modeling approach [66]. Saha et al. [63] showed that *Idh2*^{R172K} *cooperated* with mutant KRAS (*Kras*^{G12D}) to induce intrahepatic cholangio-carcinomas.

In sum, these studies demonstrate that mutant IDH cooperates with other oncogenic events to initiate cancer, consistent with the finding that *IDH*-mutant human cancers typically harbor alterations in multiple other cancer genes. In glioma, for example, *IDH* mutations are associated with missense mutations in *ATRX, TP53*, and *TERT* (diffuse astrocytomas) or codeletion of chromosome arms 1p and 19q (oligodendrogliomas; [48, 67]). In AML patients with a normal cytogenetic profile, IDH mutations are associated with mutations in *NPM1*, *FLT3-ITD*, and *DNMT3A* [68, 69].

Targeting Mutant IDH

Recent studies have begun to address the question of whether the activity of the mutant IDH enzyme remains important for the growth of

IDH-mutant cancers once they are fully established. Studies in experimental cancer models suggest that indeed this is the case with the strongest evidence coming from leukemia models. In TF-1 human erythroleukemia cells, ectopic expression of mutant IDH promotes growth factor independence, a phenotype that can be reversed with a small molecule mutant IDH inhibitor [70, 71]. Ex vivo treatment of freshly isolated *IDH*-mutant leukemic blasts with a mutant-selective IDH inhibitor induces a cellular differentiation program [70]. Pharmacological inhibition of the mutant IDH enzyme blocks colony formation of human AML cells, but not of normal CD34(+) bone marrow cells [64]. In a genetically engineered leukemia model, pharmacologic or genetic inhibition of mutant *Idh2* triggered the differentiation and death of AML cells [65], and doxycycline-induced silencing of mutant *Idh2* similarly eliminated $Idh2^{R140Q}$/*Hoxa9* or $Idh2^{R140Q}$/*Meis1a*-driven leukemia cells [60].

Data from experimental solid tumor models suggest that *IDH1*-mutant tumors remain, at least in part, dependent on the activity of the mutant enzyme. Expression of mutant $IDH1^{R132C}$ in hepatoblasts caused a differentiation block, which could be reversed by treatment with an inhibitor of mutant IDH1 [72]. In HT1080 human fibrosarcoma cells, RNAi-mediated suppression of endogenous mutant *IDH1* significantly inhibited anchorage-independent growth [73]. Knocking out the endogenous mutant *IDH1* gene similarly impaired anchorage-independent growth and *in vivo* growth of *IDH*-mutant human sarcoma cells [74]. In *IDH1*-mutant glioma cells, pharmacological blockade of the mutant enzyme impaired their anchorage-independent and *in vivo* growth [75].

The above-mentioned results in experimental models are supported by the findings of an ongoing clinical trial, which showed that the mutant IDH2 inhibitor AG-221 produces clinical responses, including complete and durable responses, in about 40% of patients with AML and MDS [76].

Using R-2-HG as a Clinical Biomarker

In addition to being responsible for the majority of biological effects associated with mutant IDH, R-2-HG represents a potentially useful clinical biomarker for the detection of *IDH*-mutant tumor cells. R-2-HG can be reliably detected in the blood of *IDH*-mutant AML patients, and measurement of R-2-HG levels can be used as an indicator of therapeutic response [77]. Despite its accumulation in *IDH*-mutant glioma tissue, elevated R-2-HG is not observed in the blood of these patients [78]. To overcome this problem, magnetic resonance spectroscopy (MRS) has been used as a means of measuring intratumoral R-2-HG levels [79, 80], which allows the detection of *IDH*-mutant tumors for both diagnostic and treatment monitoring purposes. The majority of the publications to date have used dedicated research scanners for R-2-HG detection. However, recent data suggest that clinically used MRS scanners allow sensitive detection of R-2-HG in medium to large tumors [81].

Conclusion

A remarkable body of knowledge has been generated in the few years since the first description of cancer-associated mutations in *IDH*. However, a number of key questions still remain as to the exact involvement of mutant IDH in cancer. For instance, what role does mutant *IDH* play in tumorigenesis? And how does it interact with other genetic lesions to transform cells? What are the crucial molecular alterations caused by R-2-HG? And how do they interact to transform cells or maintain tumor growth? Perhaps the most important question is, will targeted therapy against mutant IDH yield success in the clinic? With the development of numerous small molecules targeting mutant IDH, and several clinical trials currently examining their efficacy in multiple types of cancer, the future seems bright for the development of rationale therapeutic approaches for *IDH*-mutant cancers.

References

1. Warburg O. On the origin of cancer cells. Science. 1956;123(3191):309–14 PubMed PMID: 13298683. Epub 1956/02/24. eng.
2. Oermann EK, Wu J, Guan K-L, Xiong Y. Alterations of metabolic genes and metabolites in cancer. In Seminars in cell & developmental biology. 2012 Jul;23(4):370–80. PubMed PMID: 22306135. Pubmed Central PMCID: PMC3351496. English.
3. Ward PS, Thompson CB. Metabolic reprogramming: a cancer Hallmark even Warburg did not anticipate. Cancer Cell. 2012;21(3):297–308.
4. Baysal BE, Ferrell RE, Willett-Brozick JE, Lawrence EC, Myssiorek D, Bosch A, et al. Mutations in SDHD, a mitochondrial complex II gene, in hereditary paraganglioma. Science. 2000;287 (5454):848–51.
5. King A, Selak MA, Gottlieb E. Succinate dehydrogenase and fumarate hydratase: linking mitochondrial dysfunction and cancer. Oncogene. 2006;25 (34):4675–82 PubMed PMID: 16892081. English.
6. Sjoblom T, Jones S, Wood LD, Parsons DW, Lin J, Barber TD, et al. The Consensus Coding Sequences of Human Breast and Colorectal Cancers. Science (New York, NY). 2006;314(5797):268–74. English.
7. Parsons DW, Jones S, Zhang X, Lin JCH, Leary RJ, Angenendt P, et al. An Integrated Genomic Analysis of Human Glioblastoma Multiforme. Science (New York, NY). 2008;321(5897):1807–12. English.
8. Yan H, Parsons DW, Jin G, McLendon R, Rasheed BA, Yuan W, et al. IDH1 and IDH2 mutations in gliomas. New Engl J Med. 2009;360 (8):765–73. PubMed PMID: 19228619. Pubmed Central PMCID: PMC2820383. English.
9. Mardis ER, Ding L, Dooling DJ, Larson DE, McLellan MD, Chen K, et al. Recurring mutations found by sequencing an acute myeloid leukemia genome. New Engl J Med. 2009;361(11):1058–66. PubMed PMID: 19657110. Pubmed Central PMCID: PMC3201812. English.
10. Gross S, Cairns RA, Minden MD, Driggers EM, Bittinger MA, Jang HG, et al. Cancer-associated metabolite 2-hydroxyglutarate accumulates in acute myelogenous leukemia with isocitrate dehydrogenase 1 and 2 mutations. J Exp Med. 2010;207(2):339–44. PubMed PMID: 20142433. Pubmed Central PMCID: PMC2822606. English.
11. Pardanani A, Lasho TL, Finke CM, Mai M, McClure RF, Tefferi A. IDH1 and IDH2 mutation analysis in chronic- and blast-phase myeloproliferative neoplasms. Leukemia. 2010;24(6):1146–51.
12. Cairns RA, Iqbal J, Lemonnier F, Kucuk C, de Leval L, Jais J-P, et al. IDH2 mutations are frequent in angioimmunoblastic T-cell lymphoma. Blood. 2012;119(8):1901–3. PubMed PMID: 22215888. Pubmed Central PMCID: PMC3293643. English.
13. Amary MF, Bacsi K, Maggiani F, Damato S, Halai D, Berisha F, et al. IDH1 and IDH2 mutations are frequent events in central chondrosarcoma and central and periosteal chondromas but not in other mesenchymal tumours. J Pathol. 2011;224(3):334–43. PubMed PMID: 21598255. English.
14. Cerami E, Gao J, Dogrusoz U, Gross BE, Sumer SO, Aksoy BA, et al. The cBio cancer genomics portal: an open platform for exploring multidimensional cancer genomics data. Cancer Discov. 2012;2 (5):401–4. PubMed PMID: 22588877. Pubmed Central PMCID: 3956037.
15. Leonardi R, Subramanian C, Jackowski S, Rock CO. Cancer-associated isocitrate dehydrogenase mutations inactivate NADPH-dependent reductive carboxylation. J Bio Chem. 2012;287(18):14615–20. PubMed PMID: 22442146. Pubmed Central PMCID: PMC3340216. English.
16. Xu X, Zhao J, Xu Z, Peng B, Huang Q, Arnold E, et al. Structures of human cytosolic NADP-dependent isocitrate dehydrogenase reveal a novel self-regulatory mechanism of activity. J Bio Chem. 2004;279(32):33946–57. PubMed PMID: 15173171. English.
17. Dang L, White DW, Gross S, Bennett BD, Bittinger MA, Driggers EM, et al. Cancer-associated IDH1 mutations produce 2-hydroxyglutarate. Nature. 2009;462(7274):739–44.
18. Ward PS, Patel J, Wise DR, Abdel-Wahab O, Bennett BD, Coller HA, et al. The Common Feature of Leukemia-Associated IDH1 and IDH2 Mutations Is a Neomorphic Enzyme Activity Converting & alpha;-Ketoglutarate to 2-Hydroxyglutarate. Cancer Cell. 2010;17(3):225–34.
19. Jin G, Reitman ZJ, Duncan CG, Spasojevic I, Gooden DM, Rasheed BA, et al. Disruption of Wild-Type IDH1 Suppresses D-2-Hydroxyglutarate Production in IDH1-Mutated Gliomas. Cancer Res. 2013;73(2):496–501. English.
20. Lu C, Ward PS, Kapoor GS, Rohle D, Turcan S, Abdel-Wahab O, et al. IDH mutation impairs histone demethylation and results in a block to cell differentiation. Nature. 2012;483(7390):474–8.
21. Losman JA, Losman JA, Looper R, Looper R, Koivunen P, Koivunen P, et al. (R)-2-Hydroxyglutarate Is Sufficient to Promote Leukemogenesis and Its Effects Are Reversible. Science (New York, NY). 2013; English.
22. Achouri Y, Noel G, Vertommen D, Rider MH, Veiga-Da-Cunha M, Van Schaftingen E. Identification of a dehydrogenase acting on D-2-hydroxyglutarate. Biochem J. 2004;381(Pt 1):35–42. PubMed PMID: 15070399. Pubmed Central PMCID: 1133759.
23. Reitman ZJ, Sinenko SA, Spana EP, Yan H. Genetic dissection of leukemia-associated IDH1 and IDH2 mutants and D-2-hydroxyglutarate in Drosophila. Blood. 2015;125(2):336–45. PubMed PMID: 25398939. Pubmed Central PMCID: 4287640.
24. Xu W, Xu W, Yang H, Yang H, Liu Y, Liu Y, et al. Oncometabolite 2-Hydroxyglutarate is a competitive inhibitor of & alpha;-Ketoglutarate-dependent dioxygenases. CCELL. 2011;19(1):17–30.

25. McDonough MA, Loenarz C, Chowdhury R, Clifton IJ, Schofield CJ. Structural studies on human 2-oxoglutarate dependent oxygenases. Curr Opin Struct Biol. 2010;20(6):659–72.
26. Chowdhury R, Yeoh KK, Tian Y-M, Hillringhaus L, Bagg EA, Rose NR, et al. The oncometabolite 2-hydroxyglutarate inhibits histone lysine demethylases. Nature Publishing Group. 2011 Jun;12(5):463–9. PubMed PMID: 21460794. Pubmed Central PMCID: PMC3090014. English.
27. Klose RJ, Kallin EM, Zhang Y. JmjC-domain-containing proteins and histone demethylation. Nat Rev Genet. 2006;7(9):715–27.
28. Kooistra SM, Helin K. Molecular mechanisms and potential functions of histone demethylases. Nature Publishing Group. 2012;13(5):297–311.
29. Martin C, Zhang Y. The diverse functions of histone lysine methylation. Nat Rev Mol Cell Biol. 2005;6 (11):838–49. PubMed PMID: 16261189. Epub 2005/11/02. eng.
30. Guo JU, Su Y, Zhong C, Ming GL, Song H. Emerging roles of TET proteins and 5-hydroxy methylcytosines in active DNA demethylation and beyond. Cell Cycle. 2011;10(16):2662–8. PubMed PMID: 21811096. Pubmed Central PMCID: PMC3219536. Epub 2011/08/04. eng.
31. Delhommeau F, Dupont S, Della Valle V, James C, Trannoy S, Masse A, et al. Mutation in TET2 in myeloid cancers. New Eng J Med. 2009;360 (22):2289–301. PubMed PMID: 19474426. Epub 2009/05/29. eng.
32. Figueroa ME, Abdel-Wahab O, Lu C, Ward PS, Patel J, Shih A, et al. Leukemic IDH1 and IDH2 mutations result in a hypermethylation phenotype, disrupt TET2 function, and impair hematopoietic differentiation. Cancer Cell. 2010;18(6):553–67. PubMed PMID: 21130701. English.
33. Figueroa ME, Figueroa ME, Abdel-Wahab O, Abdel-Wahab O, Lu C, Lu C, et al. Leukemic IDH1 and IDH2 mutations result. A hypermethylation phenotype, disrupt TET2 function, and impair hematopoietic differentiation. CCELL. 2010;18 (6):553–67.
34. Noushmehr H, Weisenberger DJ, Diefes K, Phillips HS, Pujara K, Berman BP, et al. Identification of a CpG island methylator phenotype that defines a distinct subgroup of Glioma. Cancer Cell. 2010;17(5):510–22.
35. Turcan S, Turcan S, Rohle D, Rohle D, Goenka A, Goenka A, et al. IDH1 mutation is sufficient to establish the glioma hypermethylator phenotype. Nature. 2012;483(7390):479–83.
36. Rohle D, Popovici-Muller J, Palaskas N, Turcan S, Grommes C, Campos C, et al. An Inhibitor of Mutant IDH1 Delays Growth and Promotes Differentiation of Glioma Cells. Science (New York, NY). 2013;340 (6132):626–30. PubMed PMID: 23558169. English.
37. Koivunen P, Koivunen P, Lee S, Lee S, Duncan CG, Duncan CG, et al. Transformation by the (R)-enantiomer of 2-hydroxyglutarate linked to EGLN activation. Nature. 2012;15:1–7.
38. Bruick RK. A Conserved Family of Prolyl-4-Hydroxylases That Modify HIF. Science (New York, NY). 2001;294(5545):1337–40.
39. Epstein AC, Gleadle JM, McNeill LA, Hewitson KS, O'Rourke J, Mole DR, et al. C. elegans EGL-9 and mammalian homologs define a family of dioxygenases that regulate HIF by prolyl hydroxylation. Cell. 2001;107(1):43–54. PubMed PMID: 11595184. English.
40. Sasaki M, Sasaki M, Knobbe CB, Knobbe CB, Itsumi M, Itsumi M, et al. D-2-hydroxyglutarate produced by mutant IDH1 perturbs collagen maturation and basement membrane function. Genes & Development. 2012;26(18):2038–49. English.
41. Bleeker FE, Atai NA, Lamba S, Jonker A, Rijkeboer D, Bosch KS, et al. The prognostic IDH1(R132) mutation is associated with reduced NADP+ dependent IDH activity in glioblastoma. Acta Neuropathol. 2010,119(4).487–94. PubMed PMID. 20127344. Pubmed Central PMCID: PMC2841753. Epub 2010/02/04. eng.
42. Filomeni G, Rotilio G, Ciriolo MR. Cell signalling and the glutathione redox system. Biochem Pharmacol. 2002;64(5–6):1057–64.
43. Shi J, Zuo H, Ni L, Xia L, Zhao L, Gong M, et al. An IDH1 mutation inhibits growth of glioma cells via GSH depletion and ROS generation. Neurol Sci. 2013;35(6):839–45. English.
44. Li S, Chou AP, Chen W, Chen R, Deng Y, Phillips HS, et al. Overexpression of isocitrate dehydrogenase mutant proteins renders glioma cells more sensitive to radiation. Neuro-Oncology. 2013;15(1):57–68. English.
45. Molenaar RJ, Botman D, Smits MA, Hira VV, van Lith SA, Stap J, et al. Radioprotection of IDH1-Mutated Cancer Cells by the IDH1-Mutant Inhibitor AGI-5198. Cancer Res. 2015;75(22):4790–802.
46. Cairncross JG, Wang M, Jenkins RB, Shaw EG, Giannini C, Brachman DG, et al. Benefit from procarbazine, lomustine, and vincristine in oligodendroglial tumors is associated with mutation of IDH. J Clin Oncol: Official J Am Soc Clin Oncol. 2014;32 (8):783–90. PubMed PMID: 24516018. Pubmed Central PMCID: 3940537.
47. Labussiere M, Sanson M, Idbaih A, Delattre JY. IDH1 gene mutations: a new paradigm in glioma prognosis and therapy? Oncologist. 2010;15(2):196–9. PubMed PMID: 20133500. Pubmed Central PMCID: 3227941.
48. Cancer Genome Atlas Research N, Brat DJ, Verhaak RG, Aldape KD, Yung WK, Salama SR, et al. Comprehensive, integrative genomic analysis of diffuse lower-grade Gliomas. New Eng J Med. 2015;372(26):2481–98. PubMed PMID: 26061751. Pubmed Central PMCID: 4530011.
49. Molenaar RJ, Radivoyevitch T, Maciejewski JP, van Noorden CJ, Bleeker FE. The driver and passenger

effects of isocitrate dehydrogenase 1 and 2 mutations in oncogenesis and survival prolongation. Biochim Biophys Acta. 2014;1846(2):326–41.
50. Sasaki M, Sasaki M, Knobbe CB, Knobbe CB, Munger JC, Munger JC, et al. IDH1(R132H) mutation increases murine haematopoietic progenitors and alters epigenetics. Nature. 2012;04:1–7.
51. Tateishi K, Wakimoto H, Iafrate AJ, Tanaka S, Loebel F, Lelic N, et al. Extreme Vulnerability of IDH1 Mutant Cancers to NAD + Depletion. Cancer Cell. 2015;28(6):773–84. PubMed PMID: 26678339. Pubmed Central PMCID: 4684594.
52. Chan SM, Thomas D, Corces-Zimmerman MR, Xavy S, Rastogi S, Hong WJ, et al. Isocitrate dehydrogenase 1 and 2 mutations induce BCL-2 dependence in acute myeloid leukemia. Nat Med. 2015;21(2):178–84. PubMed PMID: 25599133. Pubmed Central PMCID: PMC4406275. Epub 2015/01/20. eng.
53. Watanabe T, Nobusawa S, Kleihues P, Ohgaki H. IDH1 mutations are early events in the development of Astrocytomas and Oligodendrogliomas. Am J Pathol. 2010;174(4):1149–53.
54. Johnson BE, Mazor T, Hong C, Barnes M, Aihara K, McLean CY, et al. Mutational Analysis Reveals the Origin and Therapy-Driven Evolution of Recurrent Glioma. Science (New York, NY). 2013; English.
55. Shlush LI, Zandi S, Mitchell A, Chen WC, Brandwein JM, Gupta V, et al. Identification of pre-leukaemic haematopoietic stem cells in acute leukaemia. Nature. 2014;12:1–13.
56. Figueroa ME, Abdel-Wahab O, Lu C, Ward PS, Patel J, Shih A, et al. Leukemic IDH1 and IDH2 mutations result in a hypermethylation phenotype, disrupt TET2 function, and impair hematopoietic differentiation. Cancer cell. 2010;18(6):553–67. PubMed PMID: 21130701. Epub 2010/12/07. eng.
57. Mylonas E, Janin M, Bawa O, Opolon P, David M, Quivoron C, et al. Isocitrate dehydrogenase (IDH)2 R140Q mutation induces myeloid and lymphoid neoplasms in mice. 2014;1–3.
58. Lu C, Lu C, Venneti S, Venneti S, Akalin A, Akalin A, et al. Induction of sarcomas by mutant IDH2. Genes Development. 2013;27(18):1986–98. English.
59. Akbay EA, Moslehi J, Christensen CL, Saha S, Tchaicha JH, Ramkissoon SH, et al. D-2-hydroxyglutarate produced by mutant IDH2 causes cardiomyopathy and neurodegeneration in mice. Genes Development. 2014 ;28(5):479–90. English.
60. Kats LM, Reschke M, Taulli R, Pozdnyakova O, Burgess K, Bhargava P, et al. Proto-Oncogenic role of mutant IDH2 in leukemia initiation and maintenance. Stem Cell. 2014;15:1–13.
61. Sasaki M, Knobbe CB, Munger JC, Lind EF, Brenner D, Brüstle A, et al. IDH1(R132H) mutation increases murine haematopoietic progenitors and alters epigenetics. Nature. 2012;04:1–7.
62. Hirata M, Sasaki M, Cairns RA, Inoue S, Puviindran V, Li WY, et al. Mutant IDH is sufficient to initiate enchondromatosis in mice. Proc Natl Acad Sci. 2015;112(9):2829–34. PubMed PMID: 25730874. Pubmed Central PMCID: PMC4352794. English.
63. Saha SK, Parachoniak CA, Ghanta KS, Fitamant J, Ross KN, Najem MS, et al. Mutant IDH inhibits HNF-4α to block hepatocyte differentiation and promote biliary cancer. Nature. 2014;02:1–18.
64. Chaturvedi A, Araujo Cruz MM, Jyotsana N, Sharma A, Yun H, Görlich K, et al. Mutant IDH1 promotes leukemogenesis in vivo and can be specifically targeted in human AML. Blood. 2013;122 (16):2877–87. PubMed PMID: 23954893. English.
65. Chen C, Chen C, Liu Y, Liu Y, Lu C, Lu C, et al. Cancer-associated IDH2 mutants drive an acute myeloid leukemia that is susceptible to Brd4 inhibition. Genes Development. 2013;27(18):1974–85. English.
66. Ogawara Y, Katsumoto T, Aikawa Y, Shima Y, Kagiyama Y, Soga T, et al. IDH2 and NPM1 Mutations Cooperate to Activate Hoxa9/Meis1 and Hypoxia Pathways in Acute Myeloid Leukemia. Cancer Res. 2015;75(10):2005–16. PubMed PMID: 25795706. Epub 2015/03/22. eng.
67. Eckel-Passow JE, Lachance DH, Molinaro AM, Walsh KM, Decker PA, Sicotte H, et al. Glioma Groups Based on 1p/19q, IDH, and TERT Promoter Mutations in Tumors. New Engl J Med. 2015;372 (26):2499–508. PubMed PMID: 26061753. Pubmed Central PMCID: 4489704.
68. Paschka P, Schlenk RF, Gaidzik VI, Habdank M, Kronke J, Bullinger L, et al. IDH1 and IDH2 mutations are frequent genetic alterations in acute myeloid leukemia and confer adverse prognosis in cytogenetically normal acute myeloid leukemia with NPM1 mutation without FLT3 internal tandem duplication. J Clini Oncol: Official J Am Soc Clini Oncol. 2010;28(22):3636–43.
69. DiNardo CD, Ravandi F, Agresta S, Konopleva M, Takahashi K, Kadia T, et al. Characteristics, clinical outcome, and prognostic significance of IDH mutations in AML. Am J Hematol. 2015;90(8):732–6. PubMed PMID: 26016821. Pubmed Central PMCID: 4612499.
70. Wang F, Travins J, DeLaBarre B, Penard-Lacronique V, Schalm S, Hansen E, et al. Targeted inhibition of mutant IDH2 in leukemia cells induces cellular differentiation. Science. 2013;340(6132):622–6.
71. Losman JA, Looper RE, Koivunen P, Lee S, Schneider RK, McMahon C, et al. (R)-2-hydroxyglutarate is sufficient to promote leukemogenesis and its effects are reversible. Science. 2013;339(6127):1621–5. PubMed PMID: 23393090. Pubmed Central PMCID: 3836459.
72. Saha SK, Parachoniak CA, Ghanta KS, Fitamant J, Ross KN, Najem MS, et al. Mutant IDH inhibits HNF-4alpha to block hepatocyte differentiation and promote biliary cancer. Nature. 2014;513

(7516):110–4. PubMed PMID: 25043045. Pubmed Central PMCID: 4499230.
73. Jin G, Pirozzi CJ, Chen LH, Lopez GY, Duncan CG, Feng J, et al. Mutant IDH1 is required for IDH1 mutated tumor cell growth. Oncotarget. 2012;3(8):774–82. PubMed PMID: 22885298. Pubmed Central PMCID: 3478455.
74. Ma S, Jiang B, Deng W, Gu ZK, Wu FZ, Li T, et al. D-2-hydroxyglutarate is essential for maintaining oncogenic property of mutant IDH-containing cancer cells but dispensable for cell growth. Oncotarget. 2015;6(11):8606–20. PubMed PMID: 25825982. Pubmed Central PMCID: PMC4496170. Epub 2015/04/01. eng.
75. Rohle D, Popovici-Muller J, Palaskas N, Turcan S, Grommes C, Campos C, et al. An inhibitor of mutant IDH1 delays growth and promotes differentiation of glioma cells. Science. 2013;340(6132):626–30. PubMed PMID: 23558169. Pubmed Central PMCID: 3985613.
76. Burris H, Mellinghoff I, Maher E, Wen P, Beeram M, Touat M, et al. Abstract PL04–05: The first reported results of AG-120, a first-in-class, potent inhibitor of the IDH1 mutant protein, in a Phase I study of patients with advanced IDH1-mutant solid tumors, including gliomas. Molecular Cancer Therapeutics. 2015, 2015;14(12 Supplement 2):PL04-5.
77. Fathi AT, Sadrzadeh H, Borger DR, Ballen KK, Amrein PC, Attar EC, et al. Prospective serial evaluation of 2-hydroxyglutarate, during treatment of newly diagnosed acute myeloid leukemia, to assess disease activity and therapeutic response. Blood. 2012;120(23):4649–52.
78. Capper D, Simon M, Langhans CD, Okun JG, Tonn JC, Weller M, et al. 2-Hydroxyglutarate concentration in serum from patients with gliomas does not correlate with IDH1/2 mutation status or tumor size. International journal of cancer Journal international du cancer. 2012;131(3):766–8.
79. Choi C, Ganji SK, DeBerardinis RJ, Hatanpaa KJ, Rakheja D, Kovacs Z, et al. 2-hydroxyglutarate detection by magnetic resonance spectroscopy in IDH-mutated patients with gliomas. Nat Med. 2012;18(4):624–9. PubMed PMID: 22281806. Pubmed Central PMCID: 3615719.
80. Andronesi OC, Kim GS, Gerstner E, Batchelor T, Tzika AA, Fantin VR, et al. Detection of 2-hydroxyglutarate in IDH-mutated glioma patients by in vivo spectral-editing and 2D correlation magnetic resonance spectroscopy. Sci Transl Med. 2012,4(116):116ra4. PubMed PMID: 22238332. Pubmed Central PMCID: 3720836.
81. De la Macarena MI, Young RJ, Rubel J, Rosenblum M, Tisnado J, Briggs S, et al. Integration of 2-hydroxyglutarate-proton magnetic resonance spectroscopy into clinical practice for disease monitoring in isocitrate dehydrogenase-mutant glioma. Neuro-oncology. 2016;18(2):283–90 PubMed PMID: 26691210. Pubmed Central PMCID: PMC4724186.

Antiangiogenic Therapy for Malignant Gliomas

11

Nancy Wang, Jonas Kloepper, Rakesh K. Jain and Tracy T. Batchelor

Background

Anti-angiogenic therapies targeting new blood vessel formation in cancer are based on the principle that solid tumors require formation of blood vessels in order to supply adequate oxygen and nutrients [1]. Endothelial cells may also secrete growth factors that further stimulate tumor growth [2]. The vascular endothelial growth factor (VEGF) pathway has been a focus of drug therapy due to its ubiquitous and increased expression in many human cancers. Bevacizumab, a recombinant, humanized, monoclonal antibody targeting the VEGF ligand A was first approved for the treatment of metastatic colorectal cancer by the United States Food and Drug Administration (FDA) in 2004 [3], followed by non-small cell lung cancer in 2006 [4], and renal cell carcinoma [5] and recurrent glioblastoma in 2009 [6]. Antiangiogenic therapy has been explored in malignant gliomas based on the rationale that these tumors express high levels of proangiogenic factors and are characterized by microvascular proliferation. This approach has received a considerable amount of attention given the limited survival following standard therapy with concurrent radiation and temozolomide followed by adjuvant temozolomide [7].

Mechanisms of Action

Angiogenesis in malignant gliomas is governed by a complex network of angiogenic factors, including VEGF (previously described as vascular permeability factor), hepatocyte growth factor (HGF), fibroblast growth factor (FGF), platelet-derived growth factor (PDGF), hypoxia inducible factor 1α, angiopoietins, interleukin-8, and others [8–13]. Angiogenesis is also constitutively activated by mitogenic pathways such as Ras/mitogen-activated protein kinase (MAPK) and phosphoinositide-3-kinase (PI3K) [14].

In the initial stages of treatment and at low doses, antiangiogenic agents are thought to normalize tumor vasculature by restoring a more normal vessel phenotype characterized by smaller vessel diameters. Normalization results in improved vessel function with reduced vascular permeability and consequently reduced

N. Wang · T.T. Batchelor
Department of Neurology, Massachusetts General Hospital, Boston, USA
e-mail: nwang6@partners.org

J. Kloepper · R.K. Jain · T.T. Batchelor
Department of Radiation Oncology, Massachusetts General Hospital, Boston, USA
e-mail: jonaskloepper@gmail.com

R.K. Jain
e-mail: jain@steele.mgh.harvard.edu

T.T. Batchelor (✉)
Department of Division of Hematology/Oncology, Massachusetts General Hospital, Boston, USA
e-mail: tbatchelor@mgh.harvard.edu

T.T. Batchelor
Stephen E. and Catherine Pappas Center for Neuro-Oncology, Yawkey 9E, Massachusetts General Hospital, 55 Fruit Street, Boston, MA 02114, USA

J. Moliterno Günel et al. (eds.), *Malignant Brain Tumors*,
DOI 10.1007/978-3-319-49864-5_11

edema [15]. These treatment benefits of VEGF pathway inhibition are apparent radiographically as the reduction of peritumoral contrast enhancement and allow for lower corticosteroid doses for vasogenic edema control. Corticosteroid use has been associated with lower OS in patients with recurrent GBM [16]. Therefore, the anti-edema effects of anti-VEGF therapy are of high importance given recent advances in immunotherapy, which can be associated with increased peritumoral edema [17–19]. Preclinical evidence also suggests that vascular normalization has the potential to alleviate hypoxia in the tumor microenvironment, thereby facilitating the infiltration of T effector cells, reducing myeloid-derived suppressor cells, and polarizing tumor-associated macrophages to an immune stimulatory M1-like phenotype [20]. Additionally, improving tumor perfusion with anti-angiogenic therapy has the potential to facilitate the delivery of cytotoxic chemotherapies. The resulting increase in oxygenation can sensitize the tumor to genotoxins, including radiation and cytotoxic chemotherapy [21, 22].

Ultimately, and according to the tumor starvation hypothesis initially proposed in 1971 by Folkman [1], antiangiogenic agents exert an antitumor effect by inducing endothelial cell apoptosis, inhibiting new blood vessel growth, and inducing the pruning of immature vessels poorly covered by perivascular cells [21–24], thereby decreasing tumor perfusion and depriving the tumor of nutrients and oxygen [1]. However, the clinical data do not support the notion that patients whose tumor perfusion decreases in response to anti-angiogenic therapies survive longer [15].

Additional mechanisms by which antiangiogenic therapy can exert antitumor effects are thought to include inhibition of Angiopoietin-2 (Ang-2) or VEGF-mediated recruitment of tumor-infiltrating monocytes and glioblastoma stem-like cells, which help regulate tumor angiogenesis and sustain tumor progression [25–29].

Clinical Trials in High Grade Glioma

Although many antiangiogenic agents have been studied in glioblastoma, bevacizumab, currently FDA approved in the United States as monotherapy for recurrent glioblastoma, is the most clinically utilized and has been subjected to a number of randomized trials (Table 11.1). Thus, bevacizumab will be the focus of this discussion. Bevacizumab binds VEGF with high affinity and specificity and was shown early on to inhibit angiogenesis and tumor growth in preclinical models of glioblastoma [30–33]. The remarkable successes and lack of dose-limiting toxicities in phase I studies in extracranial solid tumors led to its use in glioblastoma.

Bevacizumab for Recurrent Glioblastoma

Two single-arm studies evaluated the use of bevacizumab and irinotecan in 67 patients with recurrent high-grade glioma and compared the outcomes to historic controls. Radiographic response was observed in 60% of study subjects, with 6-month progression-free survival (PFS-6) of 38–46% [34, 35]. These results were in contrast to other contemporary salvage regimens that demonstrated a radiographic response of 5–10% and PFS-6 of 9–25% [36].

Two subsequent prospective phase 2 studies were conducted which led to accelerated FDA approval of bevacizumab as monotherapy for recurrent glioblastoma in 2009 [6]. In the phase 2 BRAIN study, patients were randomized to bevacizumab or bevacizumab plus irinotecan. The overall response rates (ORR) were 28.2 and 37.8%, respectively, with PFS-6 of 42.6 and 50.3%, respectively [37]. Median overall survival (OS) was 9.2 months versus 8.7 months. Older radiographic response criteria were used to assess radiographic response, and the study was not a superiority trial and allowed for crossover from single-agent bevacizumab to combination

Table 11.1 Landmark clinical trials of antiangiogenic agents for glioblastoma

Trial	Phase	Disease type	Patients (n)	Arms	Median PFS (mo)	PFS-6 (%)	Median OS (mo)	Reference
BRAIN	2	rGBM	167	BEV	4.2	42.6	9.2	[37]
				BEV + irinotecan	5.6	50.3	8.7	
NCI	2	rGBM	48	BEV	4.0	29.0	7.8	[38]
BELOB	2	rGBM	153	BEV	3.0	16.0	8.0	[63]
				Lomustine	1.0	13.0	8.0	
				BEV + lomustine	4.0	42.0	12.0	
EORTC 26101	3	rGBM	437	BEV + lomustine	4.2	NR	9.1	[64]
				Lomustine	1.5	NR	8.6	
REGAL	3	rGBM	325	Cediranib	92 days	16.0	8.0	[79]
				Cediranib + lomustine	125 days	35.0	9.4	
				Lomustine + placebo	82 days	25.0	9.8	
Enzastaurin	3	rGBM	266	Enzastaurin	1.5	11.1	6.6	[85]
				Lomustine	1.6	19	7.1	
RTOG 0825	3	nGBM	637	BEV + TMZ/XRT	10.7	NR	15.7	[72]
				TMZ/XRT	7.3	NR	16.1	
AVAGlio	3	nGBM	921	BEV + TMZ/XRT	10.6	NR	16.9	[71]
				TMZ/XRT	6.2	NR	16.8	
GLARIUS	2	nGBM (MGMT unmethylated)	170	BEV + irinotecan/XRT	9.7	71.1	16.6	[70]
				TMZ/XRT	5.9	26.2	17.3	

Abbreviations rGBM recurrent glioblastoma; nGBM newly diagnosed glioblastoma; BEV bevacizumab; TMZ temozolomide; XRT radiation therapy; NR not reported therapy. In a single-arm study of bevacizumab in 48 patients, the ORR and PFS-6 were 35 and 29%, respectively, with a median OS of 7.75 months [38]. While the FDA approved the use of bevacizumab in recurrent GBM based on these trials, the European Medicines Agency declined approval due to the lack of a non-bevacizumab control arm, modest improvement in OS, and challenges with radiographic response assessment [39]. This has led to a difference in standard of care for recurrent glioblastoma in the U.S. versus Europe.

Subsequent phase 2 trials have evaluated bevacizumab in various combinations with irinotecan, cetuximab, carboplatin, etoposide, fotemustine, sorafenib, temozolomide, erlotinib, panobinostat, and temsirolimus [37, 40–59]. There have also been trials evaluating bevacizumab and re-irradiation [60–62].

The only trial to show a survival benefit of combination therapy over bevacizumab alone was the BELOB study, a randomized phase 2 study of 148 patients with recurrent glioblastoma randomized to lomustine, bevacizumab, or both. Combination therapy resulted in a PFS-6 of 41% compared with 11 and 18% with OS at 9 months of 59% compared to 43 and 38% for lomustine and bevacizumab alone, respectively [63]. Based on these results, a phase 3 study of lomustine versus lomustine plus bevacizumab in patients with recurrent glioblastoma (EORTC 26101) was conducted, demonstrating no difference in OS with a median of 9.1 months for combination therapy versus 8.6 for lomustine alone [64]. However, there was a benefit in PFS of 4.2 months for combination therapy compared to 1.5 months for lomustine monotherapy. 35.5% of patients in the control arm of this study did cross over to receive bevacizumab.

Resistance to bevacizumab inevitably develops with resulting rapid clinical deterioration. Retrospective data has suggested that continuing bevacizumab beyond initial progression may modestly improve outcome [65]. The ongoing phase 3 TAMIGA trial (NCT01860638) aims to evaluate whether adding bevacizumab to lomustine as second-line therapy followed by standard of care for third line therapy with bevacizumab improves survival compared to lomustine alone followed by standard of care third line therapy with placebo.

In summary, clinical data to date offer only limited support for combining bevacizumab with chemotherapy in the setting of recurrent glioblastoma.

Bevacizumab for Newly Diagnosed Glioblastoma

Several single-arm phase 2 studies of bevacizumab in combination with temozolomide and radiation showed near doubling of median PFS to 13–14 months compared to historic benchmarks. However, only a modest improvement in median OS to 19–21 months was observed in these studies [66–68]. The GLARIUS study was a phase 2 trial that compared the combination of bevacizumab and radiotherapy with either irinotecan or temozolomide in newly diagnosed glioblastoma patients whose tumors expressed the DNA repair enzyme O6-methyl guanine DNA methyltransferase (MGMT). Loss of MGMT function through methylation of the gene promotor in GBM has been shown to confer increased sensitivity to therapy with the DNA alkylating agent temozolomide [69]. The GLARIUS study demonstrated a significant prolongation of PFS but no difference in OS in the bevacizumab containing arm [70]. PFS was 5.99 months in the control arm compared to 9.7 months in the bevacizumab/irinotecan arm, and median OS was 17.5 months in the control arm compared to 16.6 months in the bevacizumab/irinotecan arm. Neither therapy regimen was superior in delaying the time to deterioration in any of the pre-specified dimensions of quality of life.

Two randomized, placebo-controlled, phase 3 trials, AVAglio and RTOG 0825, investigated the addition of bevacizumab to the standard of care treatment regimen consisting of surgery and chemoradiation with temozolomide in patients with newly diagnosed glioblastoma. Both studies failed to show an improvement in OS.

In the AVAglio study, newly diagnosed glioblastoma patients were randomized to bevacizumab versus placebo in combination with standard chemoradiation. The median PFS for standard therapy plus bevacizumab was 10.6 months versus 6.2 months for standard therapy with placebo [71]. The predefined OS endpoint, however, was not met with OS of 16.8 months in the bevacizumab arm compared to 16.7 months in the placebo arm. The RTOG 0825 trial also compared bevacizumab to placebo in combination with standard therapy and demonstrated an improved PFS of 10.7 months versus 7.3 months with placebo [72]. This increase in PFS did not meet the predefined significance level of $P = 0.004$. Similar to the AVAglio trial, there was no difference in OS with a median survival of 15.7 months in the bevacizumab arm compared to 16.1 months in the placebo arm. In both studies, approximately 30–50% of controls crossed over and received bevacizumab at progression, potentially confounding the true impact on OS. While AVAglio used the revised RANO criteria to assess disease progression, RTOG 0825 used the traditional Macdonald criteria, which only evaluates enhancing disease [73, 74]. The differences in the radiographic assessments used in the AVAglio and RTOG0825 trials are laid out in detail in a publication by Chinot et al. [75].

Both trials also attempted to assess other measures of net clinical benefit, including Karnofsky performance status, corticosteroid requirement, and quality of life measures. Interestingly, the European-led AVAglio and the US-led RTOG 0825 studies showed conflicting quality of life outcomes. In the AVAglio trial, bevacizumab prolonged maintenance of Karnofsky performance status and decreased steroid utilization. Moreover, time to deterioration was prolonged in 5 pre-specified domains: global health status, physical and social functioning, motor dysfunction, and communication deficit. In contrast, the RTOG 0825 study found that bevacizumab consistently led to decreased objective and perceived cognitive function (as assessed by formal neurocognitive testing), as well as motor dysfunction and communication deficits compared to controls. The cause of the differences in quality of life outcomes is unclear, but possible reasons include different radiographic response criteria used, substantial dropout among RTOG participants, and different methods of statistical modeling.

Other Antiangiogenic Strategies

In addition to the VEGF neutralizing antibody bevacizumab, other inhibitors of the VEGF pathway as well as inhibitors of other angiogenic growth factors have also failed to show an overall survival benefit in glioblastoma. Aflibercept, a recombinant fusion protein that binds VEGF and placental growth factor (PIGF), improved survival in preclinical studies of glioblastoma but failed to meet its primary endpoint of PFS-6 in a single-arm phase 2 study of patients with recurrent glioblastoma [76, 77]. Receptor tyrosine kinase inhibitors (TKIs) that inhibit the VEGF and other angiogenic pathways have also been evaluated in glioblastoma, including cediranib, sunitinib, pazopanib, vandetanib, and sorafenib [78–83]. The only agent to reach phase 3 of clinical development was cediranib. A phase 2 study evaluating single-agent cediranib in patients with recurrent high-grade glioma showed a 27% radiographic response rate with a 6 month PFS of 26% [78]. However, a randomized, placebo-controlled, phase 3 trial of cediranib monotherapy and cediranib in combination with lomustine compared to lomustine alone failed to reach its primary endpoint of PFS prolongation [79].

Other approaches have included VEGF receptor blockade and targeting upstream pathways that lead to increased VEGF expression. A phase 2 trial of CT-322, a pegylated protein that binds and blocks VEGFR2, was terminated early due to insufficient efficacy [84]. An open label phase 2 study of the anti-VEGFR2 monoclonal antibody ramucirumab versus the anti-PDGFR monoclonal antibody IMC-3G3 has completed accrual with results pending. Enzastaurin is an oral serine/threonine kinase inhibitor that targets the proangiogenic protein kinase C and PI3K/AKT pathways. A randomized, phase 3 trial of enzastaurin versus lomustine in recurrent glioblastoma showed no difference in PFS and OS [85].

Mechanisms of Resistance

Despite promising preclinical data with antiangiogenic therapy in GBM animal models and increased PFS in patients, VEGF pathway inhibition has yet to demonstrate a survival benefit in GBM patients. Given the multiple pathways involved in tumor angiogenesis, it is perhaps not surprising that VEGF pathway inhibition alone does not durably or completely block tumor angiogenesis. There are many proposed adaptive mechanisms of resistance to anti-VEGF therapy. First, the hypoxic tumor microenvironment may trigger the release of alternative proangiogenic factors such as HGF, FGF, ANG-2, SDF1α, and interleukin-8 [29, 86–89]. Preclinical studies in GBM animal models demonstrate that dual targeting of VEGF and the alternative proangiogenic factor Ang-2 may overcome resistance to anti-VEGF monotherapy [24, 90, 91]. Second, antiangiogenic therapy may foster other modes of vessel recruitment, such as vessel co-option, intussusception, vascular mimicry, recruitment of endothelial progenitor cells, and differentiation of cancer stem-like cells into endothelial cells [92–94]. The process of vessel co-option, whereby tumors utilize native brain vessels to recruit blood supply, is under increasing investigation as an escape mechanism to antiangiogenic therapy. The molecular mechanisms of vessel co-option are still poorly understood and will yield novel approaches once the pathways involved have been identified. Third, there may be inherent insensitivity to VEGF inhibition among different tumor blood vessel subtypes with decreased anti-VEGF sensitivity in pericyte-covered tumor vessels [23, 95]. Furthermore, recruitment of bone marrow-derived cells such as monocytes and M2-skewed macrophages may rescue tumor angiogenesis through production of pro-angiogenic factors [9, 27, 96]. Lastly, studies in animal models have also shown that VEGF inhibition may induce transformation from a proneural to a more invasive mesenchymal phenotype [97, 98].

Retrospective data in high grade gliomas and prospective data in other cancers have suggested potential benefit of continuing antiangiogenic therapy past progression, suggesting that resistance is potentially epigenetically based and reversible [65, 99–101]. This becomes an important consideration in clinical trials assessing subsequent-line therapies.

Biologic and Imaging Markers

Unlike other targeted therapies, there are currently no established biomarkers that can be utilized to select patients who are more likely to respond to antiangiogenic agents. Biomarkers that have been assessed as possible predictors of increased efficacy include a 10-gene panel identified by RTOG 0825 [102], proneural transcriptional glioblastoma subtype [103], VEGF expression [104], epidermal growth factor receptor (EGFR), platelet-derived growth factor receptor a (PDGFR-a), and c-KIT [105]. However, none of these markers have been validated and none are intended for clinical practice. Other candidate biomarkers include circulating cytokines such as VEGF and sVEGFR2 [71, 106], SDH1α [107], and matrix metalloproteinases [27, 108].

Efforts have also been directed at accurately defining tumor response and progression as well as using novel imaging techniques to predict response. Unlike the Macdonald criteria, the RANO criteria account for the possible effect of antiangiogenic treatment on reducing tumor enhancement when determining disease progression [73]. Antiangiogenic therapy decreases vessel permeability, leading to a usually transient phenomenon of decreased enhancement known as "pseudoresponse". Possible imaging markers to predict tumor response include apparent diffusion coefficient [109], restriction spectrum imaging [110], dynamic contrast enhanced (DCE) and dynamic susceptibility-contrast (DSC) techniques [111, 112], vessel architectural imaging [113], and dopamine and positron emission tomography [114, 115]. Cerebral blood flow has also been investigated, with increased tumor perfusion correlating with an increase in overall survival in newly diagnosed and recurrent glioblastoma patients treated with cediranib, a pan-VEGF kinase inhibitor [105, 116].

Immunotherapy and Antiangiogenic Therapy

Responses to immunotherapy across a spectrum of cancers has led to interest in this strategy in glioblastomas despite the historical view that the central nervous system is immune-privileged due to the blood brain barrier. Preclinical data in extracranial tumors have suggested that antiangiogenic therapies increase tumor delivery of activated T cells, making the tumor more susceptible to immune attack [20]. Moreover, vascular normalization may promote an "immunosupportive tumor microenvironment" [18, 24, 90], thereby enhancing the effects of immunotherapy. There are a number of clinical trials evaluating the use of antiangiogenic therapy in combination with immune checkpoint inhibitors (pembrolizumab, MEDI4736), immune stimulants (Plerixafor), and vaccines (SL-701, rindopepimut, heat shock protein peptide complexes) in patients with glioblastoma. Preliminary results from a phase 2 trial of standard of care plus bevacizumab in combination with a dendritic cell vaccine showed improved OS in the combination group compared to the vaccine or bevacizumab alone [117]. Preliminary results from the phase 2 ReACT study of patients with EGFRvIII mutant recurrent glioblastomas found that the combination of the vaccine rindopepimut with bevacizumab prolonged median OS to 12 months versus 8.8 months for the control arm (bevacizumab plus keyhole limpet hemocyanin) [118]. PFS-6 was also significantly increased from 11% in the control arm to 27% in the experimental arm. Additionally, animal models have shown promising results in the use of antiangiogenic therapy in combination with adoptive cell transfer [119].

Future Directions

Multiple clinical trials of antiangiogenic agents in newly diagnosed and recurrent glioblastoma have failed to show an overall survival benefit. Given the existence of multiple, redundant, pro-angiogenic signal transduction pathways and the propensity of glioblastoma to develop resistance to therapeutics targeting one pathway, combination strategies are the logical next step in the development of anti-angiogenic agents. These may include combinations of multiple anti-angiogenic agents or the combination of anti-angiogenic drugs with other classes of therapeutics like immunotherapy. To better assess which patients are most likely to derive clinical benefit from antiangiogenic agents, further research on imaging and biologic markers is essential. Advances in genetically modified mouse models (GEMMs), patient-derived and stem-like cell models of glioma, and importantly, human tumor-bearing humanized mouse models will allow for more translatable preclinical studies. Additional studies are also needed to clarify the conflicting data on the benefits of anti-VEGF therapy on quality of life, an area of particular importance to patients with glioblastoma. Given retrospective data suggesting that treatment of patients with high-grade glioma with low doses of bevacizumab (5 mg/kg per week) may be superior to standard dosing, further work is needed to clarify the optimal dose and administration schedule [120]. Lastly, a better understanding of the mechanisms of resistance to antiangiogenic therapy will facilitate the development of more effective therapeutic targets and treatment strategies.

References

1. Folkman J. Tumor angiogenesis: therapeutic implications. N Engl J Med [Internet]. 1971;285 (21):1182–6. Available from: http://www.ncbi.nlm.nih.gov/pubmed/4938153.

2. Butler JM, Kobayashi H, Rafii S. Instructive role of the vascular niche in promoting tumour growth and tissue repair by angiocrine factors. Nat Rev Cancer [Internet]. Nature Publishing Group; 2010;10(2):138–46. Available from: http://www.pubmedcentral.nih.gov/articlerender.fcgi?artid=2944775&tool=pmcentrez&rendertype=abstract.
3. Hurwitz H, Fehrenbacher L, Novotny W, Cartwright T, Hainsworth J, Heim W, et al. Bevacizumab plus irinotecan, fluorouracil, and leucovorin for metastatic colorectal cancer. N Engl J Med [Internet]. 2004;350(23):2335–42. Available from: http://www.ncbi.nlm.nih.gov/pubmed/15175435.
4. Cohen MH, Gootenberg J, Keegan P, Pazdur R. FDA drug approval summary: bevacizumab (Avastin(R)) plus Carboplatin and Paclitaxel as first-line treatment of advanced/metastatic recurrent nonsquamous non-small cell lung cancer. Oncologist [Internet]. 2007;12(6):713–8. Available from: http://dx.doi.org/10.1634/theoncologist.12-6-713.
5. Summers J, Cohen MH, Keegan P, Pazdur R. FDA drug approval summary: bevacizumab plus interferon for advanced renal cell carcinoma. Oncologist [Internet]. 2010;15(1):104–11. Available from: http://www.ncbi.nlm.nih.gov/entrez/query.fcgi?cmd=Retrieve&db=PubMed&dopt=Citation&list_uids=20061402\nhttp://theoncologist.alphamedpress.org/content/15/1/104.full.pdf.
6. Cohen MH, Shen YL, Keegan P, Pazdur R. FDA drug approval summary: bevacizumab (Avastin) as treatment of recurrent glioblastoma multiforme. Oncologist. 2009;14:1131–8.
7. Stupp R, Mason WP, van den Bent MJ, Weller M, Fisher B, Taphoorn MJ, et al. Radiotherapy plus concomitant and adjuvant temozolomide for glioblastoma. N Engl J Med [Internet]. 2005;352(10):987–96. Available from: http://www.ncbi.nlm.nih.gov/pubmed/15758009.
8. Shih AH, Holland EC. Platelet-derived growth factor (PDGF) and glial tumorigenesis. Cancer Lett. 2006;232(2):139–47.
9. Du R, Lu KV, Petritsch C, Liu P, Ganss R, Passegué E, et al. HIF1alpha induces the recruitment of bone marrow-derived vascular modulatory cells to regulate tumor angiogenesis and invasion. Cancer Cell [Internet]. 2008;13(3):206–20. Available from: http://www.ncbi.nlm.nih.gov/pubmed/18328425.
10. Plate KH, Breier G, Weich HA, Risau W. Vascular endothelial growth factor is a potential tumour angiogenesis factor in human gliomas in vivo. Nature [Internet]. 1992;359(6398):845–8. Available from: http://www.ncbi.nlm.nih.gov/pubmed/1279432.
11. Reiss Y, Machein MR, Plate KH. The role of angiopoietins during angiogenesis in gliomas. Brain Pathol. 2005;15(32):311–7.
12. Brat DJ, Bellail AC, Van Meir EG. The role of interleukin-8 and its receptors in gliomagenesis and tumoral angiogenesis. Neuro Oncol [Internet]. 2005;7(2):122–33. Available from: http://www.pubmedcentral.nih.gov/articlerender.fcgi?artid=1871893&tool=pmcentrez&rendertype=abstract.
13. Schmidt NO, Westphal M, Hagel C, Ergün S, Stavrou D, Rosen EM, et al. Levels of vascular endothelial growth factor, hepatocyte growth factor/scatter factor and basic fibroblast growth factor in human gliomas and their relation to angiogenesis. Int J Cancer [Internet]. 1999;84(1):10–8. Available from: http://www.ncbi.nlm.nih.gov/pubmed/9988225.
14. Jayson GC, Kerbel R, Ellis LM, Harris AL. Antiangiogenic therapy in oncology: current status and future directions. Lancet (London, England) [Internet]. Elsevier Ltd; 2016;70(15):6171–80. Available from: http://linkinghub.elsevier.com/retrieve/pii/S0140673615010880.
15. Jain RK. Antiangiogenesis Strategies Revisited: From Starving Tumors to Alleviating Hypoxia. Cancer Cell. Elsevier Inc.; 2014;26(5):605–22.
16. Wong ET, Lok E, Gautam S, Swanson KD. Dexamethasone exerts profound immunologic interference on treatment efficacy for recurrent glioblastoma. Br J Cancer [Internet]. Nature Publishing Group; 2015;113(2):232–41. Available from: http://dx.doi.org/10.1038/bjc.2015.238.
17. Preusser M, Lim M, Hafler DA, Reardon DA, Sampson JH. Prospects of immune checkpoint modulators in the treatment of glioblastoma. Nat Rev Neurol [Internet]. Nature Publishing Group; 2015;11(9):504–14. Available from: http://www.nature.com/doifinder/10.1038/nrneurol.2015.139.
18. Garg AD, Vandenberk L, Koks C, Verschuere T, Boon L, Van Gool SW, et al. Dendritic cell vaccines based on immunogenic cell death elicit danger signals and T cell—driven rejection of high-grade glioma. Sci Transl Med. 2016;8(328):1–16.
19. Reardon DA, Gokhale PC, Klein SR, Ligon KL, Rodig SJ, Ramkissoon SH, et al. Glioblastoma Eradication Following Immune Checkpoint Blockade in an Orthotopic, Immunocompetent Model. Cancer Immunol Res [Internet]. 2015;4(February):1–12. Available from: http://cancerimmunolres.aacrjournals.org/cgi/doi/10.1158/2326-6066.CIR-15-0151.
20. Huang Y, Goel S, Duda DG, Fukumura D, Jain RK. Vascular normalization as an emerging strategy to enhance cancer immunotherapy. Cancer Res. 2013;73(10):2943–8.
21. Winkler F, Kozin SV, Tong RT, Chae SS, Booth MF, Garkavtsev I, et al. Kinetics of vascular normalization by VEGFR2 blockade governs brain tumor response to radiation: role of oxygenation, angiopoietin-1, and matrix metalloproteinases. Cancer Cell. 2004;6(6):553–63.
22. Batchelor TT, Sorensen a G, di Tomaso E, Zhang W-T, Duda DG, Cohen KS, et al. AZD2171, a pan-VEGF receptor tyrosine kinase inhibitor, normalizes tumor vasculature and alleviates edema in glioblastoma patients. Cancer Cell [Internet].

2007;11(1):83–95. Available from: http://www.ncbi.nlm.nih.gov/pubmed/17222792.
23. Benjamin LE, Golijanin D, Itin A, Pode D, Keshet E. Selective ablation of immature blood vessels in established human tumors follows vascular endothelial growth factor withdrawal. J Clin Invest. 1999;103(2):159–65.
24. Kloepper J, Riedemann L, Amoozgar Z, Seano G, Susek KH, Yu V, et al. Ang-2/VEGF bispecific antibody reprograms macrophages and resident microglia to anti-tumor phenotype and prolongs glioblastoma survival. Proc Natl Acad Sci USA. 2016 (in press).
25. Calabrese C, Poppleton H, Kocak M, Hogg TL, Fuller C, Hamner B, et al. A perivascular niche for brain tumor stem cells. Cancer Cell. 2007;11(1):69–82.
26. Folkins C, Shaked Y, Man S, Tang T, Lee CR, Zhu Z, et al. Glioma tumor stem-like cells promote tumor angiogenesis and vasculogenesis via vascular endothelial growth factor and stromal-derived factor 1. Cancer Res [Internet]. 2009;69(18):7243–51. Available from: http://www.ncbi.nlm.nih.gov/pubmed/19738068.
27. De Groot JF, Piao Y, Tran H, Gilbert M, Wu HK, Liu J, et al. Myeloid biomarkers associated with glioblastoma response to anti-VEGF therapy with aflibercept. Clin Cancer Res. 2011;17(14):4872–81.
28. De Palma M, Venneri MA, Galli R, Sergi LS, Politi LS, Sampaolesi M, et al. Tie2 identifies a hematopoietic lineage of proangiogenic monocytes required for tumor vessel formation and a mesenchymal population of pericyte progenitors. Cancer Cell. 2005;8(3):211–26.
29. Rigamonti N, Kadioglu E, Keklikoglou I, Rmili CW, Leow CC, de Palma M. Role of angiopoietin-2 in adaptive tumor resistance to VEGF signaling blockade. Cell Rep. 2014;8(3):696–706.
30. Kim KJ, Li B, Winer J, Armanini M, Gillett N, Phillips HS, et al. Inhibition of vascular endothelial growth factor-induced angiogenesis suppresses tumour growth in vivo. Nature [Internet]. 1993;362(6423):841–4. Available from: http://www.ncbi.nlm.nih.gov/pubmed/7683111.
31. Rubenstein JL, Kim J, Ozawa T, Zhang M, Westphal M, Deen DF, et al. Anti-VEGF antibody treatment of glioblastoma prolongs survival but results in increased vascular cooption. Neoplasia [Internet]. 2000;2(4):306–14. Available from: http://www.pubmedcentral.nih.gov/articlerender.fcgi?artid=1550290&tool=pmcentrez&rendertype=abstract.
32. Jahnke K, Muldoon LL, Varallyay CG, Lewin SJ, Kraemer DF, Neuwelt EA. Bevacizumab and carboplatin increase survival and asymptomatic tumor volume in a glioma model. Neuro Oncol. 2009;11:142–50.
33. Lee CG, Heijn M, di Tomaso E, Griffon-Etienne G, Ancukiewicz M, Koike C, et al. Anti-Vascular endothelial growth factor treatment augments tumor radiation response under normoxic or hypoxic conditions. Cancer Res [Internet]. 2000;60(19):5565–70. Available from: http://www.ncbi.nlm.nih.gov/entrez/query.fcgi?cmd=Retrieve&db=PubMed&dopt=Citation&list_uids=11034104.
34. Vredenburgh JJ, Desjardins A, Herndon JE, Marcello J, Reardon DA, Quinn JA, et al. Bevacizumab plus irinotecan in recurrent glioblastoma multiforme. J Clin Oncol. 2007;25(30):4722–9.
35. Vredenburgh JJ, Desjardins A, Herndon JE, Dowell JM, Reardon DA, Quinn JA, et al. Phase II trial of bevacizumab and irinotecan in recurrent malignant glioma. Clin Cancer Res. 2007;13(4):1253–9.
36. Wong ET, Hess KR, Gleason MJ, Jaeckle KA, Kyritsis AP, Prados MD, et al. Outcomes and prognostic factors in recurrent glioma patients enrolled onto phase II clinical trials. J Clin Oncol [Internet]. 1999;17(8):2572–8. Available from: http://www.ncbi.nlm.nih.gov/entrez/query.fcgi?cmd=Retrieve&db=PubMed&dopt=Citation&list_uids=10561324.
37. Friedman HS, Prados MD, Wen PY, Mikkelsen T, Schiff D, Abrey LE, et al. Bevacizumab alone and in combination with irinotecan in recurrent glioblastoma. J Clin Oncol. 2009;27(28):4733–40.
38. Kreisl TN, Kim L, Moore K, Duic P, Royce C, Stroud I, et al. Phase II trial of single-agent bevacizumab followed by bevacizumab plus irinotecan at tumor progression in recurrent glioblastoma. J Clin Oncol. 2009;27(5):740–5.
39. Wick W, Weller M, Van Den Bent M, Stupp R. Bevacizumab and recurrent malignant gliomas: a European perspective. J Clin Oncol. 2010;28(12):188–9.
40. Lee EQ, Reardon DA, Schiff D, Drappatz J, Muzikansky A, Grimm SA, et al. Phase II study of panobinostat in combination with bevacizumab for recurrent glioblastoma and anaplastic glioma. Neuro Oncol. 2015;17(6):862–7.
41. Norden AD, Young GS, Setayesh K, Muzikansky A, Klufas R, Ross GL, et al. Bevacizumab for recurrent malignant gliomas: efficacy, toxicity, and patterns of recurrence. Neurology [Internet]. 2008;70(10):779–87. Available from: http://www.ncbi.nlm.nih.gov/pubmed/18316689.
42. Francesconi AB, Dupre S, Matos M, Martin D, Hughes BG, Wyld DK, et al. Carboplatin and etoposide combined with bevacizumab for the treatment of recurrent glioblastoma multiforme. J Clin Neurosci [Internet]. Elsevier Ltd.; 2010;17(8):970–4. Available from: http://www.ncbi.nlm.nih.gov/pubmed/20541421.
43. Reardon DA, Desjardins A, Peters KB, Gururangan S, Sampson JH, McLendon RE, et al. Phase II study of carboplatin, irinotecan, and bevacizumab for bevacizumab naïve, recurrent glioblastoma. J Neurooncol [Internet]. 2012;107(1):155–64. Available from: http://www.ncbi.nlm.nih.gov/pubmed/21986722.

44. Reardon DA, Desjardins a, Vredenburgh JJ, Gururangan S, Sampson JH, Sathornsumetee S, et al. Metronomic chemotherapy with daily, oral etoposide plus bevacizumab for recurrent malignant glioma: a phase II study. Br J Cancer [Internet]. Nature Publishing Group; 2009;101(12):1986–94. Available from: http://www.pubmedcentral.nih.gov/articlerender.fcgi?artid=2795427&tool=pmcentrez&rendertype=abstract.
45. Ali SA, McHayleh WM, Ahmad A, Sehgal R, Braffet M, Rahman M, et al. Bevacizumab and irinotecan therapy in glioblastoma multiforme: a series of 13 cases. J Neurosurg [Internet]. 2008;109(2):268–72. Available from: http://www.ncbi.nlm.nih.gov/pubmed/18671639.
46. Bokstein F, Shpigel S, Blumenthal DT. Treatment with bevacizumab and irinotecan for recurrent high-grade glial tumors. Cancer. 2008;112(10):2267–73.
47. Kang TY, Jin T, Elinzano H, Peereboom D. Irinotecan and bevacizumab in progressive primary brain tumors, an evaluation of efficacy and safety. J Neurooncol. 2008;89(1):113–8.
48. Zuniga RM, Torcuator R, Jain R, Anderson J, Doyle T, Ellika S, et al. Efficacy, safety and patterns of response and recurrence in patients with recurrent high-grade gliomas treated with bevacizumab plus irinotecan. J Neurooncol. 2009;91(3):329–36.
49. Nghiemphu PL, Liu W, Lee Y, Than T, Graham C, Lai A, et al. Bevacizumab and chemotherapy for recurrent glioblastoma: a single-institution experience. Neurology. 2009;72(14):1217–22.
50. Desjardins A, Reardon DA, Coan A, Marcello J, Herndon JE, Bailey L, et al. Bevacizumab and daily temozolomide for recurrent glioblastoma. Cancer. 2012;118(5):1302–12.
51. Sathornsumetee S, Desjardins A, Vredenburgh JJ, McLendon RE, Marcello J, Herndon JE, et al. Phase II trial of bevacizumab and erlotinib in patients with recurrent malignant glioma. Neuro Oncol. 2010;12(12):1300–10.
52. Galanis E, Anderson SK, Lafky JM, Uhm JH, Giannini C, Kumar SK, et al. Phase II study of bevacizumab in combination with sorafenib in recurrent glioblastoma (N0776): a north central cancer treatment group trial. Clin Cancer Res [Internet]. 2013;19(17):4816–23. Available from: http://www.pubmedcentral.nih.gov/articlerender.fcgi?artid=3869574&tool=pmcentrez&rendertype=abstract.
53. Drappatz J, Lee EQ, Hammond S, Grimm SA, Norden AD, Beroukhim R, et al. Phase I study of panobinostat in combination with bevacizumab for recurrent high-grade glioma. J Neurooncol [Internet]. 2012;107(1):133–8. Available from: http://www.ncbi.nlm.nih.gov/pubmed/21984064.
54. Lassen U, Sorensen M, Gaziel TB, Hasselbalch B, Poulsen HS. Phase II study of bevacizumab and temsirolimus combination therapy for recurrent glioblastoma multiforme. Anticancer Res. 2013;33(4):1657–60.
55. Møller S, Grunnet K, Hansen S, Schultz H, Holmberg M, Sorensen M, et al. A phase II trial with bevacizumab and irinotecan for patients with primary brain tumors and progression after standard therapy. Acta Oncol (Madr). 2011;2012(51):797–804.
56. Soffietti R, Trevisan E, Bertero L, Cassoni P, Morra I, Fabrini MG, et al. Bevacizumab and fotemustine for recurrent glioblastoma: a phase II study of AINO (Italian Association of Neuro-Oncology). J Neurooncol. 2014;116(3):533–41.
57. Reardon DA, Desjardins A, Peters KB, Vredenburgh JJ, Gururangan S, Sampson JH, et al. Phase 2 study of carboplatin, irinotecan, and bevacizumab for recurrent glioblastoma after progression on bevacizumab therapy. Cancer [Internet]. 2011;117(23):5351–8. Available from: http://www.ncbi.nlm.nih.gov/pubmed/21590689.
58. Raizer JJ, Giglio P, Hu J, Groves M, Merrell R, Conrad C, et al. A phase II study of bevacizumab and erlotinib after radiation and temozolomide in MGMT unmethylated GBM patients. J Neurooncol. 2016;126(1):185–92.
59. Field KM, Simes J, Nowak AK, Cher L, Wheeler H, Hovey EJ, et al. Randomized phase 2 study of carboplatin and bevacizumab in recurrent glioblastoma. Neuro Oncol. 2015;17(11):1504–13.
60. Cuneo KC, Vredenburgh JJ, Sampson JH, Reardon DA, Desjardins A, Peters KB, et al. Safety and efficacy of stereotactic radiosurgery and adjuvant bevacizumab in patients with recurrent malignant gliomas. Int J Radiat Oncol Biol Phys. 2013;82(5):2018–24.
61. Cabrera AR, Cuneo KC, Vredenburgh JJ, Sampson JH, Kirkpatrick JP. Stereotactic radiosurgery and bevacizumab for recurrent glioblastoma multiforme. J Natl Compr Canc Netw [Internet]. 2012;10(6):695–9. Available from: http://www.ncbi.nlm.nih.gov/pubmed/22679114.
62. Gutin PH, Iwamoto FM, Beal K, Mohile NA, Karimi S, Hou BL, et al. Safety and efficacy of bevacizumab with hypofractionated stereotactic irradiation for recurrent malignant gliomas. Int J Radiat Oncol Biol Phys [Internet]. 2009;75(1):156–63. Available from: http://www.ncbi.nlm.nih.gov/pubmed/19167838.
63. Taal W, Oosterkamp HM, Walenkamp AME, Dubbink HJ, Beerepoot LV, Hanse MCJ, et al. Single-agent bevacizumab or lomustine versus a combination of bevacizumab plus lomustine in patients with recurrent glioblastoma (BELOB trial): A randomised controlled phase 2 trial. Lancet Oncol. 2014;15(9):943–53.
64. Wick W, Brandes A, Gorlia T, Bendszus M, Sahm F, Taal W, et al. Phase III trial exploring the combination of bevacizumab and lomustine in patients with first recurrence of a glioblastoma: the EORTC 26101 trial. Neuro Oncol [Internet]. 2015;17(Suppl. 5):v1.5–v1. Available from: http://neuro-oncology.oxfordjournals.org/cgi/doi/10.1093/neuonc/nov061.154.

65. Reardon DA, Herndon JE, Peters KB, Desjardins A, Coan A, Lou E, et al. Bevacizumab continuation beyond initial bevacizumab progression among recurrent glioblastoma patients. Br J Cancer [Internet]. Nature Publishing Group; 2012;107(9):1481–7. Available from: http://www.pubmedcentral.nih.gov/articlerender.fcgi?artid=3493761&tool=pmcentrez&rendertype=abstract.
66. Lai A, Tran A, Nghiemphu PL, Pope WB, Solis OE, Selch M, et al. Phase II study of bevacizumab plus temozolomide during and after radiation therapy for patients with newly diagnosed glioblastoma multiforme. J Clin Oncol. 2011;29(2):142–8.
67. Vredenburgh JJ, Desjardins A, Kirkpatrick JP, Reardon DA, Peters KB, Herndon JE, et al. Addition of bevacizumab to standard radiation therapy and daily temozolomide is associated with minimal toxicity in newly diagnosed glioblastoma multiforme. Int J Radiat Oncol Biol Phys. 2012;82(1):58–66.
68. Vredenburgh JJ, Desjardins A, Reardon DA, Peters KB, Herndon JE, Marcello J, et al. The addition of bevacizumab to standard radiation therapy and temozolomide followed by bevacizumab, temozolomide, and irinotecan for newly diagnosed glioblastoma. Clin Cancer Res [Internet]. 2011;17(12):4119–24. Available from: http://www.ncbi.nlm.nih.gov/pubmed/21531816.
69. Hegi ME, Diserens A-C, Gorlia T, Hamou M-F, de Tribolet N, Weller M, et al. MGMT gene silencing and benefit from temozolomide in glioblastoma. N Engl J Med. 2005;352(10):997–1003.
70. Herrlinger U, Schäfer N, Steinbach JP, Weyerbrock A, Hau P, Goldbrunner R, et al. Bevacizumab plus irinotecan versus temozolomide in newly diagnosed O6-methylguanine-DNA methyltransferase nonmethylated glioblastoma: the randomized GLARIUS trial. J Clin Oncol [Internet]. 2016; Available from: http://jco.ascopubs.org/cgi/doi/10.1200/JCO.2015.63.4691.
71. Chinot OL, Wick W, Mason W, Henriksson R, Saran F, Nishikawa R, et al. Bevacizumab plus radiotherapy-temozolomide for newly diagnosed glioblastoma. N Engl J Med [Internet]. 2014;370(8):709–22. Available from: http://www.ncbi.nlm.nih.gov/pubmed/24552318\nhttp://www.nejm.org/doi/pdf/10.1056/NEJMoa1308345.
72. Gilbert MR, Dignam JJ, Armstrong TS, Wefel JS, Blumenthal DT, Vogelbaum MA, et al. A randomized trial of bevacizumab for newly diagnosed glioblastoma. N Engl J Med [Internet]. 2014;370(8):699–708. Available from: http://www.ncbi.nlm.nih.gov/pubmed/24552317\nhttp://www.nejm.org/doi/pdf/10.1056/NEJMoa1308573.
73. Wen PY, Macdonald DR, Reardon DA, Cloughesy TF, Sorensen AG, Galanis E, et al. Updated response assessment criteria for high-grade gliomas: response assessment in neuro-oncology working group. J Clin Oncol. 2010;28(11):1963–72.
74. Macdonald DR, Cascino TL, Schold SC, Cairncross JG. Response criteria for phase II studies of supratentorial malignant glioma. J Clin Oncol [Internet]. 1990;8(7):1277–80. Available from: http://www.ncbi.nlm.nih.gov/pubmed/2358840.
75. Chinot OL, Macdonald DR, Abrey LE, Zahlmann G. Kerloëguen Y, Cloughesy TF. Response assessment criteria for glioblastoma: practical adaptation and implementation in clinical trials of antiangiogenic therapy. Curr Neurol Neurosci Rep. 2013;13(5):347.
76. Gomez-Manzano C, Holash J, Fueyo J, Xu J, Conrad CA, Aldape KD, et al. VEGF Trap induces antiglioma effect at different stages of disease. Neuro Oncol [Internet]. 2008;10(6):940–5. Available from: http://www.pubmedcentral.nih.gov/articlerender.fcgi?artid=2719008&tool=pmcentrez&rendertype=abstract.
77. De Groot JF, Lamborn KR, Chang SM, Gilbert MR, Cloughesy TF, Aldape K, et al. Phase II study of aflibercept in recurrent malignant glioma: a North American brain tumor consortium study. J Clin Oncol. 2011;29(19):2689–95.
78. Batchelor TT, Duda DG, Di Tomaso E, Ancukiewicz M, Plotkin SR, Gerstner E, et al. Phase II study of cediranib, an oral pan-vascular endothelial growth factor receptor tyrosine kinase inhibitor, in patients with recurrent glioblastoma. J Clin Oncol. 2010;28(17):2817–23.
79. Batchelor TT, Mulholland P, Neyns B, Nabors LB, Campone M, Wick A, et al. Phase III randomized trial comparing the efficacy of cediranib as monotherapy, and in combination with lomustine, versus lomustine alone in patients with recurrent glioblastoma. J Clin Oncol. 2013;31(26):3212–8.
80. Iwamoto FM, Lamborn KR, Robins HI, Mehta MP, Chang SM, Butowski NA, et al. Phase II trial of pazopanib (GW786034), an oral multi-targeted angiogenesis inhibitor, for adults with recurrent glioblastoma (North American Brain Tumor Consortium Study 06-02). Neuro Oncol. 2010;12(8):855–61.
81. Chow LQM, Eckhardt SG. Sunitinib: From rational design to clinical efficacy. J Clin Oncol. 2007;25(7):884–96.
82. Neyns B, Sadones J, Chaskis C, Dujardin M, Everaert H, Lv S, et al. Phase II study of sunitinib malate in patients with recurrent high-grade glioma. J Neurooncol. 2011;103(3):491–501.
83. Chheda MG, Wen PY, Hochberg FH, Chi AS, Drappatz J, Eichler AF, et al. Vandetanib plus sirolimus in adults with recurrent glioblastoma: results of a phase I and dose expansion cohort study. J Neurooncol. 2015;121(3):627–34.
84. Schiff D, Kesari S, De Groot J, Mikkelsen T, Drappatz J, Coyle T, et al. Phase 2 study of CT-322, a targeted biologic inhibitor of VEGFR-2 based on a domain of human fibronectin, in recurrent glioblastoma. Invest New Drugs. 2015;33(1):247–53.

85. Wick W, Puduvalli VK, Chamberlain MC, Van Den Bent MJ, Carpentier AF, Cher LM, et al. Phase III study of enzastaurin compared with lomustine in the treatment of recurrent intracranial glioblastoma. J Clin Oncol. 2010;28(7):1168–74.
86. DeLay M, Jahangiri A, Carbonell WS, Hu Y-L, Tsao S, Tom MW, et al. Microarray analysis verifies two distinct phenotypes of glioblastomas resistant to antiangiogenic therapy. Clin Cancer Res [Internet]. 2012;18(10):2930–42. Available from: http://www.ncbi.nlm.nih.gov/pubmed/22472177.
87. Lu KV, Bergers G. Mechanisms of evasive resistance to anti-VEGF therapy in glioblastoma. CNS Oncol [Internet]. 2013;2(1):49–65. Available from: http://www.pubmedcentral.nih.gov/articlerender.fcgi?artid=3673744&tool=pmcentrez&rendertype=abstract.
88. Casanovas O, Hicklin DJ, Bergers G, Hanahan D. Drug resistance by evasion of antiangiogenic targeting of VEGF signaling in late-stage pancreatic islet tumors. Cancer Cell. 2005;8(4):299–309.
89. Huang D, Ding Y, Zhou M, Rini BI, Petillo D, Qian C, et al. Interleukin-8 mediates resistance to antiangiogenic agent sunitinib in renal cell carcinoma. Cancer Res [Internet]. 2010;70(3):1063–71. Available from: http://www.ncbi.nlm.nih.gov/pubmed/20103651.
90. Peterson TE, Kirkpatrick ND, Huang Y, Farrar CT, Marijt KA, Datta M, et al. Dual inhibition of Ang-2 and VEGF receptors normalizes tumor vasculature and prolongs survival in glioblastoma by altering macrophages. Proc Natl Acad Sci USA. 2016 (in press).
91. Scholz A, Harter PN, Cremer S, Yalcin BH, Gurnik S, Yamaji M, et al. Endothelial cell-derived angiopoietin- 2 is a therapeutic target in treatment-naive and bevacizumab-resistant glioblastoma. 2015;8(1):1–19.
92. Carmeliet P, Jain RK. Molecular mechanisms and clinical applications of angiogenesis. Nature [Internet]. 2011;473(7347):298–307. Available from: http://dx.doi.org/10.1038/nature10144.
93. Wang R, Chadalavada K, Wilshire J, Kowalik U, Hovinga KE, Geber A, et al. Glioblastoma stem-like cells give rise to tumour endothelium. Nature [Internet]. Nature Publishing Group; 2010;468 (7325):829–33. Available from: http://dx.doi.org/10.1038/nature09624.
94. Ricci-Vitiani L, Pallini R, Biffoni M, Todaro M, Invernici G, Cenci T, et al. Tumour vascularization via endothelial differentiation of glioblastoma stem-like cells. Nature [Internet]. Nature Publishing Group; 2010;468(7325):824–8. Available from: http://www.ncbi.nlm.nih.gov/pubmed/21102434.
95. Sitohy B, Nagy JA, Jaminet SCS, Dvorak HF. Tumor-surrogate blood vessel subtypes exhibit differential susceptibility to anti-VEGF therapy. Cancer Res. 2011;71(22):7021–8.
96. Shojaei F, Wu X, Qu X, Kowanetz M, Yu L, Tan M, et al. G-CSF-initiated myeloid cell mobilization and angiogenesis mediate tumor refractoriness to anti-VEGF therapy in mouse models. Proc Natl Acad Sci USA. 2009;106:6742–7.
97. Piao Y, Liang J, Holmes L, Henry V, Sulman E, De Groot JF. Acquired resistance to anti-VEGF therapy in glioblastoma is associated with a mesenchymal transition. Clin Cancer Res. 2013;19(16):4392–403.
98. Lu KV, Chang JP, Parachoniak CA, Pandika MM, Aghi MK, Meyronet D, et al. VEGF inhibits tumor cell invasion and mesenchymal transition through a MET/VEGFR2 complex. Cancer Cell [Internet]. 2012;22(1):21–35. Available from: http://www.ncbi.nlm.nih.gov/pubmed/22789536.
99. Tang TC, Man S, Xu P, Francia G, Hashimoto K, Emmenegger U, et al. Development of a resistance-like phenotype to sorafenib by human hepatocellular carcinoma cells is reversible and can be delayed by metronomic UFT chemotherapy. Neoplasia [Internet]. 2010;12(11):928–40. Available from: http://www.ncbi.nlm.nih.gov/pubmed/21076618\nhttp://www.ncbi.nlm.nih.gov/pmc/articles/PMC2978915/pdf/neo1211_0928.pdf.
100. Bennouna J, Sastre J, Arnold D, Österlund P, Greil R, Van Cutsem E, et al. Continuation of bevacizumab after first progression in metastatic colorectal cancer (ML18147): A randomised phase 3 trial. Lancet Oncol. 2013;14(1):29–37.
101. von Minckwitz G, Puglisi F, Cortes J, Vrdoljak E, Marschner N, Zielinski C, et al. Bevacizumab plus chemotherapy versus chemotherapy alone as second-line treatment for patients with HER2-negative locally recurrent or metastatic breast cancer after first-line treatment with bevacizumab plus chemotherapy (TANIA): an open-label, randomised. Lancet Oncol [Internet]. 2014;15(11):1269–78. Available from: http://www.sciencedirect.com/science/article/pii/S1470204514704395.
102. Sulman EP, Won M, Blumenthal DT, Vogelbaum MA, Colman H, Jenkins RB, et al. Molecular predictors of outcome and response to bevacizumab (BEV) based on analysis of RTOG 0825, a phase III trial comparing chemoradiation (CRT) with and without BEV in patients with newly diagnosed glioblastoma (GBM). J Clin Oncol. 2013;31(Suppl. 15s):LBA2010.
103. Sandmann T, Bourgon R, Garcia J, Li C, Cloughesy T, Chinot OL, et al. Patients with proneural glioblastoma may derive overall survival benefit from the addition of bevacizumab to first-line radiotherapy and temozolomide: Retrospective analysis of the AVAglio trial. J Clin Oncol. 2015;33 (25):2735–44.
104. Sathornsumetee S, Cao Y, Marcello JE, Herndon JE, McLendon RE, Desjardins A, et al. Tumor angiogenic and hypoxic profiles predict radiographic response and survival in malignant astrocytoma patients treated with bevacizumab and irinotecan. J Clin Oncol [Internet]. 2008;26(2):271–8.

Available from: http://www.ncbi.nlm.nih.gov/pubmed/18182667.

105. Batchelor TT, Gerstner ER, Emblem KE, Duda DG, Kalpathy-Cramer J, Snuderl M, et al. Improved tumor oxygenation and survival in glioblastoma patients who show increased blood perfusion after cediranib and chemoradiation. Proc Natl Acad Sci USA [Internet]. 2013;110(47):19059–64. Available from: http://www.pubmedcentral.nih.gov/articlerender.fcgi?artid=3839699&tool=pmcentrez&rendertype=abstract.
106. Duda DG, Willett CG, Ancukiewicz M, di Tomaso E, Shah M, Czito BG, et al. Plasma soluble VEGFR-1 is a potential dual biomarker of response and toxicity for bevacizumab with chemoradiation in locally advanced rectal cancer. Oncologist [Internet]. 2010;15(6):577–83. Available from: http://eutils.ncbi.nlm.nih.gov/entrez/eutils/elink.fcgi?dbfrom=pubmed&id=20484123&retmode=ref&cmd=prlinks\nhttp://theoncologist.alphamedpress.org/cgi/doi/10.1634/theoncologist.2010-0029.
107. Duda DG, Kozin SV, Kirkpatrick ND, Xu L, Fukumura D, Jain RK. CXCL12 (SDF1α)-CXCR4/CXCR7 pathway inhibition: an emerging sensitizer for anticancer therapies? Clin Cancer Res. 2011;17(8):2074–80.
108. Tabouret E, Boudouresque F, Barrie M, Matta M, Boucard C, Loundou A, et al. Association of matrix metalloproteinase 2 plasma level with response and survival in patients treated with bevacizumab for recurrent high-grade glioma. Neuro Oncol. 2014;16(3):392–9.
109. Pope WB, Kim HJ, Huo J, Alger J, Brown MS, Gjertson D, et al. Recurrent glioblastoma multiforme: ADC histogram analysis predicts response to bevacizumab treatment. Radiology [Internet]. 2009;252(1):182–9. Available from: http://www.ncbi.nlm.nih.gov/pubmed/19561256.
110. Kothari PD, White NS, Farid N, Chung R, Kuperman JM, Girard HM, et al. Longitudinal restriction spectrum imaging is resistant to pseudoresponse in patients with high-grade gliomas treated with bevacizumab. AJNR Am J Neuroradiol [Internet]. 2013;34(9):1752–7. Available from: http://www.ncbi.nlm.nih.gov/pubmed/23578667.
111. Piludu F, Marzi S, Pace A, Villani V, Fabi A, Carapella CM, et al. Early biomarkers from dynamic contrast-enhanced magnetic resonance imaging to predict the response to antiangiogenic therapy in high-grade gliomas. Neuroradiology. 2015;57(12):1269–80.
112. O'Connor JPB, Jackson A, Parker GJM, Roberts C, Jayson GC. Dynamic contrast-enhanced MRI in clinical trials of antivascular therapies. Nat Rev Clin Oncol [Internet]. Nature Publishing Group; 2012;9(3):167–77. Available from: http://dx.doi.org/10.1038/nrclinonc.2012.2.
113. Emblem KE, Mouridsen K, Bjornerud A, Farrar CT, Jennings D, Borra RJH, et al. Vessel architectural imaging identifies cancer patient responders to anti-angiogenic therapy. Nat Med [Internet]. 2013;19(9):1178–83. Available from: http://www.ncbi.nlm.nih.gov/pubmed/23955713.
114. Chen W, Delaloye S, Silverman DHS, Geist C, Czernin J, Sayre J, et al. Predicting treatment response of malignant gliomas to bevacizumab and irinotecan by imaging proliferation with [18F] fluorothymidine positron emission tomography: a pilot study. J Clin Oncol. 2007;25(30):4714–21.
115. Harris RJ, Cloughesy TF, Pope WB, Nghiemphu PL, Lai A, Zaw T, et al. 18F-FDOPA and 18F-FLT positron emission tomography parametric response maps predict response in recurrent malignant gliomas treated with bevacizumab. Neuro Oncol. 2012;14(8):1079–89.
116. Sorensen AG, Emblem KE, Polaskova P, Jennings D, Kim H, Ancukiewicz M, et al. Increased survival of glioblastoma patients who respond to antiangiogenic therapy with elevated blood perfusion. Cancer Res. 2012;72(2):402–7.
117. Buchroithner J, Pichler J, Marosi C, Widhalm G, Seiz-Rosenhagen M, Novosielski M, et al. Vascular endothelia growth factor targeted therapy may improve the effect of dendritic cell-based cancer immune therapy. Int J Clin Pharmacol Ther [Internet]. 2014 Jan;52(1):76–7. Available from: http://www.ncbi.nlm.nih.gov/pubmed/24321210.
118. Reardon DA, Schuster J, Tran DD, Fink KL, Nabors LB, Li G, et al. ReACT: overall survival from a randomized phase II study of rindopepimut (CDX-110) plus bevacizumab in relapsed glioblastoma. J Clin Oncol. 2015;15(Suppl):2009.
119. Shrimali RK, Yu Z, Theoret MR, Chinnasamy D, Restifo NP, Rosenberg SA. Antiangiogenic agents can increase lymphocyte infiltration into tumor and enhance the effectiveness of adoptive immunotherapy of cancer. Cancer Res [Internet]. 2010;70(15):6171–80. Available from: http://www.ncbi.nlm.nih.gov/pubmed/20631075.
120. Lorgis V, Maura G, Coppa G, Hassani K, Taillandier L, Chauffert B, et al. Relation between bevacizumab dose intensity and high-grade glioma survival: a retrospective study in two large cohorts. J Neurooncol. 2012;107(2):351–8.

Immunotherapy for High-Grade Gliomas

12

Teilo H. Schaller and John H. Sampson

Introduction

Anti-cancer immunotherapies which activate the patient's own immune system have shown efficacy and specificity in a variety of cancers, promising safer and more effective therapies. FDA approval of the anti-CD20 antibody rituximab for the treatment of lymphoma, the anti-HER2 antibody herceptin for treatment of breast cancer, and breakthrough checkpoint inhibitors such as anti-CTLA4 and anti-PD-1 have validated the field of immunotherapy and herald the start of an immunotherapy age that is revolutionizing cancer treatment [1–3].

The Not-So-Privileged Blood-Brain Barrier

Traditionally, literature describing the central nervous system (CNS) portrays a limited immune response marked by the blood–brain barrier, lack of a conventional lymphatic drainage system, and low levels of T cells, antigen-presenting cells, and major histocompatibility complexes [4]. However, recent findings provide evidence that while CNS entry is limited, there is a fully developed immune response in the brain. These findings include a lymph node-like drainage system which drains CNS antigens from the cerebrospinal fluid into the cervical lymph nodes, thereby facilitating immune surveillance of the CNS [5]. In addition, evidence shows that some immune cells are fully able to migrate into the CNS, where they are involved in diseases such as multiple sclerosis, CNS infections, and are also found in gliomas [4, 6]. In addition to the not-so-privileged blood–brain barrier, angiogenesis around the growing brain tumor leads to deterioration of brain microvasculature, increasing leakage [7]. That is, barrier functions such as tight junctions between the endothelial or transcytosis mechanisms may be relaxed, allowing increased penetration by immune cells [8].

Both the inherent control of the immune system over the brain and the deterioration of the blood–brain barrier during cancer growth warrant the potential of immunotherapy to redirect and activate immune cells that specifically recognize tumor cells within the brain.

Targets for Immunotherapies

The premise of immunotherapy rests on the idea that tumor cells are foreign and that the immune system can be taught to recognize the foreign cells or that a pre-existing immune response can be augmented. In order for such recognition to take place, antigens must be found that identify a specific tumor type and elicit an immune response. Broadly speaking, there are two types

T.H. Schaller · J.H. Sampson (✉)
Department of Neurosurgery, Duke University Medical Center, DUMC 3050, 303 Research Drive, Sands Bldg. 220, Durham, NC 27710, USA
e-mail: John.sampson@duke.edu

J. Moliterno Günel et al. (eds.), *Malignant Brain Tumors*,
DOI 10.1007/978-3-319-49864-5_12

of immunologic targets, (i) tumor-associated antigens and (ii) tumor-specific antigens.

Tumor-Associated Antigens

Tumor-associated antigens (TAAs) are normal proteins that are overexpressed in tumor cells and can thereby serve to direct the immunologic response. Commonly, these antigens are lineage-differentiation antigens such as colorectal cancer antigens (CEA) [9] and alpha-fetoprotein (AFP) [10]. The major concern is that the expression of these antigens on healthy tissue, even if limited, could lead to autoimmunity if a potent immune response is elicited.

In glioblastoma, several studies have shown the overexpression of numerous proteins that could serve as immunological targets and for some antigens, clinical efficacy has been shown [11, 12]. Numerous studies have tested TAAs as potential immunotherapeutic targets for malignant brain tumors, including survivin, HER2neu, EphA2, EGFR, and telomerase [12–18].

Cancer/testis antigens (CTAs) represent a unique class of TAAs with normal expression restricted to germ cells in the testis but not in adult somatic cells. The melanoma-associated CTAs (MAGE, CAGE) are extensively expressed in a wide range of different cancers [19, 20].

An extensive expression analysis by Freitas et al. analyzed 153 cancer/testis antigens (CTAs), a class of differentiation antigens shown to be variably expressed within GBM tumors, and identified 4 CTAs (ACTL8, CTCFL, OIP5, and XAGE3) uniquely expressed within GBM tumors when compared to normal brain [21].

As with all TAAs, the question remains whether an approach targeting these antigens will yield a therapeutic window that shows efficacy yet limits adverse effects on healthy tissue expressing low levels of the antigen.

Tumor-Specific Antigens

In contrast to TAAs, which are normal proteins upregulated in cancer, tumor-specific antigens (TSAs) arise as mutations of normal proteins during the course of tumor progression and result in antigens that are exclusively expressed on malignant cells, albeit often on a subset of tumor cells. These antigens serve as prime targets for immunotherapies, as possible side effects such as cytotoxicity to healthy tissue are avoided.

In glioblastoma, a number of TSAs have been identified, of which some have already progressed into the clinic. Recent advances in genetic sequencing are rapidly identifying new mutations that identify subgroups of patients expressing a certain histologic type of brain cancer [22]. These neoantigens will need to be tested for their immunogenic potential to determine which can be used to develop future immunotherapies.

Currently, there are two TSAs that are highly prevalent and have shown immunogenicity in numerous studies. EGFRvIII is a conserved mutation of the epidermal growth factor receptor that is seen in approximately 31–50% of patients with GBM as well as in other cancers [23–28]. In those patients positive for EGFRvIII, the mutation is expressed in 37–87% of tumor cells.

A conserved mutation of isocitrate dehydrogenase type 1 (IDH1), which occurs at the critical arginine residue (Arg 132) in the catalytic pocket, results in a neomorphic enzymatic function, genetic instability, and malignant transformation [29]. This mutation, termed IDH1 (R132H), occurs in more than 70% of grade III gliomas and, from a therapeutic viewpoint, represents an ideal candidate for a tumor-specific treatment of malignant glioma [30].

In addition, viral antigens, when upregulated specifically on malignant cells, may also serve as TSAs and have the unique advantage of being intrinsically foreign to the host and thus immunogenic. Therefore, while viruses may not be exclusively restricted to tumor cells, their expression is often undetectable in normal tissue of patients harboring virus-associated cancers. Our laboratory and others have recently shown human cytomegalovirus infection and low-level viral gene expression in malignant glioma [31, 32]. Given the success and safety of cellular immunotherapeutics targeting CMV in immunocompromised patients, immunodominant CMV antigens such as immediate early 1 (IE1), phosphoprotein 65 (pp65), and glycoprotein B (gB) have been shown to be expressed in GBM tumors and represent possible tumor-specific targets for the development of immunotherapies [33–35].

Antibodies for the Treatment of Intracerebral Malignancies

Monoclonal Antibodies Target Tumor Epitopes

The development of monoclonal antibodies (mAbs) recognizing specific epitopes has been used for the immunological treatment of many diseases, including cancer [36]. By recognizing and binding to specific epitopes, mAbs expose intruding cells and target them for uptake by phagocytic cells of the immune system, such as macrophages and dendritic cells. Furthermore, mAbs can target cellular components, such as secreted proteins, and thereby interfere with cell signaling.

Advances in technology over the past decades have made it possible to produce fully human affinity-matured antibodies via phage display directed evolution, transgenic mice, or mRNA and ribosome display, thereby resolving complications associated with murine antibodies such as human anti-mouse antibody formation and cytokine release syndrome [37–41].

Although antibodies can be found in the central nervous system at physiologic levels, GBM-induced disruptions of the blood–brain barrier facilitate antibody penetration. Several studies have shown that injecting antibodies IV in GBM patients results in significant therapeutic benefit [42–45]. In murine GBM models, an antibody directed against tenascin, a component of the tumor stroma, given systemically was shown to selectively localize to the tumor [42, 43].

The epidermal growth factor receptor (EGFR) is a well-studied and versatile signal transducer that is involved in cell proliferation, differentiation, survival, and metastasis [46]. EGFR is overexpressed in a number of tumors and plays an important role in the development of high-grade gliomas, especially in glioblastoma where it is commonly (40–60% of patients) amplified up to hundreds of gene copies [47, 48]. Anti-EGFR antibodies approved for the treatment of colorectal and head and neck cancers have been shown to inhibit ligand binding, receptor dimerization, and downstream signaling [49]. Sym004, a recently developed anti-EGFR antibody with enhanced effectiveness, is being tested in a phase II trial in recurrent glioblastoma in both patients that failed and did not fail bevacizumab treatment (Table 12.1).

Bispecific Antibodies Redirect and Activate Effector Immune Cells

Various solid tumors show infiltration with T cells and increased T cell infiltration often correlates with a good clinical outcome [50]. T cell infiltration has also been shown in glioma and is increased in high-grade tumors [51]. Substantial evidence suggests that the redirection of these T cells to specifically recognize and kill tumor cells is able to eradicate well-established tumors [52, 53]. Furthermore, clinical data have shown that mABs suffer from major limitations in their mode of action, including alternative Fc glycosylation, leading to suboptimal effector cell interaction, competition with circulating IgG, and activation of inhibitory receptors [54].

Bispecific antibodies (bsABs) are capable of binding two distinct targets and can be used to link T cells to tumor cells. Bispecific T cell engagers (BiTEs) consist of two antibody-derived linked single-chain Fv fragments (scFv) that are translated in tandem. One arm of the BiTE recognizes, for instance, the CD3 epsilon subunit on the T cell and the other arm binds a tumor antigen (Fig. 12.1). Upon binding, the BiTE causes crosslinking between adjacent tumor cells and T cells, regardless of the T cell receptor recognition, leading to T cell activation, synapse formation, and tumor lysis via perforin and granzyme secretion. Following

Table 12.1 Recent clinical trials employing antibody immunotherapy for high-grade gliomas

NIH clinical trial	Type	Phase	Eligibility criteria	Primary outcome	Dosing regimen	Treatment groups
NCT02311920	Checkpt	1	Newly diagnosed GBM	Maximum safe dose	In addition to TMZ, Arm I receives anti-CTLA4 Ab ipilimumab once every 4 weeks (4 doses) followed every 3 months (4 doses), Arm II receives anti-PD1 Ab nivolumab once every 2 weeks (32 doses), and Arm III receives both Abs	Arm I: TMZ + Ipi Arm II: TMZ + Nivo Arm III: TMZ + Ipi + Nivo
NCT02526017	mAb + checkpt	1	GBM	Safety, RD, efficacy (ORR)	Arm I will receive anti-CSF1R Ab FPA008 every 2 weeks. Arm II will receive 3 mg/kg nivolumab every 2 weeks in addition to dose-escalated FPA008 every 2 weeks. Arm III uses MTD determined in Arm II and expands patient group	Arm I: mAb Arm II: mAB dose escalation + Nivo Arm III: mAB + Nivo expansion group
NCT02521090	BiTE	1/2	Recurrent and refractory GBM	Toxicity (phase I), OS (phase II)	Phase I: patients receive anti-EGFR-CD3 BiTE armed T cells IT twice weekly for 4 weeks. Phase II: patients continue to receive BiTE armed T cells IV twice weekly for 2 weeks	Single-arm
NCT02423343	Small molecule + checkpt	1/2	GBM	MTD of galunisertib combined with Nivolumab	In Arm I escalating doses of TGFβR1 kinase small molecule inhibitor galunisertib are given daily for 14 days of each 4 week cycle in combination with nivolumab every 2 weeks. Arm II will use same treatment regimen with MTD galunisertib	Cohort A: dose escalation Cohort B: expansion group
NCT02530502	Checkpt	1/2	Newly diagnosed GBM	Phase I: DLT Phase II: PFS	Focal RT over 42 days followed by TMZ on days 1–42 and anti-PD1 antibody pembrolizumab on days 1, 22, and 43 for each course for up to 6 courses	Single-arm
NCT01952769	Checkpt	1/2	Diffuse intrinsic pontine glioma	Treatment-related toxicity	Anti-PD1 antibody given biweekly. Cohort A receives two doses with increasing concentration. Cohort B concentration varies between patients	Cohort A: 2 doses Cohort B: doses of different concentration

(continued)

Table 12.1 (continued)

NIH clinical trial	Type	Phase	Eligibility criteria	Primary outcome	Dosing regimen	Treatment groups
NCT02337686	Checkpt	2	Recurrent GBM	PFS6 and immune effector:Treg ratio	Anti-PD-1 antibody pembrolizumab given once every 3 weeks (2 doses) before surgery and once every 3 weeks thereafter	Single-arm
NCT02337491	Checkpt + mAB	2	Recurrent GBM	PFS6 and MTD	Not described	Cohort A: pembrolizumab + bevacizumab Cohort B: pembrolizumab
NCT01149850	mAb	2	Newly diagnosed GBM	Overall survival	Anti-VEGF antibody bevacizumab every 2 weeks	Single-arm
NCT02540161	mAb	2	Recurrent GBM	PFS6	Anti-EGFR antibody Sym004 given every 2 weeks at 18 mg/kg	Cohort A: non-bevacizumab failures Cohort B: bevacizumab failures

Ab antibody; *BiTE* bispecific T cell engager; *Checkpt* immune checkpoint modulator; *DLT* dose-limiting toxicity; *GBM* glioblastoma; *Ipi* ipilimumab; *IT* intrathecal; *mAb* monoclonal antibody; *Nivo* nivolumab; *OS* overall survival; *MTD* maximum tolerated dose; *PFS* progression-free survival; *PFS6* 6-month progression-free survival; *ORR* objective response rate; *RD* recommended dose; *TMZ* temozolomide; *Treg* regulatory T cell

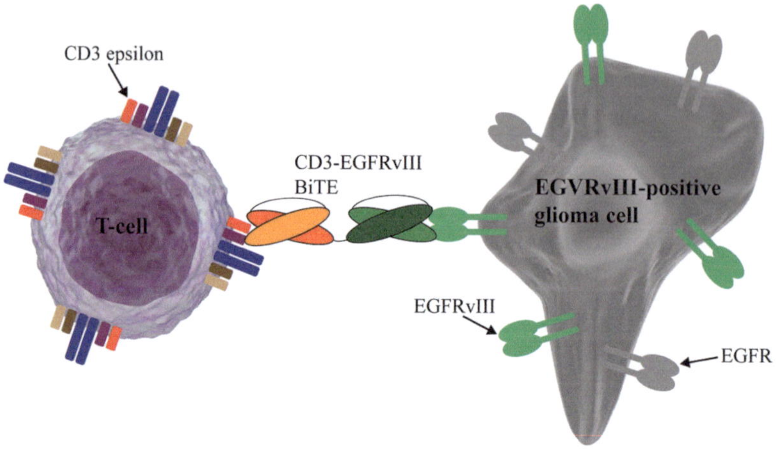

Fig. 12.1 BiTE mode of action. The anti-CD3-EGFRvIII bispecific T cell engager (BiTE) is able to bind the CD3 epsilon subunit of the T cell receptor with one of its single-chain Fv (scFv) fragments and EGFRvIII on the glioma cell with the other scFv fragment. This leads to spatially restricted crosslinking and activation of the T cell, resulting in T cell-mediated tumor cell cytotoxicity via synapse formation and the release of perforin and granzyme

BiTE-mediated tumor cell lysis, the T cells proliferate, express surface activation markers, and undergo serial rounds of killing [53, 55–57]. Furthermore, since crosslinking depends on binding to CD3 epsilon, T cell subsets implicated with tumor progression, such as Tregs, are also activated to lyse tumor cells [58, 59].

Since T cell activation requires physical linking to a tumor antigen, the immune activation is spatially and temporally restricted and highly specific for the chosen antigen. Furthermore, the small size of the BiTE results in a short half-life that allows quick regulation of antibody-mediated toxicity [60].

A recent clinical trial aims to treat patients with recurrent or refractory glioblastoma with a bispecific antibody made by the heteroconjugation of anti-EGFR and anti-CD3 antibody. Autologous activated T cells are loaded with the anti-EGFR-CD3 BiTE and injected intravenously into the patient with the goal of increasing T cell-mediated cytotoxicity toward tumor expressing EGFR [61]. The aim in this trial will be to determine whether a therapeutic window exists that will allow cell killing of EGFR over-expressing tumor cells without afflicting normal tissue (Table 12.1).

Our laboratory recently developed a BiTE produced by the heteroconjugation of an anti-EGFRvIII and anti-CD3 antibody. Experiments in mice show that systemic administration of the BiTE activates T cells in mice, resulting in extended survival and durable complete cures at rates of up to 75% [62]. Given the tumor specificity of the EGFRvIII antigen, treatment of patients with this antibody may have fewer side effects and increased efficacy.

Immune Checkpoint Modulators

The growth of a tumor is marked by significant changes to the microenvironment, leading to cancer-associated immunosuppression. This means that despite the presence of tumor-specific endogenous T cells, tumors escape destruction by upregulating inhibitory ligands that bind to inhibitory receptors on T cells, secretion of inhibitory cytokines (including TGF-beta and IL-10), and other mechanisms. This immunosuppression is particularly pronounced in glioma patients and leads to T cell dysfunction and an increase in the regulatory T cell phenotype [63–66].

Novel strategies for dealing with tumor-associated immunosuppression are the development of antagonistic mABs which block inhibitory ligands, such as CTLA-4, PD-1 and PD-L1, and agonistic mABs that stimulate the immune response by binding agonistic cell surface molecules, such as OX40 and 4-1BB (Fig. 12.2). Recent advances, in particular the FDA approval of the nivolumab–ipilimumab combination for the treatment of metastatic melanoma, highlight the powerful effect and curative potential of immune checkpoint modulators [67].

Using anti-CTLA4 antibodies, our laboratory was able to show that systemic CTLA-4 blockade leads to long-term survival in 80% of treated mice with established gliomas without eliciting experimental allergic encephalomyelitis. Furthermore, treatment resulted in the recovery of normal $CD4^{+}$ T cell counts and proliferative capacity and also suppressed increases in $CD4^{+}$ CD25+ Foxp3+ GITR+ regulatory T cell fractions [68].

The first clinical trials with anti-CTLA4 and anti-PD-1 antibodies have recently begun for the treatment of newly diagnosed and recurrent GBM and are being tested alone or in combination with other checkpoint modulators, small molecules, and mAbs (Table 12.1). In one study comparable to the recent approval of ipilimumab–nivolumab combination for melanoma, anti-CTLA4 and anti-PD-1 are being tested separately or in combination in a three-armed study in patients with newly diagnosed GBM (Table 12.1).

However, even though trials using checkpoint inhibitors and agonists or combinations thereof have shown unprecedented potential for treating various cancer types, only a certain percentage of patients respond and toxicities are significant [3, 69]. The reasons for this are still unclear but are likely to also occur in GBM, emphasizing the need for in-depth diagnosis and hinting at the future of personalized medicine where certain checkpoint modulators or combinations thereof are prescribed based on patient-specific cancer and genetic traits.

Vaccinations for Tumor Control

The goal of vaccination is to sensitize the immune system against a target antigen and thereby elicit a potent and specific immune response that includes a memory response to the target. While vaccination has been used to successfully prevent and eradicate numerous diseases such as polio, tetanus, and typhoid,

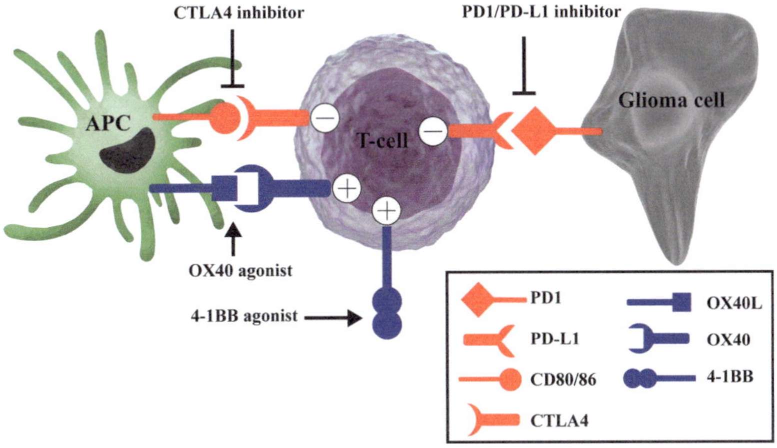

Fig. 12.2 Immune checkpoint modulators. Monoclonal antibodies directed against the immune checkpoint inhibitors CTLA4 and PD1/PD-L1 are used to prevent downregulation of T cell activity and show high potential in GBM. OX40 and 4-1BB are agonistic molecules that, when bound by an antibody, stimulate T cell activity. Both mechanisms lead to a broad upregulation of immune cell activity. *APC*, antigen-presenting cell

anti-tumor vaccinations have not shown the same efficacy and a lot of research is currently ongoing in this field.

Peptides

The major determinant for peptide vaccine-mediated immunogenicity is antigen choice. TAAs, given their expression on normal cells, usually elicit a subdued immune response due to central tolerance. On the other hand, TSAs, given their exclusive presentation on tumor cells, generally elicit a robust immune response similar to the immune response seen against antigens of infectious diseases.

The advantage of TAAs is their high frequency of expression in gliomas, making it possible to give most patients off-the-shelf synthetic tumor antigen peptides. Furthermore, by giving patients a cocktail of peptides, a broader immune response targeting multiple tumor subsets can be elicited. In contrast, TSAs are unique to the tumor and thereby peptides from these antigens may result in a highly tumor-focused immune response.

The mutated protein EGFRvIII, as discussed previously, represents an ideal target for anti-tumor immunotherapy. Our laboratory constructed a 13-amino-acid peptide spanning the vIII mutation and conjugated it to keyhole limpet hemocyanin (KLH). A phase II clinical trial showed that patients with EGFRvIII-positive newly diagnosed GBM, when vaccinated with rindopepimut, the EGFRvIII peptide, had a median survival of 26 months compared with the control historical cohort, which had a median survival of 15 months [70]. These positive results led to the start of a currently ongoing phase III clinical trial with the EGFRvIII peptide vaccine (Table 12.2).

However, given the heterogeneous nature of malignant brain tumor and peptide HLA restrictions, the drawback of single peptide vaccinations is that they may only be effective in a percentage of patients, and in the case of tumor-specific peptides only in the subset of patients expressing the mutated peptide. Trials are ongoing to determine whether combinations of multiple peptides will result in clinically effective peptide vaccination strategies (Table 12.2). Furthermore, increased research on neoantigens, antigens that spontaneously arise in individuals during the course of tumor progression, may lead to personalized solutions in which a patient's tumor is sequenced after resection and peptide vaccinations are constructed based on the mutanome. Even though major challenges remain, such as locating immunogenic mutations and quickly constructing immunogenic peptides, clinical trials employing a personalized peptide pool approach have commenced (Table 12.2).

Whole Tumor Lysate

Whole tumor lysate can be used as a source of antigen and has the advantage of providing a tumor-specific repertoire of all potentially immunogenic epitopes. The rich repertoire of tumor-associated antigens contains epitopes for both CD8+ and CD4+ T cells, which is important as the parallel presentation of MHC Class I and II antigens could result in a stronger anti-tumor response and boost CD8+ T cell memory [71]. The use of tumor lysate and its encompassing antigen repertoire could also eliminate the time-consuming task of discovering strongly immunogenic antigens.

Tumor lysates can either be obtained from autologous tumor cells, which are taken from the patient, or from an allogenic cell line. Autologous tumor cells are only useful in patient-specific anti-tumor immunotherapies while allogenic tumor cells can be stored at cell banks and vaccines can be created en masse at GMP facilities [72]. Given alone, tumor lysates are administered with a strong adjuvant hapten to provoke a strong inflammatory response and increase their immunogenicity. In a murine glioma model, a CpG-tumor lysate vaccine given subcutaneously had a cure rate of up to 55% and showed significantly longer survival times than tumor lysate or CpG alone. Given their potential to be immunosuppressive, an alternative approach, discussed below, is to create dendritic

Table 12.2 Recent clinical trials employing vaccination immunotherapy for high-grade gliomas

NIH clinical trial	Type	Phase	Eligibility criteria	Primary outcome	Dosing regimen	Treatment groups
NCT02510950	Peptide (personalized)	0	Newly diagnosed glioblastoma	Safety and tolerability, feasibility of creating vaccine	Neoantigen-specific long peptide vaccine + poly-ICLC given on cycle 1 day 1 of maintenance TMZ, then on days 3, 5, 8, 15, 22, followed by maintenance on day 22 of subsequent cycles	Single-arm
NCT02454634	Peptide	1	IDH1R132H mutated grade III–IV gliomas	Safety and tolerability (RLT), immunogenicity of IDH1 peptide	20-mer peptide with IDH1(R132H) mutation given 8 times every 2 or 4 weeks	Single-arm
NCT02287428	Peptide	1	MGMT unmethylated, newly diagnosed glioblastoma	# of adverse events, # of patients with >10 actionable peptides	Injections with personalized peptide pool (NeoVax) with 5 priming and 2 boost doses over 7 months	Single-arm
NCT02149225	Peptide (personalized)	1	Newly diagnosed glioblastoma patients	Safety study (# of AEs and SEAs), frequency of CD8 T cell specific for peptides	5–10 peptides (individually assembled, APVAC1) plus Poly-ICLC and GM-CSF given 11 times over 22 weeks. GM-CSF given along first 6 vaccinations. 2 peptides synthesized de novo (APVAC2) and given 6 months after enrollment 8 times within 10 weeks	Single-arm
NCT02049489	DC loaded with peptide antigens	1	Recurrent GBM	Safety study	At least 4 doses of DCs loaded with CD133 peptides given followed by additional vaccines for maintenance	Single-arm
NCT02010606	DC loaded with lysate	1	Newly diagnosed or recurrent GBM	Safety, adverse events, treatment-related toxicities	Autologous DCs loaded with lysate from allogeneic GBM stem-like cell line given once every week for 4 weeks followed by once every 8 weeks	Cohort A: newly diagnosed GBM Cohort B: recurrent GBM
NCT01491893	Virus	1	Recurrent supratentorial GBM	Maximum tolerated dose or optimal dose	Genetically recombinant, non-pathogenic poliovirus:rhinovirus chimera with tumor-specific conditional replication phenotype (PVSRIPO) given directly into tumor during biopsy	Single-arm
NCT01967758	Virus	1	Treated and recurrent WHO	Maximum tolerated dose	Live attenuated strain of *L. monocytogenes* expressing EGFRvII and NY = ESO-1 antigens	Arm I: low dose

(continued)

Table 12.2 (continued)

NIH clinical trial	Type	Phase	Eligibility criteria	Primary outcome	Dosing regimen	Treatment groups
			grade III/IV astrocytomas		(ADU-623) given on day 0, 21, 42, 63 (Arm I: 3E7 cfu, Arm II: 3E8 cfu, Arm III: 3E9 cfu)	Arm II: medium dose Arm III: high dose
NCT02649582	DC loaded with RNA	1/2	Newly diagnosed, histologically verified GBM	Overall survival	WT1 mRNA loaded DC vaccine given weekly for 3 weeks followed by maintenance vaccine on day 21 of every TMZ cycle	Single-arm
NCT01567202	DC loaded with lysate	2	Histologically confirmed GBM	Overall survival	8-10E6 DCs loaded with autogeneic glioma stem-like cell-associated antigens given once a week for 6 weeks	Triple-blind Arm I: DCs Arm II: placebo
NCT02366728	DC loaded with RNA	2	Newly diagnosed GBM	Overall survival	CMV pp65-loaded DC vaccines #1–3 given every two weeks followed by vaccine #4 (only Arms I–II). Td given to all during vaccine #1. Arm III patients receive basiliximab 1 week before vaccine #1–2. Before vaccine #4, Arm I receives unloaded DCs, Arm II–III Td dose	Arm I: unloaded DCs + loaded DCs Arm II: Td + loaded DCs Arm III: Td + loaded DCs + basiliximab
NCT02455557	Peptide	2	Survivin-positive GBM	Progression-free survival	Survivin-mimic peptide vaccine (SurVaxM) 1–2 weeks after chemoradiation followed by doses every 2 weekś (total of 4 doses) followed by doses every 12 weeks	Single-arm
NCT01480479	Peptide	3	Newly diagnosed EGFRvIII-positive GBM	Overall survival	EGFRvIII peptide rindopepimut or placebo given ID two times in month 1 followed by monthly injections	Arm I: rindopepimut Arm II: placebo
NCT00045968	DC loaded with lysate	3	Newly diagnosed GBM	PFS	Autologous dendritic cells pulsed with tumor lysate antigen, called DCVax-L, or autologous PBMCs (placebo) given ID twice daily on days 0, 10, 20, and at weeks 8, 16, 32, 48, 72, 96, and 120	Arm I: DCVax-L Arm II: placebo

AE adverse event; *cfu* colony-forming units; *CMV* cytomegalovirus; *DC* dendritic cell; *GBM* glioblastoma; *ID* intradermal; *lysate* tumor cell lysate; *PBMC* peripheral blood mononuclear cells; *RLT* regimen limiting toxicity; *SAE* serious adverse event; *Td* tetanus toxoid; *TMZ* temozolomide; *PFS* progression-free survival

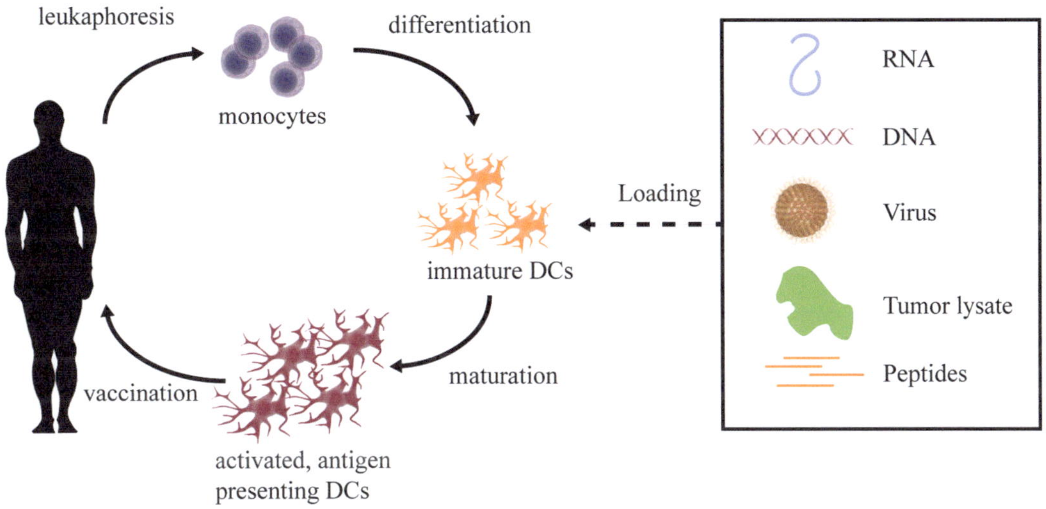

Fig. 12.3 Dendritic cell vaccine production. Patients first undergo leukapheresis to isolate PBMCs, followed by a period of differentiation to obtain immature dendritic cells (DCs). These cells are then loaded with antigens in the form of RNA, DNA, viral vectors, tumor lysate, or peptides. The DCs endogenously process the antigen and present it on their MHC molecules and, after a maturation step, the DCs are reinfused into the patient where they home to the lymph node and activate a tumor-specific immune response

cell vaccinations by pulsing dendritic cells with tumor lysate [73].

Dendritic Cells

Dendritic cells (DCs), with their powerful antigen-presenting function and unique ability to activate naïve T cells, form a crucial link between the innate and adaptive immune system. As sentinel members of the innate immune system, DCs scavenge for foreign antigens (PAMPs) and in response release cytokines. As members of the adaptive immune response, DCs take up pathogenic antigens, process them internally, and present them on their cell surface, thereby activating naïve, effector, and memory T cells and B cells, as well as maintaining tolerance against self-antigens [74]. In fact, DCs are described as the most potent endogenous activators of de novo T cell and B cell responses [75].

DC vaccination in GBM is based on the premise that patient-derived DCs can be generated *ex vivo*, stimulated to present immunogenic antigen, and reinfused into the patient where the cells will activate the adaptive immune response to destroy malignant cells (Fig. 12.3). Tumor-specific stimulation can be achieved by loading DCs with tumor cell lysate, peptides, viral vectors, DNA, or RNA [76–82].

In addition to loading DCs with the optimal tumor antigen, numerous components of the DC vaccine production process are undergoing investigation to produce potent immune responses. DCs can be matured *in vitro* to amplify the immune response using adjuvants or pro-inflammatory molecules. Though the optimal DC maturation is still under investigation, the current "gold standard" is a cytokine cocktail containing GM-CSF, IL-4, TNF-α, IL-1β, IL-6, and, in some instances, prostaglandin E2 (PGE2) [83, 84]. Subsequently, cytokines and chemokines have been used as adjuvants to increase antigen presentation and boost T cell expansion. Specifically, GM-CSF has been the most frequently used adjuvant and has shown efficacy in various systemic cancers and experimental brain tumors [85]. The therapeutic mechanism of GM-CSF involves the paracrine-mediated local release of GM-CSF at the vaccine/tumor antigen presentation interface and the resulting recruitment and activation of APCs [86]. These APCs consequently prime CD8+ and CD4+ T cells which recognize the tumor antigen, infiltrate the tumor cells, and lead to tumor regression [87].

Our laboratory has shown clinical efficacy in treating GBM patients with mRNA-transfected DCs [88]. RNA-transfected DCs have the major advantage that this approach is applicable to a wide range of patients as RNA can be amplified from a small number of tumor cells, meaning very little tumor sample is needed to prepare the therapy. In terms of safety, stimulating DCs with mRNA poses no risk of integration and is therefore a transient therapy, as compared to viral or DNA vectors [74]. In a recent randomized clinical trial, our group generated a dendritic cell vaccine using pp65 mRNA for treating glioblastoma (NCT00639639). Given its high and specific expression in glioblastoma, this viral antigen is ideal for eliciting a specific tumor response. By pre-conditioning patients with tetanus/diphtheria toxoid, lymph node homing and efficacy of the tumor antigen-specific DCs as well as patient survival was significantly increased [88]. A confirmatory double-blinded clinical trial is now testing the effects of tetanus preconditioning on survival in patients with newly diagnosed GBM (Table 12.2).

Alternatively, DCs can be pulsed with whole tumor lysate, which has a number of (theoretical) advantages over peptide loading, including the availability of the full repertoire of tumor-associated antigens, thereby allowing the DCs to "choose" the immunogenic antigen, and increasing the patient-response rate. Using autologous tumor cell lysate from each patient to load the DCs could represent an important step toward personalized medicine in the treatment of GBM. The DCVax-L vaccine (autologous dendritic cells pulsed with autologous tumor cell lysate) showed a 3-year overall survival rate, 2.5 times the usual period of survival, in a phase I/II clinical trial in newly diagnosed GBM, extended survival by 5 months or more for recurrent GBM, and is currently being tested in a blinded randomized phase III trial (Table 12.2) [89–91].

Considerations for the Future

Despite years of dedicated research, diagnosis with malignant gliomas, especially glioblastoma, remains a death sentence and places a heavy burden upon society. With a median survival of 15–17 months, traditional tumor treatments for GBM are of limited use and the need for directed therapy is dire. Recent developments in the field of immunotherapy, such as the peptide vaccine rindopepimut and the dendritic cell vaccine DCVax-L, have seen significant increases in overall survival and give hope that immunotherapy will play a major role in the treatment of malignant gliomas in the upcoming years.

The recent stunning success of checkpoint modulators, particularly the FDA approval of nivolumab–ipilimumab combination for treating metastatic melanoma, further validates immunotherapeutic approaches and is driving a number of ongoing clinical trials testing checkpoint inhibitors alone or in combination in high-grade glioma patients. However, issues such as serious toxicities and the large fraction of non-responders seen in other tumors will need to be addressed in glioma treatment.

Ultimately, long-term treatment of malignant gliomas may require approaches that combine traditional cancer therapies with various immunotherapeutics that serve to activate a tumor-specific immune response and maintain a tumor-suppressive milieu. The optimal combination of treatments could include peptides, mAbs, checkpoint modulators, and loaded DCs as well as activated immune cells and viral vectors and may require patient-specific personalization based on glioma subgroups, heterogeneity profiling, genetic sequencing, and current immune cell counts. Clinical trials testing such extensive combination approaches will need to use high-powered multi-armed approaches to discern therapeutic efficacy.

References

1. Dotan E, Aggarwal C, Smith MR. Impact of rituximab (rituxan) on the treatment of B-Cell non-hodgkin's lymphoma. P T. 2010;35(3):148–57.
2. Baselga J. Clinical trials of herceptin(R) (trastuzumab). Eur J Cancer. 2001;37(Suppl 1):18–24.
3. Kim T, Amaria RN, Spencer C, Reuben A, Cooper ZA, Wargo JA. Combining targeted therapy and immune checkpoint inhibitors in the treatment of metastatic melanoma. Cancer Biol Med. 2014;11 (4):237–46.
4. Preusser M, Lim M, Hafler DA, Reardon DA, Sampson JH. Prospects of immune checkpoint modulators in the treatment of glioblastoma. Nat Rev Neurol. 2015;11(9):504–14.
5. Louveau A, Smirnov I, Keyes TJ, Eccles JD, Rouhani SJ, Peske JD, et al. Structural and functional features of central nervous system lymphatic vessels. Nature. 2015;523(7560):337–41.
6. Ransohoff RM, Engelhardt B. The anatomical and cellular basis of immune surveillance in the central nervous system. Nat Rev Immunol. 2012;12(9):623–35.
7. Balabanov R, Dore-Duffy P. Role of the CNS microvascular pericyte in the blood-brain barrier. J Neurosci Res. 1998;53(6):637–44.
8. Banks WA, Erickson MA. The blood-brain barrier and immune function and dysfunction. Neurobiol Dis. 2010;37(1):26–32.
9. Sarobe P, Huarte E, Lasarte JJ, Borras-Cuesta F. Carcinoembryonic antigen as a target to induce anti-tumor immune responses. Curr Cancer Drug Targets. 2004;4(5):443–54.
10. He Y, Hong Y, Mizejewski GJ. Engineering alpha-fetoprotein-based gene vaccines to prevent and treat hepatocellular carcinoma: review and future prospects. Immunotherapy. 2014;6(6):725–36.
11. Tandon M, Vemula SV, Mittal SK. Emerging strategies for EphA2 receptor targeting for cancer therapeutics. Expert Opin Ther Targets. 2011;15 (1):31–51.
12. Okada H, Low KL, Kohanbash G, McDonald HA, Hamilton RL, Pollack IF. Expression of glioma-associated antigens in pediatric brain stem and non-brain stem gliomas. J Neurooncol. 2008;88 (3):245–50.
13. Fenstermaker RA, Ciesielski MJ. Challenges in the development of a survivin vaccine (SurVaxM) for malignant glioma. Expert Rev Vaccines. 2014;13 (3):377–85.
14. Liu R, Mitchell DA. Survivin as an immunotherapeutic target for adult and pediatric malignant brain tumors. Cancer Immunol Immunother. 2010;59 (2):183–93.
15. Komata T, Kanzawa T, Kondo Y, Kondo S. Telomerase as a therapeutic target for malignant gliomas. Oncogene. 2002;21(4):656–63.
16. Akiyama Y, Komiyama M, Miyata H, Yagoto M, Ashizawa T, Iizuka A, et al. Novel cancer-testis antigen expression on glioma cell lines derived from high-grade glioma patients. Oncol Rep. 2014;31 (4):1683–90.
17. Ahmed N, Salsman VS, Kew Y, Shaffer D, Powell S, Zhang YJ, et al. HER2-specific T cells target primary glioblastoma stem cells and induce regression of autologous experimental tumors. Clin Cancer Res. 2010;16(2):474–85.
18. Pedersen MW, Jacobsen HJ, Koefoed K, Hey A, Pyke C, Haurum JS, et al. Sym004: a novel synergistic anti-epidermal growth factor receptor antibody mixture with superior anticancer efficacy. Cancer Res. 2010;70(2):588–97.
19. Zendman AJ, Ruiter DJ, Van Muijen GN. Cancer/testis-associated genes: identification, expression profile, and putative function. J Cell Physiol. 2003;194(3):272–88.
20. Bolli M, Kocher T, Adamina M, Guller U, Dalquen P, Haas P, et al. Tissue microarray evaluation of melanoma antigen E (MAGE) tumor-associated antigen expression: potential indications for specific immunotherapy and prognostic relevance in squamous cell lung carcinoma. Ann Surg. 2002;236(6):785–93 (discussion 93).
21. Freitas M, Malheiros S, Stavale JN, Biassi TP, Zamuner FT, de Souza Begnami M, et al. Expression of cancer/testis antigens is correlated with improved survival in glioblastoma. Oncotarget. 2013;4(4):636–46.
22. Cancer Genome Atlas Research N. Comprehensive genomic characterization defines human glioblastoma genes and core pathways. Nature. 2008;455 (7216):1061–8.
23. Aldape KD, Ballman K, Furth A, Buckner JC, Giannini C, Burger PC, et al. Immunohistochemical detection of EGFRvIII in high malignancy grade astrocytomas and evaluation of prognostic significance. J Neuropathol Exp Neurol. 2004;63(7):700–7.
24. Frederick L, Wang XY, Eley G, James CD. Diversity and frequency of epidermal growth factor receptor mutations in human glioblastomas. Cancer Res. 2000;60(5):1383–7.
25. Wikstrand CJ, McLendon RE, Friedman AH, Bigner DD. Cell surface localization and density of the tumor-associated variant of the epidermal growth factor receptor, EGFRvIII. Cancer Res. 1997;57 (18):4130–40.
26. Wong AJ, Ruppert JM, Bigner SH, Grzeschik CH, Humphrey PA, Bigner DS, et al. Structural alterations of the epidermal growth factor receptor gene in human gliomas. Proc Natl Acad Sci USA. 1992;89 (7):2965–9.

27. Cunningham MP, Essapen S, Thomas H, Green M, Lovell DP, Topham C, et al. Coexpression, prognostic significance and predictive value of EGFR, EGFRvIII and phosphorylated EGFR in colorectal cancer. Int J Oncol. 2005;27(2):317–25.
28. Garcia de Palazzo IE, Adams GP, Sundareshan P, Wong AJ, Testa JR, Bigner DD, et al. Expression of mutated epidermal growth factor receptor by non-small cell lung carcinomas. Cancer Res. 1993;53(14):3217–20.
29. Schumacher T, Bunse L, Pusch S, Sahm F, Wiestler B, Quandt J, et al. A vaccine targeting mutant IDH1 induces antitumour immunity. Nature. 2014;512(7514):324–7.
30. Yan H, Parsons DW, Jin G, McLendon R, Rasheed BA, Yuan W, et al. IDH1 and IDH2 mutations in gliomas. N Engl J Med. 2009;360 (8):765–73.
31. Mitchell DA, Xie W, Schmittling R, Learn C, Friedman A, McLendon RE, et al. Sensitive detection of human cytomegalovirus in tumors and peripheral blood of patients diagnosed with glioblastoma. Neuro Oncol. 2008;10(1):10–8.
32. Cobbs CS, Harkins L, Samanta M, Gillespie GY, Bharara S, King PH, et al. Human cytomegalovirus infection and expression in human malignant glioma. Cancer Res. 2002;62(12):3347–50.
33. Sampson JH, Mitchell DA. Vaccination strategies for neuro-oncology. Neuro Oncol. 2015;17(Suppl 7): vii15–25.
34. Fuji S, Kapp M, Grigoleit GU, Einsele H. Adoptive immunotherapy with virus-specific T cells. Best Pract Res Clin Haematol. 2011;24(3):413–9.
35. Riddell SR, Greenberg PD. Cellular adoptive immunotherapy after bone marrow transplantation. Cancer Treat Res. 1995;76:337–69.
36. Reichert JM, Valge-Archer VE. Development trends for monoclonal antibody cancer therapeutics. Nat Rev Drug Discov. 2007;6(5):349–56.
37. Hoogenboom HR. Selecting and screening recombinant antibody libraries. Nat Biotechnol. 2005;23 (9):1105–16.
38. Lonberg N. Fully human antibodies from transgenic mouse and phage display platforms. Curr Opin Immunol. 2008;20(4):450–9.
39. Gaston RS, Deierhoi MH, Patterson T, Prasthofer E, Julian BA, Barber WH, et al. OKT3 first-dose reaction: association with T cell subsets and cytokine release. Kidney Int. 1991;39(1):141–8.
40. Hansel TT, Kropshofer H, Singer T, Mitchell JA, George AJ. The safety and side effects of monoclonal antibodies. Nat Rev Drug Discov. 2010;9(4):325–38.
41. Reynolds JC, Del Vecchio S, Sakahara H, Lora ME, Carrasquillo JA, Neumann RD, et al. Anti-murine antibody response to mouse monoclonal antibodies: clinical findings and implications. Int J Rad Appl Instrum B. 1989;16(2):121–5.
42. Bourdon MA, Coleman RE, Blasberg RG, Groothuis DR, Bigner DD. Monoclonal antibody localization in subcutaneous and intracranial human glioma xenografts: paired-label and imaging analysis. Anticancer Res. 1984;4(3):133–40.
43. Bullard DE, Adams CJ, Coleman RE, Bigner DD. In vivo imaging of intracranial human glioma xenografts comparing specific with nonspecific radiolabeled monoclonal antibodies. J Neurosurg. 1986;64 (2):257–62.
44. Scott AM, Lee FT, Tebbutt N, Herbertson R, Gill SS, Liu Z, et al. A phase I clinical trial with monoclonal antibody ch806 targeting transitional state and mutant epidermal growth factor receptors. Proc Natl Acad Sci USA. 2007;104(10):4071–6.
45. Zalutsky MR, Moseley RP, Coakham HB, Coleman RE, Bigner DD. Pharmacokinetics and tumor localization of 131I-labeled anti-tenascin monoclonal antibody 81C6 in patients with gliomas and other intracranial malignancies. Cancer Res. 1989;49 (10):2807–13.
46. Schlessinger J. Cell signaling by receptor tyrosine kinases. Cell. 2000;103(2):211–25.
47. Kang CS, Zhang ZY, Jia ZF, Wang GX, Qiu MZ, Zhou HX, et al. Suppression of EGFR expression by antisense or small interference RNA inhibits U251 glioma cell growth in vitro and in vivo. Cancer Gene Ther. 2006;13(5):530–8.
48. Watanabe K, Tachibana O, Sata K, Yonekawa Y, Kleihues P, Ohgaki H. Overexpression of the EGF receptor and p 53 mutations are mutually exclusive in the evolution of primary and secondary glioblastomas. Brain Pathol. 1996;6(3):217–23 (discussion 23-4).
49. Li S, Schmitz KR, Jeffrey PD, Wiltzius JJ, Kussie P, Ferguson KM. Structural basis for inhibition of the epidermal growth factor receptor by cetuximab. Cancer Cell. 2005;7(4):301–11.
50. Melero I, Rouzaut A, Motz GT, Coukos G. T-cell and NK-cell infiltration into solid tumors: a key limiting factor for efficacious cancer immunotherapy. Cancer Discov. 2014;4(5):522–6.
51. Lohr J, Ratliff T, Huppertz A, Ge Y, Dictus C, Ahmadi R, et al. Effector T-cell infiltration positively impacts survival of glioblastoma patients and is impaired by tumor-derived TGF-beta. Clin Cancer Res. 2011;17(13):4296–308.
52. Bargou R, Leo E, Zugmaier G, Klinger M, Goebeler M, Knop S, et al. Tumor regression in cancer patients by very low doses of a T cell-engaging antibody. Science. 2008;321(5891):974–7.
53. Hoffmann P, Hofmeister R, Brischwein K, Brandl C, Crommer S, Bargou R, et al. Serial killing of tumor cells by cytotoxic T cells redirected with a CD19-/ CD3-bispecific single-chain antibody construct. Int J Cancer. 2005;115(1):98–104.
54. Chames P, Van Regenmortel M, Weiss E, Baty D. Therapeutic antibodies: successes, limitations and hopes for the future. Br J Pharmacol. 2009;157 (2):220–33.
55. Offner S, Hofmeister R, Romaniuk A, Kufer P, Baeuerle PA. Induction of regular cytolytic T cell synapses by bispecific single-chain antibody

constructs on MHC class I-negative tumor cells. Mol Immunol. 2006;43(6):763–71.
56. Mack M, Gruber R, Schmidt S, Riethmuller G, Kufer P. Biologic properties of a bispecific single-chain antibody directed against 17-1A (EpCAM) and CD3: tumor cell-dependent T cell stimulation and cytotoxic activity. J Immunol. 1997;158(8):3965–70.
57. Dreier T, Lorenczewski G, Brandl C, Hoffmann P, Syring U, Hanakam F, et al. Extremely potent, rapid and costimulation-independent cytotoxic T-cell response against lymphoma cells catalyzed by a single-chain bispecific antibody. Int J Cancer. 2002;100(6):690–7.
58. Choi BD, Gedeon PC, Herndon JE, Archer GE, Reap EA, Sanchez-Perez L, et al. Human regulatory T cells kill tumor cells through granzyme-dependent cytotoxicity upon retargeting with a bispecific antibody. Cancer Immunol Res. 2013;1(3):163.
59. Choi BD, Gedeon PC, Sanchez-Perez L, Bigner DD, Sampson JH. Regulatory T cells are redirected to kill glioblastoma by an EGFRvIII-targeted bispecific antibody. Oncoimmunology. 2013;2(12):e26757.
60. Chames P, Baty D. Bispecific antibodies for cancer therapy: the light at the end of the tunnel? MAbs. 2009;1(6):539–47.
61. Zitron IM, Thakur A, Norkina O, Barger GR, Lum LG, Mittal S. Targeting and killing of glioblastoma with activated T cells armed with bispecific antibodies. BMC Cancer. 2013;13:83.
62. Choi BD, Kuan CT, Cai M, Archer GE, Mitchell DA, Gedeon PC, et al. Systemic administration of a bispecific antibody targeting EGFRvIII successfully treats intracerebral glioma. Proc Natl Acad Sci USA. 2013;110(1):270–5.
63. Dix AR, Brooks WH, Roszman TL, Morford LA. Immune defects observed in patients with primary malignant brain tumors. J Neuroimmunol. 1999;100(1–2):216–32.
64. Roszman T, Elliott L, Brooks W. Modulation of T-cell function by gliomas. Immunol Today. 1991;12(10):370–4.
65. Morford LA, Elliott LH, Carlson SL, Brooks WH, Roszman TL. T cell receptor-mediated signaling is defective in T cells obtained from patients with primary intracranial tumors. J Immunol. 1997;159(9):4415–25.
66. Roszman TL, Brooks WH. Immunobiology of primary intracranial tumours. III. Demonstration of a qualitative lymphocyte abnormality in patients with primary brain tumours. Clin Exp Immunol. 1980;39(2):395–402.
67. Mullard A. FDA approves first immunotherapy combo. Nat Rev Drug Discov. 2015;14(11):739.
68. Fecci PE, Ochiai H, Mitchell DA, Grossi PM, Sweeney AE, Archer GE, et al. Systemic CTLA-4 blockade ameliorates glioma-induced changes to the CD4+ T cell compartment without affecting regulatory T-cell function. Clin Cancer Res. 2007;13(7):2158–67.
69. Grimaldi AM, Marincola FM, Ascierto PA. Single versus combination immunotherapy drug treatment in melanoma. Expert Opin Biol Ther. 2015.
70. Sampson JH, Heimberger AB, Archer GE, Aldape KD, Friedman AH, Friedman HS, et al. Immunologic escape after prolonged progression-free survival with epidermal growth factor receptor variant III peptide vaccination in patients with newly diagnosed glioblastoma. J Clin Oncol. 2010;28(31):4722–9.
71. Toes RE, Ossendorp F, Offringa R, Melief CJ. CD4 T cells and their role in antitumor immune responses. J Exp Med. 1999;189(5):753–6.
72. Chiang CL, Benencia F, Coukos G. Whole tumor antigen vaccines. Semin Immunol. 2010;22(3):132–43.
73. Wu A, Oh S, Gharagozlou S, Vedi RN, Ericson K, Low WC, et al. In vivo vaccination with tumor cell lysate plus CpG oligodeoxynucleotides eradicates murine glioblastoma. J Immunother. 2007;30(8):789–97.
74. Batich KA, Swartz AM, Sampson JH. Enhancing dendritic cell-based vaccination for highly aggressive glioblastoma. Expert Opin Biol Ther. 2015;15(1):79–94.
75. Ashley DM, Faiola B, Nair S, Hale LP, Bigner DD, Gilboa E. Bone marrow-generated dendritic cells pulsed with tumor extracts or tumor RNA induce antitumor immunity against central nervous system tumors. J Exp Med. 1997;186(7):1177–82.
76. Song W, Kong HL, Carpenter H, Torii H, Granstein R, Rafii S, et al. Dendritic cells genetically modified with an adenovirus vector encoding the cDNA for a model antigen induce protective and therapeutic antitumor immunity. J Exp Med. 1997;186(8):1247–56.
77. Yamaguchi S, Tatsumi T, Takehara T, Sasakawa A, Hikita H, Kohga K, et al. Dendritic cell-based vaccines suppress metastatic liver tumor via activation of local innate and acquired immunity. Cancer Immunol Immunother. 2008;57(12):1861–9.
78. Hatfield P, Merrick AE, West E, O'Donnell D, Selby P, Vile R, et al. Optimization of dendritic cell loading with tumor cell lysates for cancer immunotherapy. J Immunother. 2008;31(7):620–32.
79. Courreges MC, Benencia F, Conejo-Garcia JR, Zhang L, Coukos G. Preparation of apoptotic tumor cells with replication-incompetent HSV augments the efficacy of dendritic cell vaccines. Cancer Gene Ther. 2006;13(2):182–93.
80. Benencia F, Courreges MC, Coukos G. Whole tumor antigen vaccination using dendritic cells: comparison of RNA electroporation and pulsing with UV-irradiated tumor cells. J Transl Med. 2008;6:21.
81. Okada H, Kalinski P, Ueda R, Hoji A, Kohanbash G, Donegan TE, et al. Induction of CD8+ T-cell responses against novel glioma-associated antigen peptides and clinical activity by vaccinations with {alpha}-type 1 polarized dendritic cells and polyinosinic-polycytidylic acid stabilized by lysine

and carboxymethylcellulose in patients with recurrent malignant glioma. J Clin Oncol. 2011;29(3):330–6.
82. Phuphanich S, Wheeler CJ, Rudnick JD, Mazer M, Wang H, Nuno MA, et al. Phase I trial of a multi-epitope-pulsed dendritic cell vaccine for patients with newly diagnosed glioblastoma. Cancer Immunol Immunother. 2013;62(1):125–35.
83. Kalinski P, Vieira PL, Schuitemaker JH, de Jong EC, Kapsenberg ML. Prostaglandin E(2) is a selective inducer of interleukin-12 p40 (IL-12p40) production and an inhibitor of bioactive IL-12p70 heterodimer. Blood. 2001;97(11):3466–9.
84. Nair S, Archer GE, Tedder TF. Isolation and generation of human dendritic cells. Curr Protoc Immunol. 2012;Chapter 7:Unit7.32.
85. Gardner TA, Elzey BD, Hahn NM. Sipuleucel-T (provenge) autologous vaccine approved for treatment of men with asymptomatic or minimally symptomatic castrate-resistant metastatic prostate cancer. Hum Vaccin Immunother. 2012;8(4):534–9.
86. Gordon EM, Levy JP, Reed RA, Petchpud WN, Liu L, Wendler CB, et al. Targeting metastatic cancer from the inside: a new generation of targeted gene delivery vectors enables personalized cancer vaccination in situ. Int J Oncol. 2008;33(4):665–75.
87. Ojima T, Iwahashi M, Nakamura M, Matsuda K, Naka T, Nakamori M, et al. The boosting effect of co-transduction with cytokine genes on cancer vaccine therapy using genetically modified dendritic cells expressing tumor-associated antigen. Int J Oncol. 2006;28(4):947–53.
88. Mitchell DA, Batich KA, Gunn MD, Huang MN, Sanchez-Perez L, Nair SK, et al. Tetanus toxoid and CCL3 improve dendritic cell vaccines in mice and glioblastoma patients. Nature. 2015;519(7543):366–9.
89. Hdeib A, Sloan AE. Dendritic cell immunotherapy for solid tumors: evaluation of the DCVax(R) platform in the treatment of glioblastoma multiforme. CNS Oncol. 2015;4(2):63–9.
90. Polyzoidis S, Ashkan K. DCVax(R)-L–developed by northwest biotherapeutics. Hum Vaccin Immunother. 2014;10(11):3139–45.
91. Bosch M, Prins R, Liau L. Abstract 2491: treatment with tumor lysate-pulsed autologous dendritic cells prolongs survival in patients with recurrent glioblastoma multiforme. Cancer Res. 2015;75:2491.

Novel Delivery Strategies

13

David S. Hersh, Aniket S. Wadajkar and Graeme F. Woodworth

Barriers to Drug Delivery

The delivery of therapeutic agents to malignant brain tumors faces unique challenges due to several physical barriers that are only found in the central nervous system (CNS). The widely studied "blood–brain barrier" (BBB) is the first obstacle encountered by drugs that are administered intravenously. The BBB is formed primarily by the specialized endothelial cells of the CNS, which are linked by tight junctions and are reinforced by a continuous, non-fenestrated basal lamina and by interactions with the surrounding glia, including pericytes and astrocytic end-foot processes [1]. The endothelial cell tight junctions of the BBB effectively limit the paracellular transport of most compounds. Furthermore, transcellular transport is typically restricted to small (less than 400 daltons), lipophilic molecules, or to nutrients and proteins that are recognized by channels or receptors on the endothelial cell surface, thereby facilitating carrier-mediated transport (CMT), receptor-mediated transcytosis (RMT), or adsorption-mediated transcytosis (AMT). While the BBB protects the CNS from neurotoxins and infectious agents, it also prevents nearly 90% of all small molecule drugs and close to 100% of all large therapeutic agents from reaching their targets [2, 3]. Although portions of many malignant brain tumors are associated with "leaky" blood vessels where there is BBB breakdown, the BBB typically remains relatively intact in regions where invading tumor cells are interspersed with healthy non-neoplastic cells [4].

The few drugs that do cross the BBB must avoid efflux transporters such as P-glycoprotein 1, a member of the ATP-binding cassette family. Efflux transporters are upregulated in certain gliomas, where they confer drug resistance properties by transporting therapeutic agents back into the vasculature [5]. Secondly, therapeutics that successfully reach the brain parenchyma must navigate the extracellular spaces (ECSs) of the brain in order to reach tumor cells in distant regions. The ECS comprises 15–20% of the total brain volume and is made up of an anisotropic, complex network of lipids, polysaccharides, and proteins. Diffusion within the ECS is limited by the width and tortuosity of the intercellular spaces, as well as by electrostatic interactions with the components of the ECS [6]. Recent efforts to

D.S. Hersh · A.S. Wadajkar · G.F. Woodworth
Department of Neurosurgery, University of Maryland School of Medicine, 22 S Greene St Suite 12D, Baltimore, MD 21201, USA
e-mail: dhersh@som.umaryland.edu

A.S. Wadajkar
e-mail: AWadajkar@smail.umaryland.edu

D.S. Hersh · A.S. Wadajkar · G.F. Woodworth
Marlene and Stewart Greenebaum Comprehensive Cancer Center, University of Maryland School of Medicine, 655 W. Baltimore Street, 8th Floor, Baltimore, MD 21201, USA

G.F. Woodworth (✉)
Department of Anatomy and Neurobiology, University of Maryland School of Medicine, 22 S Greene St Suite 12D, Baltimore, MD 21201, USA
e-mail: gwoodworth@smail.umaryland.edu

J. Moliterno Günel et al. (eds.), *Malignant Brain Tumors*,
DOI 10.1007/978-3-319-49864-5_13

accurately characterize the physicochemical properties of the brain ECS are therefore critical for designing more effective drug delivery systems [7, 8]. Interestingly, the ECS volume and structure are altered in brain tumors, with changes tending to correlate with the level of malignancy [9]. The resulting effect on diffusion is an additional obstacle to drug delivery.

Several strategies are being utilized in efforts to optimize the treatment of malignant brain tumors in spite of these barriers. Novel drug carriers including nanoparticles, viral vectors, and stem cells have been developed as vehicles for delivery to the CNS. These carriers may be delivered systemically, in which case transient BBB disruption becomes necessary. Alternatively, a variety of delivery routes have been explored that bypass the BBB, including intrathecal/intraventricular, intranasal, and direct interstitial delivery.

Novel Drug Carriers (Table 13.1)

Nanoparticles

Nanoparticle design and optimization have become a particularly promising approach in the development of novel drug carriers for therapeutic delivery to malignant brain tumors. Nanoparticles possess several unique physicochemical characteristics including small size, enhanced drug solubility, the ability for multifunctionality, a controlled drug release profile, and the potential for site-specific targeting [10]. In particular, various classes of nanoscale delivery systems—including metallic nanoparticles, polymeric nanoparticles, and liposomes—have been shown to cross the BBB via transcytotic mechanisms in numerous preclinical studies [11–14].

Metallic nanoparticles are commonly composed of inorganic materials (such as gold, silver, or iron oxide) as well as metallic allotropes of non-metals (such as carbon fullerenes). Typically smaller than polymeric nanoparticles or liposomes, metallic nanoparticles are too dense to encapsulate a drug. Nevertheless, therapeutic agents can be successfully conjugated to the surface of metallic nanoparticles for delivery to the CNS. This approach was demonstrated successfully in a preclinical glioma model [11], and recent work has shown that the application of an external magnet can further enhance the ability of the particles to cross the BBB [25]. At the clinical level, therapeutic applications of metallic nanoparticles have been primarily limited to intracranial thermotherapy [15]. In a phase II study [16], aminosilane-coated iron oxide nanoparticles were injected into the tumors of 59 patients at 2 medical centers and exposed to an alternating magnetic field, resulting in heating of the particles. Although the patients tolerated the treatment well, other technologies including magnetic resonance imaging (MRI)-guided laser interstitial thermal therapy (LITT) and MRI-guided focused ultrasound (MRgFUS) offer competing options for achieving thermal ablation.

Polymeric nanoparticles, on the other hand, are capable of carrying a wide variety of payloads, including chemotherapeutic drugs, proteins, nucleic acids, and contrast agents. Polymeric nanoparticles are characterized by a large surface area containing functional groups that can be conjugated to peptides, antibodies, or other biomolecules. The ability to tailor these surface characteristics, as well as the physicochemical properties of the nanoparticle core, makes polymeric nanoparticles popular vehicles for drug delivery to the brain [26, 27]. In particular, stabilizers such as polysorbate 80 and polyethylene glycol (PEG) can be used to coat the surface of drug-loaded nanoparticles, thereby shielding the particles from clearance and extending their circulation time [28]. Various chemotherapeutic agents, including doxorubicin [29], camptothecin [30], and paclitaxel [31], have been encapsulated within polymeric nanoparticles for the treatment of brain tumors in preclinical studies, and phase I and II studies [32, 33] have begun to explore their safety and efficacy in patients with other types of solid tumors. Nevertheless, clinical trials involving patients with brain tumors are currently lacking.

Table 13.1 Ongoing and recent clinical trials involving novel drug carriers

Carrier	Treatment	Phase	Study population	# of patients	Results	Reference
Nanoparticles	Aminosilane-coated iron oxide particles and alternating magnetic fields	I	Recurrent grade IV astrocytoma	14	• Minor or no side effects • Median maximum intratumoral temperature of 44.6 °C	[15]
		II	Recurrent grade IV astrocytoma	59	• Overall survival following first recurrence: 13.4 months • Overall survival following primary diagnosis: 23.2 months	[16]
	Liposomal doxorubicin	I	Pediatric patients with recurrent or refractory HGG	13	• No dose-limiting toxicities at 60 mg/m^2 • Grade 4 neutropenia in 2 patients at 75 mg/m^2	[17]
		II	Recurrent HGG	13	• Disease stabilization in 54% • Progression-free survival at 12 months: 15%	[18]
		II	Newly diagnosed grade IV astrocytoma	40	• Progression-free survival at 6 months: 58% • Median time to progression: 6.2 months • Overall survival: 13.4 months	[19]
	Liposomal cytarabine	II	Lymphomatous meningitis	30	• Only 1 (3%) recurrence • 50% reduction in # of injections	[20]
		II	Breast cancer with neoplastic meningitis	43	• Response (intent-to-treat): 21%[a] • Median survival: 88 days	[21]
	Rhenium nanoliposomes	I–II	Recurrent grade IV astrocytoma	N/A[b]	N/A[b]	NCT01906385

(continued)

Table 13.1 (continued)

Carrier	Treatment	Phase	Study population	# of patients	Results	Reference
Viral vectors	Adenovirus-mediated p53	I	Recurrent HGG	12	• Maximum tolerated dose was not reached • No evidence of systemic virus • Transfected cells only within 5 mm of injection site	[22]
	Recombinant adenovirus with the HSV TK gene followed by ganciclovir	I	Recurrent HGG	14	• Maximum tolerated dose was not reached • Overall median survival: 4 months • 4 patients survived >1 year	[23]
		III	Newly diagnosed grade IV astrocytoma	236	• Median time to death or reintervention: 308 versus 268 days ($p = 0.006$) • Overall survival: 497 versus 452 days ($p = 0.31$)	[24]
Stem cells	Neural stem cells with cytosine deaminase followed by oral 5-FC	I	Recurrent HGG	N/A[b]	N/A[b]	NCT01172964

5-FC 5-fluorocytosine; *HGG* high-grade glioma; *HSV* herpes simplex virus; *N/A* not applicable; *TK* thymidine kinase
[a]Liposomal cytarabine achieved comparable results to other intrathecal therapies but with one-fourth as many intrathecal injections
[b]The study is currently ongoing

Liposomes are nanoscale, self-assembled vesicles comprised of amphiphilic phospholipids that mimic the lipid bilayer of the cell membrane. As a result, liposomes are capable of carrying hydrophilic, hydrophobic, and amphoteric drug molecules and are effective at crossing the BBB [34]. Similar to polymeric nanoparticles, the surface properties of liposomes can be modified to extend their circulation time. Conjugation to hydrophilic polymers sterically stabilizes the liposomes, allowing them to avoid opsonization and uptake by the reticuloendothelial system [35]. Liposomal doxorubicin, in particular, has been used to treat patients with recurrent and/or refractory high-grade glioma (HGG) [17–19], as well as patients with brain metastases from solid tumors [36]. Other applications of liposomal delivery that are being actively explored include the intrathecal delivery of liposomal cytarabine for the treatment of neoplastic and lymphomatous meningitis [20, 21], as well as the intratumoral delivery of rhenium nanoliposomes—a novel form of brachytherapy—for the treatment of recurrent HGG (NCT01906385).

Through surface modifications and ligand conjugation, nanoparticles and liposomes that specifically target brain tumors have been developed. These nanotherapeutic agents are targeted to cell surface receptors that are expressed specifically by tumor cells, such as the epidermal growth factor receptor (EGFR) [37] and interleukin-13 (IL-13) receptor [38]. Recently, fibroblast growth factor-inducible 14 (Fn14), a member of the tumor necrosis factor receptor (TNFR) superfamily, has emerged as a novel target for GBM therapy [22]. While Fn14 levels remain low in normal brain tissue, the receptor is highly expressed by HGG—particularly the invasive cells at the rim of the tumor [39]. Nanoparticles coated with both PEG and ITEM4—a monoclonal antibody that recognizes the Fn14 receptor—were shown to specifically target tumor cells in a human xenograft model, with minimal non-specific binding to non-tumoral tissue [23]. Targeted therapeutics have the potential to reduce treatment toxicities and generate fewer side effects.

Viral Vectors

Viral vectors are biologic vehicles that have been studied extensively in the context of gene therapy, due to their innate ability to enter cells and transfer genetic material. While CNS-directed gene therapy is commonly considered a potential treatment for congenital disorders [24] and neurodegenerative diseases [40], applications in neuro-oncology have been explored as well. In particular, phase I studies have evaluated the safety and feasibility of using adenovirus as a viral vector for the delivery of p53 [41] and interferon beta [42] to patients with HGG. A particularly promising approach involves the intratumoral administration of a recombinant adenovirus carrying the herpes simplex virus (HSV) thymidine kinase (TK) gene followed by the intravenous injection of ganciclovir in patients with recurrent HGG [43]. The TK gene sensitizes the tumor cells to ganciclovir, thereby limiting the toxic effect to the neoplastic cells infected by the virus. This approach was tested in a recent phase III study [44] involving 236 patients at 38 centers in Europe, which identified a longer median time to death or reintervention in the experimental group (308 days vs. 268 days, $p = 0.006$), although overall survival remained unchanged.

Despite the advantages of viral vectors for the application of gene therapy, safety and toxicity concerns persist. Off-target biodistribution and insertional mutagenesis carry the risk of transgene overexpression, tissue damage, and tumorigenesis. Immunogenicity represents another obstacle, as clearance of the vector by the immune system reduces its efficiency as a delivery vehicle. Of note, adenovirus-associated virus (AAV) is being promoted as a safer option for viral delivery as it is non-pathogenic and non-autonomous—it can only replicate in the setting of coinfection with helper viruses. While this results in greater safety and fewer side effects, a limited amount of genetic material can be packaged within AAV. Further modification of viral vectors, as well as non-viral alternatives, is being explored for therapeutic delivery to brain tumors.

Immune and Stem Cells

As early as the 1980s, researchers recognized that immune cells are capable of crossing an intact BBB and subsequently infiltrating brain metastases [45, 46]. As a result, macrophages have been studied as a potential carrier for the delivery of nanoparticles to an experimental brain metastasis model [47]. Recently, however, focus has shifted toward the use of stem cells as alternative cellular vehicles. Neural stem cells [48] and mesenchymal stem cells [49, 50] cross the BBB effectively and migrate to primary and metastatic brain tumors, likely in response to cytokines and chemokines secreted by the tumor microenvironment. Neural stem cells, in particular, demonstrate a strong tropism for the tumor border, invasive glioma cells, and glioma stem cells [48]. Additionally, neural and mesenchymal stem cells locally suppress the immune system, thus evading immune recognition and rejection [51, 52].

Numerous preclinical studies have harnessed these unique, intrinsic features of neural and mesenchymal stem cells to deliver various therapeutic "cargo" to malignant brain tumors. Oncolytic viruses [53–55], drug-loaded nanoparticles [56, 57], and cytokines including tumor necrosis factor apoptosis-inducing ligand (TRAIL) [58–61], bone morphogenetic protein 4 (BMP4) [62], and interleukin-12 (IL-12) [63] have all been packaged within stem cells in order to enhance their delivery to tumor cells. One promising approach utilizes stem cells to deliver an enzyme—cytosine deaminase (CD)—to glioma cells, where it converts the inactive prodrug 5-fluorocytosine (5-FC) into the active chemotherapeutic compound 5-fluorouracil (5-FU) [64]. While 5-FC crosses the BBB efficiently following systemic administration, the natural tropism of stem cells for glioma cells ensures that the active drug will only be produced at sites of active tumor infiltration, thereby limiting its effect on healthy tissue. Preclinical studies [65] demonstrating the safety and efficacy of this stem cell-mediated enzyme/prodrug approach resulted in the first human study (NCT01172964) to use stem cells as a delivery vehicle for the treatment of HGG. Patients with recurrent HGG underwent intracranial injections of neural stem cells transduced with CD at the time of tumor resection or biopsy. Beginning four days later, the patients were administered oral 5-FC every 6 h for 7 days. Various doses of neural stem cells and 5-FC were tested for safety and feasibility, opening the door to further exploration of stem cell-mediated delivery for the treatment of malignant brain tumors.

Several limitations must be overcome before cell-mediated drug delivery can achieve broader use in patients. One technical challenge involves maintaining the viability of the cellular vehicle itself when dealing with cytotoxic cargo. Toxic effects of the therapeutic agent on the cell may result in premature cell death and drug release before the cell reaches its target. Nanoparticle formulations have therefore been used as a means of shielding the cell from its cargo and delaying cell death [66, 67]. Nevertheless, the lysosomal degradation of nanoparticles following endocytosis remains an issue. Spatial and temporal control over drug release from a cell vehicle therefore requires additional research. Further challenges arise from the poor loading efficiency of most cellular carriers, necessitating the delivery of large quantities of cells in order to achieve a therapeutic effect.

The largest obstacle to the clinical translation of cell-mediated delivery remains safety. Stem cells are defined, in part, by their capacity for self-renewal, which has raised concerns that stem cell therapy may induce malignant transformation. The spontaneous transformation of bone marrow-derived mesenchymal stem cells in long-term cultures has been a controversial issue [68, 69]. However, a clinical trial [70] involving the intracerebellar and intrathecal administration of neural stem cells for the treatment of ataxia telangiectasia identified one subject who developed a multifocal glioneural tumor 4 years after the treatment. Additionally, cytokines secreted by stem cells, in addition to their locally immunosuppressive effect, have been shown to promote tumor growth and metastasis in other tumor types [71, 72]. These safety concerns must be fully investigated for the success of cell-mediated delivery as a treatment strategy.

Routes of Delivery

Each of the drug carriers described above may be delivered to malignant brain tumors via several routes. Systemic administration must be coupled with strategies to cross the BBB, while other routes allow the BBB to be bypassed entirely.

Systemic Delivery

Current Strategies for Delivery Across the BBB

Numerous approaches for enhancing systemic drug delivery to the CNS have been developed over the past several decades, including intra-arterial therapy, osmotic BBB disruption, chemical BBB disruption, and manipulation of the endogenous RMT pathway. Intra-arterial delivery results in higher local drug concentrations than intravenous administration. The drug is distributed throughout the tumor capillary network and achieves a higher "area under the curve" due to the avoidance of first-pass metabolism by the liver [73]. Although typically, intra-arterial delivery is accomplished via the carotid artery, more recently cerebral angiographic techniques have been used to perform superselective intra-arterial infusions of chemotherapeutic agents [74]. Nevertheless, the administered agent must still cross the BBB in order to achieve its effect.

Transport across the BBB may occur via paracellular or transcellular routes. Osmotic BBB disruption, first proposed by Stanley Rapoport in the 1970s [75], is one mechanism for enhancing paracellular transport across the BBB. An intra-carotid infusion of a hyperosmotic agent (most commonly mannitol) is coadministered with an intra-arterial chemotherapeutic agent. The osmotic agent draws water out of the endothelial cell, produces vasodilation, and stimulates endothelial cell cytoskeletal contraction via a cadherin-dependent mechanism [76]. These processes place mechanical stress on the tight junctions linking the endothelial cells. While osmotic BBB disruption has demonstrated promising results in clinical trials [77], the technique has been associated with transient cerebral edema [78]. Additionally, non-specific disruption of the BBB takes place in areas of normal brain tissue, allowing plasma proteins to pass from the bloodstream into the parenchyma with resulting neurotoxicity [79].

Chemical BBB disruption offers a second mechanism for enhancing paracellular transport across the BBB. Intra-arterial vasoactive agents produce inflammation and destabilization of the endothelial cell membrane, resulting in transient opening of the BBB. Bradykinin, which binds to B_2 receptors on the endothelial cell membrane and activates nitric oxide synthase, is a commonly studied agent for BBB disruption, with evidence suggesting that it specifically affects the BBB in the region of a brain tumor [80, 81]. More recently, RMP-7—a synthetic bradykinin analog—has been used due to its higher potency, longer half-life, greater specificity for the B_2 receptor, and increased stability, enabling it to be delivered intravenously [82]. However, while phase I and early phase II studies [83, 84] found the combination of RMP-7 and carboplatin to be safe and effective for the treatment of refractory brain tumors, the treatment was ultimately ineffective in a larger, multicenter, placebo-controlled trial [85].

An alternative strategy for crossing the BBB involves molecular Trojan horses, which utilize the endogenous RMT pathway. Recombinant proteins or "chimeric" peptides are formed by linking a therapeutic agent that cannot typically cross the BBB on its own with a ligand or monoclonal antibody that recognizes a receptor on the endothelial cell surface. Upon binding to the receptor, the entire complex undergoes transcytosis [86]. Antibodies that recognize the transferrin receptor [87, 88] and the insulin receptor [89], both of which are found on cerebral endothelial cells, have been fused to diagnostic and therapeutic agents for delivery across the BBB in preclinical studies. Additionally, a phase I dose escalation study [90] was recently completed in which GRN1005/ANG1005, comprised of paclitaxel conjugated to a low-density lipoprotein receptor-related peptide, was administered to patients with recurrent HGG. While patients experienced toxicities including neutropenia and mucositis, there were no toxicities specific to the CNS. Furthermore, therapeutic concentrations of the drug were found in resected tumor tissue, suggesting effective transport across the BBB. Phase II trials (NCT02048059 and NCT01480583) involving patients with metastatic breast cancer are ongoing.

Ultrasound-Mediated BBB Disruption

MRI-Guided Focused Ultrasound: The Clinical Experience

Focused ultrasound is rapidly emerging as a promising tool for noninvasive disruption of the BBB. Interestingly, ultrasound was used for its therapeutic potential long before it was developed into the imaging modality that we recognize today. As early as the 1950s, Ballantine and colleagues [91] used an ultrasound beam to open the BBB in brain tissue without causing a lesion. However, the variable thickness of the skull creates beam distortions and attenuation, and prior to the 1990s, focused ultrasound could only be applied through an opening in the skull. More recently, hemispheric phased arrays of ultrasound transducers were designed together with computer software that predicts and corrects for the phase aberrations caused by the skull, enabling noninvasive focusing of the beam at points deep within the brain [92]. In addition, advanced imaging modalities—in particular, magnetic resonance thermometry—provide real-time monitoring of temperature changes at the skull, along the beam path, and at the focal point, allowing appropriate adjustments to be made [93].

Focused ultrasound produces a high rate of energy deposition at the focal point, resulting in spatial intensities that are orders of magnitude higher than in the prefocal region. Heat is released, and temperatures can reach up to 60 °C, at which point coagulative necrosis occurs [94]. This mechanism is being harnessed in clinical trials for the noninvasive ablation of deep brain targets in the thalamus and basal ganglia for the treatment of essential tremor and Parkinson's disease. However, ultrasound also produces non-thermal, mechanical effects, including cavitation, acoustic radiation forces, and acoustic streaming. Cavitation refers to the oscillation of micron-sized gas-filled bubbles in response to the positive and negative components of the ultrasound beam. The diameter of the bubbles varies with the pressure field—at lower amplitudes, stable oscillation (i.e., non-inertial cavitation) occurs, but as the pressure amplitude increases, the bubbles become unstable and collapse (i.e., inertial cavitation). The latter process produces shock waves and high-velocity jets, which place mechanical stress on the adjacent tissue [95]. Acoustic radiation forces refer to the unidirectional forces that occur along the beam path as a result of the momentum that is transferred from the ultrasound beam to a reflecting or absorbing surface [96]. Radiation forces that occur in a liquid medium produce acoustic streaming, which may enhance convection [97].

Whereas continuous ultrasound exposures are typically used for thermal ablation, pulsed exposures with short duty cycles apply ultrasound energy at lower rates, producing temperature elevations of only 4–5 °C, allowing the mechanical effects of ultrasound to play a larger role. Kullervo Hynynen, Nathan McDannold, and colleagues [98] showed for the first time in 2001 that focused ultrasound could be used to noninvasively disrupt the BBB without damaging the surrounding tissue. Importantly, they introduced the concept of using intravenous lipid or albumin-encased gas microbubbles, 1–5 μm in diameter. The microbubbles cluster near capillary walls, where they undergo stable cavitation in the presence of low frequencies and pressure amplitudes. The resulting oscillations place stress on the endothelial tight junctions that form the BBB, localizing the effects of ultrasound to the vasculature at the focal point [99]. Microbubbles lower the threshold for cavitation and reduce the amount of energy needed to achieve BBB opening, thereby minimizing the risk of heating at the skull or damage along the beam path. In addition to the paracellular route generated by microbubble cavitation, recent evidence suggests that sonication may also promote transcellular transport across the BBB by upregulating proteins involved in transcytosis, such as caveolin-1 and caveolin-2 [100]. The resulting disruption of the BBB typically persists for 4–6 h [101].

Numerous preclinical studies have demonstrated that focused ultrasound can be used to facilitate the delivery of various agents across the BBB, including liposome-encapsulated doxorubicin [102–104], methotrexate [105], carmustine [106], temozolomide [107], and the monoclonal antibody trastuzumab [108, 109]. Immunotherapy agents (e.g., interleukin-12) [110], stem cells [111], and gene therapy vectors [112–114] have been successfully delivered across the BBB with ultrasound technology, as well. Ultrasound-induced opening of the BBB was demonstrated to be safe in two recent studies [115, 116] involving repeated BBB disruption in the central visual field targets and basal ganglia of non-human primates. Long-term neurological deficits were not identified.

The first phase I study (NCT02343991) of MRgFUS for opening of the BBB is currently ongoing. Brain tumor patients are administered microbubbles and undergo sonication, followed by the intravenous administration of liposomal doxorubicin. The patients are subsequently taken to the OR for resection of the tumor, with careful tissue sampling in the region of ultrasound application to measure the concentration of doxorubicin as well as in adjacent regions. The first patient to enroll in the study was recently treated successfully, without adverse effects.

Limitations of Focused Ultrasound

The potential for focused ultrasound to open the BBB *noninvasively* is particularly attractive. Nevertheless, transcranial focused ultrasound currently requires the application of a stereotactic frame, similar to deep brain stimulation and Gamma Knife radiosurgery. Although this can be performed on an outpatient basis, the inherent risks of any frame-based procedure apply, including pin site infection. In contrast to focused ultrasound ablation for the treatment of movement disorders, which entails only a single treatment, current chemotherapy regimens typically involve complex dosing schemes. Given the transient nature of ultrasound-induced BBB disruption, sonication would be required prior to each individual treatment—a complicated matter when a stereotactic frame is involved. Furthermore, the need for complete hair removal in order to achieve acoustic coupling is a source of hesitation for some patients, and the use of MRI to localize and monitor the targeted region precludes patients with pacemakers and certain metallic implants. Technological limitations exist, as well—while transcranial focused ultrasound has been optimized to treat small, focal targets in deep brain regions such as the thalamus and basal ganglia, it remains to be seen whether regions adjacent to the skull can be included within the treatment envelope, as well as whether the BBB can be opened in large volumes of brain tissue, such as the 2-cm rim surrounding a brain tumor, within a reasonable time frame.

Future Directions

In addition to addressing the limitations described above, researchers have been developing novel microbubbles to be used with focused ultrasound. The surface of a microbubble can be modified with ligands that recognize and bind to tumor-specific antigens, thereby increasing the specificity of the microbubble for tumor vessels. Additionally, a microbubble can be used to encapsulate a therapeutic agent, only releasing the drug upon exposure to ultrasound. As a proof of principle, carmustine-loaded microbubbles were recently shown to facilitate improved circulation and reduced clearance of the drug and improved survival in a murine tumor model [117, 118]. A vascular endothelial growth factor (VEGF) ligand was subsequently conjugated to the drug-loaded microbubbles, resulting in targeting of the drug's effects to regions of tumor-induced angiogenesis [119]. Further advances in drug carriers, combined with ultrasound-induced BBB opening, will contribute significantly to effective drug delivery to malignant brain tumors.

Intrathecal and Intraventricular Delivery

As an alternative to opening or modulating the BBB, bypassing the BBB itself has become a common strategy. Early attempts to circumvent the BBB as well as the blood–cerebrospinal fluid (CSF) barrier involved delivering therapeutic agents directly into the CSF via the lumbar arachnoid space (intrathecal delivery) or ventricular system (intraventricular delivery). Intra-CSF administration is typically accomplished via lumbar puncture or through an indwelling, subcutaneous ventricular access device, such as an Ommaya or Rickham reservoir. However, rapid CSF turnover, as well as limited diffusion across the ependymal layer and into interstitial spaces, limits the efficacy of intrathecal or intraventricular administration for the treatment of parenchymal disease [120]. As a result, drug delivery to the CSF is generally reserved for treating meningeal diseases, including neoplastic meningitis and meningeal gliomatosis [121–125].

Intranasal Delivery

Intranasal Delivery: The Clinical Experience

Another route that has been garnering attention for its potential to noninvasively bypass the BBB involves intranasal delivery. Intranasal administration has been investigated previously as a means of achieving *systemic* distribution, due to the porous endothelial membrane and large surface area of nasal blood vessels, the rapid onset following administration, and the ability to avoid first-pass metabolism [126]. More recently, however, nasal administration has also been recognized as a strategy for delivering therapeutic agents directly to the CNS.

Following intranasal administration of a substance, transport must first take place across the olfactory and respiratory epithelia in the nasal passages. This may occur via intracellular pathways (including endocytosis into the olfactory sensory neurons and transcytosis across sustentacular cells) as well as extracellular pathways involving paracellular transport to the lamina propria. Paracellular transport may be facilitated by cell turnover within the nasal epithelium, which produces rearrangements of the epithelial tight junctions [127]. Local mechanical injury occurring during intranasal delivery may also allow larger substances to cross the nasal mucosa [128]. Substances that reach the lamina propria are then absorbed into the systemic circulation, drain via nasal lymphatics to the deep cervical lymph nodes, or travel along olfactory and trigeminal nerve endings to the olfactory bulb or the brain stem, respectively. Recent work examining the transport rate of [^{125}I]-insulin growth factor-1 (IGF-1) from the nares to the CNS has suggested that substances are carried by bulk flow within the perineural spaces of the olfactory and trigeminal nerves to points of entry into the brain [129]. From there, the substances distribute to distant sites within the CNS via communication with the CSF of the subarachnoid space or bulk flow within the perivascular spaces of cerebral blood vessels, a process driven by arterial pulsations related to the cardiac cycle [130, 131].

A number of preclinical studies have explored the intranasal administration of various therapeutic agents for the treatment of malignant brain tumors. Carboplatin-loaded polycaprolactone nanoparticles [132], methotrexate [133], neural stem cells [134], mesenchymal stem cells [135], telomerase inhibitors [136], and small interfering RNA-based therapies [137] have been successfully delivered intranasally in various murine models of glioma. In humans, intranasal delivery has primarily been studied for cardiovascular, endocrine, and neurocognitive agents, including vasopressin [138], angiotensin II [139], cholecystokinin [140], insulin [141], and oxytocin [142]. The only known study involving an antitumoral therapy was a phase I–II study [143] that examined the intranasal delivery of perillyl alcohol, a compound with previously identified anticancer activity through a poorly characterized, transforming growth factor-β (TGF-β) and/or Ras-dependent mechanism. Perillyl alcohol had been shown to have some efficacy in other solid tumors, but oral administration resulted in a variety of gastrointestinal side effects [144, 145]. Adults with recurrent HGG were administered an inhalational formulation of perillyl alcohol 4× daily through the nose. None of the patients in the study reported any toxicities associated with the treatment. However, further studies will be needed to study the efficacy of this treatment.

Limitations of Intranasal Delivery

One challenge in the study of intranasal delivery is that small animal models are not particularly representative of nasal anatomy and physiology in humans. Approximately 50% of the total surface area of the nose consists of olfactory epithelium in rats, whereas it is only 3–8% of the total surface area in humans [128]. Therapeutic agents that were successfully delivered to the CNS via the intranasal route in murine models may therefore fail in clinical trials. Other limitations are related to the low pH and relatively low permeability of the nasal mucosa. As a result, intranasal drug delivery is mainly limited to potent drugs that are delivered in small volumes. Higher volumes are likely to cause nasal irritation or injury. Active mucociliary clearance represents yet another obstacle to efficient intranasal delivery [127]. New drug formulations and carriers are therefore being explored in order to optimize the use of the intranasal route for the treatment of malignant brain tumors.

Interstitial Delivery

While intrathecal, intraventricular, and intranasal delivery bypasses the BBB, interstitial delivery represents the most direct option for intraparenchymal treatment. The current options for the interstitial delivery of therapeutic agents include implantable interstitial wafers and catheter-based convection-enhanced delivery (CED).

Interstitial Wafers

Carmustine Interstitial Wafer: The Clinical Experience

In 1976, Robert Langer and Judah Folkman revolutionized the drug delivery world by successfully incorporating macromolecules into non-inflammatory, biodegradable polymers [146]. These polymers can be safely implanted into biologic tissues, where subsequent degradation facilitates the sustained release of the biochemically active macromolecules. By modifying the chemical composition of the polymer, the kinetics of polymer degradation and macromolecule release can be closely regulated. Throughout the 1980s and 1990s, Langer partnered with Henry Brem and his colleagues at the Johns Hopkins University in order to translate this work from the bench to the operating room. Their efforts culminated in the clinical application of interstitial chemotherapy in the form of carmustine-loaded wafers, which currently remains the only FDA-approved locally delivered treatment for HGG.

The carmustine interstitial wafer (CIW) is comprised of the polyanhydride polymer poly [1,3-bis-(p-carboxyphenoxy propane)-co-(sebacic anhydride)] (CPP:SA) loaded with 3.8% carmustine (bis-chloroethylnitrosourea (BCNU)), a member of the nitrosourea family of chemotherapeutic agents [147]. At the time that CIW was being developed, intravenous BCNU was a standard treatment for HGG at many centers. The systemic administration of nitrosoureas had been shown to have a modest effect on survival [148], but BCNU has a short half-life and has been associated with side effects that include pulmonary fibrosis, myelosuppression, and hepatic dysfunction [149]. BCNU therefore represented a good choice to be incorporated into the hydrophobic matrix of the wafer, which would increase its half-life, increase local delivery of the drug to the residual tumor cells at the margin of the resection cavity, facilitate sustained release of the drug over 2–3 weeks, and decrease off-target effects.

Initial clinical trials [147] examined CIW implantation in patients with recurrent gliomas who had completed radiation therapy. A phase I–II study enrolled 21 patients with recurrent grade III or grade IV astrocytomas, who underwent tumor resection followed by implantation of up to 8 wafers. Three concentrations of BCNU were studied: 1.93, 3.85, and 6.35% by weight. Patients tolerated the interstitial treatment at all 3 doses, and there were no adverse reactions to the BCNU wafers themselves. The intermediate dose of BCNU, 3.85% by weight, was studied in a subsequent phase III study [150]—a prospective, randomized, placebo-controlled trial involving 27 centers and a total of 222 patients with recurrent grade III or grade IV astrocytomas. The study demonstrated a median survival of 31 weeks versus 23 weeks for patients receiving CIW versus placebo, respectively (hazard ratio = 0.67, $p = 0.006$), and the 6-month survival of patients with GBM was 50% higher in the treatment group relative to placebo ($p = 0.02$). The following year, in 1996, the FDA approved CIW for patients with recurrent HGG.

A second set of clinical trials focused on the use of CIW at the time of initial diagnosis.

A phase I study [151] involving 21 patients with grade IV and 1 patient with grade III astrocytoma established the safety of implanting CIW during the initial tumor resection, followed by radiation therapy. A phase III prospective, multicenter, randomized, double-blind trial [152] involving 32 patients identified a median survival of 58 weeks versus 40 weeks for the treatment and placebo groups, respectively ($p = 0.012$). A subsequent phase III study [153] confirmed the survival benefit in a larger group of patients, enrolling 240 patients and establishing a median survival of 13.9 months in the treatment group versus 11.6 months in the placebo group, with a 29% risk reduction ($p = 0.03$) over the course of 30 months. A follow-up study [154] confirmed that on long-term follow-up (i.e., 3 years after implantation), the survival advantage was maintained. The success of these clinical trials prompted the FDA to approve CIW for patients with newly diagnosed HGG in 2003.

CIW was the first major advance in HGG therapy since 1978, when radiation therapy was adopted into the standard adjuvant treatment of HGG [149]. In 2005, however, a second agent was added to the neuro-oncologist's armamentarium, when a phase III study by Roger Stupp and colleagues [155] demonstrated the safety and efficacy of a postoperative chemoradiation treatment strategy using orally delivered temozolomide and fractionated radiation therapy together over 6 weeks followed by maintenance temozolomide for six months. This regimen improved median survival from 12.1 to 14.6 months compared to radiation alone. Following this study, clinicians and researchers have explored the safety and efficacy of combining CIW with postoperative radiotherapy and temozolomide. Typically, chemoradiation is not initiated until 2–4 weeks following surgical resection or biopsy to allow for recovery and healing; CIW therefore offers a theoretical bridge to the chemoradiation treatments, providing sustained release of BCNU during the intervening period. A number of retrospective studies [156–163] and two prospective, observational studies [164, 165] have supported a role for multimodal therapy and have encouraged efforts for a randomized phase III study.

Limitations of Interstitial Wafers

Despite the survival advantage offered by CIW, some clinicians have been hesitant to implement interstitial wafers into their practice due to concerns that there is an increased risk of perioperative complications. Theoretical risks of CIW include seizures, cerebral edema, intracranial abscess, CSF leak, wound infection, impaired wound healing, and wafer migration. The phase III study that established the role of CIW in the initial treatment of HGG found similar rates of adverse events in the treatment and placebo arms of the trial, with two exceptions: CSF leak (5% in the treatment group vs. 0.8% in the placebo group) and delayed intracranial hypertension (9.1% in the treatment group vs. 1.7% in the placebo group) [153]. As a result, CIW has only been recommended for circumstances in which a watertight dural closure can be obtained; additionally, patients are monitored for cerebral edema and treated with high-dose corticosteroids postoperatively. Nevertheless, reported rates of adverse events remain highly variable. While one meta-analysis [166] associated CIW with a complication rate of 42.7%, a recent study [167] identified similar complication rates among patients with and without CIW wafers, even when combined with chemoradiation.

Interstitial chemotherapy is also limited by restricted distribution and rapid clearance of the free drug within and from the brain. Initial preclinical studies [168] in rabbits were promising, demonstrating that 3 days after wafer implantation, the effective depth of penetration of BCNU (defined as the distance from the polymer at which the concentration was 10% of its maximum value) was 10–12 mm. Given the evidence that the majority of HGG recurrences occur within 2 cm of the initial resection cavity, these data were felt to be encouraging. The limited distribution of BCNU is likely due to a combination of factors, including high interstitial pressure compared to pressure within the tumor resection cavity, the narrow width and high tortuosity of the brain ECS, and rapid clearance or partitioning into nearby cells. Nevertheless, experiments in non-human primates demonstrated high doses of BCNU (in the millimolar range) 3 mm from the wafer, as well as significant doses (in the micromolar range) throughout the entire brain. Importantly, 7 days following implantation, significant doses of BCNU persisted 1–2 cm from the wafer [169]. Postoperative edema may contribute to the convective flow of BCNU, allowing greater distribution than with diffusion alone. Additionally, while the lipophilicity of the drug contributes to rapid partitioning and/or clearance, it is possible that this same property allows BCNU to circulate within the blood and/or CSF and reenter the brain parenchyma at sites distant from the wafer [170].

Future Directions

Although CIW is the only local treatment approved for use in humans, a variety of therapeutic agents are being incorporated into polymer wafers and hydrogels for preclinical testing, including methotrexate [171], doxorubicin [171], carboplatin [172], 5-fluorouracil [173], ardipusilloside I [174], and butylidenephthalide [175, 176]. Additionally, biomaterial advances have resulted in improved polymers, new wafer designs, and most recently, implantable microchips consisting of multiple, discrete, drug-containing reservoirs [177]. Microchips enable controlled release via two mechanisms. On the one hand, each reservoir can be sealed with a polymer membrane; the composition and molecular mass of the polymer determine its rate of degradation, thereby allowing the contents of that reservoir to be released at a predefined point in time [178]. Alternatively, a metallic membrane can be incorporated and subsequently disintegrated by electrothermal ablation [179]. A resorbable polymer microchip containing BCNU and a microelectromechanical (MEMS) microchip containing temozolomide have both demonstrated efficacy in a 9L rat gliosarcoma model [180, 181], and the first clinical trial of an implantable microchip for drug delivery (for the treatment of osteoporosis) was recently completed [182]. Incorporating microchip technology into the treatment of malignant brain tumors would potentially allow more precise temporal control over the local delivery of chemotherapeutics.

Convection-Enhanced Delivery

CED: The Clinical Experience

A second strategy for interstitial delivery involves infusing a therapeutic agent directly into the region of interest via one or multiple stereotactically placed catheters. In 1994, Bobo et al. [183] described the underlying principles of CED—the continuous infusion of a therapeutic agent under pressure generates bulk flow. As a result, the distribution of the infusate is pressure driven, in contrast to therapeutic agents that are delivered via interstitial wafers or bolus injections, where the volume of distribution (V_d) is dictated by diffusion—a process dependent on the concentration gradient. Whereas interstitial wafers result in a high concentration of drug in the immediately adjacent region followed by a steep drop-off, CED has been promoted for the ability to generate more constant concentrations over larger distances. Nevertheless, the experience with CED has shown that a number of factors influence the V_d, including the infusion volume (V_i), infusion flow rate, tissue parameters (e.g., the size of the ECS), and infusate parameters (e.g., molecular size and charge) [184].

Numerous phase I and phase II clinical trials have explored the safety and efficacy of CED for the delivery of various compounds. The ideal agent does not cross the BBB easily (thereby reducing its rate of clearance from the brain), specifically targets neoplastic cells, and is associated with non-CNS toxicities that preclude its systemic administration. Conventional chemotherapeutic agents that fit this description include topotecan and carboplatin, and preliminary phase I studies [185–187] suggest that CED allows these agents to be delivered at therapeutic concentrations while avoiding toxicity. The vast majority of studies, however, have explored the use of CED for the delivery of more exotic therapies that target a variety of tumor-specific antigens. These include antisense oligonucleotides that inhibit TGF-β2 [188], immunostimulating oligodeoxynucleotides containing CpG motifs [189], liposomal gene therapy vectors [190], and monoclonal antibodies conjugated to radioactive isotopes [191].

Targeted immunotoxins represent the most heavily studied class of compounds delivered via CED. Toxins in current use are obtained from either *Corynebacterium diphtheria* or *Pseudomonas aeruginosa* and modified by replacing the toxin's native targeting mechanisms with tumor-specific ligands that recognize the transferrin receptor, interleukin-4 (IL-4) receptor, IL-13 receptor, or EGFR. Phase I and II studies have included TP-38 (Pseudomonas exotoxin fused with EGFR) [192], NBI-3001 (Pseudomonas exotoxin linked to IL-4) [193, 194], and TF-CRM107 (diphtheria toxin fused to transferrin C) [195, 196]. TF-CRM107, in particular, demonstrated a 50% decrease in tumor volume in 9 of 15 patients in an initial phase I trial; less impressive results in a subsequent phase II trial, however, resulted in the termination of a planned phase III trial.

As a result, the only CED agent to reach a phase III study has been cintredekin besudotox (CB), a Pseudomonas toxin fused with recombinant human IL-13. Phase I studies [197, 198] initially identified maximum tolerate infusate concentrations of 0.5 μg/mL, delivered via CED for 96 h. These parameters were then tested in the PRECISE trial [199], a phase III study in which patients were randomized 2:1 to receive CB versus CIW. The trial, which recruited 296 patients from 52 centers, was unfortunately deemed a failure, as it did not result in a statistically significant difference in median overall survival between the groups. Of note, there *was* a significant improvement in progression-free survival (17.7 vs. 11.4 weeks, $p = 0.0008$), but this was not a prespecified end point of the study. While trying to explain the negative outcome of the trial, some have pointed to flaws in its statistical design, while others have emphasized a subsequent analysis showing that, on average, the "coverage volume" included only 20% of the 2-cm rim around the resection cavity [200]. Suboptimal catheter positioning (only 51% of the catheters were accurately positioned) and the inability to accurately track the drug distribution in real time likely contributed to the poor distribution of CB [201].

Limitations of CED

The outcome of the PRECISE trial highlights some of the inherent limitations of CED in its current form. In the absence of real-time imaging to track the distribution of infusate, numerous factors can alter the geometry and V_d in unpredictable ways. For example, leakage into the subarachnoid space and/or the ventricles can result in diminished concentrations at the region of interest, as well as a higher prevalence of toxicities, including chemical meningitis. Optimizing catheter placement is therefore critical in ensuring adequate distribution. Additionally, even when catheter positioning is appropriate, the tissue characteristics in and adjacent to a tumor are often heterogeneous and difficult to predict. Of note, the tumor is often characterized by a higher interstitial pressure than the surrounding tissue [202]; the pressure gradient therefore shunts the infusate away from the tumor.

Another process that reduces the effective V_d involves "backflow" or "reflux" along the catheter. Preclinical studies [203] have shown that with larger cannula size, there is more trauma to the tissue upon insertion of the catheter. If the surrounding tissue is not tightly sealed around the catheter, the infusate will travel along the path of least resistance—along the catheter itself, instead of into the tissue. Similarly, high infusion rates promote reflux, although conversely, infusion rates that are *too* low allow the infusate to be cleared before adequate concentrations can accumulate. Optimizing the rate of infusion often requires finding a balance between the two extremes [204].

Future Directions

Since the early CED trials, a number of advances in the realms of engineering, mathematical modeling, and imaging have dramatically changed the landscape of tumor treatment with CED. Of note, CED was initially performed with simple, one-port catheters. However, a variety of more advanced catheters are now available. Reflux-free catheters involve different variations of a "stepped" cannula design, which allows for a small catheter tip while maintaining ease of placement [205, 206]. Multiple port catheters are characterized by multiple openings, although studies have shown that the infusate is, in reality, only delivered from the most proximal port [184]. Porous hollow fiber catheters have walls that consist of millions of pores with diameters of 0.45 μm in order to increase the surface area exposed to the infusate [207]. Balloon-tipped catheters incorporate a balloon proximal to the tip of the catheter, which can be expanded to fill the resection cavity and prevent reflux during the infusion. Early results in a canine model are promising [208].

In addition to newer catheter designs, being able to predict the distribution of the infusate ahead of time would have significant implications for planning catheter placement and infusion volumes. Rigorous mathematical modeling and computational methods have begun to account for the anisotropy and heterogeneity of the human brain, particularly in the setting of tumor infiltration [209–212]. Until such models are perfected, however, the only way to know the spatial distribution of the infusate is through real-time imaging. MRI has been used to monitor the distribution of liposomes delivered via CED by incorporating gadolinium–diethylene triamine pentaacetic acid (Gd-DTPA) into the liposome construct [213]. Alternatively, Gd-DTPA can be coinfused with the therapeutic agent during CED [214]. For those who would prefer to visualize the therapeutic agent itself, iron oxide nanoparticles can be imaged directly with MRI, thus enabling real-time adjustments to the flow rate if reflux occurs [215].

Despite these advances, drug distribution following CED remains limited by the physical constraints of the narrow and anisotropic brain ECS. Strategies to increase the "effective pore size" of the brain ECS include using enzymes to degrade the extracellular matrix (ECM) [216] and dilating the brain ECS by coinfusing a hyperosmotic solution [216–218]. Applying ultrasound energy to brain tissue has emerged as another potential strategy for modifying the ECS and has been shown to increase the dispersion of locally delivered dyes (e.g., Evans blue dye), ^{3}H-labeled molecules of various sizes, and drugs (i.e., BCNU) in the brain parenchyma [219–222]. These ultrasound-based effects are likely secondary to radiation forces that contribute to the convective flow produced during CED [220], in addition to mechanical effects that alter the structure of the brain ECS, resulting in greater brain tissue permeability [222]. By increasing the pore sizes within the ECS, ultrasound has the potential to facilitate the delivery of larger therapeutic agents with bigger payloads.

As CED technology undergoes further refinement, it may also become useful to provide prolonged infusions over longer time frames. Currently, CED requires patients to remain hospitalized, with infusions taking place via an externalized catheter. Chronic therapies could be provided in an outpatient setting, however, through implantable ports. One such system involves connecting the port to a subcutaneous pump in a manner comparable to intrathecal pumps used for chronic pain and spasticity [223]. An alternative model uses a transcutaneous port which can be accessed for an intermittent delivery regimen, similar to an Ommaya reservoir [187]. These newer designs will enable more widespread use of CED.

Conclusion

In summary, unique physical and biological features of the CNS present significant barriers to the effective delivery of therapeutic agents to malignant brain tumors. As a result, clinicians and researchers have developed novel methods for packaging and delivering treatments to the CNS. Nanoparticle carriers, viral vectors, stem cell-mediated delivery, MRgFUS, interstitial wafers, and catheter-based CED are all in varying stages of clinical development and testing. The success and failure of each of these strategies will help guide new directions for research, with the ultimate goal of improving the survival and quality of life of patients with malignant brain tumors.

References

1. Obermeier B, Daneman R, Ransohoff RM. Development, maintenance and disruption of the blood-brain barrier. Nat Med. 2013;19(12):1584–96.
2. Pardridge WM. Drug transport across the blood-brain barrier. J Cereb Blood Flow Metab. 2012;32(11):1959–72.
3. Pardridge WM. The blood-brain barrier: bottleneck in brain drug development. NeuroRx. 2005;2(1):3–14.
4. Wen PY, Kesari S. Malignant gliomas in adults. N Engl J Med. 2008;359(5):492–507.
5. Henson JW, Cordon-Cardo C, Posner JB. P-glycoprotein expression in brain tumors. J Neurooncol. 1992;14(1):37–43.
6. Sykova E, Nicholson C. Diffusion in brain extracellular space. Physiol Rev. 2008;88(4):1277–340.
7. Thorne RG, Nicholson C. In vivo diffusion analysis with quantum dots and dextrans predicts the width of brain extracellular space. Proc Natl Acad Sci U S A. 2006;103(14):5567–72.
8. Nance EA, Woodworth GF, Sailor KA, Shih TY, Xu Q, Swaminathan G, et al. A dense poly(ethylene glycol) coating improves penetration of large polymeric nanoparticles within brain tissue. Sci Transl Med. 2012;4(149):149ra19.
9. Vargova L, Homola A, Zamecnik J, Tichy M, Benes V, Sykova E. Diffusion parameters of the extracellular space in human gliomas. Glia. 2003;42(1):77–88.
10. Karim R, Palazzo C, Evrard B, Piel G. Nanocarriers for the treatment of glioblastoma multiforme: current state-of-the-art. J Control Release. 2016.
11. Cheng Y, Dai Q, Morshed RA, Fan X, Wegscheid ML, Wainwright DA, et al. Blood-brain barrier permeable gold nanoparticles: an efficient delivery platform for enhanced malignant glioma therapy and imaging. Small. 2014;10(24):5137–50.
12. Zensi A, Begley D, Pontikis C, Legros C, Mihoreanu L, Wagner S, et al. Albumin nanoparticles targeted with Apo E enter the CNS by transcytosis and are delivered to neurones. J Control Release. 2009;137(1):78–86.
13. Huwyler J, Wu D, Pardridge WM. Brain drug delivery of small molecules using immunoliposomes. Proc Natl Acad Sci U S A. 1996;93(24):14164–9.
14. Beduneau A, Saulnier P, Benoit JP. Active targeting of brain tumors using nanocarriers. Biomaterials. 2007;28(33):4947–67.
15. Maier-Hauff K, Rothe R, Scholz R, Gneveckow U, Wust P, Thiesen B, et al. Intracranial thermotherapy using magnetic nanoparticles combined with external beam radiotherapy: results of a feasibility study on patients with glioblastoma multiforme. J Neurooncol. 2007;81(1):53–60.
16. Maier-Hauff K, Ulrich F, Nestler D, Niehoff H, Wust P, Thiesen B, et al. Efficacy and safety of intratumoral thermotherapy using magnetic iron-oxide nanoparticles combined with external beam radiotherapy on patients with recurrent glioblastoma multiforme. J Neurooncol. 2011;103(2):317–24.
17. Chastagner P, Devictor B, Geoerger B, Aerts I, Leblond P, Frappaz D, et al. Phase I study of non-pegylated liposomal doxorubicin in children with recurrent/refractory high-grade glioma. Cancer Chemother Pharmacol. 2015;76(2):425–32.
18. Fabel K, Dietrich J, Hau P, Wismeth C, Winner B, Przywara S, et al. Long-term stabilization in patients with malignant glioma after treatment with liposomal doxorubicin. Cancer. 2001;92(7):1936–42.
19. Ananda S, Nowak AK, Cher L, Dowling A, Brown C, Simes J, et al. Phase 2 trial of temozolomide and pegylated liposomal doxorubicin in the treatment of patients with glioblastoma multiforme following concurrent radiotherapy and chemotherapy. J Clin Neurosci. 2011;18(11):1444–8.
20. Spina M, Chimienti E, Martellotta F, Vaccher E, Berretta M, Zanet E, et al. Phase 2 study of intrathecal, long-acting liposomal cytarabine in the prophylaxis of lymphomatous meningitis in human immunodeficiency virus-related non-Hodgkin lymphoma. Cancer. 2010;116(6):1495–501.
21. Jaeckle KA, Phuphanich S, Bent MJ, Aiken R, Batchelor T, Campbell T, et al. Intrathecal treatment of neoplastic meningitis due to breast cancer with a slow-release formulation of cytarabine. Br J Cancer. 2001;84(2):157–63.
22. Perez JG, Tran NL, Rosenblum MG, Schneider CS, Connolly NP, Kim AJ, et al. The TWEAK receptor Fn14 is a potential cell surface portal for targeted delivery of glioblastoma therapeutics. Oncogene. 2015.
23. Schneider CS, Perez JG, Cheng E, Zhang C, Mastorakos P, Hanes J, et al. Minimizing the non-specific binding of nanoparticles to the brain enables active targeting of Fn14-positive glioblastoma cells. Biomaterials. 2015;42:42–51.
24. Biffi A. Gene therapy for lysosomal storage disorders: a good start. Hum Mol Genet. 2015.
25. Kong SD, Lee J, Ramachandran S, Eliceiri BP, Shubayev VI, Lal R, et al. Magnetic targeting of nanoparticles across the intact blood-brain barrier. J Control Release. 2012;164(1):49–57.
26. Vergoni AV, Tosi G, Tacchi R, Vandelli MA, Bertolini A, Costantino L. Nanoparticles as drug delivery agents specific for CNS: in vivo biodistribution. Nanomedicine. 2009;5(4):369–77.
27. Barbu E, Molnar E, Tsibouklis J, Gorecki DC. The potential for nanoparticle-based drug delivery to the brain: overcoming the blood-brain barrier. Expert Opin Drug Deliv. 2009;6(6):553–65.

28. Gref R, Domb A, Quellec P, Blunk T, Muller RH, Verbavatz JM, et al. The controlled intravenous delivery of drugs using PEG-coated sterically stabilized nanospheres. Adv Drug Deliv Rev. 1995;16(2–3):215–33.
29. Ambruosi A, Khalansky AS, Yamamoto H, Gelperina SE, Begley DJ, Kreuter J. Biodistribution of polysorbate 80-coated doxorubicin-loaded [14C]-poly(butyl cyanoacrylate) nanoparticles after intravenous administration to glioblastoma-bearing rats. J Drug Target. 2006;14(2):97–105.
30. Sawyer AJ, Saucier-Sawyer JK, Booth CJ, Liu J, Patel T, Piepmeier JM, et al. Convection-enhanced delivery of camptothecin-loaded polymer nanoparticles for treatment of intracranial tumors. Drug Deliv Transl Res. 2011;1(1):34–42.
31. Geldenhuys W, Mbimba T, Bui T, Harrison K, Sutariya V. Brain-targeted delivery of paclitaxel using glutathione-coated nanoparticles for brain cancers. J Drug Target. 2011;19(9):837–45.
32. Zuckerman JE, Gritli I, Tolcher A, Heidel JD, Lim D, Morgan R, et al. Correlating animal and human phase Ia/Ib clinical data with CALAA-01, a targeted, polymer-based nanoparticle containing siRNA. Proc Natl Acad Sci U S A. 2014;111(31):11449–54.
33. Weiss GJ, Chao J, Neidhart JD, Ramanathan RK, Bassett D, Neidhart JA, et al. First-in-human phase 1/2a trial of CRLX101, a cyclodextrin-containing polymer-camptothecin nanopharmaceutical in patients with advanced solid tumor malignancies. Invest New Drugs. 2013;31(4):986–1000.
34. Samad A, Sultana Y, Aqil M. Liposomal drug delivery systems: an update review. Curr Drug Deliv. 2007;4(4):297–305.
35. Gabizon A, Martin F. Polyethylene glycol-coated (pegylated) liposomal doxorubicin. Rationale for use in solid tumours. Drugs. 1997;54(Suppl 4):15–21.
36. Caraglia M, Addeo R, Costanzo R, Montella L, Faiola V, Marra M, et al. Phase II study of temozolomide plus pegylated liposomal doxorubicin in the treatment of brain metastases from solid tumours. Cancer Chemother Pharmacol. 2006;57(1):34–9.
37. Bouras A, Kaluzova M, Hadjipanayis CG. Radiosensitivity enhancement of radioresistant glioblastoma by epidermal growth factor receptor antibody-conjugated iron-oxide nanoparticles. J Neurooncol. 2015;124(1):13–22.
38. Thaci B, Brown CE, Binello E, Werbaneth K, Sampath P, Sengupta S. Significance of interleukin-13 receptor alpha 2-targeted glioblastoma therapy. Neuro Oncol. 2014;16(10):1304–12.
39. Winkles JA. The TWEAK-Fn14 cytokine-receptor axis: discovery, biology and therapeutic targeting. Nat Rev Drug Discov. 2008;7(5):411–25.
40. During MJ, Kaplitt MG, Stern MB, Eidelberg D. Subthalamic GAD gene transfer in Parkinson disease patients who are candidates for deep brain stimulation. Hum Gene Ther. 2001;12(12):1589–91.
41. Lang FF, Bruner JM, Fuller GN, Aldape K, Prados MD, Chang S, et al. Phase I trial of adenovirus-mediated p53 gene therapy for recurrent glioma: biological and clinical results. J Clin Oncol. 2003;21(13):2508–18.
42. Eck SL, Alavi JB, Judy K, Phillips P, Alavi A, Hackney D, et al. Treatment of recurrent or progressive malignant glioma with a recombinant adenovirus expressing human interferon-beta (H5.010CMVhIFN-beta): a phase I trial. Hum Gene Ther. 2001;12(1):97–113.
43. Smitt PS, Driesse M, Wolbers J, Kros M, Avezaat C. Treatment of relapsed malignant glioma with an adenoviral vector containing the herpes simplex thymidine kinase gene followed by ganciclovir. Mol Ther. 2003;7(6):851–8.
44. Westphal M, Yla-Herttuala S, Martin J, Warnke P, Menei P, Eckland D, et al. Adenovirus-mediated gene therapy with sitimagene ceradenovec followed by intravenous ganciclovir for patients with operable high-grade glioma (ASPECT): a randomised, open-label, phase 3 trial. Lancet Oncol. 2013;14(9):823–33.
45. Strik HM, Stoll M, Meyermann R. Immune cell infiltration of intrinsic and metastatic intracranial tumours. Anticancer Res. 2004;24(1):37–42.
46. Schackert G, Simmons RD, Buzbee TM, Hume DA, Fidler IJ. Macrophage infiltration into experimental brain metastases: occurrence through an intact blood-brain barrier. J Natl Cancer Inst. 1988;80(13):1027–34.
47. Choi MR, Bardhan R, Stanton-Maxey KJ, Badve S, Nakshatri H, Stantz KM, et al. Delivery of nanoparticles to brain metastases of breast cancer using a cellular Trojan horse. Cancer Nanotechnol. 2012;3(1–6):47–54.
48. Aboody KS, Brown A, Rainov NG, Bower KA, Liu S, Yang W, et al. Neural stem cells display extensive tropism for pathology in adult brain: evidence from intracranial gliomas. Proc Natl Acad Sci U S A. 2000;97(23):12846–51.
49. Smith CL, Chaichana KL, Lee YM, Lin B, Stanko KM, O'Donnell T, et al. Pre-exposure of human adipose mesenchymal stem cells to soluble factors enhances their homing to brain cancer. Stem Cells Transl Med. 2015;4(3):239–51.
50. Pendleton C, Li Q, Chesler DA, Yuan K, Guerrero-Cazares H, Quinones-Hinojosa A. Mesenchymal stem cells derived from adipose tissue vs bone marrow: in vitro comparison of their tropism towards gliomas. PLoS ONE. 2013;8(3):e58198.
51. Pluchino S, Zanotti L, Rossi B, Brambilla E, Ottoboni L, Salani G, et al. Neurosphere-derived multipotent precursors promote neuroprotection by an immunomodulatory mechanism. Nature. 2005;436(7048):266–71.
52. Jones BJ, McTaggart SJ. Immunosuppression by mesenchymal stromal cells: from culture to clinic. Exp Hematol. 2008;36(6):733–41.

53. Ahmed AU, Thaci B, Alexiades NG, Han Y, Qian S, Liu F, et al. Neural stem cell-based cell carriers enhance therapeutic efficacy of an oncolytic adenovirus in an orthotopic mouse model of human glioblastoma. Mol Ther. 2011;19(9):1714–26.
54. Thaci B, Ahmed AU, Ulasov IV, Tobias AL, Han Y, Aboody KS, et al. Pharmacokinetic study of neural stem cell-based cell carrier for oncolytic virotherapy: targeted delivery of the therapeutic payload in an orthotopic brain tumor model. Cancer Gene Ther. 2012;19(6):431–42.
55. Tyler MA, Ulasov IV, Sonabend AM, Nandi S, Han Y, Marler S, et al. Neural stem cells target intracranial glioma to deliver an oncolytic adenovirus in vivo. Gene Ther. 2009;16(2):262–78.
56. Roger M, Clavreul A, Huynh NT, Passirani C, Schiller P, Vessieres A, et al. Ferrociphenol lipid nanocapsule delivery by mesenchymal stromal cells in brain tumor therapy. Int J Pharm. 2012;423 (1):63–8.
57. Li L, Guan Y, Liu H, Hao N, Liu T, Meng X, et al. Silica nanorattle-doxorubicin-anchored mesenchymal stem cells for tumor-tropic therapy. ACS Nano. 2011;5(9):7462–70.
58. Sasportas LS, Kasmieh R, Wakimoto H, Hingtgen S, van de Water JA, Mohapatra G, et al. Assessment of therapeutic efficacy and fate of engineered human mesenchymal stem cells for cancer therapy. Proc Natl Acad Sci U S A. 2009;106(12):4822–7.
59. Menon LG, Kelly K, Yang HW, Kim SK, Black PM, Carroll RS. Human bone marrow-derived mesenchymal stromal cells expressing S-TRAIL as a cellular delivery vehicle for human glioma therapy. Stem Cells. 2009;27 (9):2320–30.
60. Bagci-Onder T, Wakimoto H, Anderegg M, Cameron C, Shah K. A dual PI3 K/mTOR inhibitor, PI-103, cooperates with stem cell-delivered TRAIL in experimental glioma models. Cancer Res. 2011;71(1):154–63.
61. Choi SA, Hwang SK, Wang KC, Cho BK, Phi JH, Lee JY, et al. Therapeutic efficacy and safety of TRAIL-producing human adipose tissue-derived mesenchymal stem cells against experimental brainstem glioma. Neuro Oncol. 2011;13(1):61–9.
62. Li Q, Wijesekera O, Salas SJ, Wang JY, Zhu M, Aprhys C, et al. Mesenchymal stem cells from human fat engineered to secrete BMP4 are nononcogenic, suppress brain cancer, and prolong survival. Clin Cancer Res. 2014;20(9):2375–87.
63. Ryu CH, Park SH, Park SA, Kim SM, Lim JY, Jeong CH, et al. Gene therapy of intracranial glioma using interleukin 12-secreting human umbilical cord blood-derived mesenchymal stem cells. Hum Gene Ther. 2011;22(6):733–43.
64. Kosaka H, Ichikawa T, Kurozumi K, Kambara H, Inoue S, Maruo T, et al. Therapeutic effect of suicide gene-transferred mesenchymal stem cells in a rat model of glioma. Cancer Gene Ther. 2012;19 (8):572–8.
65. Aboody KS, Najbauer J, Metz MZ, D'Apuzzo M, Gutova M, Annala AJ, et al. Neural stem cell-mediated enzyme/prodrug therapy for glioma: preclinical studies. Sci Transl Med. 2013;5 (184):184ra59.
66. Steinfeld U, Pauli C, Kaltz N, Bergemann C, Lee HH. T lymphocytes as potential therapeutic drug carrier for cancer treatment. Int J Pharm. 2006;311(1–2):229–36.
67. Nowacek AS, Miller RL, McMillan J, Kanmogne G, Kanmogne M, Mosley RL, et al. NanoART synthesis, characterization, uptake, release and toxicology for human monocyte-macrophage drug delivery. Nanomedicine (Lond). 2009;4(8):903–17.
68. Rosland GV, Svendsen A, Torsvik A, Sobala E, McCormack E, Immervoll H, et al. Long-term cultures of bone marrow-derived human mesenchymal stem cells frequently undergo spontaneous malignant transformation. Cancer Res. 2009;69 (13):5331–9.
69. Bernardo ME, Zaffaroni N, Novara F, Cometa AM, Avanzini MA, Moretta A, et al. Human bone marrow derived mesenchymal stem cells do not undergo transformation after long-term in vitro culture and do not exhibit telomere maintenance mechanisms. Cancer Res. 2007;67(19):9142–9.
70. Amariglio N, Hirshberg A, Scheithauer BW, Cohen Y, Loewenthal R, Trakhtenbrot L, et al. Donor-derived brain tumor following neural stem cell transplantation in an ataxia telangiectasia patient. PLoS Med. 2009;6(2):e1000029.
71. Karnoub AE, Dash AB, Vo AP, Sullivan A, Brooks MW, Bell GW, et al. Mesenchymal stem cells within tumour stroma promote breast cancer metastasis. Nature. 2007;449(7162):557–63.
72. Djouad F, Plence P, Bony C, Tropel P, Apparailly F, Sany J, et al. Immunosuppressive effect of mesenchymal stem cells favors tumor growth in allogeneic animals. Blood. 2003;102(10):3837–44.
73. Eckman WW, Patlak CS, Fenstermacher JD. A critical evaluation of the principles governing the advantages of intra-arterial infusions. J Pharmacokinet Biopharm. 1974;2(3):257–85.
74. Rajappa P, Krass J, Riina HA, Boockvar JA, Greenfield JP. Super-selective basilar artery infusion of bevacizumab and cetuximab for multiply recurrent pediatric ependymoma. Interv Neuroradiol. 2011;17(4):459–65.
75. Rapoport SI, Hori M, Klatzo I. Reversible osmotic opening of the blood-brain barrier. Science. 1971;173(4001):1026–8.
76. Rapoport SI. Osmotic opening of the blood-brain barrier: principles, mechanism, and therapeutic applications. Cell Mol Neurobiol. 2000;20(2):217–30.
77. Doolittle ND, Miner ME, Hall WA, Siegal T, Jerome E, Osztie E, et al. Safety and efficacy of a multicenter study using intraarterial chemotherapy in conjunction with osmotic opening of the blood-brain barrier for the treatment of patients

with malignant brain tumors. Cancer. 2000;88 (3):637–47.
78. Rapoport SI, Fredericks WR, Ohno K, Pettigrew KD. Quantitative aspects of reversible osmotic opening of the blood-brain barrier. Am J Physiol. 1980;238(5):R421–31.
79. Nadal A, Fuentes E, Pastor J, McNaughton PA. Plasma albumin is a potent trigger of calcium signals and DNA synthesis in astrocytes. Proc Natl Acad Sci U S A. 1995;92(5):1426–30.
80. Nakano S, Matsukado K, Black KL. Increased brain tumor microvessel permeability after intracarotid bradykinin infusion is mediated by nitric oxide. Cancer Res. 1996;56(17):4027–31.
81. Matsukado K, Sugita M, Black KL. Intracarotid low dose bradykinin infusion selectively increases tumor permeability through activation of bradykinin B2 receptors in malignant gliomas. Brain Res. 1998;792(1):10–5.
82. Bartus RT, Elliott P, Hayward N, Dean R, McEwen EL, Fisher SK. Permeability of the blood brain barrier by the bradykinin agonist, RMP-7: evidence for a sensitive, auto-regulated, receptor-mediated system. Immunopharmacology. 1996;33(1–3):270–8.
83. Warren KE, Patel MC, Aikin AA, Widemann B, Libucha M, Adamson PC, et al. Phase I trial of lobradimil (RMP-7) and carboplatin in children with brain tumors. Cancer Chemother Pharmacol. 2001;48(4):275–82.
84. Gregor A, Lind M, Newman H, Grant R, Hadley DM, Barton T, et al. Phase II studies of RMP-7 and carboplatin in the treatment of recurrent high grade glioma. RMP-7 European Study Group. J Neurooncol. 1999;44(2):137–45.
85. Prados MD, Schold SJS, Fine HA, Jaeckle K, Hochberg F, Mechtler L, et al. A randomized, double-blind, placebo-controlled, phase 2 study of RMP-7 in combination with carboplatin administered intravenously for the treatment of recurrent malignant glioma. Neuro Oncol. 2003;5(2):96–103.
86. Pardridge WM. Drug and gene targeting to the brain with molecular Trojan horses. Nat Rev Drug Discov. 2002;1(2):131–9.
87. Shin SU, Friden P, Moran M, Olson T, Kang YS, Pardridge WM, et al. Transferrin-antibody fusion proteins are effective in brain targeting. Proc Natl Acad Sci U S A. 1995;92(7):2820–4.
88. Yu YJ, Zhang Y, Kenrick M, Hoyte K, Luk W, Lu Y, et al. Boosting brain uptake of a therapeutic antibody by reducing its affinity for a transcytosis target. Sci Transl Med. 2011;3(84):84ra44.
89. Boado RJ, Hui EK, Lu JZ, Sumbria RK, Pardridge WM. Blood-brain barrier molecular trojan horse enables imaging of brain uptake of radioiodinated recombinant protein in the rhesus monkey. Bioconjug Chem. 2013;24(10):1741–9.
90. Drappatz J, Brenner A, Wong ET, Eichler A, Schiff D, Groves MD, et al. Phase I study of GRN1005 in recurrent malignant glioma. Clin Cancer Res. 2013;19(6):1567–76.
91. Ballantine HT Jr, Bell E, Manlapaz J. Progress and problems in the neurological applications of focused ultrasound. J Neurosurg. 1960;17:858–76.
92. Hynynen K, Jolesz FA. Demonstration of potential noninvasive ultrasound brain therapy through an intact skull. Ultrasound Med Biol. 1998;24(2):275–83.
93. Cline HE, Hynynen K, Hardy CJ, Watkins RD, Schenck JF, Jolesz FA. MR temperature mapping of focused ultrasound surgery. Magn Reson Med. 1994;31(6):628–36.
94. Haar GT, Coussios C. High intensity focused ultrasound: physical principles and devices. Int J Hyperthermia. 2007;23(2):89–104.
95. Krasovitski B, Frenkel V, Shoham S, Kimmel E. Intramembrane cavitation as a unifying mechanism for ultrasound-induced bioeffects. Proc Natl Acad Sci U S A. 2011;108(8):3258–63.
96. Hancock HA, Smith LH, Cuesta J, Durrani AK, Angstadt M, Palmeri ML, et al. Investigations into pulsed high-intensity focused ultrasound-enhanced delivery: preliminary evidence for a novel mechanism. Ultrasound Med Biol. 2009;35(10):1722–36.
97. Frenkel V, Gurka R, Liberzon A, Shavit U, Kimmel E. Preliminary investigations of ultrasound induced acoustic streaming using particle image velocimetry. Ultrasonics. 2001;39(3):153–6.
98. Hynynen K, McDannold N, Vykhodtseva N, Jolesz FA. Noninvasive MR imaging-guided focal opening of the blood-brain barrier in rabbits. Radiology. 2001;220(3):640–6.
99. Sheikov N, McDannold N, Sharma S, Hynynen K. Effect of focused ultrasound applied with an ultrasound contrast agent on the tight junctional integrity of the brain microvascular endothelium. Ultrasound Med Biol. 2008;34(7):1093–104.
100. Deng J, Huang Q, Wang F, Liu Y, Wang Z, Wang Z, et al. The role of caveolin-1 in blood-brain barrier disruption induced by focused ultrasound combined with microbubbles. J Mol Neurosci. 2012;46(3):677–87.
101. Park J, Zhang Y, Vykhodtseva N, Jolesz FA, McDannold NJ. The kinetics of blood brain barrier permeability and targeted doxorubicin delivery into brain induced by focused ultrasound. J Control Release. 2012;162(1):134–42.
102. Kovacs Z, Werner B, Rassi A, Sass JO, Martin-Fiori E, Bernasconi M. Prolonged survival upon ultrasound-enhanced doxorubicin delivery in two syngenic glioblastoma mouse models. J Control Release. 2014;187:74–82.
103. Treat LH, McDannold N, Vykhodtseva N, Zhang Y, Tam K, Hynynen K. Targeted delivery of doxorubicin to the rat brain at therapeutic levels using MRI-guided focused ultrasound. Int J Cancer. 2007;121(4):901–7.
104. Treat LH, McDannold N, Zhang Y, Vykhodtseva N, Hynynen K. Improved anti-tumor effect of

liposomal doxorubicin after targeted blood-brain barrier disruption by MRI-guided focused ultrasound in rat glioma. Ultrasound Med Biol. 2012;38(10):1716–25.
105. Mei J, Cheng Y, Song Y, Yang Y, Wang F, Liu Y, et al. Experimental study on targeted methotrexate delivery to the rabbit brain via magnetic resonance imaging-guided focused ultrasound. J Ultrasound Med. 2009;28(7):871–80.
106. Liu HL, Hua MY, Yang HW, Huang CY, Chu PC, Wu JS, et al. Magnetic resonance monitoring of focused ultrasound/magnetic nanoparticle targeting delivery of therapeutic agents to the brain. Proc Natl Acad Sci U S A. 2010;107(34):15205–10.
107. Wei KC, Chu PC, Wang HY, Huang CY, Chen PY, Tsai HC, et al. Focused ultrasound-induced blood-brain barrier opening to enhance temozolomide delivery for glioblastoma treatment: a preclinical study. PLoS ONE. 2013;8(3):e58995.
108. Park EJ, Zhang YZ, Vykhodtseva N, McDannold N. Ultrasound-mediated blood-brain/blood-tumor barrier disruption improves outcomes with trastuzumab in a breast cancer brain metastasis model. J Control Release. 2012;163(3):277–84.
109. Kinoshita M, McDannold N, Jolesz FA, Hynynen K. Noninvasive localized delivery of Herceptin to the mouse brain by MRI-guided focused ultrasound-induced blood-brain barrier disruption. Proc Natl Acad Sci U S A. 2006;103(31):11719–23.
110. Chen PY, Hsieh HY, Huang CY, Lin CY, Wei KC, Liu HL. Focused ultrasound-induced blood-brain barrier opening to enhance interleukin-12 delivery for brain tumor immunotherapy: a preclinical feasibility study. J Transl Med. 2015;13:93.
111. Burgess A, Ayala-Grosso CA, Ganguly M, Jordao JF, Aubert I, Hynynen K. Targeted delivery of neural stem cells to the brain using MRI-guided focused ultrasound to disrupt the blood-brain barrier. PLoS ONE. 2011;6(11):e27877.
112. Huang Q, Deng J, Xie Z, Wang F, Chen S, Lei B, et al. Effective gene transfer into central nervous system following ultrasound-microbubbles-induced opening of the blood-brain barrier. Ultrasound Med Biol. 2012;38(7):1234–43.
113. Wang S, Olumolade OO, Sun T, Samiotaki G, Konofagou EE. Noninvasive, neuron-specific gene therapy can be facilitated by focused ultrasound and recombinant adeno-associated virus. Gene Ther. 2015;22(1):104–10.
114. Hsu PH, Wei KC, Huang CY, Wen CJ, Yen TC, Liu CL, et al. Noninvasive and targeted gene delivery into the brain using microbubble-facilitated focused ultrasound. PLoS ONE. 2013;8(2):e57682.
115. McDannold N, Arvanitis CD, Vykhodtseva N, Livingstone MS. Temporary disruption of the blood-brain barrier by use of ultrasound and microbubbles: safety and efficacy evaluation in rhesus macaques. Cancer Res. 2012;72(14):3652–63.
116. Downs ME, Buch A, Sierra C, Karakatsani ME, Teichert T, Chen S, et al. Long-term safety of repeated blood-brain barrier opening via focused ultrasound with microbubbles in non-human primates performing a cognitive task. PLoS ONE. 2015;10(5):e0125911.
117. Ting CY, Fan CH, Liu HL, Huang CY, Hsieh HY, Yen TC, et al. Concurrent blood-brain barrier opening and local drug delivery using drug-carrying microbubbles and focused ultrasound for brain glioma treatment. Biomaterials. 2012;33(2):704–12.
118. Fan CH, Ting CY, Chang YC, Wei KC, Liu HL, Yeh CK. Drug-loaded bubbles with matched focused ultrasound excitation for concurrent blood-brain barrier opening and brain-tumor drug delivery. Acta Biomater. 2015;15:89–101.
119. Fan CH, Ting CY, Liu HL, Huang CY, Hsieh HY, Yen TC, et al. Antiangiogenic-targeting drug-loaded microbubbles combined with focused ultrasound for glioma treatment. Biomaterials. 2013;34(8):2142–55.
120. Blasberg RG, Patlak C, Fenstermacher JD. Intrathecal chemotherapy: brain tissue profiles after ventriculocisternal perfusion. J Pharmacol Exp Ther. 1975;195(1):73–83.
121. Fleischhack G, Jaehde U, Bode U. Pharmacokinetics following intraventricular administration of chemotherapy in patients with neoplastic meningitis. Clin Pharmacokinet. 2005;44(1):1–31.
122. Beauchesne P. Intrathecal chemotherapy for treatment of leptomeningeal dissemination of metastatic tumours. Lancet Oncol. 2010;11(9):871–9.
123. Platini C, Long J, Walter S. Meningeal carcinomatosis from breast cancer treated with intrathecal trastuzumab. Lancet Oncol. 2006;7(9):778–80.
124. Ochiai H, Campbell SA, Archer GE, Chewning TA, Dragunsky E, Ivanov A, et al. Targeted therapy for glioblastoma multiforme neoplastic meningitis with intrathecal delivery of an oncolytic recombinant poliovirus. Clin Cancer Res. 2006;12(4):1349–54.
125. Witham TF, Fukui MB, Meltzer CC, Burns R, Kondziolka D, Bozik ME. Survival of patients with high grade glioma treated with intrathecal thiotriethylenephosphoramide for ependymal or leptomeningeal gliomatosis. Cancer. 1999;86(7):1347–53.
126. Costantino HR, Illum L, Brandt G, Johnson PH, Quay SC. Intranasal delivery: physicochemical and therapeutic aspects. Int J Pharm. 2007;337(1–2):1–24.
127. Lochhead JJ, Thorne RG. Intranasal delivery of biologics to the central nervous system. Adv Drug Deliv Rev. 2012;64(7):614–28.
128. Pardridge WM. Blood-brain barrier delivery. Drug Discov Today. 2007;12(1–2):54–61.
129. Thorne RG, Pronk GJ, Padmanabhan V, Frey WH 2nd. Delivery of insulin-like growth factor-I to the rat brain and spinal cord along olfactory and trigeminal pathways following intranasal administration. Neuroscience. 2004;127(2):481–96.

130. Lochhead JJ, Wolak DJ, Pizzo ME, Thorne RG. Rapid transport within cerebral perivascular spaces underlies widespread tracer distribution in the brain after intranasal administration. J Cereb Blood Flow Metab. 2015;35(3):371–81.
131. Hadaczek P, Yamashita Y, Mirek H, Tamas L, Bohn MC, Noble C, et al. The "perivascular pump" driven by arterial pulsation is a powerful mechanism for the distribution of therapeutic molecules within the brain. Mol Ther. 2006;14(1):69–78.
132. Alex AT, Joseph A, Shavi G, Rao JV, Udupa N. Development and evaluation of carboplatin-loaded PCL nanoparticles for intranasal delivery. Drug Deliv. 2015:1–10.
133. Shingaki T, Inoue D, Furubayashi T, Sakane T, Katsumi H, Yamamoto A, et al. Transnasal delivery of methotrexate to brain tumors in rats: a new strategy for brain tumor chemotherapy. Mol Pharm. 2010;7(5):1561–8.
134. Reitz M, Demestre M, Sedlacik J, Meissner H, Fiehler J, Kim SU, et al. Intranasal delivery of neural stem/progenitor cells: a noninvasive passage to target intracerebral glioma. Stem Cells Transl Med. 2012;1(12):866–73.
135. Balyasnikova IV, Prasol MS, Ferguson SD, Han Y, Ahmed AU, Gutova M, et al. Intranasal delivery of mesenchymal stem cells significantly extends survival of irradiated mice with experimental brain tumors. Mol Ther. 2014;22(1):140–8.
136. Hashizume R, Ozawa T, Gryaznov SM, Bollen AW, Lamborn KR, Frey WH 2nd, et al. New therapeutic approach for brain tumors: Intranasal delivery of telomerase inhibitor GRN163. Neuro Oncol. 2008;10(2):112–20.
137. Kanazawa T, Morisaki K, Suzuki S, Takashima Y. Prolongation of life in rats with malignant glioma by intranasal siRNA/drug codelivery to the brain with cell-penetrating peptide-modified micelles. Mol Pharm. 2014;11(5):1471–8.
138. Pietrowsky R, Struben C, Molle M, Fehm HL, Born J. Brain potential changes after intranasal versus intravenous administration of vasopressin: evidence for a direct nose-brain pathway for peptide effects in humans. Biol Psychiatry. 1996;39(5):332–40.
139. Derad I, Willeke K, Pietrowsky R, Born J, Fehm HL. Intranasal angiotensin II directly influences central nervous regulation of blood pressure. Am J Hypertens. 1998;11(8 Pt 1):971–7.
140. Denecke H, Meyer F, Feldkamp J, Fritzen R, Pietrowsky R. Repetitive intranasal administration of cholecystokinin potentiates its central nervous effects. Physiol Behav. 2004;83(1):39–45.
141. Kern W, Born J, Schreiber H, Fehm HL. Central nervous system effects of intranasally administered insulin during euglycemia in men. Diabetes. 1999;48(3):557–63.
142. Rilling JK, DeMarco AC, Hackett PD, Thompson R, Ditzen B, Patel R, et al. Effects of intranasal oxytocin and vasopressin on cooperative behavior and associated brain activity in men. Psychoneuroendocrinology. 2012;37(4):447–61.
143. da Fonseca CO, Schwartsmann G, Fischer J, Nagel J, Futuro D, Quirico-Santos T, et al. Preliminary results from a phase I/II study of perillyl alcohol intranasal administration in adults with recurrent malignant gliomas. Surg Neurol. 2008;70 (3):259–66; discussion 66–7.
144. Azzoli CG, Miller VA, Ng KK, Krug LM, Spriggs DR, Tong WP, et al. A phase I trial of perillyl alcohol in patients with advanced solid tumors. Cancer Chemother Pharmacol. 2003;51 (6):493–8.
145. Bailey HH, Levy D, Harris LS, Schink JC, Foss F, Beatty P, et al. A phase II trial of daily perillyl alcohol in patients with advanced ovarian cancer: Eastern Cooperative Oncology Group Study E2E96. Gynecol Oncol. 2002;85(3):464–8.
146. Langer R, Folkman J. Polymers for the sustained release of proteins and other macromolecules. Nature. 1976;263(5580):797–800.
147. Brem H, Mahaley MS Jr, Vick NA, Black KL, Schold SC Jr, Burger PC, et al. Interstitial chemotherapy with drug polymer implants for the treatment of recurrent gliomas. J Neurosurg. 1991;74(3):441–6.
148. Stewart LA. Chemotherapy in adult high-grade glioma: a systematic review and meta-analysis of individual patient data from 12 randomised trials. Lancet. 2002;359(9311):1011–8.
149. Walker MD, Alexander E Jr, Hunt WE, MacCarty CS, Mahaley MS Jr, Mealey J Jr, et al. Evaluation of BCNU and/or radiotherapy in the treatment of anaplastic gliomas. A cooperative clinical trial. J Neurosurg. 1978;49(3):333–43.
150. Brem H, Piantadosi S, Burger PC, Walker M, Selker R, Vick NA, et al. Placebo-controlled trial of safety and efficacy of intraoperative controlled delivery by biodegradable polymers of chemotherapy for recurrent gliomas. The Polymer-brain Tumor Treatment Group. Lancet. 1995;345 (8956):1008–12.
151. Brem H, Ewend MG, Piantadosi S, Greenhoot J, Burger PC, Sisti M. The safety of interstitial chemotherapy with BCNU-loaded polymer followed by radiation therapy in the treatment of newly diagnosed malignant gliomas: phase I trial. J Neurooncol. 1995;26(2):111–23.
152. Valtonen S, Timonen U, Toivanen P, Kalimo H, Kivipelto L, Heiskanen O, et al. Interstitial chemotherapy with carmustine-loaded polymers for high-grade gliomas: a randomized double-blind study. Neurosurgery. 1997;41(1):44–8; discussion 8–9.
153. Westphal M, Hilt DC, Bortey E, Delavault P, Olivares R, Warnke PC, et al. A phase 3 trial of local chemotherapy with biodegradable carmustine (BCNU) wafers (Gliadel wafers) in patients with primary malignant glioma. Neuro Oncol. 2003;5 (2):79–88.

154. Westphal M, Ram Z, Riddle V, Hilt D, Bortey E, Executive Committee of the Gliadel Study G. Gliadel wafer in initial surgery for malignant glioma: long-term follow-up of a multicenter controlled trial. Acta Neurochir (Wien). 2006;148 (3):269–75; discussion 75.
155. Stupp R, Mason WP, van den Bent MJ, Weller M, Fisher B, Taphoorn MJ, et al. Radiotherapy plus concomitant and adjuvant temozolomide for glioblastoma. N Engl J Med. 2005;352(10):987–96.
156. McGirt MJ, Than KD, Weingart JD, Chaichana KL, Attenello FJ, Olivi A, et al. Gliadel (BCNU) wafer plus concomitant temozolomide therapy after primary resection of glioblastoma multiforme. J Neurosurg. 2009;110(3):583–8.
157. Menei P, Metellus P, Parot-Schinkel E, Loiseau H, Capelle L, Jacquet G, et al. Biodegradable carmustine wafers (Gliadel) alone or in combination with chemoradiotherapy: the French experience. Ann Surg Oncol. 2010;17(7):1740–6.
158. Pan E, Mitchell SB, Tsai JS. A retrospective study of the safety of BCNU wafers with concurrent temozolomide and radiotherapy and adjuvant temozolomide for newly diagnosed glioblastoma patients. J Neurooncol. 2008;88(3):353–7.
159. Bock HC, Puchner MJ, Lohmann F, Schutze M, Koll S, Ketter R, et al. First-line treatment of malignant glioma with carmustine implants followed by concomitant radiochemotherapy: a multicenter experience. Neurosurg Rev. 2010;33(4):441–9.
160. Barr JG, Grundy PL. The effects of the NICE Technology Appraisal 121 (gliadel and temozolomide) on survival in high-grade glioma. Br J Neurosurg. 2012;26(6):818–22.
161. Pavlov V, Page P, Abi-Lahoud G, Nataf F, Dezamis E, Robin A, et al. Combining intraoperative carmustine wafers and Stupp regimen in multimodal first-line treatment of primary glioblastomas. Br J Neurosurg. 2015;29(4):524–31.
162. Noel G, Schott R, Froelich S, Gaub MP, Boyer P, Fischer-Lokou D, et al. Retrospective comparison of chemoradiotherapy followed by adjuvant chemotherapy, with or without prior gliadel implantation (carmustine) after initial surgery in patients with newly diagnosed high-grade gliomas. Int J Radiat Oncol Biol Phys. 2012;82(2):749–55.
163. Lechapt-Zalcman E, Levallet G, Dugue AE, Vital A, Diebold MD, Menei P, et al. O(6) -methylguanine-DNA methyltransferase (MGMT) promoter methylation and low MGMT-encoded protein expression as prognostic markers in glioblastoma patients treated with biodegradable carmustine wafer implants after initial surgery followed by radiotherapy with concomitant and adjuvant temozolomide. Cancer. 2012;118 (18):4545–54.
164. Duntze J, Litre CF, Eap C, Theret E, Debreuve A, Jovenin N, et al. Implanted carmustine wafers followed by concomitant radiochemotherapy to treat newly diagnosed malignant gliomas: prospective, observational, multicenter study on 92 cases. Ann Surg Oncol. 2013;20(6):2065–72.
165. Salmaggi A, Milanesi I, Silvani A, Gaviani P, Marchetti M, Fariselli L, et al. Prospective study of carmustine wafers in combination with 6-month metronomic temozolomide and radiation therapy in newly diagnosed glioblastoma: preliminary results. J Neurosurg. 2013;118(4):821–9.
166. Bregy A, Shah AH, Diaz MV, Pierce HE, Ames PL, Diaz D, et al. The role of Gliadel wafers in the treatment of high-grade gliomas. Expert Rev Anticancer Ther. 2013;13(12):1453–61.
167. Chaichana KL, Kone L, Bettegowda C, Weingart JD, Olivi A, Lim M, et al. Risk of surgical site infection in 401 consecutive patients with glioblastoma with and without carmustine wafer implantation. Neurol Res. 2015;37(8):717–26.
168. Grossman SA, Reinhard C, Colvin OM, Chasin M, Brundrett R, Tamargo RJ, et al. The intracerebral distribution of BCNU delivered by surgically implanted biodegradable polymers. J Neurosurg. 1992;76(4):640–7.
169. Fung LK, Ewend MG, Sills A, Sipos EP, Thompson R, Watts M, et al. Pharmacokinetics of interstitial delivery of carmustine, 4-hydroperoxycyclophosphamide, and paclitaxel from a biodegradable polymer implant in the monkey brain. Cancer Res. 1998;58(4):672–84.
170. Fleming AB, Saltzman WM. Pharmacokinetics of the carmustine implant. Clin Pharmacokinet. 2002;41(6):403–19.
171. Bouhadir KH, Alsberg E, Mooney DJ. Hydrogels for combination delivery of antineoplastic agents. Biomaterials. 2001;22(19):2625–33.
172. Olivi A, Ewend MG, Utsuki T, Tyler B, Domb AJ, Brat DJ, et al. Interstitial delivery of carboplatin via biodegradable polymers is effective against experimental glioma in the rat. Cancer Chemother Pharmacol. 1996;39(1–2):90–6.
173. Sun ZJ, Chen C, Sun MZ, Ai CH, Lu XL, Zheng YF, et al. The application of poly (glycerol-sebacate) as biodegradable drug carrier. Biomaterials. 2009;30(28):5209–14.
174. Dang H, Wang J, Cheng JX, Wang PY, Wang Y, Cheng LF, et al. Efficacy of local delivery of ardipusilloside I using biodegradable implants against cerebral tumor growth. Am J Cancer Res. 2015;5(1):243–54.
175. Harn HJ, Lin SZ, Lin PC, Liu CY, Liu PY, Chang LF, et al. Local interstitial delivery of z-butylidenephthalide by polymer wafers against malignant human gliomas. Neuro Oncol. 2011;13 (6):635–48.
176. Yen SY, Chen SR, Hsieh J, Li YS, Chuang SE, Chuang HM, et al. Biodegradable interstitial release polymer loading a novel small molecule targeting Axl receptor tyrosine kinase and reducing brain tumour migration and invasion. Oncogene. 2015.

177. Santini JT Jr, Richards AC, Scheidt RA, Cima MJ, Langer RS. Microchip technology in drug delivery. Ann Med. 2000;32(6):377–9.
178. Richards Grayson AC, Choi IS, Tyler BM, Wang PP, Brem H, Cima MJ, et al. Multi-pulse drug delivery from a resorbable polymeric microchip device. Nat Mater. 2003;2(11):767–72.
179. Maloney JM, Uhland SA, Polito BF, Sheppard NF Jr, Pelta CM, Santini JT Jr. Electrothermally activated microchips for implantable drug delivery and biosensing. J Control Release. 2005;109(1–3):244–55.
180. Kim GY, Tyler BM, Tupper MM, Karp JM, Langer RS, Brem H, et al. Resorbable polymer microchips releasing BCNU inhibit tumor growth in the rat 9L flank model. J Control Release. 2007;123(2):172–8.
181. Masi BC, Tyler BM, Bow H, Wicks RT, Xue Y, Brem H, et al. Intracranial MEMS based temozolomide delivery in a 9L rat gliosarcoma model. Biomaterials. 2012;33(23):5768–75.
182. Farra R, Sheppard NF, Jr., McCabe L, Neer RM, Anderson JM, Santini JT, Jr., et al. First-in-human testing of a wirelessly controlled drug delivery microchip. Sci Transl Med. 2012;4(122):122ra21.
183. Bobo RH, Laske DW, Akbasak A, Morrison PF, Dedrick RL, Oldfield EH. Convection-enhanced delivery of macromolecules in the brain. Proc Natl Acad Sci U S A. 1994;91(6):2076–80.
184. Raghavan R, Brady ML, Rodriguez-Ponce MI, Hartlep A, Pedain C, Sampson JH. Convection-enhanced delivery of therapeutics for brain disease, and its optimization. Neurosurg Focus. 2006;20(4):E12.
185. Bruce JN, Fine RL, Canoll P, Yun J, Kennedy BC, Rosenfeld SS, et al. Regression of recurrent malignant gliomas with convection-enhanced delivery of topotecan. Neurosurgery. 2011;69(6):1272–9; discussion 9–80.
186. Anderson RC, Kennedy B, Yanes CL, Garvin J, Needle M, Canoll P, et al. Convection-enhanced delivery of topotecan into diffuse intrinsic brainstem tumors in children. J Neurosurg Pediatr. 2013;11(3):289–95.
187. Barua NU, Hopkins K, Woolley M, O'Sullivan S, Harrison R, Edwards RJ, et al. A novel implantable catheter system with transcutaneous port for intermittent convection-enhanced delivery of carboplatin for recurrent glioblastoma. Drug Deliv. 2016;23(1):167–73.
188. Bogdahn U, Hau P, Stockhammer G, Venkataramana NK, Mahapatra AK, Suri A, et al. Targeted therapy for high-grade glioma with the TGF-beta2 inhibitor trabedersen: results of a randomized and controlled phase IIb study. Neuro Oncol. 2011;13(1):132–42.
189. Carpentier A, Metellus P, Ursu R, Zohar S, Lafitte F, Barrie M, et al. Intracerebral administration of CpG oligonucleotide for patients with recurrent glioblastoma: a phase II study. Neuro Oncol. 2010;12(4):401–8.
190. Voges J, Reszka R, Gossmann A, Dittmar C, Richter R, Garlip G, et al. Imaging-guided convection-enhanced delivery and gene therapy of glioblastoma. Ann Neurol. 2003;54(4):479–87.
191. Patel SJ, Shapiro WR, Laske DW, Jensen RL, Asher AL, Wessels BW, et al. Safety and feasibility of convection-enhanced delivery of Cotara for the treatment of malignant glioma: initial experience in 51 patients. Neurosurgery. 2005;56(6):1243–52; discussion 52–3.
192. Sampson JH, Akabani G, Archer GE, Berger MS, Coleman RE, Friedman AH, et al. Intracerebral infusion of an EGFR-targeted toxin in recurrent malignant brain tumors. Neuro Oncol. 2008;10(3):320–9.
193. Weber F, Asher A, Bucholz R, Berger M, Prados M, Chang S, et al. Safety, tolerability, and tumor response of IL4-Pseudomonas exotoxin (NBI-3001) in patients with recurrent malignant glioma. J Neurooncol. 2003;64(1–2):125–37.
194. Weber FW, Floeth F, Asher A, Bucholz R, Berger M, Prados M, et al. Local convection enhanced delivery of IL4-Pseudomonas exotoxin (NBI-3001) for treatment of patients with recurrent malignant glioma. Acta Neurochir Suppl. 2003;88:93–103.
195. Laske DW, Youle RJ, Oldfield EH. Tumor regression with regional distribution of the targeted toxin TF-CRM107 in patients with malignant brain tumors. Nat Med. 1997;3(12):1362–8.
196. Weaver M, Laske DW. Transferrin receptor ligand-targeted toxin conjugate (Tf-CRM107) for therapy of malignant gliomas. J Neurooncol. 2003;65(1):3–13.
197. Kunwar S, Prados MD, Chang SM, Berger MS, Lang FF, Piepmeier JM, et al. Direct intracerebral delivery of cintredekin besudotox (IL13-PE38QQR) in recurrent malignant glioma: a report by the Cintredekin Besudotox Intraparenchymal Study Group. J Clin Oncol. 2007;25(7):837–44.
198. Vogelbaum MA, Sampson JH, Kunwar S, Chang SM, Shaffrey M, Asher AL, et al. Convection-enhanced delivery of cintredekin besudotox (interleukin-13-PE38QQR) followed by radiation therapy with and without temozolomide in newly diagnosed malignant gliomas: phase 1 study of final safety results. Neurosurgery. 2007;61(5):1031–7; discussion 7–8.
199. Kunwar S, Chang S, Westphal M, Vogelbaum M, Sampson J, Barnett G, et al. Phase III randomized trial of CED of IL13-PE38QQR vs Gliadel wafers for recurrent glioblastoma. Neuro Oncol. 2010;12(8):871–81.
200. Sampson JH, Archer G, Pedain C, Wembacher-Schroder E, Westphal M, Kunwar S, et al. Poor drug distribution as a possible explanation for the results of the PRECISE trial. J Neurosurg. 2010;113(2):301–9.

201. Mueller S, Polley MY, Lee B, Kunwar S, Pedain C, Wembacher-Schroder E, et al. Effect of imaging and catheter characteristics on clinical outcome for patients in the PRECISE study. J Neurooncol. 2011;101(2):267–77.
202. Jain RK. Barriers to drug delivery in solid tumors. Sci Am. 1994;271(1):58–65.
203. Chen MY, Lonser RR, Morrison PF, Governale LS, Oldfield EH. Variables affecting convection-enhanced delivery to the striatum: a systematic examination of rate of infusion, cannula size, infusate concentration, and tissue-cannula sealing time. J Neurosurg. 1999;90(2):315–20.
204. Morrison PF, Chen MY, Chadwick RS, Lonser RR, Oldfield EH. Focal delivery during direct infusion to brain: role of flow rate, catheter diameter, and tissue mechanics. Am J Physiol. 1999;277(4 Pt 2): R1218–29.
205. Krauze MT, Saito R, Noble C, Tamas M, Bringas J, Park JW, et al. Reflux-free cannula for convection-enhanced high-speed delivery of therapeutic agents. J Neurosurg. 2005;103(5):923–9.
206. Gill T, Barua NU, Woolley M, Bienemann AS, Johnson DE, Sullivan SO, et al. In vitro and in vivo testing of a novel recessed-step catheter for reflux-free convection-enhanced drug delivery to the brain. J Neurosci Methods. 2013;219(1):1–9.
207. Oh S, Odland R, Wilson SR, Kroeger KM, Liu C, Lowenstein PR, et al. Improved distribution of small molecules and viral vectors in the murine brain using a hollow fiber catheter. J Neurosurg. 2007;107(3):568–77.
208. Olson JJ, Zhang Z, Dillehay D, Stubbs J. Assessment of a balloon-tipped catheter modified for intracerebral convection-enhanced delivery. J Neurooncol. 2008;89(2):159–68.
209. Raghavan R, Brady M. Predictive models for pressure-driven fluid infusions into brain parenchyma. Phys Med Biol. 2011;56(19):6179–204.
210. Linninger AA, Somayaji MR, Erickson T, Guo X, Penn RD. Computational methods for predicting drug transport in anisotropic and heterogeneous brain tissue. J Biomech. 2008;41(10):2176–87.
211. Linninger AA, Somayaji MR, Mekarski M, Zhang L. Prediction of convection-enhanced drug delivery to the human brain. J Theor Biol. 2008;250 (1):125–38.
212. Linninger AA, Somayaji MR, Zhang L, Smitha Hariharan M, Penn RD. Rigorous mathematical modeling techniques for optimal delivery of macromolecules to the brain. IEEE Trans Biomed Eng. 2008;55(9):2303–13.
213. Saito R, Bringas JR, McKnight TR, Wendland MF, Mamot C, Drummond DC, et al. Distribution of liposomes into brain and rat brain tumor models by convection-enhanced delivery monitored with magnetic resonance imaging. Cancer Res. 2004;64 (7):2572–9.
214. Sampson JH, Brady M, Raghavan R, Mehta AI, Friedman AH, Reardon DA, et al. Colocalization of gadolinium-diethylene triamine pentaacetic acid with high-molecular-weight molecules after intracerebral convection-enhanced delivery in humans. Neurosurgery. 2011;69(3):668–76.
215. Hadjipanayis CG, Machaidze R, Kaluzova M, Wang L, Schuette AJ, Chen H, et al. EGFRvIII antibody-conjugated iron oxide nanoparticles for magnetic resonance imaging-guided convection-enhanced delivery and targeted therapy of glioblastoma. Cancer Res. 2010;70(15):6303–12.
216. Neeves KB, Sawyer AJ, Foley CP, Saltzman WM, Olbricht WL. Dilation and degradation of the brain extracellular matrix enhances penetration of infused polymer nanoparticles. Brain Res. 2007;1180:121–32.
217. Kume-Kick J, Mazel T, Vorisek I, Hrabetova S, Tao L, Nicholson C. Independence of extracellular tortuosity and volume fraction during osmotic challenge in rat neocortex. J Physiol. 2002;542(Pt 2):515–27.
218. Mamot C, Nguyen JB, Pourdehnad M, Hadaczek P, Saito R, Bringas JR, et al. Extensive distribution of liposomes in rodent brains and brain tumors following convection-enhanced delivery. J Neurooncol. 2004;68(1):1–9.
219. Lewis GK Jr, Olbricht WL, Lewis GK Sr. Acoustically enhanced Evans blue dye perfusion in neurological tissues. J Acoust Soc Am. 2008;2 (1):20001–200017.
220. Lewis GK Jr, Schulz ZR, Pannullo SC, Southard TL, Olbricht WL. Ultrasound-assisted convection-enh anced delivery to the brain in vivo with a novel transducer cannula assembly: laboratory investigation. J Neurosurg. 2012;117(6):1128–40.
221. Olbricht W, Sistla M, Ghandi G, Lewis G Jr, Sarvazyan A. Time-reversal acoustics and ultrasound-assisted convection-enhanced drug delivery to the brain. J Acoust Soc Am. 2013;134 (2):1569–75.
222. Liu Y, Paliwal S, Bankiewicz KS, Bringas JR, Heart G, Mitragotri S, et al. Ultrasound-enhanced drug transport and distribution in the brain. AAPS PharmSciTech. 2010;11(3):1005–17.
223. Sonabend AM, Stuart RM, Yun J, Yanagihara T, Mohajed H, Dashnaw S, et al. Prolonged intracerebral convection-enhanced delivery of topotecan with a subcutaneously implantable infusion pump. Neuro Oncol. 2011;13(8):886–93.
224. Strasser JF, Fung LK, Eller S, Grossman SA, Saltzman WM. Distribution of 1,3-bis (2-chloroethyl)-1-nitrosourea and tracers in the rabbit brain after interstitial delivery by biodegradable polymer implants. J Pharmacol Exp Ther. 1995;275(3):1647–55.

Radiation Therapy for Malignant Gliomas: Current Options

14

Laura E.G. Warren, Marc R. Bussiére and Helen A. Shih

Introduction

Based on data from 2008 to 2012, the estimated average annual age-adjusted incidence rate of malignant primary brain tumors is 7.23 per 100,000 [1]. Malignant gliomas are the most common subtype, comprising 80% of patients with malignant primary brain tumors. These tumors are most often highly aggressive, invasive, and carry a poor prognosis. Other chapters in this book are dedicated to the epidemiology, pathology, diagnosis, and prognosis of malignant gliomas. It is worth re-emphasizing that over the past decade increasing attention has been paid to genomic analysis of malignant gliomas as patients with histologically identical tumors could have very different outcomes. In particular, three specific molecular markers have undergone extensive study: 1p/19q chromosomal codeletion, O^6-methylguanine methyltransferase (*MGMT*) promoter methylation, and mutations of isocitrate dehydrogenase (*IDH*) 1 and 2 [2–5]. Recent studies have confirmed that in particular *IDH* mutations and 1p/19q codeletion correlated better with clinical outcomes than did histologic classification. This chapter will focus on the role of radiotherapy in the management of malignant gliomas, with discussion of the impact of molecular genetic factors on treatment recommendations.

L.E.G. Warren · M.R. Bussiére · H.A. Shih (✉)
Department of Radiation Oncology, Massachusetts General Hospital, 30 Fruit Street, Boston, MA 02114-2696, USA
e-mail: hshih@mgh.harvard.edu

Glioblastoma

The standard of care for patients with glioblastoma (GBM) is maximum safe resection followed by adjuvant radiation therapy and chemotherapy. Surgical resection can alleviate mass effect, achieve cytoreduction, and provide tissue for histopathologic and molecular characterization. More extensive surgical resection is associated with improved outcomes in several retrospective analyses [6–9]. However, if gross total or subtotal resection cannot safely be performed, biopsy is necessary for diagnostic confirmation of glioblastoma unless the tumor is in an area where even if a biopsy would result in severe neurologic deficits. In addition to extent of surgical resection, younger age, lack of corticosteroid use at baseline, higher Karnofsky Performance Status (KPS), and better mental status are associated with improved outcomes [10, 11].

Adjuvant radiation therapy is an integral component of the multimodality management of GBM given its demonstrated improvement on local control and survival. The survival benefit of adjuvant fractionated adjuvant radiation therapy (RT) compared to supportive care or to single or multiagent chemotherapy for patients with glioblastoma was demonstrated in five randomized controlled trials performed in the 1970s–1980s [12–16]. With the inclusion of RT, the median survival improved 16–24 weeks

J. Moliterno Günel et al. (eds.), *Malignant Brain Tumors*,
DOI 10.1007/978-3-319-49864-5_14

Table 14.1 Early studies in malignant glioma analyzing the role for adjuvant chemotherapy, radiation therapy, or both compared to supportive care alone following surgery for patients with malignant gliomas

	No patients	Histology	Extent of resection	Median overall survival by group (months)			
				Supportive care (mo)	Chemo[a] (mo)	Radiation[b] (mo)	ChemoRT[a] (mo)
BTSG 69–01 [13] (1978)	303	90% GBM, 9% AA, 1% other HGG	5% biopsy only; otherwise varied	3.2	4.2	8.1	8.0
BTSG 72–01 [14] (1980)	467	84% GBM, 11% AA, 5% other HGG	"Definitive surgical intervention"	–	5.5	8.3	9.7 (semust.) 11.7 (BCNU)
SGSG [12] (1981)	118	Grades III and IV astrocytoma	"Large tumor resection"	5.2	–	10.8	10.8
University Hospital, Lund, Sweden [16] (1991)	171	53% Grade III, 42% Grade III–IV, 4% Grade IV	35% gross total resection	–	10.5	–	15.5

[a]Chemotherapy Regimen: BTSG 69-01: BCNU; BTSG 72-01: Semustine for chemo alone group and BCNU or semustine for chemoRT groups; SGSG: Bleomycin; Swedish: Procarbazine, Vincristine, Lomustine (CCNU)
[b]RT Regimen: BTSG 69-01 and BTSG 72-01: 50-60 Gy to the whole brain; SGSG: 45 Gy to supratentorial brain; Swedish: 58 Gy to ipsilateral hemisphere, 50 Gy to contralateral hemisphere

compared to supportive care or chemotherapy alone (Table 14.1). A pooled analysis of these five trials and one additional contemporary trial that failed to show a survival benefit with the addition of RT [17] demonstrated a relative risk of death of 0.81 (95% CI, 0.74–0.88, p <0.001) with the addition of RT [18]. The addition of chemotherapy to RT in the Brain Tumor Study Group (BTSG) and Scandinavian Glioblastoma Study Group (SGSG) studies did not significantly improve overall survival [12–14]. The value of chemotherapy in addition to RT was demonstrated, however, in a meta-analysis which showed a 5% increase in two-year overall survival with the addition of chemotherapy [19].

In addition to RT, adjuvant temozolomide (TMZ) has become standard of care based on a landmark study by Stupp et al. [20] demonstrating a median survival benefit of 2.5 months with the addition of TMZ concomitant with and adjuvant to RT after debulking surgery for glioblastoma. Median overall survival at two years was also improved from 10 to 26%. The benefit of TMZ is most pronounced in patients with *MGMT* promoter methylation; in this patient population, median survival improved from 15.3 months (95% CI, 13.0–20.9) to 21.7 months (95% CI, 17.4–30.4) (p = 0.007) [21]. The *MGMT* gene encodes a DNA-repair protein that removes alkyl groups from the O^6 position of guanine, an important site of DNA alkylation. Chemotherapy-induced lesions, especially O^6-methylguanine, trigger cytotoxicity and apoptosis if left unrepaired. High levels of *MGMT* activity in cancer cells can decrease the therapeutic efficacy of alkylating agents [21]. However, promoter methylation leads to silencing of this gene, which prevents DNA damage repair. TMZ improves overall survival even for those patients with unmethylated *MGMT* albeit to a much smaller degree than in patients harboring *MGMT* promoter methylation [22]. *MGMT* promoter methylation has also been shown to be an independent favorable prognostic factor. Induction TMZ was proposed for patients with newly diagnosed glioblastoma given these data demonstrating the significant benefit of TMZ. A phase II trial by Chinot et al. [23] gave patients with inoperable newly diagnosed glioblastoma TMZ in a 7-day on/7-day off regimen for 28 days for up to 4 cycles prior to delivery of conventional RT. At a median follow-up of 6 months, median progression-free and overall survival was shorter than other published reports [20]. Based on these data, the standard of care for GBM remains maximal safe surgical resection followed by adjuvant concurrent chemoradiation then adjuvant chemotherapy.

Molecular analyses may play an increasingly important role in treatment recommendations for patients with glioblastoma. This is particularly relevant given recent studies that demonstrate that gliomas can be classified based on *TERT* promoter mutations, *IDH* mutations, and 1p/19q codeletion. This classification method identifies groups with distinct ages at diagnosis, overall survival, and association with germ line variants [24]. This methodology is particularly relevant given poor histopathologic reproducibility among pathologists when classifying gliomas, particularly for tumors with oligodendroglial components [25].

Management of Malignant Glioma in the Elderly

Management of high-grade glioma, specifically glioblastoma, in the elderly and in patients with poor performance status is a specific research focus. This research is motivated by a concern that long courses of RT or combined modality therapy may not be tolerable in this patient population. Keime-Guibert et al. [26] examined patients randomized to either fractionated RT (50 Gy in 28 fractions) and supportive care or supportive care only, which consisted of treatment with corticosteroids and anticonvulsant agents, physical and psychological support, and management by a palliative care team. Patients were 70 years of age or older with a newly diagnosed anaplastic astrocytoma or glioblastoma and a KPS 70 or greater. Eighty-five patients were enrolled, and the trial was discontinued at the first interim analysis based on results demonstrating superiority of RT and supportive care when compared to supportive care alone. At a median follow-up of 21 weeks, the median survival was 29.1 weeks (95% confidence interval (CI), 25.4–34.9 weeks) with RT and supportive care compared to 16.9 weeks (95% CI, 13.4–21.4 weeks) with supportive care alone ($p = 0.002$). Importantly, the investigators also examined differences in KPS, health-related quality of life, and cognition and did not find significant differences between the two treatment arms. These results demonstrate the benefit of RT for anaplastic astrocytomas or GBM in an elderly patient population with good performance status.

Two studies examined shorter-course RT in elderly patients or those with worse performance status. One Canadian study by Roa et al. [27] randomized patients to standard (60 Gy in 30 fractions) versus hypofractionated (40 Gy in 15 fractions) RT in 100 patients equal to or older than 60 years old with histologically confirmed GBM and a KPS of 50 or greater. The investigators did not see a statistically significant difference in overall survival between the two regimens with a similar median survival of 5.1 months in the standard RT arm and 5.6 months in the hypofractionated arm ($p = 0.57$). Another prospective study by the Nordic Clinical Brain Tumour Study Group randomized patients older than age 60 to one of three regimens: six monthly cycles of TMZ, standard fractionated RT (60 Gy in 30 fractions), or hypofractioned RT (34 Gy in 10 fractions). [28] For patients ages 60–70, there was no difference in overall survival. However, for patients older than 70, treatment with either TMZ or hypofractionated RT resulted in improved overall survival when compared with standard fractionation RT. Temozolomide alone was shown to be non-inferior compared to standard fractionation RT in patients older than 65 with glioblastoma or anaplastic astrocytoma in NOA-08, a phase 3 randomized trial [29]. *MGMT* promoter methylation was independently associated with improved overall survival. Event-free survival was dependent on *MGMT* promoter methylation status; those patients with promoter methylation had improved overall survival if they were randomized to TMZ compared to RT; the inverse was also true for those without promoter methylation. These results together suggest that for elderly patients or patients with a poor performance status with newly diagnosed glioblastoma or anaplastic astrocytoma, hypofractionated radiation therapy or temozolomide alone may be considered. *MGMT* status can help guide the choice between TMZ and RT monotherapy.

Anaplastic Astrocytoma

Three histologic subtypes of WHO grade III anaplastic gliomas are described by the WHO 2007 classification system: anaplastic astrocytoma (AA), anaplastic oligodendroglioma (AO), and anaplastic oligoastrocytoma/mixed anaplastic glioma (AOA). *MGMT* promoter methylation has been identified as a prognostic marker in patients with grade III gliomas; it is unclear whether it is also a predictive factor as it is in patients with glioblastoma [30]. As astrocytic tumors tend to behave more aggressively than oligodendroglial tumors, the recommended approach to AA is maximum safe resection typically followed by adjuvant radiation therapy, with or without concurrent TMZ. This approach is extrapolated from the management of GBM. Although patients with AA were only a small proportion of the total numbers of patients, the trials from the 1970s and 1980s described above that demonstrated a survival benefit with the addition of adjuvant RT following surgery as compared to chemotherapy or supportive care alone support the use of RT in this patient population [13, 14]. Although there are no data to guide the optimal dose and/or RT schedule in treating patients with grade III gliomas, many radiation oncologists choose to use a dose of 59.4 Gy in 1.8 Gy fractions for grade III tumors in comparison to 60 Gy in 2 Gy fractions like for glioblastoma. The rationale is that the biologic dose reduction and smaller fraction size may lead to reduced late normal tissue toxicity for patients with more favorable prognoses.

The role for adjuvant chemotherapy for patients with AA is less definitive than in patients with glioblastomas. Often recommendations are made based on molecular features that suggest the tumor will behave more like a lower or higher grade tumor. Before the introduction of TMZ, procarbazine, lomustine, and vincristine (PCV) chemotherapy was most often prescribed. Recently presented results from NRG Oncology/Radiation Therapy Oncology Group (RTOG) 9813, a randomized phase III study, demonstrate similar overall survival but decreased toxicity, most related to bone marrow toxicity, when utilizing radiation therapy and TMZ as compared to radiation therapy and nitrosourea-based chemotherapy for patients with AA [31].

The recently closed CATNON trial is a randomized Phase III trial of anaplastic glioma without 1p/19q loss of heterozygosity (Clinicaltrials.gov, NCT00626990). The purpose of the trial is to study the impact of temozolomide concomitant with and adjuvant to RT in this patient population. This study will help elucidate the optimal treatment of anaplastic glioma by taking into account both histology and genotype. Until these results are available, knowledge of clinical and molecular prognostic factors and extrapolation from data from studies of higher and lower grade tumors will help guide the optimal therapy in patients with AA.

Anaplastic Oligodendroglioma

Anaplastic oligodendrogliomas and mixed anaplastic oligoastrocytomas generally have a better prognosis than AA, with a median survival of at least 3–15 years compared with 2–3 years, respectively. Based on molecular analysis, these tumors have been characterized by a greater likelihood of harboring specific molecular markers, including co-deletion of 1p/19q chromosomes, which is a favorable prognostic feature associated with improved response to treatment and better survival [32]. These tumors are also more likely to show mutations in IDH.

RTOG 9402, a phase III trial randomizing patients with pure AO or AOA to induction PCV chemotherapy plus RT versus RT alone, showed no difference in overall survival for the entire cohort. However, the median survival of those with co-deleted 1p/19q tumors treated with PCV and RT was twice as long as patients receiving RT alone (14.7 vs. 7.3 years; $p = 0.03$) [33]. European Organization for the Research and Treatment of Cancer (EORTC) 26951 similarly randomized patients with AO or AOA to RT with or without adjuvant PCV. Overall survival in the RT/PCV treatment arm was significantly longer for all patients (42.0 vs. 30.6 months) and there was a trend toward greater benefit from adjuvant PCV in the patients with a 1p/19q codeletion [34].

At most centers, similarly to anaplastic astrocytoma and glioblastoma, TMZ has replaced PCV chemotherapy secondary to reduced toxicity and ease of administration; there are no randomized trials comparing these two agents. Further complicating the sequencing of therapy is that PCV chemotherapy cannot safely be given concurrently with RT; therefore, it was given before or after RT in the published trials. Therefore, if the decision is made to extrapolate these data and use TMZ as an alternative chemotherapy, the question arises whether TMZ should be given prior to RT, following RT, or concurrent to and following RT. The optimal sequence of RT and chemotherapy remains unknown; the most common approach is RT with concurrent and adjuvant TMZ. For patients with mixed oligodendroglial and astrocytic components, often the presence or absence of the 1p/19q co-deletion and *MGMT* status are used to guide the decision on whether to include chemotherapy with RT.

Given the concerns about the neurocognitive toxicities of radiation therapy and the chemosensitivity of anaplastic oligodendrogliomas to chemotherapy, some practitioners have chosen to utilize chemotherapy alone in the post-operative adjuvant setting and utilize RT only as salvage therapy [35]. The NOA-04 trial randomized patients with grade III anaplastic gliomas to PCV chemotherapy versus RT versus TMZ following surgical resection; if unacceptable toxicity or disease progression occurred, patients who had previously received RT received chemotherapy whereas those who had only received chemotherapy received RT [30]. Patients randomized to upfront RT or chemotherapy had similar outcomes with regard to median time to treatment failure. Long-term results that were presented recently in abstract form confirm a similar efficacy of these different approaches [36]. The CODEL trial, which is sponsored by the Alliance for Clinical Trials in Oncology (Clinicaltrials.gov, NCT00887146), is currently accruing and randomizing patients to RT with concomitant and adjuvant TMZ, RT with adjuvant PCV chemotherapy, or TMZ alone for patients with 1p/19q co-deleted anaplastic glioma or low-grade glioma. Initially, RT alone was one of the randomized treatment protocols; however, based on the results from RTOG 9402 and EORTC 26951, this arm was discontinued. The results from this trial will help elucidate the optimal treatment approach for patients with 1p/19q co-deleted tumors.

Low-Grade Gliomas

Low-grade gliomas are a heterogeneous group of intracranial and spinal tumors that occur primarily in children and young adults. As defined by the WHO grading system, these tumors are grades I-II/IV. Molecular and genetic analyses are increasingly helpful in understanding the clinical behavior of these tumors. The known negative prognostic factors include age greater than 40, astrocytoma histology, persistent neurologic symptoms, new symptoms after an asymptomatic period, high Ki-67 (>3%), and crossing the midline [37, 38]. This section will only address the role for radiation therapy in adults with grade II gliomas, including astrocytomas, oligodendrogliomas, and mixed oligoastrocytomas given the breadth of management approaches to low-grade gliomas across histologies and patient populations.

The role for immediate post-operative radiation therapy in grade II gliomas is less clear than in patients with higher grade gliomas. EORTC 22845 was a phase 3 trial that randomized 311 patients to early RT (54 Gy in 1.8 Gy daily fractions), defined as a maximum of eight weeks between surgical resection and the start of RT, or

RT at the time of clinical and/or radiographic progression [39]. All patients underwent maximal debulking surgery at diagnosis. While progression-free survival was improved with early RT (55% vs. 35%, p <0.0001), median overall survival was similar across the arms (7.2 vs. 7.4 years in the early versus no early RT, p = 0.9). Importantly, early RT did not significantly increase the risk of transformation to high-grade glioma. Seizures were better controlled in the early radiotherapy group but a full quality of life analysis was not performed so the impact of RT on other measures is unknown. This trial is often used as justification to postpone RT until disease progression.

If adjuvant RT is recommended, two trials examined the impact of dose escalation on outcomes. EORTC 22844 randomized 379 patients with supratentorial low-grade glioma to either 45 Gy or 59.4 Gy of RT post-operatively. There was no significant difference in overall survival or disease-free survival between the 2 arms; however, patients in the high-dose arm reported significantly worse levels of functioning and more symptom burden following RT [40, 41]. An Intergroup trial conduced by the National Central Cancer Treatment Group (NCCTG)/ RTOG/Eastern Cooperative Oncology Group (ECOG) randomized 203 patients with low-grade glioma to either 50.4 Gy or 64.8 Gy post-operative RT [42]. Similar to EORTC 22844, this study showed no overall survival or disease-free survival benefit and increased toxicity with increased RT dose. Grade 3–5 radionecrosis was more common in the high-dose arm (5% vs. 2.5%). Taken together, the EORTC 22844, EORTC 22845, and the Intergroup trials suggest that the decision to recommend adjuvant RT should be made after review of a patient's risk factors, clinical status, and discussion with the patient about the risks and benefits. For patients with more favorable risk factors, initial observation after surgery with RT reserved for salvage therapy may be reasonable. For older patients with unresected disease or unfavorable features, immediate adjuvant therapy should be considered. In those patients in whom adjuvant radiation therapy is recommended, most radiation oncologists recommend 50.4–54 Gy in 1.8 Gy daily fractions to balance efficacy and toxicity.

With regard to the addition of chemotherapy to early RT, RTOG 9802 randomized patients with grade 2 gliomas with KPS 50 or greater and high-risk features, defined as age 40 years old or older or 18–39 with a less than gross total resection, to adjuvant RT alone versus RT followed by six cycles of PCV [43]. The first published report demonstrated that there was a trend toward improved progression-free survival patients with the addition of PCV chemotherapy (5-year progression-free survival: 63% vs. 46%, p = 0.06); 5-year overall survival was not significantly different (72% vs. 63%, p = 0.13). However, on post hoc analysis, for 2-year survivors the addition of PCV to RT did confer a survival advantage. More recent results presented in abstract form demonstrate improved median survival (13.3 vs. 7.8 years, p = 0.03) and progression-free survival (10.4 years vs. 4.0 years, p = 0.002) at a median follow-up of 11.9 years with the addition of PCV [44]. The role for chemotherapy alone was investigated in EORTC 22033, which randomized high-risk low-grade gliomas to either 12 cycles of post-operative dose-intense TMZ or RT (50.4 Gy) [45]. Preliminary results at a median follow-up of 3.8 years suggest no difference in progression-free survival between the two arms. 1p deletion was a positive prognostic factor irrespective of treatment. Patients with 1p-intact tumors showed a trend toward worse progression-free survival with TMZ alone (30 vs. 41 months, p = 0.06). Final results from this study as well as the CODEL trial discussed above will hopefully help elucidate the best initial adjuvant therapy for patients with 1p/19q co-deleted tumors.

Radiation Planning, Treatment Fields, and Dose

Quality magnetic resonance imaging (MRI) is critical to radiation treatment planning. Although computed tomography (CT) can visualize the tumor, MRI is significantly more sensitive to the extent of the tumor as well as its associated findings, including peri-tumoral edema. The most useful sequences on MRI are T1- and T2-weighed images. Glioblastomas are nearly always heterogeneously enhancing on T1-weighted images following administration of gadolinium contrast; anaplastic gliomas are more variably enhancing. T2-weighted fluid attenuation inversion recovery (FLAIR) images are the most useful series for full visualization of tumor-associated edema for high-grade gliomas. Low-grade gliomas most often are non-enhancing, thus, the FLAIR sequence is often the best sequence by which to visualize the tumor. Ideally, the extent of tumor resection and determination of residual disease should be assessed by performing a post-operative MRI within 24–48 h of surgery. By performing this study within this time period, residual tumor can be distinguished from post-surgical effects.

In the pre-CT and MRI era, whole brain irradiation was usually employed as adjuvant RT for malignant glioma. However, studies demonstrated that the majority of recurrences were within a few centimeters of the pre-surgical tumor [46, 47]. With the added impetus to reduce treatment-related toxicity of whole brain radiation therapy (WBRT), subsequent trials confirmed no benefit to whole brain irradiation compared to more focal irradiation [48]. Additionally, with the development of image-based RT planning, more localized RT was feasible. Utilization of both MRI and CT data for treatment planning is now standard of care [49]. Based on the tendency for malignant gliomas to infiltrate adjacent brain tissue, potential expansion across the midline via the corpus callosum should be considered when defining treatment volumes. The value of utilizing F-18 fluorodeoxyglucose (FDG) PET for definition of treatment volumes, particularly the boost volume, has been of recent interest. However, studies have not demonstrated improved survival with the use of FDG PET compared to historical controls [50, 51]. The value of PET for patients with glioblastoma continues to be investigated, particularly with regard to its potential role in assessing early treatment response or recurrence.

A typical RT plan involves an initial course of targeting the T2 hyperintense volume plus a 1–2 cm margin to encompass potential microscopic disease and treating this target volume to 45–50 Gy. This first course is followed by a boost to the T1 post-contrast tumor plus a 2–2.5 cm margin to a total dose of 60 Gy using 30 fractions of 2 Gy. Alternatively, the T1 enhancing and T2 hyperintense disease can be treated as a single volume with a margin to 60 Gy (see Fig. 14.1). A total dose of 60 Gy is the standard of care based on several studies that showed improved survival with dose escalation to 60 Gy [52–54].

Several other studies examined the utility of dose escalation beyond 60 Gy for glioblastoma using a variety of techniques including 3D conformal RT, [55] stereotactic radiosurgery, [56] brachytherapy, [57, 58] and particle therapy [59, 60]. However, even up to doses as high as 90 Gy, tumor recurrence often occurs in-field [59, 61] and dose escalation with brachytherapy failed to show a survival benefit in a randomized trial [57]. Radiation necrosis often proves the limiting factor preventing dose escalation to a larger volume and/or to a boost volume. Given the technical complexity of brachytherapy and the emergence of stereotactic techniques, interest in brachytherapy has declined in favor of stereotactic radiosurgery (SRS) or stereotactic radiation therapy (SRT). SRS and SRT will be discussed in more detail in the next section. Given continued poor outcomes with conventional radiation therapy and lack of efficacy of dose escalation, several other approaches have been studied, including hyperfractionation, [62, 63] without evidence of improved survival with altered fractionation. The doses for anaplastic gliomas are extrapolated from the glioblastoma trials and most often are 59.4 Gy in 1.8 Gy per fraction. An acceptable dose range for low-grade gliomas is 45–54 Gy; the most often prescribed dose is 54 Gy in 30 fractions.

The use of 3D conformal RT versus intensity-modulated RT (IMRT) is often decided upon based on tumor location. IMRT is an advanced type of radiation therapy that modulates the intensity of the radiation of each beam

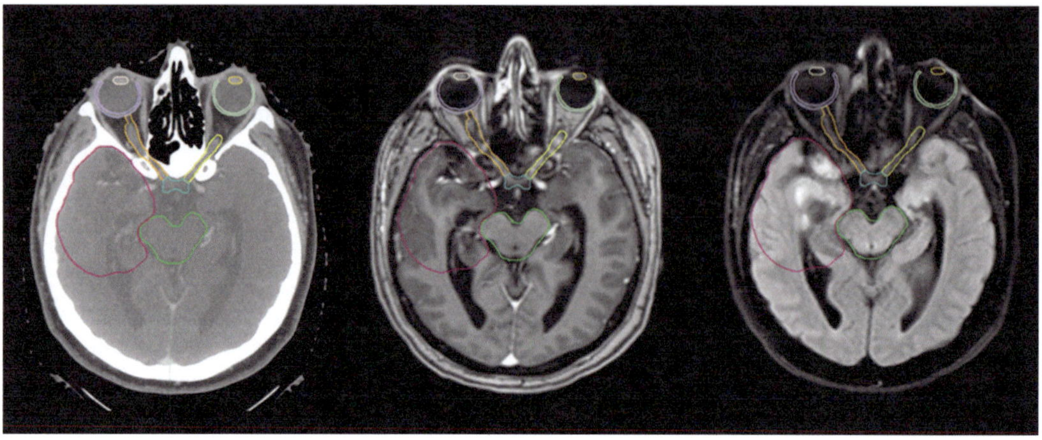

Fig. 14.1 Clinical target volume (CTV) is outlined (*pink*) on representative slices at the same level from the planning computed tomography (CT), T1-weighted post-gadolinium, and T2-weighted FLAIR magnetic resonance imaging (MRI) series, respectively, from *left* to *right*. The planning CT is fused with the pre- and post-operative MRI images to aid with contouring of the target volume and neighboring critical structures. The lenses, retinae, optic nerves, optic chiasm, and brainstem are seen on this representative slice

during treatment by utilizing computer algorithms to simultaneously optimize the tumor dose and minimize dose to normal structures. Dosimetric planning studies have shown superior target coverage and increased dose sparing to neighboring normal structures with the use of IMRT [64, 65]. IMRT is most beneficial when the tumor abuts critical radiation-sensitive structures such as the optic chiasm, optic nerves, pituitary gland, and/or brainstem. Figures 14.2 and 14.3 demonstrate the capacity of IMRT to increase the dose homogeneity and reduce the dose to critical normal structures. However, level I evidence examining clinical endpoints is lacking to support the use of IMRT over 3D conformal radiation therapy.

Role for Stereotactic Radiosurgery and Stereotactic Radiation Therapy

SRS and SRT are techniques that use an external stereotactic localization system to precisely aim at small targets typically within the cranium. Because of the combination of high precision targeting a small volume, high doses of radiation can often be safely delivered. When delivering the dose in one treatment (or up to five), the term SRS is used. When the stereotactic planning and delivery system is used with more traditional low dose per day fractionation, the term SRT is employed. SRS and SRT allow for limited dose to the adjacent normal structures by utilizing multiple radiation beams, often with arcs, accurate localization of the lesion, and reproducibility of patient positioning using more stringent immobilization techniques. Using this technique, treatment precision and accuracy are within 1–1.5 mm with either frame-based or frameless approaches, the latter made possible by more advanced real time image guidance [66–68]. In comparison to conventionally fractionated treatment, the target volume with SRS is defined by residual or recurrent T1-enhancing tumor.

Given that glioblastoma usually recurs within the original treatment field after conventional doses of RT, studies were undertaken to assess the value of dose escalation with stereotactic radiosurgery for newly diagnosed malignant gliomas. One prospective study examined the utilization of a radiosurgery boost given 2–4 weeks after conventional RT for patients with glioblastoma and anaplastic astrocytoma [69]. The median radiosurgery boost was 12 Gy

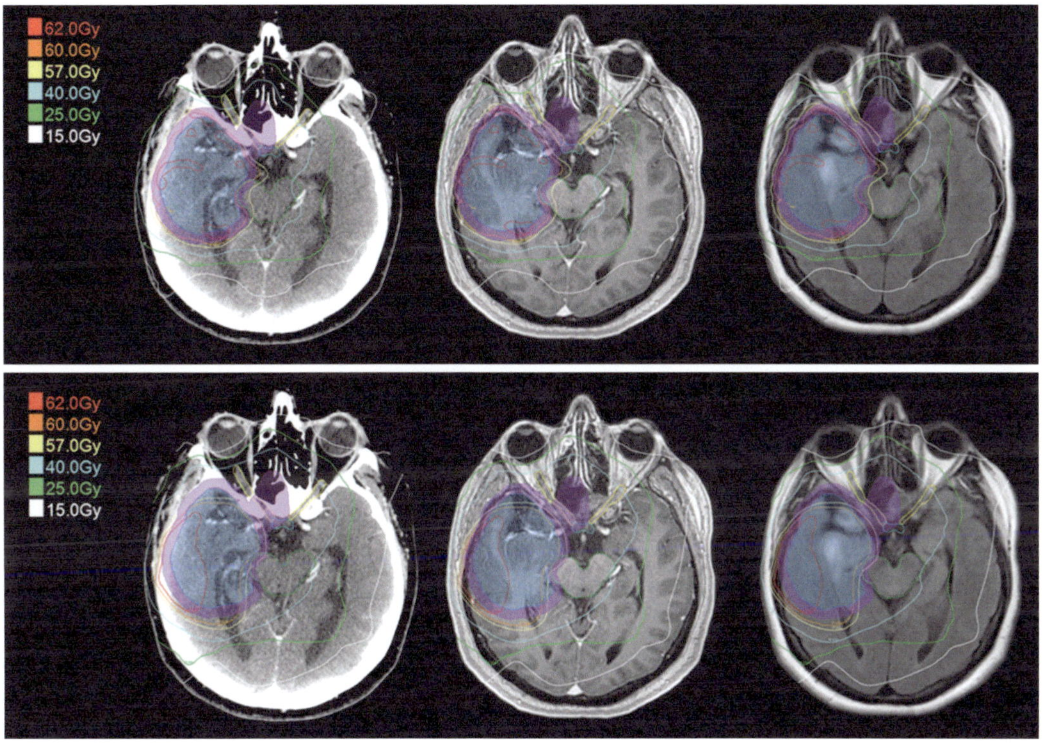

Fig. 14.2 A comparison of intensity-modulated radiation therapy (IMRT) and 3-dimensional conformal radiation therapy (3DCRT) for the same patient as in Fig. 1 with a resected glioblastoma. The *top row* is the IMRT plan as seen on the computed tomography (CT), T1-weighted post-gadolinium and T2-weighted FLAIR magnetic resonance images, respectively, from *left* to *right*. The *bottom row* is the corresponding 3DCRT plan. The clinical target volume (*blue*) was expanded by 3 mm to create the planning target volume (PTV) seen in *pink*. The PTV was prescribed 60 Gy in 30 fractions. The area receiving 62 Gy, also known as the "hot spot," is visibly larger in the 3DCRT plan

(Range: 10–25 Gy) after 59.4 Gy of conventional RT. At a median follow-up of 19 months, 76% of patients were still alive; of those who died, 67% of patients died of recurrent disease, 22% died of treatment complications, and 11% died of intercurrent disease. The authors concluded that radiosurgery was a useful adjunct to other treatment modalities. Several other prospective trials suggested a benefit with the additional of stereotactic radiosurgery when compared to historic controls [70, 71]. However, a prospective randomized trial, RTOG 9305, did not confirm a survival benefit with SRS boost delivered prior to standard external beam radiation therapy [56]. Of note, in this study there was no difference in patterns of failure between the two arms with 93% of patients failing locally, defined as recurrent or persistent tumor located within 2 cm of the enhancing edge of the post-operative lesion.

Hypofractionated stereotactic radiotherapy (hSRT) combines SRT with intermediate dose per fraction and typically a limited number of fractions. Utilization of the stereotactic approach enables reduction of normal tissue dose and hopefully corresponding toxicity. RTOG 0023 was a prospective Phase II trial examining the feasibility, toxicity, and efficacy of an integrated stereotactic boost of either 20 or 28 Gy delivered in 4 fractions as part of initial management for resected glioblastoma. No significant survival benefit was seen with this dose-intense regimen [72]. A subsequent randomized trial, EORTC 22972-26991/MRC BR10, attempted to

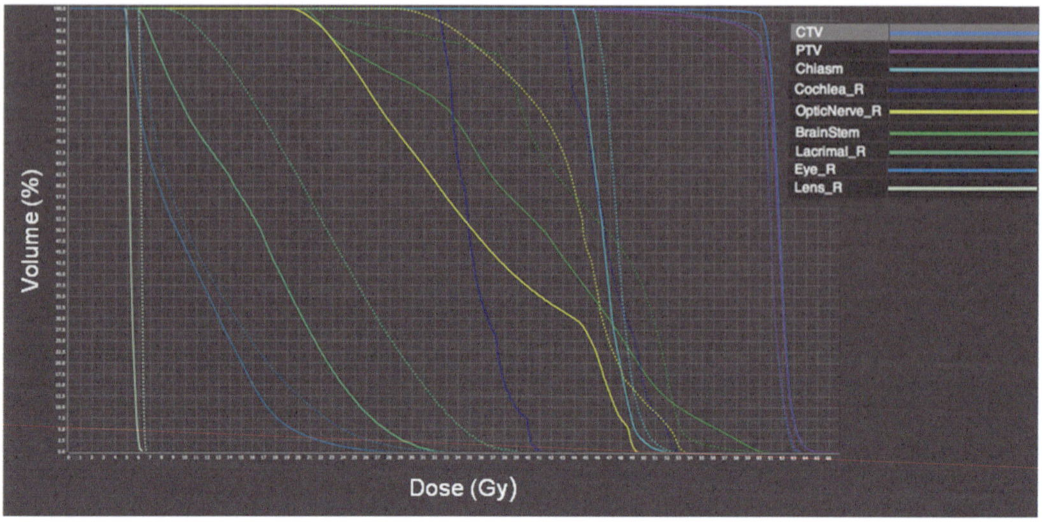

Fig. 14.3 A dose–volume histogram (DVH) allows for evaluation of the dose received by the target volumes and critical normal structures. This dose–volume histogram compares the doses delivered by an intensity-modulated radiation therapy plan (IMRT, *solid lines*) as compared to a three-dimensional conformation radiation therapy plan (3DCRT, *dashed lines*). The vertical axis represents the proportion (%) of the total volume of a structure receiving a particular dose, which is represented on the horizontal axis. Coverage of the clinical target volume (CTV), and planning target volume (PTV) is improved and doses to the critical normal structures are lower with use of IMRT

randomize patients with high-grade gliomas to conventional radiation therapy with or without fractionated stereotactic boost but was closed early due to poor accrual [73]. Published results found acute and late toxicities of the stereotactic boost to be low but no definitive conclusions regarding the value of the stereotactic boost could be reached given the small number of patients enrolled.

Toxicities of Radiation Therapy

During radiation therapy, common potential acute toxicities include fatigue, skin erythema, headache, alopecia, loss of appetite, nausea, and more rarely seizures or vomiting. Long-term effects of radiation may include ongoing fatigue, cataracts, vision loss, hearing loss, xerostomia, RT-induced leukoencephalopathy, endocrinopathies, and neurocognitive impairments. Brain necrosis secondary to RT is dose-dependent, rare but serious and may require corticosteroids or surgical intervention in the more severe symptomatic cases. The risk of radiation-associated secondary malignancy following irradiation of the central nervous system is estimated to be 1–3% twenty years following RT and generally occurring to those who received radiation delivered during childhood or young adulthood [74–76].

Radiation and Recurrent Disease

Recurrent disease can be treated with resection, re-irradiation, second-line chemotherapy, or experimental therapy on a clinical trial. Consideration of resection is dependent on the location of the recurrence and tumor volume and may be most appropriate for patients with a reasonable performance status and symptomatic disease that would benefit from a debulking surgical procedure. Re-irradiation for malignant gliomas is only feasible for a minority of patients due to concerns about normal tissue tolerance. The time interval between initial RT and re-irradiation is particularly important given the concern that treatment-related toxicities are inversely proportional to the interval between initial and re-irradiation. There are no prospective randomized trials defining the standard of care with regard to re-irradiation. Retrospective studies utilizing fractionated RT [77], SRT [78], or SRS [79] demonstrated tolerability and seeming efficacy. Several retrospective and prospective studies examined the role of brachytherapy for recurrent or progressive glioblastomas; the investigators concluded that brachytherapy both at the time of re-resection using inflatable balloon catheters [80, 81] or permanent seed implants [82] were safe and efficacious. One significant concern with re-irradiation delivered via brachytherapy in particular is radiation necrosis, which can be associated with significant morbidity and even mortality [83, 84].

With regard to systemic agents, both PCV and TMZ have activity in patients who have failed initial treatment; however, salvage chemotherapy only offers modest benefits with progression-free survival rates of 20–30% at six months. Bevacizumab is approved for relapsed disease based on phase II data showing it is well-tolerated and active given with or without irinotecan for recurrent glioblastoma [85]. Several studies have researched the potential of combining re-irradiation with systemic therapies. One study examined re-irradiation to a total dose of 36 Gy in 18 fractions with or without APG101, a CD95 ligand-binding fusion protein, for patients with recurrent glioblastoma measuring 1–4 cm in size. It demonstrated a progression-free survival rate at six months of only 3.8% with re-irradiation alone but 20.7% with combination therapy [86]. Other studies have examined the combination of bevacizumab with radiation therapy for recurrent malignant gliomas and found this combination to be safe and well-tolerated [87–89]. RTOG 12-05 is a Phase II randomized trial currently accruing that is examining bevacizumab alone versus bevacizumab with re-irradiation for patients with recurrent glioblastoma. The role for re-irradiation for recurrent anaplastic gliomas should be considered on an individual basis with particular attention paid to patient preference, performance status, time since prior therapies, and anatomic location. The prior radiation dose to critical structures, in particular the optic nerves, optic chiasm, and brainstem must be taken into account when considering a safe cumulative dose. Enrollment on clinical trials is recommended.

Conclusions and Future Directions

Unfortunately, the prognosis remains poor for patients with malignant gliomas despite robust investigation into multimodality therapies. A number of additional ongoing studies are utilizing advanced radiation modalities, vaccines, novel chemotherapies, and targeted agents to try to improve patient outcomes. Maximum safe resection with adjuvant concomitant RT and TMZ followed by TMZ remains the standard of care for patients with glioblastoma. Increasingly for patients with Grade II and Grade III gliomas molecular data is guiding management with regard to the role for RT and chemotherapy. How best to incorporate genomic data into prognostication and treatment recommendations is under investigation and will likely change standard approaches to malignant gliomas in the future.

References

1. Ostrom QT, Gittleman H, Fulop J, et al. CBTRUS statistical report: primary brain and central nervous system tumors diagnosed in the United States in 2008–2012. Neuro Oncol. 2015;17 Suppl 4:iv1–iv62.
2. Parsons DW, Jones S, Zhang X, et al. An integrated genomic analysis of human glioblastoma multiforme. Science. 2008;321:1807–12.
3. Yan H, Parsons DW, Jin G, et al. IDH1 and IDH2 mutations in gliomas. N Engl J Med. 2009;360: 765–73.
4. Smith JS, Alderete B, Minn Y, et al. Localization of common deletion regions on 1p and 19q in human gliomas and their association with histological subtype. Oncogene. 1999;18:4144–52.
5. Smith JS, Perry A, Borell TJ, et al. Alterations of chromosome arms 1p and 19q as predictors of survival in oligodendrogliomas, astrocytomas, and mixed oligoastrocytomas. J Clin Oncol. 2000;18: 636–45.
6. Grabowski MM, Recinos PF, Nowacki AS, et al. Residual tumor volume versus extent of resection: predictors of survival after surgery for glioblastoma. J Neurosurg. 2014;121:1115–23.

7. Lacroix M, Abi-Said D, Fourney DR, et al. A multivariate analysis of 416 patients with glioblastoma multiforme: prognosis, extent of resection, and survival. J Neurosurg. 2001;95:190–8.
8. Mirimanoff R-O, Gorlia T, Mason W, et al. Radiotherapy and temozolomide for newly diagnosed glioblastoma: recursive partitioning analysis of the EORTC 26981/22981-NCIC CE3 phase III randomized trial. J Clin Oncol. 2006;24:2563–9.
9. Simpson JR, Horton J, Scott C, et al. Influence of location and extent of surgical resection on survival of patients with glioblastoma multiforme: results of three consecutive Radiation Therapy Oncology Group (RTOG) clinical trials. Int J Radiat Oncol Biol Phys. 1993;26:239–44.
10. Gorlia T, van den Bent MJ, Hegi ME, et al. Nomograms for predicting survival of patients with newly diagnosed glioblastoma: prognostic factor analysis of EORTC and NCIC trial 26981-22981/CE.3. *Lancet*. Oncol. 2008;9:29–38.
11. Curran WJ, Scott CB, Horton J, et al. Recursive partitioning analysis of prognostic factors in three Radiation Therapy Oncology Group malignant glioma trials. J Natl Cancer Inst. 1993;85:704–10.
12. Kristiansen K, Hagen S, Kollevold T, et al. Combined modality therapy of operated astrocytomas grade III and IV. Confirmation of the value of postoperative irradiation and lack of potentiation of bleomycin on survival time: a prospective multicenter trial of the Scandinavian Glioblastoma Study Grou. Cancer. 1981;47:649–52.
13. Walker MD, Alexander E, Hunt WE, et al. Evaluation of BCNU and/or radiotherapy in the treatment of anaplastic gliomas. A Cooperative Clini Trial J Neurosurg. 1978;49:333–43.
14. Walker MD, Green SB, Byar DP, et al. Randomized comparisons of radiotherapy and nitrosoureas for the treatment of malignant glioma after surgery. N Engl J Med. 1980;303:1323–9.
15. Andersen AP. Postoperative irradiation of glioblastomas. Results in a randomized series. Acta Radiol Oncol Radiat Phys Biol. 1978;17:475–84.
16. Sandberg-Wollheim M, Malmström P, Strömblad LG, et al. A randomized study of chemotherapy with procarbazine, vincristine, and lomustine with and without radiation therapy for astrocytoma grades 3 and/or 4. Cancer. 1991;68:22–9.
17. Shapiro WR, Young DF. Treatment of malignant glioma. A controlled study of chemotherapy and irradiation. Arch Neurol. 1976;33:450–94.
18. Laperriere N, Zuraw L, Cairncross G. Radiotherapy for newly diagnosed malignant glioma in adults: a systematic review. Radiother Oncol. 2002;64: 259–73.
19. Stewart LA. Chemotherapy in adult high-grade glioma: a systematic review and meta-analysis of individual patient data from 12 randomised trials. Lancet (London, England). 2002;359:1011–8.
20. Stupp R, Mason WP, van den bent M, et al. Radiotherapy plus concomitant and adjuvant temozolomide for glioblastoma. N Engl J Med. 2005;352:987–996.
21. Hegi ME, Diserens A-C, Gorlia T, et al. MGMT gene silencing and benefit from temozolomide in glioblastoma. N Engl J Med. 2005;352:997–1003.
22. Hegi ME, Liu L, Herman JG, et al. Correlation of O6-methylguanine methyltransferase (MGMT) promoter methylation with clinical outcomes in glioblastoma and clinical strategies to modulate MGMT activity. J Clin Oncol. 2008;26:4189–99.
23. Chinot OL, Barrié M, Fuentes S, et al. Correlation between O6-methylguanine-DNA methyltransferase and survival in inoperable newly diagnosed glioblastoma patients treated with neoadjuvant temozolomide. J Clin Oncol. 2007;25:1470–5.
24. Eckel-Passow JE, Lachance DH, Molinaro AM, et al. Glioma groups based on 1p/19q, IDH, and TERT promoter mutations in Tumors. N Engl J Med. 2015;372:2499–508.
25. Giannini C, Scheithauer BW, Weaver AL, et al. Oligodendrogliomas: reproducibility and prognostic value of histologic diagnosis and grading. J Neuropathol Exp Neurol. 2001;60:248–62.
26. Keime-Guibert F, Chinot O, Taillandier L, et al. Radiotherapy for glioblastoma in the elderly. N Engl J Med. 2007;356:1527–35.
27. Roa W, Brasher PM a, Bauman G, et al. Abbreviated course of radiation therapy in older patients with glioblastoma multiforme: a prospective randomized clinical trial. J Clin Oncol 2004;22:1583–8.
28. Malmström A, Grønberg BH, Marosi C, et al. Temozolomide versus standard 6-week radiotherapy versus hypofractionated radiotherapy in patients older than 60 years with glioblastoma: The Nordic randomised, phase 3 trial. Lancet Oncol. 2012;13:916–26.
29. Wick W, Platten M, Meisner C, et al. Temozolomide chemotherapy alone versus radiotherapy alone for malignant astrocytoma in the elderly: the NOA-08 randomised, phase 3 trial. Lancet Oncol. 2012;13:707–15.
30. Wick W, Hartmann C, Engel C, et al. NOA-04 randomized phase III trial of sequential radiochemotherapy of anaplastic glioma with Procarbazine, Lomustine, and Vincristine or Temozolomide. J Clin Oncol. 2009;27:5874–80.
31. Chang S, Zhang P, Cairncross J, et al. Results of NRG oncology/RTOG 9813: a phase III randomized study of radiation therapy (RT) and temozolomide (TMZ) versus RT and nitrosourea (NU) therapy for anaplastic astrocytoma (AA). J Clin Oncol. 2015;33.
32. Cairncross JG, Ueki K, Zlatescu MC, et al. Specific genetic predictors of chemotherapeutic response and survival in patients with anaplastic oligodendrogliomas. J Natl Cancer Inst. 1998;90:1473–9.
33. Cairncross G, Wang M, Shaw E, et al. Phase III trial of chemoradiotherapy for anaplastic oligodendroglioma: Long-term results of RTOG 9402. J Clin Oncol. 2013;31:337–43.

34. van den Bent MJ, Brandes AA, Taphoorn MJB, et al. Adjuvant procarbazine, lomustine, and vincristine chemotherapy in newly diagnosed anaplastic oligodendroglioma: long-term follow-up of EORTC brain tumor group study 26951. J Clin Oncol. 2013;31:344–50.
35. Taliansky-Aronov A, Bokstein F, Lavon I, et al. Temozolomide treatment for newly diagnosed anaplastic oligodendrogliomas: a clinical efficacy trial. J Neurooncol. 2006;79:153–7.
36. Wick W, Roth P, Wiestler B, et al. Long-term analysis of the NOA-04 randomized phase III trial of sequential radiochemotherapy of anaplastic glioma with PCV or temozolomide. ASCO Meet Abstr. 2015;33:2001.
37. Pignatti F, van den Bent M, Curran D, et al. Prognostic factors for survival in adult patients with cerebral low-grade glioma. J Clin Oncol. 2002;20:2076–84.
38. Montine TJ, Vandersteenhoven JJ, Aguzzi A, et al. Prognostic significance of Ki-67 proliferation index in supratentorial fibrillary astrocytic neoplasms. Neurosurgery 1994;34:674–8; discussion 678–9.
39. Van Den Bent MJ, Afra D, De Witte O, et al. Long-term efficacy of early versus delayed radiotherapy for low-grade astrocytoma and oligodendroglioma in adults: the EORTC 22845 randomised trial. Lancet. 2005;366:985–90.
40. Karim ABMF, Maat B, Hatlevoll R, et al. A randomized trial on dose-response in radiation therapy of low-grade cerebral glioma: European organization for research and treatment of cancer (EORTC) study 22844. Int J Radiat Oncol Biol Phys. 1996;36: 549–56.
41. Kiebert GM, Curran D, Aaronson NK, et al. Quality of life after radiation therapy of cerebral low-grade gliomas of the adult: results of a randomised phase III trial on dose response (EORTC trial 22844). EORTC Radiotherapy Co-operative Group. Eur J Cancer. 1998;34:1902–9.
42. Shaw E, Arusell R, Scheithauer B, et al. Prospective randomized trial of low-versus high-dose radiation therapy in adults with supratentorial low-grade glioma: initial report of a North Central Cancer Treatment Group/Radiation Therapy Oncology Group/Eastern Cooperative Oncology Group Study. J Clin Oncol. 2002;20:2267–76.
43. Shaw EG, Wang M, Coons SW, et al. Randomized trial of radiation therapy plus procarbazine, lomustine, and vincristine chemotherapy for supratentorial adult low-grade glioma: Initial results of RTOG 9802. J Clin Oncol. 2012;30:3065–70.
44. Mehta MP, Won M, Shaw EG, et al. Mature Survival Data from RTOG 9802: a Phase III Study of Radiation Therapy (RT) With or Without Procarbazine, CCNU, and Vincristine (PCV) for adult patients with high-risk Low-Grade Glioma (LGG). Int J Radiat Oncol. 2014;90:S37–8.
45. Baumert B, Mason W, Ryan G, et al. Temozolomide chemotherapy versus radiotherapy in molecularly characterized (1p loss) low-grade glioma: a randomized phase III intergroup study by the EORTC/NCIC-CTG/TROG/MRC-CTU (EORTC 22033-26033). J Clin Oncol. 2013;31S:2007.
46. Massey V, Wallner KE. Patterns of second recurrence of malignant astrocytomas. Int J Radiat Oncol Biol Phys. 1990;18:395–8.
47. Wallner KE, Galicich JH, Krol G, et al. Patterns of failure following treatment for glioblastoma multiforme and anaplastic astrocytoma. Int J Radiat Oncol Biol Phys. 1989;16:1405–9.
48. Shapiro WR, Green SB, Burger PC, et al. Randomized trial of three chemotherapy regimens and two radiotherapy regimens and two radiotherapy regimens in postoperative treatment of malignant glioma. Brain Tumor Cooperative Group Trial 8001. J Neurosurg. 1989;71:1–9.
49. Thornton AF, Sandler HM, Ten Haken RK, et al. The clinical utility of magnetic resonance imaging in 3-dimensional treatment planning of brain neoplasms. Int J Radiat Oncol Biol Phys. 1992;24:767–75.
50. Gross MW, Weber WA, Feldmann HJ, et al. The value of F-18-fluorodeoxyglucose PET for the 3-D radiation treatment planning of malignant gliomas. Int J Radiat Oncol Biol Phys. 1998;41:989–95.
51. Douglas JG, Stelzer KJ, Mankoff DA, et al. [F-18]-fluorodeoxyglucose positron emission tomography for targeting radiation dose escalation for patients with glioblastoma multiforme: clinical outcomes and patterns of failure. Int J Radiat Oncol Biol Phys. 2006;64:886–91.
52. Chang CH, Horton J, Schoenfeld D, et al. Comparison of postoperative radiotherapy and combined postoperative radiotherapy and chemotherapy in the multidisciplinary management of malignant gliomas. A joint Radiation Therapy Oncology Group and Eastern Cooperative Oncology Group study. Cancer. 1983;52:997–1007.
53. Walker MD, Strike TA, Sheline GE. An analysis of dose-effect relationship in the radiotherapy of malignant gliomas. Int J Radiat Oncol Biol Phys. 1979;5:1725–31.
54. Bleehen NM, Stenning SP. A, Medical Research Council trial of two radiotherapy doses in the treatment of grades 3 and 4 astrocytoma. The Medical Research Council Brain Tumour Working Party. Br J Cancer. 1991;64:769–74.
55. Tsien C, Moughan J, Michalski JM, et al. Phase I three-dimensional conformal radiation dose escalation study in newly diagnosed glioblastoma: Radiation Therapy Oncology Group Trial 98-03. Int J Radiat Oncol Biol Phys. 2009;73:699–708.
56. Souhami L, Seiferheld W, Brachman D, et al. Randomized comparison of stereotactic radiosurgery followed by conventional radiotherapy with carmustine to conventional radiotherapy with carmustine for patients with glioblastoma multiforme: report of Radiation Therapy Oncology Group 93-05

protocol. Int J Radiat Oncol Biol Phys. 2004;60: 853–60.
57. Selker RG, Shapiro WR, Burger P, et al. The Brain Tumor Cooperative Group NIH Trial 87-01: a randomized comparison of surgery, external radiotherapy, and carmustine versus surgery, interstitial radiotherapy boost, external radiation therapy, and carmustine. Neurosurgery. 2002;51:343–55; discussion 355–7.
58. Laperriere NJ, Leung PM, McKenzie S, et al. Randomized study of brachytherapy in the initial management of patients with malignant astrocytoma. Int J Radiat Oncol Biol Phys. 1998;41:1005–11.
59. Fitzek MM, Thornton AF, Rabinov J, et al. Accelerated fractionated proton/photon irradiation to 90 cobalt gray equivalent for glioblastoma multiforme: results of a phase II prospective trial. J Neurosurg. 1999;91:251–60.
60. Mizoe J-E, Tsujii H, Hasegawa A, et al. Phase I/II clinical trial of carbon ion radiotherapy for malignant gliomas: combined X-ray radiotherapy, chemotherapy, and carbon ion radiotherapy. Int J Radiat Oncol Biol Phys. 2007;69:390–6.
61. Lee SW, Fraass BA, Marsh LH, et al. Patterns of failure following high-dose 3-D conformal radiotherapy for high-grade astrocytomas: a quantitative dosimetric study. Int J Radiat Oncol Biol Phys. 1999;43:79–88.
62. Prados MD, Wara WM, Sneed PK, et al. Phase III trial of accelerated hyperfractionation with or without difluromethylornithine (DFMO) versus standard fractionated radiotherapy with or without DFMO for newly diagnosed patients with glioblastoma multiforme. Int J Radiat Oncol Biol Phys. 2001;49:71–7.
63. Scott CB, Scarantino C, Urtasun R, et al. Validation and predictive power of Radiation Therapy Oncology Group (RTOG) recursive partitioning analysis classes for malignant glioma patients: a report using RTOG 90-06. Int J Radiat Oncol Biol Phys. 1998;40:51–5.
64. MacDonald SM, Ahmad S, Kachris S, et al. Intensity Modulated Radiation Therapy (IMRT) Versus Three Dimensional Conformal Radiation Therapy (3DCRT) for the Treatment of High Grade Glioma: A Dosimetric Comparison. J Appl Clin Med Phys. 2007;8.
65. Hermanto U, Frija EK, Lii MJ, et al. Intensity-modulated radiotherapy (IMRT) and conventional three-dimensional conformal radiotherapy for high-grade gliomas: does IMRT increase the integral dose to normal brain? Int J Radiat Oncol Biol Phys. 2007;67:1135–44.
66. Lutz W, Winston KR, Maleki N. A system for stereotactic radiosurgery with a linear accelerator. Int J Radiat Oncol Biol Phys. 1988;14:373–81.
67. Yeung D, Palta J, Fontanesi J, et al. Systematic analysis of errors in target localization and treatment delivery in stereotactic radiosurgery (SRS). Int J Radiat Oncol Biol Phys. 1994;28:493–8.
68. Chang SD, Main W, Martin DP, et al. An analysis of the accuracy of the CyberKnife: a robotic frameless stereotactic radiosurgical system. Neurosurgery. 2003;52:140–6; discussion 146–7.
69. Loeffler JS, Alexander E, Shea WM, et al. Radiosurgery as part of the initial management of patients with malignant gliomas. J Clin Oncol. 1992;10:1379–85.
70. Mehta MP, Masciopinto J, Rozental J, et al. Stereotactic radiosurgery for glioblastoma multiforme: report of a prospective study evaluating prognostic factors and analyzing long-term survival advantage. Int J Radiat Oncol Biol Phys. 1994;30:541–9.
71. Smith KA, Ashby LS, Gonzalez LF, et al. Prospective trial of gross-total resection with Gliadel wafers followed by early postoperative Gamma Knife radiosurgery and conformal fractionated radiotherapy as the initial treatment for patients with radiographically suspected, newly diagnosed glioblas. J Neurosurg. 2008;109(Suppl):106–17.
72. Cardinale R, Won M, Choucair A, et al. A phase II trial of accelerated radiotherapy using weekly stereotactic conformal boost for supratentorial glioblastoma multiforme: RTOG 0023. Int J Radiat Oncol Biol Phys. 2006;65:1422–8.
73. Baumert BG, Brada M, Bernier J, et al. EORTC 22972-26991/MRC BR10 trial: fractionated stereotactic boost following conventional radiotherapy of high grade gliomas. Clinical and quality-assurance results of the stereotactic boost arm. Radiother Oncol. 2008;88:163–72.
74. Sznajder L, Abrahams C, Parry DM, et al. Multiple schwannomas and meningiomas associated with irradiation in childhood. Arch Intern Med. 1996;156:1873–8.
75. Ron E, Modan B, Boice JD, et al. Tumors of the brain and nervous system after radiotherapy in childhood. N Engl J Med. 1988;319:1033–9.
76. Brada M, Ford D, Ashley S, et al. Risk of second brain tumour after conservative surgery and radiotherapy for pituitary adenoma. BMJ. 1992;304: 1343–6.
77. Combs SE, Thilmann C, Edler L, et al. Efficacy of fractionated stereotactic reirradiation in recurrent gliomas: long-term results in 172 patients treated in a single institution. J Clin Oncol. 2005;23:8863–9.
78. Fogh SE, Andrews DW, Glass J, et al. Hypofractionated stereotactic radiation therapy: an effective therapy for recurrent high-grade gliomas. J Clin Oncol. 2010;28:3048–53.
79. Patel M, Siddiqui F, Jin J-Y, et al. Salvage reirradiation for recurrent glioblastoma with radiosurgery: radiographic response and improved survival. J Neurooncol. 2009;92:185–91.
80. Chan TA, Weingart JD, Parisi M, et al. Treatment of recurrent glioblastoma multiforme with GliaSite brachytherapy. Int J Radiat Oncol Biol Phys. 2005;62:1133–9.
81. Tatter SB, Shaw EG, Rosenblum ML, et al. An inflatable balloon catheter and liquid 125I radiation source (GliaSite Radiation Therapy System) for treatment of recurrent malignant glioma: multicenter

safety and feasibility trial. J Neurosurg. 2003;99:297–303.
82. Larson DA, Suplica JM, Chang SM, et al. Permanent iodine 125 brachytherapy in patients with progressive or recurrent glioblastoma multiforme. Neuro. Oncol. 2004;6:119–26.
83. Scharfen CO, Sneed PK, Wara WM, et al. High activity iodine-125 interstitial implant for gliomas. Int J Radiat Oncol Biol Phys. 1992;24:583–91.
84. Chamberlain MC, Barba D, Kormanik P, et al. Concurrent cisplatin therapy and iodine 125 brachytherapy for recurrent malignant brain tumors. Arch Neurol. 1995;52:162–7.
85. Friedman HS, Prados MD, Wen PY, et al. Bevacizumab alone and in combination with irinotecan in recurrent glioblastoma. J Clin Oncol. 2009;27: 4733–40.
86. Wick W, Fricke H, Junge K, et al. A phase II, randomized, study of weekly APG101 + reirradiation versus reirradiation in progressive glioblastoma. Clin Cancer Res. 2014;20:6304–13.
87. Gutin PH, Iwamoto FM, Beal K, et al. Safety and efficacy of bevacizumab with hypofractionated stereotactic irradiation for recurrent malignant gliomas. Int J Radiat Oncol Biol Phys. 2009;75:156–63.
88. Niyazi M, Ganswindt U, Schwarz SB, et al. Irradiation and bevacizumab in high-grade glioma retreatment settings. Int J Radiat Oncol Biol Phys. 2012;82:67–76.
89. Hundsberger T, Brügge D, Putora PM, et al. Re-irradiation with and without bevacizumab as salvage therapy for recurrent or progressive high-grade gliomas. J Neurooncol. 2013;112:133–9.

Glioma Radiosensitizers: Exciting New Developments and Directions

15

Christopher D. Corso and Ranjit S. Bindra

Introduction

Systemic therapies are often given with radiation (RT) or other DNA damaging agents concurrently to enhance local control for solid tumors with high local recurrence rates, including malignant brain tumors such as glioblastoma (GBM). This approach capitalizes on synergistic interactions between the agents and is referred to as chemo- or radiosensitization [1]. To this end, temozolomide (TMZ) is given concurrently as a radiosensitizer as part of the current standard of care for GBM following surgical resection [2, 3]. Furthermore, approximately 50% of GBM tumors are found to have silencing of the O(6)-methylguanine-DNA methyltransferase (*MGMT*) gene via promoter hypermethylation [4]. MGMT is a key DNA repair protein that is required for the resolution of TMZ-induced DNA damage, and thus these tumors exhibit increased sensitivity to this agent.

Ionizing radiation and many chemotherapies produce double strand breaks (DSBs) which can lead to death in actively dividing cells if they cannot be repaired prior to progression of the cell cycle. Mammalian cells utilize two main pathways to repair DSBs: homologous recombination (HR) and non-homologous end joining (NHEJ). While HR utilizes homologous DNA sequences as a repair template, NHEJ processes and re-ligates the DSB ends [5]. Emerging data suggest that DSB repair proteins are viable targets for chemo- and radiosensitization, especially for GBM. The rationale for this approach is supported by several key findings: (1) many gliomas have altered or dysregulated DNA repair activity as a result of mutations in PTEN, EGFR, and other genes [6–8], which renders them susceptible to inhibition of the remaining intact DNA repair pathways [9]; (2) actively dividing tumor cells exhibit replication stress and are susceptible to agents which disrupt genomic integrity [10–12]; and (3) DSB repair pathways are critical for the repair of DSBs induced by RT and other DNA damaging agents [5].

Here, we discuss several exciting new directions in the development of malignant glioma radiosensitizers which act via inhibition of key DSB repair pathways. In particular, we highlight ongoing translational research efforts and ongoing clinical trials related to the development of inhibitors targeting the ataxia telangiectasia mutated (ATM) and ataxia telangiectasia and Rad3 related (ATR) axes, as well as a key G2/M checkpoint protein, Wee1. Finally, we discuss a unique bench-to-bedside trial at our institution which is testing novel DSB repair inhibitor in recurrent GBM.

C.D. Corso · R.S. Bindra (✉)
Department of Therapeutic Radiology, Yale University School of Medicine, 15 York Street, Hunter 313C, New Haven, CT 06520, USA
e-mail: ranjit.bindra@yale.edu

J. Moliterno Günel et al. (eds.), *Malignant Brain Tumors*,
DOI 10.1007/978-3-319-49864-5_15

ATM and ATR as Targets for Radiosensitization

As discussed above, DSBs lead to activation of DNA damage response (DDR) pathways which are mediated, in part, by ATM and ATR as well as two downstream kinases, checkpoint kinases 1 (Chk1) and 2 (Chk2) [13]. After activation, ATM and ATR upregulate cell cycle checkpoint pathways, which induce cell cycle arrest and DNA repair. By transiently arresting or delaying the cell cycle, they provide the necessary time for the repair of a lesion prior to DNA replication and mitosis, where unrepaired lesions can lead to mitotic cell death. It is has been shown that expression of DSB repair genes is often altered in human gliomas and other cancers, leading to dependence on the remaining intact repair DDR pathways [14, 15]. Thus, ATM and ATR signaling pathways provide attractive points of intervention for inhibition of radiation-induced DNA cell cycle arrest which can potentiate the efficacy of cancer treatment and lead to radiosensitization.

Overview of the ATM-Chk2 Axis

DSBs are sensed by the heterotrimeric Mre11/Rad50/NBS1 (MRN) complex which serves as an activation platform for the DNA damage checkpoint kinase ATM [16, 17]. In undamaged cells, quiescent ATM exists as homodimers, which dissociate into active monomers upon activation [18]. Inactive ATM auto-phosphorylates at Ser1981 and subsequently phosphorylates histone variant H2AX (γH2AX) proximal to the DNA break. Phosphorylation of H2AX leads to further enhancement of ATM binding and allows the DNA damage signal to spread along the chromatin [16]. Activated ATM phosphorylates hundreds of proteins including p53, c-Abl, BRCA1, and NBS1 which further propagates the DNA damage signal into numerous cellular pathways and processes [19].

ATM coordinates DNA repair primarily via homologous recombination (HR) which is a relatively error-free method of DSB repair that uses a homologous sister chromatid as a template for repair [20]. ATM is responsible for recruitment of HR proteins such as Mre11 and CtIP (CtBP Interacting Protein) which leads to creation of 3′ single-stranded nucleotide overhangs, followed by replication protein A (RPA) and RAD51 nucleofilament formation [21, 22]. The nucleofilament mediates the homology search, strand invasion, and formation of the D-loop, leading to promotion of DNA synthesis. A full review of ATM involvement in DNA repair is beyond the scope of this work; however, a recent review provides excellent discussion on this topic [23].

An important effector of ATM signaling is checkpoint kinase 2 (Chk2), which is phosphorylated at residue Thr68 by ATM following DSB formation [24]. Once activated, Chk2 is thought to dissociate from sites of damage and disperse as a monomer throughout the nucleus to phosphorylate over 20 substrates involved in apoptosis, gene transcription, and cell cycle progression [25]. In the presence of DSBs, Chk2 arrests the cell cycle by several mechanisms including through phosphorylation and cytoplasmic-translocation of Cdc25C phosphatase [19]. In the cytoplasm, Cdc25C can no longer dephosphorylate and activate the cyclinB1/cyclin-dependent kinase 1 (Cdk1) complex, maintaining Cdk1 in an inert form and preventing progression into mitosis [26]. Chk2 also phosphorylates p53 to promote p21 accumulation and G_2/M arrest. Through similar molecular mechanisms, Chk2 activation can also lead to G_1/S arrest in the presence of DSBs.

Overview of the ATR-Chk1 Axis

In the classical model, ATM and ATR were thought to act on different types of DNA breaks: ATM was activated in response to DSBs, whereas ATR was thought to act in response to single-strand breaks (SSBs). Studies now show that in fact, ATR responds to single-stranded regions of DNA generated at stalled replications forks, but it also appears to be activated in the presence of single-strand DNA (ssDNA) generated by processing of DSBs [27]. The activation of ATR in the presence of DSBs requires both ATM and the nuclease activity of Mre11 to generate ssDNA coated with RPA that is necessary for ATR recruitment [27, 28]. ATR, like ATM, has a large number of molecular substrates. ATR appears to exert its effects on cell cycle arrest primarily through the phosphorylation of checkpoint kinase 1 (Chk1) [29]. Chk1 has an effect on S-phase progression through inhibition of Cdc25 phosphatases and regulation of cyclin-dependent kinases [30]. Chk1 also plays a role in preventing cellular progression into mitosis with unrepaired DNA damage through sequestration of Cdc25C into the cytoplasm and degradation of Cdc25A which maintains Cdk1 in its inactive state resulting in G_2/M arrest [30, 31]. Importantly, it appears that IR-induced G_2/M-phase arrest involves the cooperation of ATR and ATM, since double deletion of ATR and ATM eliminates nearly all IR-induced delay [32]. While the activation of ATM occurs essentially irrespective of the cell cycle phase, ATR is primarily activated in the S and G_2 phase, suggesting that ATR activation is regulated by ATM in a cell cycle-dependent manner [27].

Small Molecule ATM and ATR Inhibitors as Glioma Radiosensitizers

GBM is a highly radioresistant tumor that tends to recur locally despite aggressive surgery and chemo-radiation. One explanation for this nearly eventual recurrence following an initial response to treatment is that GBMs appear to exhibit upregulation of the DNA damage response. This is supported by an analysis of multiple human glioma cell lines by Bartkova and colleagues, in which constitutive activation of the DDR pathway and upregulation of the ATM-Chk2 axis was observed at increased levels in GBM when compared to lower grade gliomas [33].

Other investigators have suggested that high rates of local failure may be attributed to failure to sterilize a subpopulation of radioresistant GBM cancer stem cells (CSCs), which are cells that are capable of repopulating a GBM tumor in vivo. In one study, Bao and colleagues demonstrated that CD133-positive cancer stem cells exhibited radioresistance due to preferential activation of the DDR and an increase in DNA repair capacity when compared to CD133-negative cells [34]. This radioresistance was overcome with an inhibitor of Chk1 and Chk2, suggesting that targeting DDR pathways in CSCs could provide an important therapeutic strategy for malignant brain cancers [34].

Recently, it was demonstrated that primary GBM cells grown in stem cell conditions exhibited increased radioresistance relative to differentiated cell populations originating from the same parental tumor [9]. The stem-like cells exhibited enhanced G_2/M checkpoint activation and DSB repair following IR relative to their differentiated tumor cell counterparts. The observed radioresistance was capable of being overcome by treatment with the ATM inhibitor KU-55933, which produced potent radiosensitization of the GBM CSCs [9]. ATR and Chk1 are also expressed at high levels in GBM stem-like cells under basal conditions, which exhibit rapid Chk1 activation in response to IR [9]. Combined inhibition of PARP and ATR using olaparib and VE-821 resulted in profound radiosensitization of the GBM CSCs, which exceeded the effect of ATM inhibition alone [9].

There have been many other studies demonstrating the efficacy of ATM and ATR inhibitors in malignant glioma models both in vitro and in vivo. One group found that ATM inhibition with KU-55933 led to improved radiosensitization when compared with a DNA-PK inhibitor in glioma stem cells and led to prolonged survival for mice with intracranial xenografts [35]. The ATM inhibitor KU-60019 was also shown to cause radiosensitization of mutant p53 human glioma cells when delivered via intracranial convection-enhanced delivery [36]. ATR inhibition with VE-821 was shown to be effective in inhibiting the growth of cancer cells in 3-D spheroid models of glioblastoma [37]. These studies, among others, provide evidence that inhibition of ATM and ATR may represent an effective therapeutic strategy moving forward for targeting even the most radioresistant subpopulations of GBM.

Wee1 as a Target for Radiosensitization

Another molecule that has emerged as a key G_2/M checkpoint regulator is Wee1 kinase [38]. As discussed above, Wee1 is phosphorylated by Chk1 in response to DNA damage. Wee1 blocks entry into mitosis by catalyzing inhibitory phosphorylation of the Tyr15 residue on Cdk1. Inhibition of Cdk1 leads to inactivation of the Cdc2/cyclin B complex that leads to G_2/M cell cycle arrest [39]. This checkpoint plays a key role in repairing DNA damage prior to entry into mitosis. Inhibition of Wee1 has been shown to abrogate G_2/M arrest and propel cells into premature mitosis which can ultimately lead to cell death via mitotic catastrophe or apoptosis [40]. Inhibition of Wee1 through pyrido-pyrimidine derivatives such as PD0166285, or via siRNA knockdown has been shown to sensitize multiple cancer cell lines to radiation and other DNA damaging agents [40–42]. The sensitization effect is most pronounced in p53-deficient cells which exhibit increased reliance on the G_2/M checkpoint due to disruption of the p53 mediated G_1 checkpoint [41]. Consistent with the concept of synthetic lethality, if a cell harbors an inherent G_1/S deficiency and then undergoes induced disruption of the G_2/M checkpoint, unrepaired DNA damage will lead to enhanced cell killing.

Preclinical efficacy of the Wee1 inhibitor MK-1775 as a radiosensitizer was initially studied in p53-deficient mouse xenograft models [43]. Bridges et al. demonstrated that oral administration of MK-1775 enhanced xenograft tumor response when combined with daily fractionated radiation in mice bearing p53-null lung cancer xenografts. Others have since shown that inhibition of Wee1 is also effective in p53 wild-type tumor models, including a pediatric high-grade glioma xenograft model where MK-1775 combined with radiation was shown to confer a survival benefit when compared to radiation alone [44].

The successful preclinical studies led to clinical trial testing in humans. Recently, Do et al. published a phase I trial which examined the safety of MK-1775 monotherapy [45]. The drug exhibited a half-life of approximately 11 h and common toxicities included myelosuppression and diarrhea. Interestingly, archival tissue from five patients confirmed TP53 mutations, though no responses were observed in these patients.

There are currently two ongoing clinical trials that are studying the efficacy of Wee1 inhibitors with radiation in CNS tumors. In the ABTC1202 trial, MK-1775 is being combined with radiation and temozolomide for newly diagnosed or recurrent GBM (NCT01849146). In another ongoing Phase I trial, MK-1775 is being studied together with local radiation for pediatric patients with diffuse intrinsic pontine glioma (NCT01922076). Whether the combination of radiation and MK-1775 is effective in humans remains to be seen, since MK-1775 was recently reported to have limited blood brain barrier penetration in mouse xenograft models of GBM [46].

Drug Repurposing to Rapidly Developing Novel Radiosensitizers: A Case Study

As illustrated by the recent formation of the National Center for Advancing Translational Sciences (NCATS) program, *Discovering New Therapeutic Uses for Existing Molecules*, there is great interest in identifying new disease indications for existing drugs. This approach, referred to as "drug repurposing," is advantageous because such agents have already cleared key developmental milestones, and thus they can rapidly enter into clinical trials [47]. Our laboratory recently identified a calcium channel blocker, mibefradil dihydrochloride, as a GBM radiosensitizer in a screen for novel DNA repair inhibitors. Mibefradil was previously FDA-approved to treat hypertension, and we subsequently repurposed it as a GBM radiosensitizer in an investigator-initiated Phase I trial for recurrent GBM at our institution. Interim results from this study indicate that mibefradil can be combined safely with RT, and we have observed several promising treatment responses. The novel application of mibefradil at our institution is outlined below.

We executed a high-throughput, cell-based screen for novel DSB repair inhibitors, using a unique assay that we developed which measures NHEJ and HR in living cells. This screen identified mibefradil as a potent NHEJ repair inhibitor, and we demonstrated that it could induce substantial radiosensitization in glioma tumor cells in vitro, at levels similar to that induced by TMZ. This work was recently published [48]. Radiosensitization by mibefradil was independently confirmed by another laboratory in vivo using a rat C6 glioma model [49]. Ongoing work in our laboratory using a variety of orthogonal approaches indicates that mibefradil targets a sub-pathway of NHEJ which also repairs TMZ damage, with greatest activity in replicating cells. Collectively, these data identified mibefradil as a novel DSB repair inhibitor and a glioma radiosensitizer.

Based on our finding that mibefradil inhibits NHEJ and radiosensitizes glioma tumor cells, we recently designed a single center, open-label Phase I trial testing this drug as a radiosensitizer in recurrent GBM (NCT02202993). This is a standard 3 + 3 drug dose escalation trial with a fixed 30 Gy RT dose in 5 fractions. The hypofractionated RT scheme is based on previous re-irradiation protocols utilizing larger fraction sizes (50–52). A subset of eligible subjects are offered the option to participate in a translational research sub-study that administers mibefradil for 5 days prior to planned surgery, and a sample of resected tissue is sent for analysis of mibefradil brain tissue concentrations, using optimized protocols that we established with collaborators at the Massachusetts General Hospital (53).

Our trial opened for enrollment in August 2014 with a target accrual of 24 subjects. Preliminary results in the first 12 patients show that mibefradil can be safely combined with RT. No evidence of radionecrosis was observed, and the combination therapy was generally well tolerated in all patients. Interim results indicate a median progression-free survival (PFS) and overall survival (OS) of 5.3 and 12.8 months, respectively. These results compare favorably to historical controls, a finding which suggests an expected median PFS and OS of 1.8–2.1 and 5.8–7.7 months, respectively (54, 55). Several intriguing cases of local control were observed in our study patients, including complete responses (CRs) at the treated sites. Moreover, results from 2 translational-surgical sub-study subjects have demonstrated mibefradil brain tumor tissue concentrations up to 3.5 micromolar in contrast-enhancing tumor tissue, and up to 0.788 μM in non-enhancing tissue. These levels are well within the range of concentrations required for radiosensitization in vitro (56, 57). While this is a Phase I trial with primary safety endpoints, these data are nonetheless promising for potential efficacy.

Conclusions and Future Directions

Taken together, these data highlight the emerging promise of targeting key DSB repair pathways as a strategy for glioma radiosensitization. While only a few DSB repair targets have been discussed here, it should be noted that there a number of drugs in preclinical or clinical development which are being tested as potential glioma radiosensitizers, which either directly or indirectly target other key DSB repair proteins and pathways. Examples include the development of poly(ADP)-ribose polymerase (PARP) inhibitors and histone deacetylase inhibitors. One of the greatest concerns for radiosensitizer development is the therapeutic index, since radiosensitization of surrounding normal tissue may negate any potential gain in local control for this disease. Conventional wisdom has specified that NHEJ inhibitors, while known to induce potent radiosensitization, may inadvertently target quiescent normal tissue in the brain. However, this paradigm is now being challenged, with DNA-PK inhibitors in clinical trials as radiosensitizers for extracranial solid tumors (e.g., NCT02516813). Regardless, the HR pathway is preferentially utilized in replicating tumor cells, and inhibitors of this pathway may also represent ideal glioma radiosensitizers with a favorable therapeutic index.

References

1. Seiwert TY, Salama JK, Vokes EE. The concurrent chemoradiation paradigm–general principles. Nat Clin Pract Oncol. 2007;4(2):86–100.
2. Stupp R, Mason WP, van den Bent MJ, Weller M, Fisher B, Taphoorn MJ, et al. Radiotherapy plus concomitant and adjuvant temozolomide for glioblastoma. New Engl J Med. 2005;352(10):987–96.
3. Stupp R, Hegi ME, Mason WP, van den Bent MJ, Taphoorn MJ, Janzer RC, et al. Effects of radiotherapy with concomitant and adjuvant temozolomide versus radiotherapy alone on survival in glioblastoma in a randomised phase III study: 5-year analysis of the EORTC-NCIC trial. Lancet Oncol. 2009;10 (5):459–66.
4. Hegi ME, Diserens AC, Gorlia T, Hamou MF, de Tribolet N, Weller M, et al. MGMT gene silencing and benefit from temozolomide in glioblastoma. New Engl J Med. 2005;352(10):997–1003.
5. Ciccia A, Elledge SJ. The DNA damage response: making it safe to play with knives. Mol Cell. 2010;40 (2):179–204.
6. Bassi C, Ho J, Srikumar T, Dowling RJ, Gorrini C, Miller SJ, et al. Nuclear PTEN controls DNA repair and sensitivity to genotoxic stress. Science. 2013;341 (6144):395–9.
7. Mukherjee B, McEllin B, Camacho CV, Tomimatsu N, Sirasanagandala S, Nannepaga S, et al. EGFRvIII and DNA double-strand break repair: a molecular mechanism for radioresistance in glioblastoma. Cancer Res. 2009;69(10):4252–9.
8. Squatrito M, Holland EC. DNA damage response and growth factor signaling pathways in gliomagenesis and therapeutic resistance. Cancer Res. 2011;71 (18):5945–9.
9. Ahmed SU, Carruthers R, Gilmour L, Yildirim S, Watts C, Chalmers AJ. Selective inhibition of parallel DNA damage response pathways optimizes radiosensitization of glioblastoma stem-like cells. Cancer Res. 2015;75(20):4416–28.
10. Aziz K, Nowsheen S, Pantelias G, Iliakis G, Gorgoulis VG, Georgakilas AG. Targeting DNA damage and repair: embracing the pharmacological era for successful cancer therapy. Pharmacol Ther. 2012;133 (3):334–50.
11. Curtin NJ. DNA repair dysregulation from cancer driver to therapeutic target. Nat Rev Cancer. 2012;12 (12):801–17.
12. Huhn D, Bolck HA, Sartori AA. Targeting DNA double-strand break signalling and repair: recent advances in cancer therapy. Swiss Med Wkly. 2013;143.
13. Awasthi P, Foiani M, Kumar A. ATM and ATR signaling at a glance. J Cell Sci. 2015;128(23):4255–62.
14. Srivastava M, Raghavan SC. DNA double-strand break repair inhibitors as cancer therapeutics. Chem Biol. 2015;22(1):17–29.
15. Squatrito M, Brennan CW, Helmy K, Huse JT, Petrini JH, Holland EC. Loss of ATM/Chk2/p53 pathway components accelerates tumor development and contributes to radiation resistance in gliomas. Cancer Cell. 2010;18(6):619–29.
16. Matt S, Hofmann TG. The DNA damage-induced cell death response: a roadmap to kill cancer cells. Cell Mol Life Sci. 2016.
17. Lee JH, Mand MR, Deshpande RA, Kinoshita E, Yang SH, Wyman C, et al. Ataxia telangiectasia-mutated (ATM) kinase activity is regulated by ATP-driven conformational changes in the Mre11/Rad50/Nbs1 (MRN) complex. J Biol Chem. 2013;288(18):12840–51.
18. Bakkenist CJ, Kastan MB. DNA damage activates ATM through intermolecular autophosphorylation and dimer dissociation. Nature. 2003;421 (6922):499–506.
19. Matsuoka S, Ballif BA, Smogorzewska A, McDonald ER 3rd, Hurov KE, Luo J, et al. ATM and ATR substrate analysis reveals extensive protein networks responsive to DNA damage. Science. 2007;316 (5828):1160–6.
20. Kocher S, Rieckmann T, Rohaly G, Mansour WY, Dikomey E, Dornreiter I, et al. Radiation-induced double-strand breaks require ATM but not Artemis for homologous recombination during S-phase. Nucleic Acids Res. 2012;40(17):8336–47.
21. Sartori AA, Lukas C, Coates J, Mistrik M, Fu S, Bartek J, et al. Human CtIP promotes DNA end resection. Nature. 2007;450(7169):509–14.
22. Mazon G, Mimitou EP, Symington LS. SnapShot: homologous recombination in DNA double-strand break repair. Cell. 2010;142(4):646, e1.
23. Panier S, Durocher D. Push back to respond better: regulatory inhibition of the DNA double-strand break response. Nat Rev Mol Cell Biol. 2013;14(10):661–72.
24. Ahn JY, Schwarz JK, Piwnica-Worms H, Canman CE. Threonine 68 phosphorylation by ataxia telangiectasia mutated is required for efficient activation of Chk2 in response to ionizing radiation. Cancer Res. 2000;60(21):5934–6.
25. Lukas C, Falck J, Bartkova J, Bartek J, Lukas J. Distinct spatiotemporal dynamics of

mammalian checkpoint regulators induced by DNA damage. Nat Cell Biol. 2003;5(3):255–60.
26. Takizawa CG, Morgan DO. Control of mitosis by changes in the subcellular location of cyclin-B1-Cdk1 and Cdc25C. Curr Opin Cell Biol. 2000;12(6):658–65.
27. Jazayeri A, Falck J, Lukas C, Bartek J, Smith GC, Lukas J, et al. ATM- and cell cycle-dependent regulation of ATR in response to DNA double-strand breaks. Nat Cell Biol. 2006;8(1):37–45.
28. Duursma AM, Driscoll R, Elias JE, Cimprich KA. A role for the MRN complex in ATR activation via TOPBP1 recruitment. Mol Cell. 2013;50(1):116–22.
29. Liu Q, Guntuku S, Cui XS, Matsuoka S, Cortez D, Tamai K, et al. Chk1 is an essential kinase that is regulated by Atr and required for the G(2)/M DNA damage checkpoint. Genes Dev. 2000;14(12):1448–59.
30. Sanchez Y, Wong C, Thoma RS, Richman R, Wu Z, Piwnica-Worms H, et al. Conservation of the Chk1 checkpoint pathway in mammals: linkage of DNA damage to Cdk regulation through Cdc25. Science. 1997;277(5331):1497–501.
31. Peng CY, Graves PR, Thoma RS, Wu Z, Shaw AS, Piwnica-Worms H. Mitotic and G2 checkpoint control: regulation of 14-3-3 protein binding by phosphorylation of Cdc25C on serine-216. Science. 1997;277(5331):1501–5.
32. Brown EJ, Baltimore D. Essential and dispensable roles of ATR in cell cycle arrest and genome maintenance. Genes Dev. 2003;17(5):615–28.
33. Bartkova J, Hamerlik P, Stockhausen MT, Ehrmann J, Hlobilkova A, Laursen H, et al. Replication stress and oxidative damage contribute to aberrant constitutive activation of DNA damage signalling in human gliomas. Oncogene. 2010;29(36):5095–102.
34. Bao S, Wu Q, McLendon RE, Hao Y, Shi Q, Hjelmeland AB, et al. Glioma stem cells promote radioresistance by preferential activation of the DNA damage response. Nature. 2006;444(7120):756–60.
35. Lim YC, Roberts TL, Day BW, Stringer BW, Kozlov S, Fazry S, et al. Increased sensitivity to ionizing radiation by targeting the homologous recombination pathway in glioma initiating cells. Mol Oncol. 2014;8(8):1603–15.
36. Biddlestone-Thorpe L, Sajjad M, Rosenberg E, Beckta JM, Valerie NC, Tokarz M, et al. ATM kinase inhibition preferentially sensitizes p53-mutant glioma to ionizing radiation. Clin Cancer Res. 2013;19(12):3189–200.
37. Pires IM, Olcina MM, Anbalagan S, Pollard JR, Reaper PM, Charlton PA, et al. Targeting radiation-resistant hypoxic tumour cells through ATR inhibition. Br J Cancer. 2012;107(2):291–9.
38. Russell P, Nurse P. Negative regulation of mitosis by wee1+ , a gene encoding a protein kinase homolog. Cell. 1987;49(4):559–67.
39. Mueller S, Haas-Kogan DA. WEE1 kinase as a target for cancer therapy. J Clin Oncol Off J Am Soc Clin Oncol. 2015;33(30):3485–7.
40. Wang Y, Decker SJ, Sebolt-Leopold J. Knockdown of Chk1, Wee1 and Myt1 by RNA interference abrogates G2 checkpoint and induces apoptosis. Cancer Biol Ther. 2004;3(3):305–13.
41. Wang Y, Li J, Booher RN, Kraker A, Lawrence T, Leopold WR, et al. Radiosensitization of p53 mutant cells by PD0166285, a novel G(2) checkpoint abrogator. Cancer Res. 2001;61(22):8211–7.
42. Behdad A, Perry A. Central nervous system primitive neuroectodermal tumors: a clinicopathologic and genetic study of 33 cases. Brain Pathol. 2010;20(2):441–50.
43. Bridges KA, Hirai H, Buser CA, Brooks C, Liu H, Buchholz TA, et al. MK-1775, a novel Wee1 kinase inhibitor, radiosensitizes p53-defective human tumor cells. Clin Cancer Res. 2011;17(17):5638–48.
44. Mueller S, Hashizume R, Yang X, Kolkowitz I, Olow AK, Phillips J, et al. Targeting Wee1 for the treatment of pediatric high-grade gliomas. Neuro-Oncology. 2014;16(3):352–60.
45. Do K, Wilsker D, Ji J, Zlott J, Freshwater T, Kinders RJ, et al. Phase I study of single-agent AZD1775 (MK-1775), a Wee1 kinase inhibitor, in patients with refractory solid tumors. J Clin Oncol Off J Am Soc Clin Oncol. 2015;33(30):3409–15.
46. Pokorny JL, Calligaris D, Gupta SK, Iyekegbe DO Jr, Mueller D, Bakken KK, et al. The efficacy of the Wee1 inhibitor MK-1775 combined with temozolomide is limited by heterogeneous distribution across the blood-brain barrier in glioblastoma. Clin Cancer Res. 2015;21(8):1916–24.
47. Pantziarka P, Bouche G, Meheus L, Sukhatme V, Sukhatme VP. Repurposing drugs in your medicine cabinet: untapped opportunities for cancer therapy? Future oncology. 2015;11(2):181–4.
48. Goglia AG, Delsite R, Luz AN, Shahbazian D, Salem AF, Sundaram RK, et al. Identification of novel radiosensitizers in a high-throughput, cell-based screen for DSB repair inhibitors. Mol Cancer Ther. 2014.
49. Sheehan JP, Xu Z, Popp B, Kowalski L, Schlesinger D. Inhibition of glioblastoma and enhancement of survival via the use of mibefradil in conjunction with radiosurgery. J Neurosurg. 2013;118(4):830–7.
50. Omuro A, Beal K, Gutin P, Karimi S, Correa DD, Kaley TJ, et al. Phase II study of bevacizumab, temozolomide, and hypofractionated stereotactic radiotherapy for newly diagnosed glioblastoma. Clin Cancer Res Off J Am Assoc Cancer Res. 2014;20(19):5023–31.
51. Shapiro LQ, Beal K, Goenka A, Karimi S, Iwamoto FM, Yamada Y, et al. Patterns of failure after concurrent bevacizumab and hypofractionated stereotactic radiation therapy for recurrent high-grade glioma. Int J Radiat Oncol Biol Phys. 2013;85(3):636–42.
52. Fogh SE, Andrews DW, Glass J, Curran W, Glass C, Champ C, et al. Hypofractionated stereotactic radiation therapy: an effective therapy for recurrent

high-grade gliomas. J Clin Oncol Off J Am Soc Clin Oncol. 2010;28(18):3048–53.
53. Holdhoff M, Supko JG, Gallia GL, Hann CL, Bonekamp D, Ye X, et al. Intratumoral concentrations of imatinib after oral administration in patients with glioblastoma multiforme. J Neurooncol. 2010;97(2):241–5.
54. Gorlia T, Stupp R, Brandes AA, Rampling RR, Fumoleau P, Dittrich C, et al. New prognostic factors and calculators for outcome prediction in patients with recurrent glioblastoma: a pooled analysis of EORTC brain tumour group phase I and II clinical trials. Eur J Cancer. 2012;48(8):1176–84.
55. Clarke JL, Ennis MM, Yung WK, Chang SM, Wen PY, Cloughesy TF, et al. Is surgery at progression a prognostic marker for improved 6-month progression-free survival or overall survival for patients with recurrent glioblastoma? Neuro-Oncology. 2011;13(10):1118–24.
56. Goglia AG, Delsite R, Luz AN, Shahbazian D, Salem AF, Sundaram RK, et al. Identification of novel radiosensitizers in a high-throughput, cell-based screen for DSB repair inhibitors. Mol Cancer Ther. 2015;14(2):326–42.
57. Keir ST, Friedman HS, Reardon DA, Bigner DD, Gray LA. Mibefradil, a novel therapy for glioblastoma multiforme: cell cycle synchronization and interlaced therapy in a murine model. J Neurooncol. 2013;111(2):97–102.

Part IV

Tumor-Specific Approach

16 Infiltrative Glioma

Ghazaleh Tabatabai

Introduction

Infiltrative glioma includes astrocytoma, oligodendroglioma, and until recently mixed gliomas of World Health Organization (WHO) grades II and III. All these tumors have in common that they might lead to malignant progression. Even patients with the same histological diagnosis and WHO grade, however, have very different outcome showing that histological diagnosis and WHO grade do not suffice to reflect the full spectrum of heterogeneity. Recent molecular analyses that are discussed below will certainly change this. Yet, all randomized clinical trials so far enrolled patients mainly based on histological diagnoses, and molecular markers that had been discovered during the conduction of the trial were then assessed in subsequent retrospective analyses. Therefore, the first part of the chapter summarizes clinical evidence based on the clinical trials. Then, recent advancements in prognostic and predictive factors are briefly discussed regarding their impact on current clinical decision-making outside clinical trials and potential future clinical trial concepts.

G. Tabatabai (✉)
Interdisciplinary Division of Neuro-Oncology, Departments of Neurology & Stroke and Neurosurgery, Hertie Institute for Clinical Brain Research, University Hospital Tübingen, Eberhard Karls University Tübingen, Hoppe-Seyler-Strasse 3, 72076 Tübingen, Germany
e-mail: ghazaleh.tabatabai@uni-tuebingen.de

J. Moliterno Günel et al. (eds.), *Malignant Brain Tumors*,
DOI 10.1007/978-3-319-49864-5_16

Clinical Presentation, Diagnostic Workup and Unfavorable Risk Factors

Most patients present with seizures or focal neurological deficits or headaches. MRI shows intraparenchymal lesions; most of lower grade tumors do not show contrast enhancement but turn up on fluid-attenuated inversion recovery (FLAIR) or T2-weighted sequences.

Several clinical criteria had been discussed to define clinical risk factors at initial presentation. Since these criteria were mainly defined in the pre-molecular era, their limitation from today's perspective is certainly the lack of novel molecular markers (see below). In addition, the defining clinical criteria used in clinical trials so far are different; therefore, it is important to take this into account when comparing outcomes across clinical trials. For example, criteria defined by Pignatti and coauthors defined the following five criteria as unfavorable prognostic indicators in patients with low-grade glioma: (i) age >40, (ii) histology of astrocytoma, (iii) tumor maximal diameter >6 cm, (iv) tumors crossing midline structures, and (v) focal neurologic deficits/seizures. A high-risk low-grade glioma was defined by the presence of three of these five factors warranting postoperative radiation therapy (see below) [1]. These factors were validated in the NCCT86-72-51 trial by correlating the Pignatti score-derived definition of high-risk *vs* low-risk glioma with median overall survival (MOS) and MOS was 3.9 years in the high-risk group and 10.8 years in the low-risk group. Of note, completeness of resection, mini-mental status examination (MMSE) scores and deletions of 1p and 19q were evaluated in addition to the Pignatti criteria in this trial. Multivariate analyses indicated that tumor size >5 cm, histological diagnosis of astrocytoma, and MMSE score <27 were correlated with worse clinical outcome. A co-deletion of 1p and 19q was correlated with a better outcome, but it has to be taken into account that the 1p and 19q status was only available in 66/203 patients in this trial [2].

A pooled analysis of the EORTC 22844 and EORTC 22845 with subsequent validation in the RTOG 9802 and NCCTG trial showed that focal neurological deficits, astrocytoma histology, tumor size >5 cm are correlated with poor PFS and OS [3].

Neurosurgical Resection

Surgery has a dual aim of mass reduction and tissue asservation for histological and (nowadays) molecular diagnostics. Depending on neuroanatomical location and patients' comorbidity, the safety of maximal resection can be assessed. In fact, whenever possible, this should be taken into account. It might be helpful to include epilepsy surgery approaches in the planning of surgical resection of infiltrative gliomas, because symptomatic seizures might be substantially reduced with surgery alone [4]. Early maximal safe resection is attempted in many centers.

Chemotherapy: PCV and Temozolomide

A postoperative treatment with chemotherapy alone instead of radiation therapy was assessed in the EORTC 22033-26033 trial (WHO grade II tumors) and in the NOA-04 trial (anaplastic gliomas) [5]. Among the rationale for this therapeutic strategy was to defer radiation therapy because of potential radiation-induced neurotoxicity. This was not only considered relevant for patients with low-grade glioma but also for anaplastic glioma.

The chemotherapy regimen tested in comparison with radiation therapy (50.4 Gy) alone in patients with low-grade glioma with the EORTC 22033 trial was temozolomide in a dose-dense regimen (21/28, 75 mg/m^2). First data after a median follow-up of 3.75 years showed no difference in PFS (40-month PFS with TMZ alone versus 47 months in the RT group).

Current molecular subgroup analyses of the EORTC 22033 indicate that 1p deletion was a overall favorable prognostic marker. The presence of IDH1 mutation and intact 1p and 19q seemed to predict better PFS for RT. Median overall survival has not yet been reached; therefore, these results are still premature. Of note, the statistical design of this trial is not a non-inferiority design; thus, it remains to be clarified based on the mature data to which extent equal measures for PFS and OS really reflect equality of TMZ compared with RT [6].

The polychemotherapy regimen including procarbazine, lomustine/CCNU, and vincristine (PCV) was available before temozolomide, and therefore, many early clinical trials used this chemotherapy regimen.

In the NOA-04 trial, patients with anaplastic glioma received either chemotherapy or RT as postoperative treatment. The chemotherapy arm was further divided into PCV or TMZ. Apart from this, no direct comparative trials have been conducted to compare TMZ with PCV directly head to head. Patients in the NOA-04 trial with anaplastic astrocytoma (52.6%) or anaplastic oligodendroglioma (47.4%) were randomized to receive initial radiation therapy up to 54–60 Gy (Arm A) or 4 cycles of PCV (Arm B1) or 8 cycles of TMZ (Arm B2). The randomization was performed at 2:1:1 between study arms A: B1:B2. Primary endpoint was time to treatment failure; further analyses included PFS, OS, and correlation of molecular markers with clinical outcome. The first results were reported in 2009 [7], and at that time, the analysis did not demonstrate any difference in clinical efficacy measures between initial chemotherapy and radiation therapy. A long-term clinical follow-up of the intention-to-treat population and the biomarker group was presented at the *ASCO* Annual

Meeting in 2015 [8]. The long-term follow-up did not support a differential efficacy of initial TMZ or PCV versus initial RT. Most astrocytic tumors in this trial were CIMP^{neg}, and hypermethylation of *MGMT* was predictive of benefit for PFS in arms B1 and B2, i.e., PCV and TMZ. This finding had been previously suggested in a study within the biomarker cohort of the NOA-04 trial with known *MGMT* and *IDH1* status [9]. The study investigated the impact of *IDH1* mutation on the prognostic or predictive role of *MGMT* gene promoter methylation or co-deletion of 1p/19q, and PFS was used as primary clinical endpoint. All results of the NOA-04 biomarker cohort (n = 183) were validated in two independent validation cohorts, the German Glioma Network (n = 75) and the NOA-08 trial (n = 34), respectively. A predictive role of *MGMT* gene promoter methylation for a benefit from chemotherapy (but not RT) was confined to patients with *IDH1* wild-type tumors. In *IDH1*-mutated tumors, MGMT gene promoter methylation correlated with prolonged PFS in all treatment groups, i.e., chemotherapy alone or in combination with RT or RT alone, indicating a prognostic role in this setting. However, 1p/19q co-deletion did not distinguish a prognostic from a predictive role of MGMT methylation. Thus, for clinical decision-making in infiltrative glioma, a combined assessment of *IDH1* and *MGMT* status will be helpful (Fig. 16.1).

Radiation Therapy

In randomized clinical trials (Table 16.1), different doses and regimes of radiation therapy (RT) have been applied: higher dose (59.4 Gy, 64.8 Gy) or—in grade II gliomas—lower dose (45 Gy, 50.4 Gy). The randomized multicenter phase III trial EORTC 22844 [10] investigated the impact of low-dose versus high-dose radiation therapy in patients with low-grade gliomas. The primary endpoint was median overall survival. Importantly, quality of life was assessed in both arms too. There was no difference in median overall survival, but quality of life was better in the low-dose radiation group. Another trial group compared different radiation dosages: In the NCCTG/RTOG/ECOG trial, high-dose (64.8 Gy) versus low-dose RT was investigated. Median overall survival was similar, but patients in the high-dose group had significant reduction of scores in the mini-mental status examination. Both trials suggest, therefore, that low-dose RT leads to similar progression-free and overall survival with more stable quality of life and mini-mental status examinations. In WHO grade II tumors, the next arising question was whether the onset of RT after complete resection could be delayed. This question was addressed in the EORTC 22845 trial, where RT, a dosage of 54 Gy, was either administered immediately after resection or at next tumor progression. Median progression-free survival after immediate RT was 5.3 years compared with 3.4 years with delayed RT. Yet, median overall survival was not significantly different (7.4 years in immediate RT versus 7.2 years in delayed RT) [11]. A similar patient population is represented in a subgroup of the RTOG 9802 trial, i.e., patients (n = 111) under the age of 40 years and with macroscopic complete resection as verified by postoperative MRI. These patients did not receive any further therapy after resection, and 48% had progression at 5 years after resection [12].

Combining Radiation Therapy with PCV or Temozolomide

Combinations of RT with chemotherapy have been investigated in grade II and grade III glioma, and RT was either combined with PCV (usually in earlier trials) or TMZ.

The RTOG 9802 trial compared a sequential therapy of RT (54 Gy) followed by PCV (maximum 6 cycles) versus RT (54 Gy) alone in patients with low-grade glioma with clinical risk factors (defined in this trial as age >40 years or subtotal resection). Both PFS and MOS were significantly prolonged with RT → PCV, mainly in patients with histology of oligodendroglioma. The authors' conclusion was that RT followed by PCV is superior to RT alone in patients with

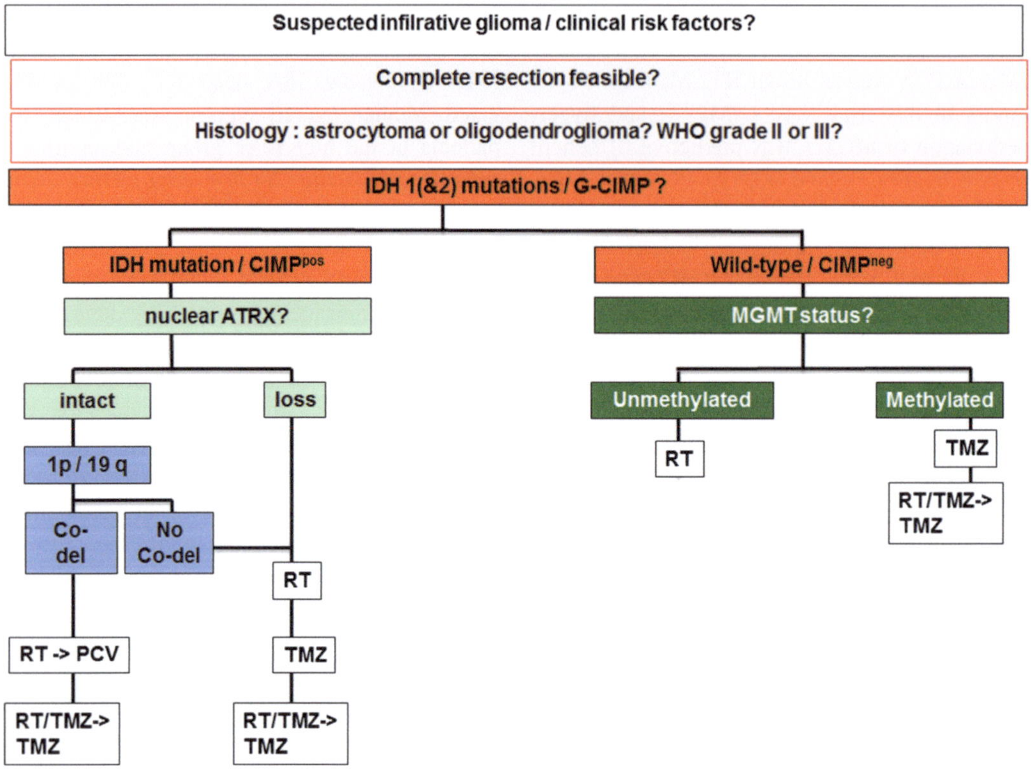

Fig. 16.1 Schematic overview of a possible clinical decision algorithm outside clinical trials for infiltrative glioma. *IDH* isocitrate dehydrogenase; *ATRX* alpha thalassemia mental retardation X-linked; *MGMT* O^6 methylguanine methyltransferase; *G-CIMP* glioma-CpG island methylator phenotype; *RT* radiation therapy; *TMZ* temozolomide; *PCV* procarbazine, lomustine/CCNU, and vincristine

low-grade glioma, age >40 or incomplete resection leading to practice change in clinical routine [13].

Progressive Disease

At progression, all three therapeutic modalities surgery, chemotherapy, or RT will in principle be reconsidered. The choice of treatment modality depends on several clinical factors including patient's wish, KPS, neuroanatomical site of progression, latency between first RT and a potential second RT, chemotherapy regimen at primary diagnosis, and treatment-related toxicities. The impact of re-resection has not been prospectively evaluated; subgroup analysis of glioblastoma trials suggests that re-resection is beneficial only if complete re-resection at progression is feasible [14]. If a postoperative watchful waiting strategy was considered and safe maximal re-resection is not feasible, RT will be evaluated. For patients who have a progression of their disease after RT → PCV, salvage chemotherapy with TMZ is considered.

Neurocognition and Quality of Life

Since many otherwise healthy young patients are often affected, and treatment regimens lead to a significant prolongation of the life span, the preservation of quality of life and neurocognitive functioning is of utmost importance.

Neurocognition at diagnosis has not been widely explored in clinical trials, but only longitudinal assessments of patients enable the detection of subtle deficits during therapy. On the

Table 16.1 Randomized clinical phase III trials in gliomas grade II and grade III

Trial	Study population	Study treatment
EORTC 22844	Low-grade glioma WHO grade II	After surgery RT 45 Gy versus 59.4 Gy
EORTC 22845	Low-grade glioma WHO grade II	After surgery RT versus watchful waiting
EORTC 22033	Low-grade glioma WHO grade II	Registration after surgery Enrollment at progression RT versus TMZ (21/28)
RTOG 9802	Low-grade glioma WHO grade II Incomplete resection	RT versus RT → PCV
NOA-04	Anaplastic glioma WHO grade III	RT versus chemotherapy (4 × PCV vs. 8 × TMZ5/28)
EORTC 26951	Anaplastic glioma WHO grade III	RT versus RT → PCV
RTOG 9402	Anaplastic glioma WHO grade III	RT/PCV versus RT
EORTC 26053	Anaplastic glioma WHO grade III No co-deletion of 1p and 19q	RT versus RT/TMZ versus RT/TMZ → 12 × TMZ RT → 12 × TMZ

RT radiation; *TMZ* temozolomide; *PCV* procarbazine; *CCNU* vincristine

other hand, it might be difficult to clearly attribute the occurrence of deficits to a certain (therapy-induced) cause. At diagnosis, for example, cognitive deficits are usually attributed to the tumor or to tumor-related seizures or depressed mood alterations resulting from the diagnosis or anticonvulsive medication. Certainly, further factors including genetic susceptibility, lifestyle, and sleeping disorders have a profound influence on cognition [15]. Consequently, any measured changes in neurocognitive deficits during therapy need to be carefully assessed.

Worsening of neurocognition can transiently occur after neurosurgical resection [16], and comparison of treatment-induced alterations in neurocognitive function in different trials might be difficult due to different test batteries in different series. Moreover, longitudinal assessments of MMSE scores do not integrate all neurocognitive modalities and are therefore rather insensitive for detecting subtle deficits. In the RTOG 9802 trial, MMSE assessments were assessed at baseline and then yearly up to 5 years. There was no difference between treatment arms [15].

Refinement of Treatment Strategies in Clinical Practice Based on Comprehensive Molecular Diagnostics?

As outlined above, most clinical phase III trials (Table 16.1) started at a timepoint before the recent advancements in molecular biomarkers. The study populations were therefore mainly based on histological diagnosis and histology-based grading of tumors. Besides the well-accepted high interobserver variability in classification and grading of glioma based on morphology alone, even clinical trials with central pathology review show different clinical courses in patients with same histological diagnoses. The longitudinal follow-up analyses of the NOA-04, the EORTC 26951, and the RTOG 9402 impressively demonstrate that molecular diagnosis is superior to histological diagnosis for defining the course of the disease and for predicting a benefit from therapy. This lesson does definitely not imply that histology is outdated and replaced by molecular diagnosis but rather demonstrates that a multilayer diagnostic workup including morphology, histology-based grading, and molecular diagnostics is a necessity (and not a luxury anymore).

The most commonly used molecular markers for further categorizing infiltrative gliomas include IDH/G-CIMP, MGMT, 1p/19q, ATRX, and TERT. A suggestion for clinical algorithm for therapy decision outside clinical trials is outlined in Fig. 16.1.

The question on the optimal treatment of anaplastic gliomas without 1p/19q co-deletion, i.e., mainly anaplastic astrocytoma (as anaplastic oligodendroglioma harbor 1p/19 q co-deletion), was addressed in the EORTC 26053 CATNON trial (Principal investigator: Martin van den Bent). In this 4-arm trial, patients were randomized to (i) RT alone, (ii) RT plus concomitant TMZ, (iii) RT followed by 12 cycles of TMZ (5/28) maintenance therapy, and (iv) RT plus concomitant TMZ followed by 12 cycles of TMZ maintenance therapy. Recruitment was finalized in July 2015.

Perspectives on Future Therapeutic Strategies in Infiltrative Glioma

Current trials investigating targeted strategies against *IDH1* mutations, e.g., the NOA-16 trial (NCT02454634) using a peptide vaccination, or trials using an *IDH1* inhibitor will lead to important insights for extending currently available postoperative treatment options like RT, TMZ, and PCV.

Clinical trials with immune checkpoint inhibitors nivolumab or pembrolizumab are currently ongoing in glioblastoma (NCT02017717, NCT02617589, NCT02667587). It might be interesting to investigate safety and efficacy of combining immune checkpoint blockade in *IDH* wild-type *MGMT*-unmethylated infiltrative glioma with RT.

Further rare actionable mutations are present, e.g., BRAF mutations or EGFRvIII calling for investigating vemurafenib or dabrafenib in BRAF-mutated infiltrative gliomas, potentially combined with MEK inhibitors (like in malignant melanomas). Therapeutic strategies targeting EGFRvIII have been investigated in several clinical trials, most recently in a peptide vaccination phase III trial in EGFRvIII-positive glioblastoma (NCT01480479).

All potential novel approaches that will be tested in clinical trials need to be thoroughly evaluated for effects on patient-reported outcome and assessments on neurocognitive functioning to ensure that an extension of progression-free or overall survival is accompanied by a preservation of quality of life and neurocognition.

References

1. Pignatti F, van den Bent M, Curran D, Debruyne C, Sylvester R, Therasse P, Afra D, Cornu P, Bolla M, Vecht C, Karim AB. European Organization for Research and Treatment of Cancer Brain Tumor Cooperative Group; European Organization for Research and Treatment of Cancer Radiotherapy Cooperative Group. Prognostic factors for survival in adult patients with cerebral low-grade glioma. J Clin Oncol. 2002;20:2076–84.
2. Daniels TB, Brown PD, Felten SJ, Wu W, Buckner JC, Arusell RM, Curran WJ, Abrams RA, Schiff D, Shaw EG. Validation of EORTC prognostic factors for adults with low-grade glioma. Int J Radiat Oncol Biol Phys. 2011;81:218–24.
3. Gorlia T, Wu W, Wang M, Baumert BG, Mehta M, Buckner JC, Shaw E, Brown P, Stupp R, Galanis E, Lacombe D, van den Bent MJ. New validated prognostic models and prognostic calculators in patients with low-grade gliomas diagnosed by central pathology review: a pooled analysis of EORTC/RTOG/NCCTG phase III clinical trials. Neuro Oncol. 2013;15:1568–79.
4. Hollon T, Hervey-Jumber SL, Sagher O, Orringer DA. Advances in the surgical management of low-grade glioma. Semin Radiat Oncol. 2015;25:181–8.
5. Wick W, Hartmann C, Engel C, Stoffels M, Felsberg J, Stockhammer F, et al. NOA-04 randomized phase III trial of sequential radiochemotherapy of anaplastic glioma with procarbazine, lomustine, and vincristine or temozolomide. J Clin Oncol. 2009;27 (35):5874–80.
6. Baumert BG, Hegi ME, Mason WP, Ryan G, Hoang-Xuan K, Bromberg JE, et al. Radiotherapy in relation to temozolomide: subgroup analysis of molecular markers of the randomized phase III study by the EORTC/NCIC-CTG/TROG/MRC-CTU (EORTC 22033–26033) in patients with a high risk low-grade glioma. J Clin Oncol. 2015;33(suppl; abstr 2006).

7. Wick W, Hartmann C, Engel C, Stoffels M, Felsberg J, Stockhammer F, et al. NOA-04 randomized phase III trial of sequential radiochemotherapy of anaplastic glioma with procarbazine, lomustine, and vincristine or temozolomide. J Clin Oncol. 2009;27(35):5874–80.
8. Wick W, Roth P, Wiestler B, Hartmann C, Hau P, Nakamura M, et al. Long-term analysis of the NOA-04 randomized phase III trial of sequential radiochemotherapy of anaplastic glioma with PCV or temozolomide. J Clin Oncol. 2015;33(suppl; abstr 2001).
9. Wick W, Meisner C, Hentschel B, Platten M, Schilling A, Wiestler B, et al. Prognostic or predictive value of MGMT promoter methylation in gliomas depends on IDH1 mutation. Neurology. 2013;81:1515–22.
10. Kiebert GM, Curran D, Aaronson NK, Bolla M, Menten J, Rutten EH, et al. Quality of life after radiation therapy of cerebral low-grade gliomas of the adult: results of a randomised phase III trial on dose response (EORTC 22844). EORTC Radiotherapy Cooperative Group. Eur J Cancer 1990. 1998;34:1902–9.
11. van den Bent MJ, Afra D, de Witte O, Ben Hassel M, Schraub S, Hoang-Xuan K, et al. EORTC radiotherapy and brain tumor groups and the uk medical research council long-term efficacy of early versus delayed radiotherapy for low-grade astrocytoma and oligodendroglioma in adults: the EORTC 22845 randomised trial. Lancet. 2005;366:985–90.
12. Shaw EG, Berkey B, Coons SW, Bullard D, Brachman D, Buckner JC, Stelzer KJ, Barger GR, Brown PD, Gilbert MR, Mehta M. Recurrence following neurosurgeon-determined gross-total resection of adult supratentorial low-grade glioma: results of a prospective clinical trial. Br J Neurosurg. 2008;109:835–41.
13. van den Bent MJ. Practice changing mature results of RTOG study 9802: another positive PCV trial makes adjuvant chemotherapy part of standard of care in low-grade glioma. Neuro Oncol. 2014;16:1570–4.
14. Suchorska B, Weller M, Tabatabai G, Senft C, Hau P, Sabel MC, et al. Complete resection of contrast-enhancing tumor volume is associated with improved survival in recurrent glioblastoma-results from the DIRECTOR trial. Neuro Oncol. 2016.
15. Prabhu RS, Won M, Shaw EG, Hu C, Brachman DG, Buckner JC, Stelzer KJ, Barger GR, Brown PD, Gilbert MR, Mehta MP. Effect of the addition of chemotherapy to radiotherapy on cognitive function in patients with low-grade glioma: secondary analysis of RTOG 98-02. J Clin Oncol. 2014;32:535–41.
16. Wu AS, Witgert ME, Lang FF, Xiao L, Bekele BN, Meyers CA, Ferson D, Wefel JS. Neurocognitive function before and after surgery for insular gliomas J Neurosurg. 2011;115(6):1115–25.

17 Tumor-Specific Approach: Oligodendroglioma (IDH1 Mutated, 1p/19q Deleted)

Charles Marc Leyrer, Erin Murphy and Manmeet Ahluwalia

Introduction

Oligodendroglioma (OD) is a histologic subtype of gliomas representing approximately ~5% of CNS gliomas. Of the 77,670 CNS tumors estimated for 2016, ODs are estimated to comprise 490 of them [1]. The majority of these tumors are World Health Organization (WHO) grade II; however, >10% are grade III disease requiring nuclear atypia, brisk mitotic activity, endothelial proliferation, and/or necrosis [2]. Oligodendrogliomas tend to develop in younger patients in the 4th to 5th decade of life and have a long natural history given their slower progression than other malignant gliomas. However, regardless of treatment, the risk of recurrence is high and ~70% will undergo anaplastic transformation in their lifetime [3]. These histologic changes are thought to occur gradually over time which can make it difficult to determine when treatment is required. The current treatment paradigm involves a combination of maximum safe resection followed by observation or further treatment with radiation therapy and/or chemotherapy.

The choice and timing of the most appropriate adjuvant therapy is currently changing to strike a balance between optimal survival and minimizing toxicities. Previously, decisions were based mostly on clinical factors; however, there is a myriad of new molecular factors that aid in our decision making [4, 5]. These factors will likely help select patients who may, or may not, require more intensive therapy [6].

Overview

Origin/History

There is very little data on the exact etiology of ODs with no significant inheritance pattern. These tumors typically arise within the cerebral hemispheres, and specifically the frontal lobe, with a higher incidence in African Americans and males in the 5th and 6th decades of life [1, 7]. These tumors are rarely associated with genetic syndromes (i.e., Lynch syndrome, Li–Fraumeni syndrome, neurofibromatosis type 1) and even rarer to be the hallmark of these syndromes [8]. Oligodendrogliomas are thought to have improved outcomes compared to other similar glial tumors, such as astrocytoma, and are increasingly identified as requiring a thoughtful treatment approach [8]. The diagnosis of ODs requires a combination of neuroimaging, histopathology, and molecular characterization.

C.M. Leyrer (✉) · E. Murphy
9500 Euclid Ave./T-28, Cleveland, OH 44195, USA
e-mail: leyrerc@ccf.org

E. Murphy
e-mail: murphye3@ccf.org

M. Ahluwalia
Mail Code S73 9500 Euclid Avenue,
Cleveland, OH, USA
e-mail: ahluwam@ccf.org

J. Moliterno Günel et al. (eds.), *Malignant Brain Tumors*,
DOI 10.1007/978-3-319-49864-5_17

Neuroimaging

Gliomas are typically initially identified on magnetic resonance imaging (MRI), usually after a symptomatic presentation. They are classically hyperintense on T2-weighted and fluid-attenuated inversion recovery (FLAIR) sequences with little mass effect or vasogenic edema [9]. Contrast enhancement on CT and MRI was initially thought to be a hallmark of high-grade disease and regarded as a sampling error if a low-grade tumor was identified. Newer evaluations are showing it is possible that contrast enhancement may be present in roughly half of low-grade ODs and was not significant for low- versus high-grade disease [10, 11]. Oligodendrogliomas with contrast enhancement have worse outcomes when compared to their non-enhancing counterparts [12–14].

Oligodendrogliomas can be distinguished from other gliomas by their tendency to present with seizures on initial diagnosis as it can be seen in over 80% of cases [15]. While gliomas tend to originate from the frontal/temporal lobes and grow along white matter tracts, the type of seizure can indicate the location of the greatest lesion load with generalized tonic–clonic seizures showing in the mesial frontal regions and partial seizures located more caudolaterally in the orbitofrontal and temporal lobes [16, 17]. Seizures were initially thought to be a favorable prognostic factor for ODs; however, this has not been replicated in larger trials by EORTC [18]. The reason is complicated by the fact that patients with seizures tend to be without neurological deficits possibly due to the location of the lesion or it could be the association with seizures and 1p/19q codeleted tumors which is one of the most significant recent advancements in molecular genetics and tumor evaluation [19].

Newer imaging techniques may aid in further determining higher risk disease. Amino acid uptake of [F-18] fluoroethyltyrosine ([17] F-FET) PET with a diffuse pattern on MRI correlated with a higher risk of transformation and death in low-grade glioma compared to a circumscribed pattern [20]. MR spectroscopy is being utilized to aid in identification of isocitrate dehydrogenase (IDH)-mutated tumors based on elevated protein levels and may be able to aid in distinguishing ODs from astrocytomas [21, 22]. While these newer imaging techniques may inform our management decisions, pathologic examination remains critical in the diagnosis.

Histology

The classification is still largely based on histopathologic features which centers on the 2007 World Health Organization classification [2]. These cells resemble oligodendroglia and are called anaplastic if they have focal or diffuse features which infer a worse prognosis. According to the WHO 2007 classification, the type of tumor must first be differentiated as astrocytic, oligodendroglial, or mixed. These tumors are then classified as grade II (low-grade), grade III (anaplastic), or grade IV (glioblastoma). Features used to make this differentiation include mitotic activity, microvascular proliferation, nuclear atypia, and necrosis [7]. Accurate diagnosis can be hampered by the fact that a biopsy alone may result in sampling error and the innate heterogeneity of gliomas [23, 24].

Oligodendroglioma cells are characteristically round and uniform with clear nuclear membranes. Occasionally seen is a clear perinuclear halo which is due to how the tumor is fixed with formalin. The perinuclear halo in combination with the round membrane appears similar to a fried egg and is classically associated with ODs. Oligodendrogliomas are usually evenly spaced in a honeycomb- or 'chicken wire'-like pattern with various branching capillaries. Calcifications are common in $\sim$20% of low-grade gliomas and can be suggestive of ODs [25].

Oligodendroglioma Versus Astrocytoma

Even with histologic characterization, it can be difficult to identify ODs as we are limited in immunohistochemical identifiers specific to ODs [26]. Glial fibrillary acidic protein (GFAP) is occasionally expressed by these cells which can aid in diagnosis; however, it has not been associated with a significant prognostic value [27]. Olig2 and neuronal intermediate filament alpha-internexin (INA) expression were thought to be helpful in distinguishing ODs given their association in development. Yet recent publications have shown they do not provide the accuracy necessary to classify ODs from its astrocytoma counterparts [28–31]. INA expression has been associated with 1p/19q codeletion along with the absence of phosphorylated cyclic-AMP responsive element binding protein (p-CREB) expression as it is associated with astrocytoma histology [30–32]. These markers will require further study to fully assess their value as they are still very early in evaluation.

Molecular Characterization

The advancement of molecular genetics has allowed for further classification of gliomas and is playing a larger role given its prognostic value. The exact clinical prognostic significance for ODs is limited as the majority of data available are from research encompassing ODs, mixed oligoastrocytomas, and astrocytomas [18, 33]. The most commonly used prognostic models are the EORTC model and RPA for low-grade gliomas developed by Bauman et al. [18, 34]. The EORTC prognostic model was based on analysis of EORTC 22844 and 22845 which identified a number of prognostic factors including age ≥40 years, tumor diameter >6 cm, tumor crossing midline, neurologic deficits at diagnosis, and astrocytoma histology. The RPA classification categorizes tumors to four different risk groups based on KPS, age at diagnosis, and presence/absence of contrast enhancement.

The association of OD and loss of heterozygosity for chromosome arms 1p and 19q was initially reported in 1994 and has since shown to have a significant prognostic significance [35, 36]. Patients with 1p/19q codeletion have significantly longer median and progression-free survival compared to their counterparts with preserved 1p and 19q. The majority of tumors showing 1p/19q codeletion are thought to be due to a single unbalanced translocation event between arms 1 and 19 at centromere (q10;p10) rather than smaller deletions [37]. This may explain why tumors require both 1p and 19q loss for a better predictive outcome rather than 1p or 19q alone [38, 39]. In further evaluation, 1p/19q codeletion has since been shown to be predictive of treatment response in large prospective randomized studies and associated with improved overall survival and improved response to PCV chemotherapy [35, 40–42].

A second major discovery was the association of IDH mutation with 1p/19q and can correlate with tumor type as IDH1 mutations are mostly found at codon 132 in astrocytic tumors and IDH2 mutations at codon 172 in oligodendroglial tumors [43]. Newer studies now believe that IDH mutations may be one of the initial events of early tumor mutations and are created prior to 1p/19q deletion. These mutations can drive gliomas toward OD subtype unlike tumor protein 53 (TP53) and alpha-thalassemia/mental retardation syndrome, X-linked (ATRX) mutations which are associated with the astrocytoma histology [44]. Both IDH1 and IDH2 are associated with improved outcomes in oligodendroglial tumors [45]. However, attempts to associate IDH-mutated astrocytomas with improved PFS and OS have not held for IDH1-mutated tumors [46, 47].

Of recent interest are two mutations which are rarely found together: telomerase reverse transcriptase (TERT) and alpha–thalassemia/mental retardation syndrome, X-linked (ATRX) [48]. ATRX is associated with telomere maintenance, and a mutation is typically associated with astrocytoma histology where IDH is mutated and 1p/19q is intact [49–51]. Recent molecular analysis of the NOA-04 clinical trial showed improved survival in anaplastic astrocytomas tumors which were ATRX mutated [49]. TERT is required to maintain telomere length, and mutations result in increased telomerase activity. It is most commonly found in high-grade disease, but it can present in oligodendrogliomas with 1p/19q codeletion. When absent in 1p/19q codeleted tumors or the mutation is present in

1p/19q non-codeleted or IDH wild-type tumors, it carries a poor prognosis which some compare to glioblastomas [52–54].

The investigation and sequencing of 1p/19q deleted tumors led to the discovery of two inactivating mutations in a homologue of Dropsophilia Capicua (CIC) on 19q and far-upstream binding protein 1 (FUBP1) on 1p [55]. Both CIC and FUBP1 are associated with tumor suppressor activity and are present in 46 and 24% of grade II/III oligodendrogliomas, respectively, but rarely in mixed oligoastrocytomas or astrocytomas [55, 56]. The impact of these mutations on prognosis is indeterminate at this time; however, they may play a role, in conjunction with ATRX, in better defining astrocytic versus oligodendroglial tumors [57].

Another factor to consider is O6-methylguanine-DNA-methyltransferase (MGMT), which is an important DNA repair enzyme which acts to prevent errors during DNA replication. In higher grade tumors, MGMT promotor methylation has been associated with improved prognosis and with increased sensitivity to alkylating chemotherapies such as temozolomide [58]. MGMT methylation is closely associated with IDH mutation status and whether it is the former or the latter that is important in prognosis is difficult to determine. It may play a larger role is in IDH wild-type tumors where patients with MGMT methylation were shown to have a more favorable prognosis [53, 59, 60].

Current Management

Our treatment approaches in the past have been based on grade of tumor and classic prognostic factors. However, with new molecular prognostic information of these tumors, the treatment approaches will likely change in near future. Historically, approach to treatment for grade III tumors was a combination of maximal safe resection followed by radiation and/or chemotherapy, which has yielded median survival times of 12–14 years in patients with WHO grade III 1p/19q codeletion [61]. Similarly, treatment approaches for grade II tumors start with maximal safe resection followed by observation or adjuvant therapies based on the classic prognostic factors. Although the outcomes may be better in WHO grade II patients, the risk of recurrence is still high [8]. Initial management is generally focused on symptom control including antiepileptic drugs for seizures, steroids for vasogenic edema, and occasionally surgical drainage or decompression if there is significant obstruction or intracranial pressure [62]. With improved imaging and prognostic factors, physicians are increasingly considering delayed treatment given the long and indolent history of these tumors with good prognostic factors once the initial symptoms are controlled. However we await randomized data to help guide treatment such as the ongoing CATNON and CODEL trials. CODEL [NCT00887146] will attempt to evaluate TMZ versus PCV concurrent with radiation and if radiation can be delayed with TMZ alone. In patients who are 1p/19q codeleted, CATNON [NCT00626990] has recently closed and is focused the role of concurrent and/or adjuvant TMZ with radiation.

Surgery

First-line management generally utilizes surgery at diagnosis as it has many additional benefits above tumor debulking as it can be utilized to improve symptom control and provide tissue which can better predict outcomes and aid in treatment management. Given the long natural history of these tumors and high risk of recurrence, even with GTR, some have considered up-front observation with the idea that this may improve a patient's quality of life without an impact on overall survival if they are followed closely [63, 64]. While this may be an option with a more carefully selected patient population, recent studies are showing improved survival in patients with earlier surgical intervention [5, 65]. A recent evaluation in Norway of two centers, one which favored biopsy and another favoring early resection of LGGs, showed improved OS in patients at the center with earlier surgical intervention. Also of concern is evidence that these tumors will continue to grow over time and can complicate future treatments given the increase in size [66]. In patients presenting with seizures, surgery is important not only as a means of symptom control, but also has been shown to impact overall survival [65].

Surgery can range anywhere from biopsy to complete resection with aggressiveness of surgery dependent on a multitude of factors including patient age/performance status, tumor involvement of eloquent brain areas, amount and feasibility of tumor reduction with aggressive surgery, and time since last intervention [67]. While there are no randomized trials evaluating extent of resection, there is increasing evidence that correlates a more aggressive surgical intervention with improved outcomes among low-grade tumors [68–71]. This is especially true in larger tumors or patients presenting with seizure as GTR can improve seizure control over STR by almost double (43–79%) [72]. When compared to GTR, patients with a STR have up to 1.4 and 4.9 times the risk of recurrence and death, respectively [68]. However, there is an inverse correlation between the increasing size of a lesion and the decrease in extent of resection [18].

The data involving extent of resection are limited in ODs as the majority of previous studies included low- and high-grade tumors or mixed oligoastrocytomas/astrocytomas. The more protracted course and increased chemosensitivity of ODs may allow for less aggressive early surgical intervention. El-Hateer et al. [19] had previously shown an OS and PFS benefit with > 90% resection, but when evaluating solely tumors with OD subtype, they were unable to show a benefit with increased extent of resection at presentation which has been supported in other evaluations [14, 73, 74].

As we attempt to better determine which patients require more extensive resection, molecular genetics are becoming important even in surgical evaluation. Patients with IDH wild-type tumors tend to be more infiltrative on MRI compared to their counterpart IDH-mutated tumors which tend to be more localized and often presenting with seizures [75, 76]. Conversely, IDH-mutated tumors are associated with a more complete surgical resection, even in enhancing disease [77]. With the aid of utilizing improved imaging techniques such as awake craniotomy, functional MRI mapping, and intraoperative MRI (as outlined in previous chapters), we may be able to obtain a safer and more extensive resection. There may be a subset of OD patients who would not benefit with significant surgical resection at presentation; however, this population is difficult to define without a prospective evaluation.

Radiation Therapy

Historically, radiotherapy followed surgery either within weeks from completion or delayed and utilized at time of recurrence/progression. Radiation acts by causing DNA damage and subsequent apoptosis of active tumors cells but is non-discriminatory and also damages normal surrounding brain tissue. The acute side effects such as fatigue, headaches, dizziness, nausea, vomiting, and seizure can resolve; however, the concern comes with long-term clinical side effects such as neurocognitive changes, reduced quality of life, and radiation necrosis [78, 79]. Careful consideration is given to the timing of radiotherapy especially given the longer life span associated with these tumors.

Treatment of gliomas, specifically ODs, is usually a dose to 45–54 Gy in 1.8–2.0 Gy/fractions. Attempts at escalating beyond these doses were performed in prospective randomized trials. EORTC 22844 showed there was no benefit to dose escalation of 59.4 Gy over 45 Gy at 1.8 Gy/fraction with similar 5-year OS (59% with high doses vs. 58% with lower doses) and PFS (50% vs. 47%) [70]. Given that the majority of recurrences occur within the radiation field, further dose escalation was evaluated by the combined efforts of NCCTG, RTOG, and EORTC. They compared radiation doses of 50.4 and 64.8 Gy at 1.8 Gy/fraction [11]. Again, there was no significant improvement in OS (65% vs. 72% in the low-dose group) while also showing a significant increase in risk of grade 3–5 radiation

necrosis from
2.5 to 5%.

Given the slow progression of ODs, some have questioned the role of radiation therapy immediately following surgery as radiation can be an effective salvage therapy. EORTC 22845 was a large phase 3 trial which attempted to evaluate this question of radiation alone after surgery or delayed until progression [3]. After 7 years of follow-up, there was a benefit in 5-year PFS of 55% with early RT and 35% with delayed RT but no benefit in 5-year overall survival (68.4% vs. 65.7%) as most patients in the observation arm received salvage radiotherapy. Quality of life and cognitive toxicity were not evaluated in this trial, but there was a benefit in seizure control if RT was received after surgical intervention.

With the introduction of stereotactic radiosurgery (SRS), some institutions have utilized SRS in select cases of both initial and recurrent treatment. The benefit of SRS is the theoretical ability to decrease radiation dose to normal tissues surrounding the tumor. In the up-front setting, current reviews show that these treatments are well tolerated; however, they have been unable to show a clear advantage over standard treatment outcomes [80]. While patients did have favorable short-term and long-term outcomes, the patients selected can be biased by tumor location, size, and patient performance [81–83]. SRS may be advantageous in recurrent tumors who have previously received radiation as these patients can sometimes be limited in further treatment options. Reirradiation has been shown to be well tolerated in a small subset of patients with recurrent low- and high-grade disease, but the exact fractionation and timing is unclear [84, 85].

There is still concern for the long-term impact of radiation with some retrospective series showing evidence that RT can be associated with increased late neurotoxicity [86–88]. It may be more appropriate to identify patients at high risk with poor prognostic factors who may better benefit from early intervention with RT. One of these subsets may be subtotally resected tumors as they are at higher risk for earlier progression, 1p/19q intact patients as they are less susceptible to chemotherapy, and possibly IDH wild-type tumors [69, 89].

Chemotherapy

In the few years with increasing recognition of the chemosensitivity associated with ODs and 1p/19q, chemotherapy has played a significant role in the management of this disease. The association of 1p/19q with chemosensitivity was shown to be significant in anaplastic ODs and oligoastrocytomas after the long-term results of RTOG 9402 was published [61]. While chemotherapy did not influence median survival in combination with radiation in non-deleted tumors (2.6 vs. 2.7 years), there was a significant improvement if procarbazine, lomustine, and vincristine (PCV) were given concurrently with RT (14.7 vs. 7.3 years). Given the increasing role of IDH status in gliomas, this was retrospectively validated in RTOG 9402 and, again, there was an overall survival benefit to combined chemotherapy and radiotherapy in IDH-mutated tumors but not in IDH wild-type tumors [90].

In low-grade gliomas specifically, the results of the phase III study RTOG 9802 did show a significant benefit in PFS and initially no OS benefit with the addition of concurrent PCV chemotherapy to RT in high-risk patients (age >40 or STR) [91]. However, with longer follow-up, there was a significant OS benefit ($p = 0.002$) with a 10-year overall survival of 40% with RT alone versus 60% with addition of PCV chemotherapy [92]. These results, unfortunately, did not include molecular analysis which was shown to be such an important factor in RTOG 9402. While the role of 1p/19q and IDH status is a known prognostic marker, its role in chemosensitivity is not as clearly defined as in anaplastic gliomas. Still, recent data are promising.

Reviews have shown longer PFS and improved response to chemotherapy in tumors with 1p/19q codeletion [93–95]. In a study of 132 patients with a known IDH status, there was an association with IDH mutation with improved overall survival and chemosensitivity with temozolomide [96]. The methylation status of MGMT has also been shown to be a predictor of response to chemotherapy in low-grade disease [97]. The majority of this data are limited in size, population, and extent of analysis and as such questions still remain if these markers can predict response to chemotherapy on their own or, instead, predicting response to treatment. Hopefully, upcoming prospective trials by RTOG, EORTC, and ECOG will shed light on this question as they are also hoping to answer the other important question of the use of temozolomide.

PCV Versus Temozolomide

While PCV was used in the earlier large published prospective trials, temozolomide is gaining increased use over the historically proven PCV. When undergoing treatment with temozolomide, patients with low-grade gliomas are able to maintain their quality of life in all realms [98]. It can be given safely and has been shown to have an improved response in 1p/19q codeleted tumors with favorable outcomes [99–102]. While the role for treatment in higher grade disease is more certain, the role in low-grade gliomas is still under active investigation and will hopefully be answered in the coming years given the already early results.

RTOG 0424 evaluated high-risk patients undergoing RT with concurrent and adjuvant temozolomide which has shown an improved three-year overall survival of 73.1% compared to historical controls in EORTC 22844 and 22845 [103]. While limited by the comparison to historical controls, EORTC 22033–26033 will attempt to answer the difficult question of radiation versus temozolomide after surgical resection with 1p status included in the stratification. Still early in analysis, patients with 1p intact who received temozolomide trended toward a worse PFS, while those with 1p deleted had an improved OS [104]. While long-term follow-up is required, early results show that 1p/19q status may allow for stratification into different treatment algorithms. The ECOG-E3F05 will further attempt to define the role of temozolomide as it investigates concurrent and adjuvant treatment with RT versus radiation alone in low-grade glioma patients with tumor progression or uncontrolled symptoms.

Even if results prove to have better outcomes, there may be those who advocate for temozolomide. The reasoning is due to the toxicity and complexity of administration of PCV chemotherapy. Recent studies have shown up to 38% of patients are forced to discontinue PCV versus 8% for TMZ and 9% refused to continue PCV versus 4% for TMZ [105]. This does not account for patients who required dose reduction, treatment interruptions (both impairing treatment outcomes) or had more severe toxicities such as debilitating fatigue, neuropathy, and even death. PCV chemotherapy also requires three agents given over 6–8 weeks of varying dose and intensity. This can be further complicated by non-compliant patients, given the complexity of the schedule, who already have difficulty with the cognitive effects of their disease, surgery, and/or radiation. TMZ is an oral agent which is given at a relatively simpler dosing schedule at more regular intervals. There has already been a large shift by a number of large institutions away from PCV to TMZ chemotherapy given the belief that TMZ will be similar to PCV in terms of outcomes and it may be difficult for some to shift back if PCV has improved outcomes [106].

Future Chemotherapies

In brain cells, IDH1 and IDH2 are very similar in their effect where they catalyze the reversible conversion of isocitrate to alpha-ketoglutarate (aKG). When IDH is mutated, this pathway is disrupted and instead it generates D-2-hydroxyglutarate (D2HG) which can be >100 times more when compared to normal cells [107]. Elevated levels of D2HG are believed to disrupt the normal function of aKG-dependent enzymes. This in turn leads to several detrimental downstream effects including increasing levels of DNA methylation by inhibition of TET hydroxylase along with disruption of histone demethylase and prolyl hydroxylase leading to abnormal collagen maturation [107–109]. It is suggested that this process, and the downstream effects, may be one of the key events in tumorigenesis [110, 111]. By disrupting the conversion of isocitrate to aKG, it also disrupts the normal pathway by which the cell can create NADPH which can further impair cellular activity and may be the reason IDH has a significant prognostic value [112]. Tumor cells account for this by attempting to balance the metabolic shift by increasing conversion of other metabolites, such as glutamine and glutamate to aKG by glutaminase and glutamate dehydrogenase (GDH) [113, 114].

Ways to disrupt this pathway and the compensatory mechanisms by which it recovers are becoming an increasing area of research as novel targeted agents for gliomas. Glutaminase inhibition with small interfering RNA (siRNA) or molecular inhibitors have already shown promise with increased sensitivity in IDH-mutated tumors [114]. Multiple compounds have been developed which specifically inhibit IDH-mutated tumors by inhibiting IDH1 R132H (AGI 5198, IDH305, AG-120, and AG-881) and IDH2 R140Q (AGI 6780 and AG-881) as these are the more common sites of IDH mutations [115, 116]. Also, undergoing phase I evaluation is a peptide vaccine specifically targeting the IDH1 R132H mutation (NCT02454634) with idea to provoke an immune response to the IDH1-mutated tumors. While the exact benefit is unclear, early mouse models have shown impaired growth in IDH1-mutated gliomas with both inhibitor compounds and IDH1 peptide vaccine [117].

Given the ability to detect 2-hydroxyglutarate (2HG) on proton MR spectroscopy, there is increasing evidence of the correlation between 2HG detection on imaging and IDH1 mutation status [118, 119]. The prognostic significance of IDH status may have a significant impact on the future of surgical planning and management. This imaging may be able to aid in biopsy targeting and risk stratification before a surgical resection, and we may be able to identify a subset of patients who can be observed prior to resection. It has already been shown as a sufficient way to monitor treatment response to the recent inhibitors AGI 5198/6780 and may be an important aspect of future trials as it can be difficult to assess response on normal CT/MRI imaging [120].

References

1. Ostrom QT, Gittleman H, Fulop J, Liu M, Blanda R, Kromer C, et al. CBTRUS statistical report: primary brain and central nervous system tumors diagnosed in the United States in 2008–2012. Neuro-oncology. 2015;17 Suppl 4:iv1–iv62. PubMed PMID: 26511214. Pubmed Central PMCID: 4623240.
2. Louis DN, Ohgaki H, Wiestler OD, Cavenee WK, Burger PC, Jouvet A, et al. The 2007 WHO classification of tumours of the central nervous system. Acta neuropathologica. 2007;114(2):97–109. PubMed PMID: 17618441. Pubmed Central PMCID: 1929165.
3. van den Bent MJ, Afra D, de Witte O, Ben Hassel M, Schraub S, Hoang-Xuan K, et al. Long-term efficacy of early versus delayed radiotherapy for low-grade astrocytoma and oligodendroglioma in adults: the EORTC 22845 randomised trial. Lancet. 2005;366(9490):985-90. PubMed PMID: 16168780.
4. Weller M, Stupp R, Hegi ME, van den Bent M, Tonn JC, Sanson M, et al. Personalized care in neuro-oncology coming of age: why we need MGMT and 1p/19q testing for malignant glioma patients in clinical practice. Neuro-oncology. 2012;14 Suppl 4:iv100–8. PubMed PMID: 23095825. Pubmed Central PMCID: 3480248.
5. Jakola AS, Myrmel KS, Kloster R, Torp SH, Lindal S, Unsgard G, et al. Comparison of a strategy favoring early surgical resection vs a strategy favoring watchful waiting in low-grade gliomas. JAMA. 2012;308(18):1881–8.
6. Engelhard HH, Stelea A, Mundt A. Oligodendroglioma and anaplastic oligodendroglioma: clinical features, treatment, and prognosis. Surg Neurol. 2003;60(5):443–56.
7. Louis DN, Ohgaki H, Wiestler OD, Cavenee WK. World Health Organization Classification of Tumours. Lyon: IARC Press; 2007. p. 312.
8. Goodenberger ML, Jenkins RB. Genetics of adult glioma. Cancer genetics. 2012;205(12):613–21.
9. Schomas DA, Laack NN, Rao RD, Meyer FB, Shaw EG, O'Neill BP, et al. Intracranial low-grade gliomas in adults: 30-year experience with long-term follow-up at Mayo Clinic. Neuro-oncology. 2009;11(4):437–45. PubMed PMID: 19018039. Pubmed Central PMCID: 2743224.

10. Forst DA, Nahed BV, Loeffler JS, Batchelor TT. Low-grade gliomas. The oncologist. 2014;19(4):403–13. PubMed PMID: 24664484. Pubmed Central PMCID: 3983820.
11. White ML, Zhang Y, Kirby P, Ryken TC. Can tumor contrast enhancement be used as a criterion for differentiating tumor grades of oligodendrogliomas? AJNR Am J Neuroradiol. 2005;26(4):784–90.
12. Shaw E, Arusell R, Scheithauer B, O'Fallon J, O'Neill B, Dinapoli R, et al. Prospective randomized trial of low- versus high-dose radiation therapy in adults with supratentorial low-grade glioma: initial report of a North Central Cancer Treatment Group/Radiation Therapy Oncology Group/Eastern Cooperative Oncology Group study. J Clini Oncol: Official J Am Soc Clini Oncol. 2002;20(9):2267–76.
13. Vaquero J, Zurita M, Morales C, Coca S. Prognostic significance of tumor-enhancement and angiogenesis in oligodendroglioma. Acta Neurol Scand. 2002;106(1):19–23.
14. Shaw EG, Scheithauer BW, O'Fallon JR, Tazelaar HD, Davis DH. Oligodendrogliomas: the Mayo Clinic experience. J Neurosurg. 1992;76(3):428–34.
15. Lebrun C, Fontaine D, Ramaioli A, Vandenbos F, Chanalet S, Lonjon M, et al. Long-term outcome of oligodendrogliomas. Neurology. 2004;62(10):1783–7.
16. Daumas-Duport C, Varlet P, Tucker ML, Beuvon F, Cervera P, Chodkiewicz JP. Oligodendrogliomas. Part I: Patterns of growth, histological diagnosis, clinical and imaging correlations: a study of 153 cases. J Neurooncol. 1997;34(1):37–59.
17. Wieshmann UC, Milinis K, Paniker J, Das K, Jenkinson MD, Brodbelt A, et al. The role of the corpus callosum in seizure spread: MRI lesion mapping in oligodendrogliomas. Epilepsy Res. 2015;109:126–33.
18. Duffau H, Capelle L. Preferential brain locations of low-grade gliomas. Cancer. 2004;100(12):2622–6.
19. Pignatti F, van den Bent M, Curran D, Debruyne C, Sylvester R, Therasse P, et al. Prognostic factors for survival in adult patients with cerebral low-grade glioma. J Clini Oncol:Official J Am Soc Clini Oncol. 2002;20(8):2076–84.
20. El Hateer H, Souhami L, Robergc D, Macstro RD, Leblanc R, Eldebawy E, et al. Low-grade oligodendroglioma: an indolent but incurable disease? Clini Article J Neurosurg. 2009;111(2):265–71.
21. Floeth FW, Pauleit D, Sabel M, Stoffels G, Reifenberger G, Riemenschneider MJ, et al. Prognostic value of O-(2-18F-fluoroethyl)-L-tyrosine PET and MRI in low-grade glioma. J Nucl Med:Official Publ Soc Nucl Med. 2007;48(4):519–27.
22. Chen R, Ravindra VM, Cohen AL, Jensen RL, Salzman KL, Prescot AP, et al. Molecular features assisting in diagnosis, surgery, and treatment decision making in low-grade gliomas. Neurosurg Focus. 2015;38(3):E2.
23. Chawla S, Oleaga L, Wang S, Krejza J, Wolf RL, Woo JH, et al. Role of proton magnetic resonance spectroscopy in differentiating oligodendrogliomas from astrocytomas. J Neuroimaging:Official J Am Soc Neuroimaging. 2010;20(1):3–8.
24. van den Bent MJ. Interobserver variation of the histopathological diagnosis in clinical trials on glioma: a clinician's perspective. Acta neuropathologica. 2010;120(3):297–304. PubMed PMID: 20644945. Pubmed Central PMCID: 2910894.
25. Giannini C, Scheithauer BW, Weaver AL, Burger PC, Kros JM, Mork S, et al. Oligodendrogliomas: reproducibility and prognostic value of histologic diagnosis and grading. J Neuropathol Exp Neurol. 2001;60(3):248–62.
26. Pirzkall A, Nelson SJ, McKnight TR, Takahashi MM, Li X, Graves EE, et al. Metabolic imaging of low-grade gliomas with three-dimensional magnetic resonance spectroscopy. Int J Radiat Oncol Biol Phys. 2002;53(5):1254–64.
27. Perry A. Oligodendroglial neoplasms: current concepts, misconceptions, and folklore. Adv Anat Pathol. 2001;8(4):183–99.
28. Kros JM, Van Eden CG, Stefanko SZ, Batenburg M, van der Kwast TH. Prognostic implications of glial fibrillary acidic protein containing cell types in oligodendrogliomas. Cancer. 1990;66(6):1204–12 PubMed PMID: 2205356.
29. Takei H, Yogeswaren ST, Wong KK, Mehta V, Chintagumpala M, Dauser RC, et al. Expression of oligodendroglial differentiation markers in pilocytic astrocytomas identifies two clinical subsets and shows a significant correlation with proliferation index and progression free survival. J Neurooncol. 2008;86(2):183–90.
30. Preusser M, Budka H, Rossler K, Hainfellner JA. OLIG2 is a useful immunohistochemical marker in differential diagnosis of clear cell primary CNS neoplasms. Histopathology. 2007;50(3):365–70.
31. Eigenbrod S, Roeber S, Thon N, Giese A, Krieger A, Grasbon-Frodl E, et al. alpha-Internexin in the diagnosis of oligodendroglial tumors and association with 1p/19q status. J Neuropathol Exp Neurol. 2011;70(11):970–8.
32. Ducray F, Mokhtari K, Criniere E, Idbaih A, Marie Y, Dehais C, et al. Diagnostic and prognostic value of alpha internexin expression in a series of 409 gliomas. Eur J Cancer. 2011;47(5):802–8.
33. Barresi V, Mondello S, Branca G, Rajan TS, Vitarelli E, Tuccari G. p-CREB expression in human gliomas: potential use in the differential diagnosis between astrocytoma and oligodendroglioma. Hum Pathol. 2015;46(2):231–8.
34. Kitange GJ, Templeton KL, Jenkins RB. Recent advances in the molecular genetics of primary gliomas. Curr Opin Oncol. 2003;15(3):197–203.
35. Bauman G, Lote K, Larson D, Stalpers L, Leighton C, Fisher B, et al. Pretreatment factors predict overall survival for patients with low-grade

glioma: a recursive partitioning analysis. Int J Radiat Oncol Biol Phys. 1999;45(4):923–9.
36. Cairncross JG, Ueki K, Zlatescu MC, Lisle DK, Finkelstein DM, Hammond RR, et al. Specific genetic predictors of chemotherapeutic response and survival in patients with anaplastic oligodendrogliomas. J Natl Cancer Inst. 1998;90(19):1473–9.
37. Reifenberger J, Reifenberger G, Liu L, James CD, Wechsler W, Collins VP. Molecular genetic analysis of oligodendroglial tumors shows preferential allelic deletions on 19q and 1p. Am J Pathol. 1994;145(5):1175 Pubmed Central PMCID: 1887413.
38. Jenkins RB, Blair H, Ballman KV, Giannini C, Arusell RM, Law M, et al. A t(1;19)(q10;p10) mediates the combined deletions of 1p and 19q and predicts a better prognosis of patients with oligodendroglioma. Cancer Res. 2006;66(20):9852–61.
39. Idbaih A, Marie Y, Pierron G, Brennetot C, Hoang-Xuan K, Kujas M, et al. Two types of chromosome 1p losses with opposite significance in gliomas. Annals Neurology. 2005;58(3):483–7.
40. Polivka J Jr, Polivka J, Repik T, Rohan V, Hes O, Topolcan O. Co-deletion of 1p/19q as Prognostic and Predictive Biomarker for Patients in West Bohemia with Anaplastic Oligodendroglioma. Anticancer Res. 2016;36(1):471–6.
41. Wick W, Hartmann C, Engel C, Stoffels M, Felsberg J, Stockhammer F, et al. NOA-04 randomized phase III trial of sequential radiochemotherapy of anaplastic glioma with procarbazine, lomustine, and vincristine or temozolomide. J Clini Oncol:Official J Am Soc Clini Oncol. 2009;27(35):5874–80.
42. van den Bent MJ, Brandes AA, Taphoorn MJ, Kros JM, Kouwenhoven MC, Delattre JY, et al. Adjuvant procarbazine, lomustine, and vincristine chemotherapy in newly diagnosed anaplastic oligodendroglioma: long-term follow-up of EORTC brain tumor group study 26951. J Clini Oncol: Official J Am Soc Clini Oncol. 2013;31(3):344–50.
43. Intergroup Radiation Therapy Oncology Group T, Cairncross G, Berkey B, Shaw E, Jenkins R, Scheithauer B, et al. Phase III trial of chemotherapy plus radiotherapy compared with radiotherapy alone for pure and mixed anaplastic oligodendroglioma: Intergroup Radiation Therapy Oncology Group Trial 9402. J Clini Oncol:Official J Am Soc Clin Oncol. 2006;24(18):2707–14.
44. Wang XW, Ciccarino P, Rossetto M, Boisselier B, Marie Y, Desestret V, et al. IDH mutations: genotype-phenotype correlation and prognostic impact. BioMed Res Int. 2014;2014:540236. PubMed PMID: 24877111. Pubmed Central PMCID: 4022066.
45. Wesseling P, van den Bent M, Perry A. Oligodendroglioma: pathology, molecular mechanisms and markers. Acta neuropathologica. 2015;129(6):809–27. PubMed PMID: 25943885. Pubmed Central PMCID: 4436696.
46. van den Bent MJ, Dubbink HJ, Marie Y, Brandes AA, Taphoorn MJ, Wesseling P, et al. IDH1 and IDH2 mutations are prognostic but not predictive for outcome in anaplastic oligodendroglial tumors: a report of the European Organization for Research and Treatment of Cancer Brain Tumor Group. Clini Cancer Res:An Official J Am Assoc Cancer Res. 2010;16(5):1597–604.
47. Thon N, Eigenbrod S, Kreth S, Lutz J, Tonn JC, Kretzschmar H, et al. IDH1 mutations in grade II astrocytomas are associated with unfavorable progression-free survival and prolonged postrecurrence survival. Cancer. 2012;118(2):452–60.
48. Ahmadi R, Stockhammer F, Becker N, Hohlen K, Misch M, Christians A, et al. No prognostic value of IDH1 mutations in a series of 100 WHO grade II astrocytomas. J Neurooncol. 2012;109(1):15–22.
49. Ohgaki H, Kleihues P. Population-based studies on incidence, survival rates, and genetic alterations in astrocytic and oligodendroglial gliomas. J Neuropathol Exp Neurol. 2005;64(6):479–89.
50. Wiestler B, Capper D, Holland-Letz T, Korshunov A, von Deimling A, Pfister SM, et al. ATRX loss refines the classification of anaplastic gliomas and identifies a subgroup of IDH mutant astrocytic tumors with better prognosis. Acta Neuropathol. 2013;126(3):443–51.
51. Kannan K, Inagaki A, Silber J, Gorovets D, Zhang J, Kastenhuber ER, Heguy A, Petrini JH, Chan TA, Huse JT. Whole-exome sequencing identifies ATRX mutation as a key molecular determinant in lower-grade glioma. Oncotarget. 2012;3(10):1194–203 PubMed PMID: 23104868. Pubmed Central PMCID: 3717947.
52. Brandner S, von Deimling A. Diagnostic, prognostic and predictive relevance of molecular markers in gliomas. Neuropathol Appl Neurobiol. 2015;41(6):694–720.
53. Arita H, Narita Y, Fukushima S, Tateishi K, Matsushita Y, Yoshida A, et al. Upregulating mutations in the TERT promoter commonly occur in adult malignant gliomas and are strongly associated with total 1p19q loss. Acta Neuropathol. 2013;126(2):267–76.
54. Labussiere M, Di Stefano AL, Gleize V, Boisselier B, Giry M, Mangesius S, et al. TERT promoter mutations in gliomas, genetic associations and clinico-pathological correlations. British journal of cancer. 2014;111(10):2024-32. PubMed PMID: 25314060. Pubmed Central PMCID: 4229642.
55. Koelsche C, Sahm F, Capper D, Reuss D, Sturm D, Jones DT, et al. Distribution of TERT promoter mutations in pediatric and adult tumors of the nervous system. Acta Neuropathol. 2013;126(6):907–15.
56. Bettegowda C, Agrawal N, Jiao Y, Sausen M, Wood LD, Hruban RH, et al. Mutations in CIC and FUBP1 contribute to human oligodendroglioma. Science. 2011;333(6048):1453–5. PubMed PMID: 21817013. Pubmed Central PMCID: 3170506.

57. Jiao Y, Killela PJ, Reitman ZJ, Rasheed AB, Heaphy CM, de Wilde RF, et al. Frequent ATRX, CIC, FUBP1 and IDH1 mutations refine the classification of malignant gliomas. Oncotarget. 2012;3 (7):709–22. PubMed PMID: 22869205. Pubmed Central PMCID: 3443254.
58. Yip S, Butterfield YS, Morozova O, Chittaranjan S, Blough MD, An J, et al. Concurrent CIC mutations, IDH mutations, and 1p/19q loss distinguish oligodendrogliomas from other cancers. J Pathol. 2012;226(1):7–16. PubMed PMID: 22072542. Pubmed Central PMCID: 3246739.
59. Hegi ME, Diserens AC, Gorlia T, Hamou MF, de Tribolet N, Weller M, et al. MGMT gene silencing and benefit from temozolomide in glioblastoma. N Eng J Med. 2005;352(10):997–1003.
60. Leu S, von Felten S, Frank S, Vassella E, Vajtai I, Taylor E, et al. IDH/MGMT-driven molecular classification of low-grade glioma is a strong predictor for long-term survival. Neuro-oncology. 2013;15(4):469–79. PubMed PMID: 23408861. Pubmed Central PMCID: 3607260.
61. Wick W, Meisner C, Hentschel B, Platten M, Schilling A, Wiestler B, et al. Prognostic or predictive value of MGMT promoter methylation in gliomas depends on IDH1 mutation. Neurology. 2013;81(17):1515–22.
62. Cairncross G, Wang M, Shaw E, Jenkins R, Brachman D, Buckner J, et al. Phase III trial of chemoradiotherapy for anaplastic oligodendroglioma: long-term results of RTOG 9402. J Clini Oncol:Official J Am Soc Clini Oncol. 2013;31(3):337–43. PubMed PMID: 23071247. Pubmed Central PMCID: 3732012.
63. Sarmiento JM, Venteicher AS, Patil CG. Early versus delayed postoperative radiotherapy for treatment of low-grade gliomas. Cochrane Database Syst Rev. 2015;6:CD009229. PubMed PMID: 26118544. Pubmed Central PMCID: 4506130.
64. Reijneveld JC, Sitskoorn MM, Klein M, Nuyen J, Taphoorn MJ. Cognitive status and quality of life in patients with suspected versus proven low-grade gliomas. Neurology. 2001;56(5):618–23.
65. van Veelen ML, Avezaat CJ, Kros JM, van Putten W, Vecht C. Supratentorial low grade astrocytoma: prognostic factors, dedifferentiation, and the issue of early versus late surgery. J Neurol Neurosurg Psychiatry. 1998 May;64(5):581–7. PubMed PMID: 9598670. Pubmed Central PMCID: 2170094.
66. Afra D, Osztie E, Sipos L, Vitanovics D. Preoperative history and postoperative survival of supratentorial low-grade astrocytomas. Br J Neurosurg. 1999;13(3):299–305.
67. Mandonnet E, Delattre JY, Tanguy ML, Swanson KR, Carpentier AF, Duffau H, et al. Continuous growth of mean tumor diameter in a subset of grade II gliomas. Annals of neurology. 2003;53(4):524–8.
68. Sawaya R, Hammoud M, Schoppa D, Hess KR, Wu SZ, Shi WM, et al. Neurosurgical outcomes in a modern series of 400 craniotomies for treatment of parenchymal tumors. Neurosurgery. 1998;42 (5):1044–55; discussion 55-6. PubMed PMID: 9588549.
69. Claus EB, Horlacher A, Hsu L, Schwartz RB, Dello-Iacono D, Talos F, et al. Survival rates in patients with low-grade glioma after intraoperative magnetic resonance image guidance. Cancer. 2005;103(6):1227–33.
70. Smith JS, Chang EF, Lamborn KR, Chang SM, Prados MD, Cha S, et al. Role of extent of resection in the long-term outcome of low-grade hemispheric gliomas. J Clini Oncol:Official J Am Soc Clin Oncol. 2008;26(8):1338–45.
71. Karim AB, Maat B, Hatlevoll R, Menten J, Rutten EH, Thomas DG, et al. A randomized trial on dose-response in radiation therapy of low-grade cerebral glioma: European Organization for Research and Treatment of Cancer (EORTC) Study 22844. Int J Radiat Oncol Biol Phys. 1996;36(3): 549–56.
72. Nicolato A, Gerosa MA, Fina P, Iuzzolino P, Giorgiutti F, Bricolo A. Prognostic factors in low-grade supratentorial astrocytomas: a uni-multivariate statistical analysis in 76 surgically treated adult patients. Surg Neurol. 1995;44(3): 208–21; discussion 21-3. PubMed PMID: 8545771.
73. Englot DJ, Han SJ, Berger MS, Barbaro NM, Chang EF. Extent of surgical resection predicts seizure freedom in low-grade temporal lobe brain tumors. Neurosurgery. 2012;70(4):921–8; discussion 8. PubMed PMID: 21997540.
74. Lebrun C, Fontaine D, Bourg V, Ramaioli A, Chanalet S, Vandenbos F, et al. Treatment of newly diagnosed symptomatic pure low-grade oligodendrogliomas with PCV chemotherapy. Eur J Neurol. 2007;14(4):391–8.
75. Maiuri F, Del Basso De Caro ML, Iaconetta G, Peca C, Esposito M, de Divitiis E. Prognostic and survival-related factors in patients with well-differentiated oligodendrogliomas. Zentralblatt fur Neurochirurgie. 2006;67(4):204-9. PubMed PMID: 17106834.
76. Stockhammer F, Misch M, Helms HJ, Lengler U, Prall F, von Deimling A, et al. IDH1/2 mutations in WHO grade II astrocytomas associated with localization and seizure as the initial symptom. Seizure. 2012;21(3):194–7.
77. Metellus P, Coulibaly B, Colin C, de Paula AM, Vasiljevic A, Taieb D, et al. Absence of IDH mutation identifies a novel radiologic and molecular subtype of WHO grade II gliomas with dismal prognosis. Acta Neuropathol. 2010;120(6): 719–29.
78. Juratli TA, Cahill DP, McCutcheon IE. Determining optimal treatment strategy for diffuse glioma: the emerging role of IDH mutations. Expert Rev Anticancer Ther. 2015;15(6):603–6.
79. Surma-aho O, Niemela M, Vilkki J, Kouri M, Brander A, Salonen O, et al. Adverse long-term

effects of brain radiotherapy in adult low-grade glioma patients. Neurology. 2001;56(10):1285–90.
80. Douw L, Klein M, Fagel SS, van den Heuvel J, Taphoorn MJ, Aaronson NK, et al. Cognitive and radiological effects of radiotherapy in patients with low-grade glioma: long-term follow-up. Lancet Neurol. 2009;8(9):810–8.
81. Roberge D, Souhami L, Olivier A, Leblanc R, Podgorsak E. Hypofractionated stereotactic radiotherapy for low grade glioma at McGill University: long-term follow-up. Technol Cancer Res Treat. 2006;5(1):1–8.
82. Combs SE, Schulz-Ertner D, Thilmann C, Edler L, Debus J. Fractionated stereotactic radiation therapy in the management of primary oligodendroglioma and oligoastrocytoma. Int J Radiat Oncol Biol Phys. 2005;62(3):797–802.
83. Lee DH, Kim EY, Park S, Phi JH, Kim SK, Cho BK, et al. Reclosure of surgically induced spinal open neural tube defects by the intraamniotic injection of human embryonic stem cells in chick embryos 24 hours after lesion induction. J Neurosurg. 2006;105(2 Suppl):127–33.
84. Heppner PA, Sheehan JP, Steiner LE. Gamma knife surgery for low-grade gliomas. Neurosurgery. 2005;57(6):1132–9; discussion. PubMed PMID: 16331161.
85. Shepherd SF, Laing RW, Cosgrove VP, Warrington AP, Hines F, Ashley SE, et al. Hypofractionated stereotactic radiotherapy in the management of recurrent glioma. Int J Radiat Oncol Biol Phys. 1997;37(2):393–8.
86. Kano H, Niranjan A, Khan A, Flickinger JC, Kondziolka D, Lieberman F, et al. Does radiosurgery have a role in the management of oligodendrogliomas? J Neurosurg. 2009;110(3):564–71.
87. Correa DD, Shi W, Thaler HT, Cheung AM, DeAngelis LM, Abrey LE. Longitudinal cognitive follow-up in low grade gliomas. J Neurooncol. 2008;86(3):321–7.
88. Taphoorn MJ, Schiphorst AK, Snoek FJ, Lindeboom J, Wolbers JG, Karim AB, et al. Cognitive functions and quality of life in patients with low-grade gliomas: the impact of radiotherapy. Annals Neurol. 1994;36(1):48–54.
89. Olson JD, Riedel E, DeAngelis LM. Long-term outcome of low-grade oligodendroglioma and mixed glioma. Neurology. 2000;54(7):1442–8.
90. Shaw EG, Berkey B, Coons SW, Bullard D, Brachman D, Buckner JC, et al. Recurrence following neurosurgeon-determined gross-total resection of adult supratentorial low-grade glioma: results of a prospective clinical trial. J Neurosurg. 2008;109(5):835–41. PubMed PMID: 18976072. Pubmed Central PMCID: 3833272.
91. Cairncross JG, Wang M, Jenkins RB, Shaw EG, Giannini C, Brachman DG, et al. Benefit from procarbazine, lomustine, and vincristine in oligodendroglial tumors is associated with mutation of IDH. J Clini Oncol:Official J Am Soc Clini Oncol. 2014 Mar 10;32(8):783-90. PubMed PMID: 24516018. Pubmed Central PMCID: 3940537.
92. Shaw EG, Wang M, Coons SW, Brachman DG, Buckner JC, Stelzer KJ, et al. Randomized trial of radiation therapy plus procarbazine, lomustine, and vincristine chemotherapy for supratentorial adult low-grade glioma: initial results of RTOG 9802. J Clini Oncol:Official J Am Soc Clini Oncol. 2012;30(25):3065–70. PubMed PMID: 22851558. Pubmed Central PMCID: 3732006.
93. al. JCBe. Phase III study of radiation therapy (RT) with or without procarbazine, CCNU, and vincristine (PCV) in low-grade glioma: RTOG 9802 with Alliance, ECOG, and SWOG. ASCO Annual Meeting; Chicago, Illinois2014.
94. Kouwenhoven MC, Kros JM, French PJ, Biemond-ter Stege EM, Graveland WJ, Taphoorn MJ, et al. 1p/19q loss within oligodendroglioma is predictive for response to first line temozolomide but not to salvage treatment. Eur J Cancer. 2006;42(15):2499–503.
95. Kujas M, Lejeune J, Benouaich-Amiel A, Criniere E, Laigle-Donadey F, Marie Y, et al. Chromosome 1p loss: a favorable prognostic factor in low-grade gliomas. Annals Neurology. 2005;58 (2):322–6.
96. Iwamoto FM, Nicolardi L, Demopoulos A, Barbashina V, Salazar P, Rosenblum M, et al. Clinical relevance of 1p and 19q deletion for patients with WHO grade 2 and 3 gliomas. J Neurooncol. 2008;88(3):293–8.
97. Houillier C, Wang X, Kaloshi G, Mokhtari K, Guillevin R, Laffaire J, et al. IDH1 or IDH2 mutations predict longer survival and response to temozolomide in low-grade gliomas. Neurology. 2010;75(17):1560–6.
98. Everhard S, Kaloshi G, Criniere E, Benouaich-Amiel A, Lejeune J, Marie Y, et al. MGMT methylation: a marker of response to temozolomide in low-grade gliomas. Annals Neurology. 2006;60 (6):740–3.
99. Liu R, Solheim K, Polley MY, Lamborn KR, Page M, Fedoroff A, et al. Quality of life in low-grade glioma patients receiving temozolomide. Neuro-oncology. 2009;11(1):59–68. PubMed PMID: 18713953. Pubmed Central PMCID: 2718960.
100. Kaloshi G, Benouaich-Amiel A, Diakite F, Taillibert S, Lejeune J, Laigle-Donadey F, et al. Temozolomide for low-grade gliomas: predictive impact of 1p/19q loss on response and outcome. Neurology. 2007;68(21):1831–6.
101. Kesari S, Schiff D, Drappatz J, LaFrankie D, Doherty L, Macklin EA, et al. Phase II study of protracted daily temozolomide for low-grade gliomas in adults. Clini Cancer Res:An Official J Am Assoc Cancer Res. 2009;15(1):330–7.
102. Pouratian N, Gasco J, Sherman JH, Shaffrey ME, Schiff D. Toxicity and efficacy of protracted low

dose temozolomide for the treatment of low grade gliomas. J Neurooncol. 2007;82(3):281–8.
103. Hoang-Xuan K, Capelle L, Kujas M, Taillibert S, Duffau H, Lejeune J, et al. Temozolomide as initial treatment for adults with low-grade oligodendrogliomas or oligoastrocytomas and correlation with chromosome 1p deletions. J Clini Oncol: Official J Am Soc Clinical Oncol. 2004;22(15): 3133–8.
104. Fisher BJ, Lui J, Macdonald DR, Lesser GJ, Coons S, Brachman D, et al. A phase II study of a temozolomide-based chemoradiotherapy regimen for high-risk low-grade gliomas: Preliminary results of RTOG 0424. 2013.
105. Baumert BG, Mason WP, Ryan G, Bromberg JE, Bent MJVD, Hoang-Xuan K, et al. Temozolomide chemotherapy versus radiotherapy in molecularly characterized (1p loss) low-grade glioma: a randomized phase III intergroup study by the EORTC/NCIC-CTG/TROG/MRC-CTU (EORTC 22033-26033). 2013.
106. Lassman AB. Procarbazine, lomustine and vincristine or temozolomide: which is the better regimen? CNS Oncol. 2015;4(5):341–6.
107. Panageas KS, Iwamoto FM, Cloughesy TF, Aldape KD, Rivera AL, Eichler AF, et al. Initial treatment patterns over time for anaplastic oligodendroglial tumors. Neuro-oncology. 2012;14 (6):761–7. PubMed PMID: 22661585. Pubmed Central PMCID: 3367843.
108. Waitkus MS, Diplas BH, Yan H. Isocitrate dehydrogenase mutations in gliomas. Neuro-oncology. 2016 ;18(1):16–26. PubMed PMID: 26188014. Pubmed Central PMCID: 4677412.
109. Sasaki M, Knobbe CB, Itsumi M, Elia AJ, Harris IS, Chio, II, et al. D-2-hydroxyglutarate produced by mutant IDH1 perturbs collagen maturation and basement membrane function. Genes Dev. 2012;26(18):2038–49. PubMed PMID: 22925884. Pubmed Central PMCID: 3444730.
110. Chowdhury R, Yeoh KK, Tian YM, Hillringhaus L, Bagg EA, Rose NR, et al. The oncometabolite 2-hydroxyglutarate inhibits histone lysine demethylases. EMBO reports. 2011;12(5):463–9. PubMed PMID: 21460794. Pubmed Central PMCID: 3090014.
111. Watanabe T, Nobusawa S, Kleihues P, Ohgaki H. IDH1 mutations are early events in the development of astrocytomas and oligodendrogliomas. Am J Pathol. 2009;174(4):1149–53. PubMed PMID: 19246647. Pubmed Central PMCID: 2671348.
112. Lai A, Kharbanda S, Pope WB, Tran A, Solis OE, Peale F, et al. Evidence for sequenced molecular evolution of IDH1 mutant glioblastoma from a distinct cell of origin. J Clinical Oncol:Official J Am Soc Clini Oncol. 2011;29(34):4482-90. PubMed PMID: 22025148. Pubmed Central PMCID: 3236649.
113. Dang L, White DW, Gross S, Bennett BD, Bittinger MA, Driggers EM, et al. Cancer-associated IDH1 mutations produce 2-hydroxyglutarate. Nature. 2010;465(7300):966. PubMed PMID: 20559394. Pubmed Central PMCID: 3766976.
114. Chen R, Nishimura MC, Kharbanda S, Peale F, Deng Y, Daemen A, et al. Hominoid-specific enzyme GLUD2 promotes growth of IDH1R132H glioma. Proc Nat Acad Sci United States of Am. 2014;111(39):14217–22. PubMed PMID: 25225364. Pubmed Central PMCID: 4191757.
115. Seltzer MJ, Bennett BD, Joshi AD, Gao P, Thomas AG, Ferraris DV, et al. Inhibition of glutaminase preferentially slows growth of glioma cells with mutant IDH1. Cancer Res. 2010;70 (22):8981–7. PubMed PMID: 21045145. Pubmed Central PMCID: 3058858.
116. Popovici-Muller J, Saunders JO, Salituro FG, Travins JM, Yan S, Zhao F, et al. Discovery of the first potent inhibitors of mutant IDH1 that lower tumor 2-HG in Vivo. ACS Med Chem Lett. 2012;3 (10):850–5. PubMed PMID: 24900389. Pubmed Central PMCID: 4025665.
117. Wang F, Travins J, DeLaBarre B, Penard-Lacronique V, Schalm S, Hansen E, et al. Targeted inhibition of mutant IDH2 in leukemia cells induces cellular differentiation. Science. 2013;340(6132): 622–6.
118. Schumacher T, Bunse L, Pusch S, Sahm F, Wiestler B, Quandt J, et al. A vaccine targeting mutant IDH1 induces antitumour immunity. Nature. 2014;512(7514):324–7.
119. Choi C, Ganji SK, DeBerardinis RJ, Hatanpaa KJ, Rakheja D, Kovacs Z, et al. 2-hydroxyglutarate detection by magnetic resonance spectroscopy in IDH-mutated patients with gliomas. Nature Med. 2012;18(4):624–9. PubMed PMID: 22281806. Pubmed Central PMCID: 3615719.
120. Elkhaled A, Jalbert LE, Phillips JJ, Yoshihara HA, Parvataneni R, Srinivasan R, et al. Magnetic resonance of 2-hydroxyglutarate in IDH1-mutated low-grade gliomas. Sci Transl Med. 2012;4 (116):116ra5. PubMed PMID: 22238333. Pubmed Central PMCID:

18 Glioblastoma

Hans-Georg Wirsching and Michael Weller

Epidemiology

Incidence and Survival

Approximately half of all malignant primary brain tumors are glioblastomas (46.1%), but compared to other cancer entities, the annual incidence of 3.2 per 100,000 is low [1]. For example, in the USA, 172 per 100,000 women per year are diagnosed with breast cancer [1], and the estimated incidence proportion of brain metastases in women with breast cancer lies around 5.1% [2]. Males are affected 1.6-fold more often than females, and Whites are affected approximately 2-fold more often than Blacks, but no major geographical differences in the distribution of new diagnoses of glioblastoma have been reported [1]. Age-adjusted annual incidence rates of glioblastoma increase with age to peak at 15.2 per 100,000 in patients aged 75–84 [1].

The median age at diagnosis is 64 and survival rates decrease with age (Fig. 18.1). Approximately one-third of children and adolescents with glioblastoma survive for two years, as opposed to only 3.3% of patients aged 75 or older [1]. Despite the better prognosis of younger glioblastoma patients, no curative therapies exist for either old or young patients. Patients aged 65–70 years or older are underrepresented or have even been excluded from most clinical trials in glioblastoma patients due to their particularly poor prognosis and concerns of dropouts from long-lasting therapy regimens due to general health impairment. In reverse, these limitations prompted several clinical trials designed to overcome these limitations by the implementation of simplified and shorter therapy regimens in elderly patients [3], as discussed further below.

Endogenous Risk Factors

The cell of origin of glioblastoma is thought to be a neural stem cell (Box 18.1), but risk factors yielding malignant transformation of these cells remain largely elusive. Endogenous risk factors for glioblastoma other than age include a small minority of below 1% of glioblastomas that arise in patients with hereditary cancer syndromes, such as the Li-Fraumeni syndrome commonly caused by mutations in the tumor suppressor gene *TP53*, neurofibromatosis types I and II caused by mutations in the *NF1* and *NF2* genes, or the Turcot syndrome caused by mutations in the DNA repair gene *APC* [4, 5]. Glioblastomas in these mostly young patients are usually preceded by the diagnosis of World Health Organization (WHO) grade II or III gliomas. Families with more than one family member affected by

H.-G. Wirsching · M. Weller (✉)
Department of Neurology, University Hospital Zurich, Frauenklinikstrasse 26, 8091 Zurich, Switzerland
e-mail: michael.weller@usz.ch

H.-G. Wirsching
e-mail: hans-georg.wirsching@usz.ch

J. Moliterno Günel et al. (eds.), *Malignant Brain Tumors*,
DOI 10.1007/978-3-319-49864-5_18

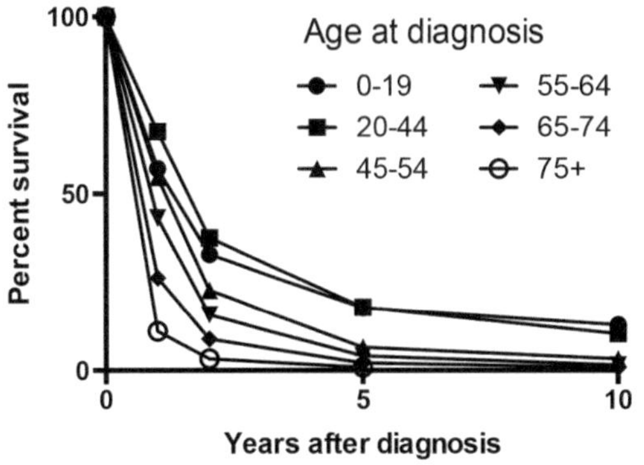

Fig. 18.1 Survival rates of glioblastoma patients by age groups [1]

glioblastoma are rare, thus challenging the search for susceptibility gene loci. Although a twofold risk for glioma has been reported in first-degree relatives of affected individuals [6], the familial risk association is low in consideration of the low overall glioma risk. Consequently, no high penetrance gene variants associated with glioma risk have been identified by genome-wide linkage studies among family members [7, 8]. Population-based genome-wide association studies identified five single nucleotide polymorphism (SNP) risk alleles for gliomagenesis in four genes: *TP53* (odds ratio [OR] 2.70, allele frequency [AF] 0.01), *EGFR* (2 risk alleles: OR 1.20 and 1.25, AF 0.28 and 0.83), *TERT* (OR 1.35, AF 0.50), and *RTEL1* (OR 1.40, AF 0.75) [9]. Of these, *TERT* and *RTEL1* are both involved in the maintenance of telomeres and the identified risk alleles are strongly associated with older age at diagnosis and histological classification as glioblastoma [10]. These studies indicate that a distinct telomerase-associated pathomechanism is associated with the development of glioblastomas in elderly patients. The low penetrance of any risk alleles suggests that the pathophysiology of gliomas follows polygenic patterns and that these patterns follow distinct evolutionary sequences [11, 12], as discussed in more detail in Chap. 2.

Box 18.1. The Cell of Origin of Glioblastomas

The brain is the micro-anatomically by far most complex organ of the human body. Its composition of hundreds of different cell types poses the question of the cell of origin of glioblastomas. DNA is most sensitive to mutational stress during replication, but most brain cells enter a definite post-mitotic state until adulthood. A small pool of brain cells termed neural stem and progenitor cells (NSPC) retains the ability to replicate which may play a role in learning and memory as well as tissue repair after injury. Consequently, NSPC have been suggested as the most likely origin of glioblastomas [13]. In adults, NSPC have been identified in the subventricular zones lining the lateral ventricles [14], in the subcortical white matter [15] and in the hippocampi of the temporal lobes [16]. In line with the hypothesis that NSPC are the cells of origin in gliomagenesis, the majority of adult gliomas arise in supratentorial brain areas that harbor NSPC, particularly in the frontal (25.8%), temporal (19.7%), and parietal (12.2%) lobes, contrasted by lower frequencies of gliomas arising from the spinal chord (4.3%), brainstem (4.2%), cerebellum (2.9%), or occipital lobe (3.2%) [17].

Atopic disease is an endogenous factor that is associated with reduced risk for gliomas. A risk reduction by approximately 40% has been determined in a meta-analysis of 3450 patients diagnosed with glioma from eight observational studies [18]. Analyses of 911 immune function genes in germ line DNA of 1054 glioblastoma patients and 2384 controls revealed an association of glioblastoma with the *IL2-RA* gene encoding the regulatory T-cell (T-reg) marker CD25 [19]. The physiologic function of T-regs is to limit T-cell responses and thereby prevent autoimmunity, and lower T-reg levels are observed in patients with atopic disease. In contrast, in preclinical glioblastoma models higher frequencies of T-regs decrease survival and contribute to the immunosuppressive microenvironment that prevents immunologic antitumor responses [20, 21]. The challenges that T-reg and other immunosuppressants pose to upcoming immunotherapy approaches against gliomas are discussed in more detail in Chap. 12.

Exogenous Risk Factors

Exogenous risk factors for the development of glioblastomas are widely elusive. No association with exposure to cancerogenic agents or smoking has been reported. Risk associations of brain cancer and gliomas with ionizing irradiation have been studied, but data on the more specific association with glioblastoma have not been reported. In a cohort of 105,427 atomic bomb survivors including 56 patients with gliomas, a linear dose–risk relationship with an excess relative risk (ERR) of 0.56/Gy (95% confidence interval [CI] -0.2-2.0) has been reported for gliomas at moderate dose levels with a time lag of more than 15 years, and this relationship was less pronounced with increasing age at exposure [22]. In a population-based study in 14,361 long-term survivors of childhood primary brain tumors, high-dose irradiation (30–44.9 Gy) yielded an excess absolute risk of 19.3 per 10,000 patient years for the diagnosis of gliomas ($N = 40$, including 10 glioblastomas) [23]. A third population-based study investigated the long-term risk for brain tumors during a median follow-up period of 40 years after radiotherapy of the skull. A total of 10,834 patients were treated for tinea capitis during childhood with up to 6 Gy. Comparison with 5392 siblings as well as a matched population group yielded an ERR of 2.6 (95% CI 0.8–8.6) for any gliomas and the ERR for "high grade gliomas," referring to anaplastic gliomas or glioblastomas, followed linear kinetics at 1.98/Gy (95% CI 0.73–4.69) [24, 25]. Doses of diagnostic computed tomography (CT) scans of the brain reach doses in the range of 30–40 mGy and should be considered too low to increase glioma risk, but recent epidemiology studies with a maximum follow-up in the range of 20 years suggest that the relatively higher biological activity of low-energy x-radiation from CT scans may yet yield relevant effects: In a population-based study among 176,587 children receiving diagnostic CT scans, the ERR for gliomas was 0.019/mGy [26] and a case–control study reported an increased risk for gliomas among patients with a positive family history for any cancer that received >3 repeat CT scans (OR 3.74, 95% CI 1.24–11.28) [27]. A third population-based study in 11 million people in Australia including 680,000 children and adolescents exposed to diagnostic CT scans defined an incidence rate ratio of 2.44 (95% CI 2.12–2.81) for brain cancer based on 210 patients exposed to brain CT that suffered from brain cancer subsequently and these values decreased with increasing age at first exposure [28], but the specific risk for glioblastoma was not reported.

The spread of mobile phone use at the end of the 1990s prompted extensive studies of brain tumor risk, but no definite association of mobile phone use with gliomagenesis has been reported [9, 29]. Occupational exposure to extremely low-frequency electric fields was studied over decades, including one study following 20,141 Swiss railway workers for 30 years [30] and one Dutch study following 120,852 people with high exposure to electric fields for 17 years [31], but no association with lifetime risk for glioblastoma or other brain cancers was observed. The INTEROCC study including 2054 glioma cases and 5601 controls likewise reported no association of exposure to extremely low-frequency electric fields with lifetime glioma risk, but there was an association of glioma risk with exposure 1–4 years prior to diagnosis [32].

Viral oncogenesis and particularly an oncogenetic or oncomodulatory role for cytomegalovirus (CMV) in gliomagenesis have been postulated, because some of the CMV gene products interact with glioblastoma core signaling pathways, but experimental evidence to confirm this role for CMV is scarce [33, 34].

Screening and Prevention

Biomarkers for detecting glioblastomas in a systematic screening program are not established and concerns exist about the wide use of magnetic resonance imaging (MRI), because detection of incidental imaging changes of unclear clinical significance may yield unnecessary operations [35]. Low incidence rates of glioblastomas would yield high rates of false-positive MRI lesions, whereas rapid growth renders the time window for detection in the range of a few weeks to months [36]. The recent identification of single nucleotide polymorphism (SNP) risk alleles sheds light on the perspective of a genetic blood test to estimate glioblastoma risk [36]. Such a test would be less resource-intense than MRI and could preselect high-risk patients for MRI to reduce the rate of false-positive MRI, but clinical risk factors that could add to such a genetic risk assessment are elusive, thus disabling preventive measures [36]. Detection of smaller tumors facilitates safe resection and thereby improves outcome in selected study populations [37–39], but, finally, there is a lack of evidence to support the notion that earlier detection and earlier treatment of glioblastoma improve outcome.

Diagnosis and Disease Monitoring

Clinical Presentation

Tumor location, epilepsy, and the extent of edema and tissue destruction determine the disease course. Therefore, there is no typical clinical presentation of glioblastoma. Despite the fatal prognosis of glioblastoma, quality of life and cognitive functioning may be preserved or improved by the standard treatment options discussed further below, even in the frail elderly population, but once first-line treatments have failed, decline of quality of life and cognition is usually rapid and may be severe [40–43].

In adults, approximately half of all glioblastomas infiltrate multiple lobes and multifocal growth occurs in approximately 5% [44]. Approximately 20% of all patients with glioblastoma initially present with sensorimotor symptoms, and initial growth in the speech-dominant, i.e., mostly the left hemisphere yields aphasia as the presenting symptom in approximately 5% of glioblastoma patients [45].

Transient aphasia and transient sensorimotor deficits termed Todd's paresis may result from epilepsy, particularly from seizures that evolve from the temporal lobes [46]. Epilepsy precedes the initial diagnosis of glioblastoma in 24–68% of patients and develops in additional 19–38% later during the course of the disease [46–49]. Epilepsy at diagnosis is associated with longer survival, probably because tumors are diagnosed earlier during the disease course, as indicated by an association with smaller tumor size, and because epilepsy is associated with younger age as well as cortical location, thereby yielding good surgical resectability [45, 46]. Anticancer effects of anti-convulsant drugs have been proposed, particularly for valproic acid [50], but pooled analyses of prospectively collected data of 1896 patients from four recent clinical trials do not support this hypothesis [51].

Less than one-third of all patients with glioblastoma initially present with headaches [45], mostly as a result of increased intracranial pressure that typically presents at night or at awakening with a dull character. Other symptoms of increased intracranial pressure including dizziness, fatigue, nausea, vomiting, and neurocognitive slowing may be present at diagnosis. Almost generally, these symptoms evolve during the disease course. Symptoms of increased intracranial pressure may be ameliorated by the use of steroids, typically dexamethasone at up to 12 mg daily as single dose in the morning [52].

Diagnosis of frontal lobe glioblastomas may be delayed, because frontal tumors can mimic psychogenic disorders or may be mistaken for the physiologic aging process by presenting with mood disorders or personality changes. However, survival of patients with frontal lobe glioblastoma is longer compared to patients with glioblastomas arising from the parietal or temporal lobes [53], probably due to an association with favorable prognostic features such as younger age, mutations in the genes encoding isocitrate dehydrogenase (*IDH*) 1 and 2 [54, 55], and higher rates of complete resection of contrast-enhancing tumor [56].

Leptomeningeal dissemination of glioblastoma cells may cause headache and mimic spinal disease such as painful nerve root compression or myelitis. Clinical suspicion and diagnosis of leptomeningeal dissemination are rare and, if at all, usually occur late during the disease course [57], but in one autopsy study 5 of 25 patients had leptomeningeal metastases [58]. Risk factors reported from the few systematic studies on leptomeningeal dissemination in glioblastoma include incomplete or multiple resections, ventricular entry or proximity of the tumor to the ventricular system, younger age, male gender, and gains at the 1p36 chromosomal region [59–63].

Glioblastomas arising from the brain stem typically present with combinations of cranial nerve palsies, dysphagia, or occlusive hydrocephalus. Brain stem glioblastomas are rare in adults, but account for the majority of pediatric glioblastomas [64].

Glioblastomas exhibit a particular tropism to the brain and only few anecdotal cases of distant organ metastases, mostly to lung, pleura, lymph nodes, bone, and liver, have been reported [65]. Consequently, follow-up scans of the entire body are dispensable in glioblastoma patients and transplantation of organs from donors with glioblastoma is per se feasible, because the risk of cancer transmission is minimal [66, 67]. However, organ donation requires sudden intracranial events such as hemorrhage that lead to brain death, or gradual death of intubated patients to enable non-heart-beating organ donation [68], but both modes of death are uncommon in glioblastoma, because patients mostly die as a consequence of gradual decline in a home or hospice setting.

Imaging

New onset neurological symptoms are commonly followed by MRI as part of a neurological work-up. CT may be performed when MRI is not available or not possible, e.g., because of cardiac pacemakers or other metallic implants, or when acute hemorrhage is suspected, but the sensitivity of CT to detect glioblastoma-specific changes is inferior to MRI. On MRI, glioblastomas typically appear as diffuse masses that are characterized by contrast enhancement at the margin that marks disruption of the blood–brain barrier. Furthermore, hypointensity on T2-weighted images at the tumor core marks necrosis, and hyperintensity on T2-weighted and fluid-attenuated inversion recovery (FLAIR) images of the surrounding brain parenchyma is a correlate of edema or non-contrast-enhancing tumor tissue (Fig. 18.2).

Radiographic diagnostics of glioblastoma have been refined by diffusion/perfusion- and

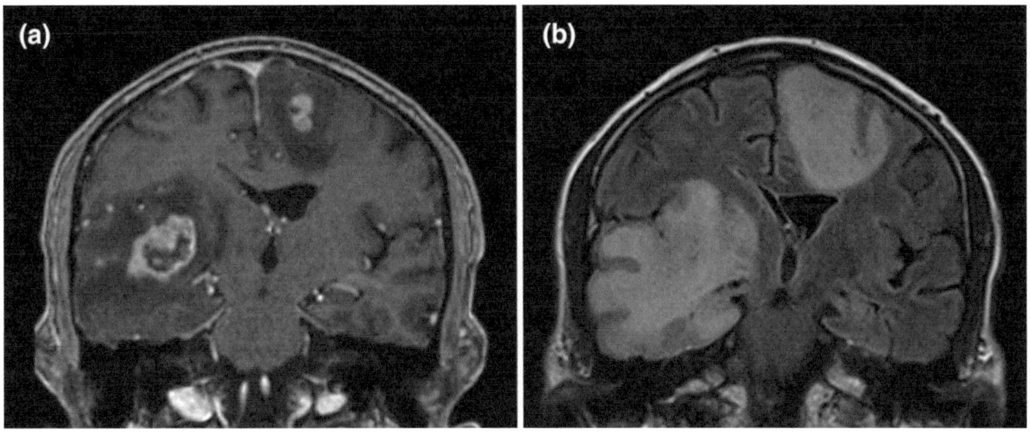

Fig. 18.2 Neuroimaging features of glioblastoma. Magnetic resonance imaging (MRI), T1-weighted gadolinium-enhanced (**a**), fluid-attenuated inversion recovery (FLAIR, **b**).

susceptibility-weighted MRI sequences, T1 contrast subtraction maps, and MR spectroscopy, and tractography or functional MRI has been implemented in many centers to improve maximal safe resection [69]. Overall, advances in imaging technology have improved the discrimination of glioblastoma from other contrast-enhancing lesions such as metastases, from non-brain tumors, primary central nervous system lymphomas, or abscess or inflammatory lesions [70–74]. Detection of the oncometabolite 2-hydroxyglutarate, which is metabolized by mutant isocitrated dehydrogenase (IDH), may enable the diagnosis of IDH-mutated glioblastoma by MR spectroscopy [75]. Positron emission tomography (PET) utilizing amino acid tracers, typically O-(2-[18F]fluoroethyl)-L-tyrosine (FET), is increasingly applied to identify hot spots of increased metabolism and presumably highest tumor grade before biopsies [76]. The developments of imaging technology are discussed in more detail in Chap. 1, but we emphasize that despite these advances, the appearance of glioblastoma on imaging scans can vary considerably, thus making tissue-based diagnosis yet indispensible [77].

Histopathology

The definite diagnosis of glioblastoma is made by histology. Glioblastomas are assigned to the highest grade of the 2007 World Health Organization (WHO) classification of primary brain tumors, i.e., grade IV, which is defined by the presence of necrosis and microvascular proliferation. Other signs of malignancy shared with anaplastic gliomas, which are assigned WHO grade III, include anaplasia, high mitotic rates, and invasiveness [78]. Furthermore, two rare histopathological glioblastoma variants, giant cell glioblastoma and gliosarcoma, have been included as distinct tumor entities in the 2007 WHO classification of primary brain tumors and account for approximately 2% of all WHO grade IV gliomas [78]. Extensive lymphocytic infiltration is present in giant cell glioblastoma, but a putative clinical significance of this feature, e.g., for the application of immunotherapy approaches, is not known. The multinucleated phenotype of giant cell glioblastoma is associated with the loss of *TP53* and high expression levels of aurora B [79]. Giant cell glioblastoma is associated with slightly better prognosis than glioblastoma when adjusting for age, gender, race, tumor size, surgical extent, and radiation therapy use (HR = 0.76, 95% CI 0.59–0.97) [80]. Gliosarcomas may resemble meningiomas macroscopically and are characterized by a prominent mesenchymal metaplastic histological appearance. Extracranial metastases occur more frequently and the prognosis of gliosarcoma is probably slightly worse compared to glioblastoma (HR = 1.17, 95% CI 1.05–1.31) [81].

Recently, overlap of the genomic and epigenetic characteristics of central nervous system primitive neuroectodermal tumors (CNS-PNET) and a distinct molecular glioblastoma subtype that is characterized by point mutations in G34 of histone H3.3 have been identified in a cohort of 81 G34-mutant CNS tumors, thus suggesting that CNS-PNET and G34-mutant glioblastomas comprise a single biological entity [82]. Other histopathologic glioblastoma variants that have been suggested include small cell astrocytoma, fibrillary glioblastoma, and granular cell astrocytoma [83], but the biological significance of these histopathological diagnoses is less clear. Glioblastomas that are preceded by the histological diagnosis of WHO grade II or grade III gliomas are termed secondary glioblastoma, but the molecular marker-based classification of gliomas discussed further below and in more detail in Chap. 2 has widely substituted this terminology and will complement the next edition of the WHO classification of primary brain tumors [36].

Molecular Classification

The evolving landscape of molecular heterogeneity of glioblastoma currently defines at least 7 molecular subtypes based on the integrated analyses of genomic, epigenetic, and gene expression data [12, 54], but treatment concepts that take these molecular classifications into account are yet to be established. It is also of note that the biomarker with the strongest impact on clinical decision making, i.e., hypermethylation of the promoter of the O6-methylguanyl DNA methyltransferase (*MGMT*) gene, was not detected as a distinguishing feature of the molecular glioblastoma subtypes that were identified by unsupervised integrative analyses of (epi-) genome-wide analyses. MGMT is a DNA repair protein that counteracts DNA alkylation by chemotherapy and *MGMT* gene silencing due to promoter methylation predicts benefit from alkylating chemotherapy in glioblastoma [84–87].

Besides *MGMT* testing, a rough dual prognostic categorization of glioblastoma based on the presence of distinct point mutations of *IDH-1* or *-2* has entered clinical practice [36]. *IDH-1* or *-2* mutations are early events during the evolution of glioblastoma that are strongly associated with younger age and longer overall survival, and these glioblastomas commonly evolve from histopathological WHO grade II or grade III gliomas [88, 89]. *IDH* mutations are present in approximately 5–10% of all glioblastomas and are virtually absent in patients aged 65 years or older. The most common *IDH* mutation making up approximately 90% of all *IDH* mutations in glioblastoma is $IDH1^{R132H}$, which can be detected by immunohistochemistry [90], but detection of other *IDH1* or *IDH2* mutations requires gene sequencing.

In 2010, four glioblastoma subtypes termed proneural, neural, classical, and mesenchymal were defined based on the differential expression of 840 genes in 200 glioblastoma samples, and *IDH* mutant glioblastoma was identified as a subgroup of the prognostically favorable proneural gene expression subtype [91]. Subsequent methylome-wide analyses of 210 glioblastoma samples that included 59 pediatric glioblastomas identified six glioblastoma subtypes of which only *IDH* mutant tumors retained the favorable prognosis of the proneural gene expression pattern [54], and these *IDH* mutant glioblastomas can be further subclassified based on a distinct epigenetic pattern designated glioma CpG island methylator phenotype (G-CIMP) [92, 93]. *IDH* mutant glioblastomas that do not exhibit the G-CIMP gene methylation pattern are instead characterized by the activation of cell cycle genes as a result of cyclin-dependent kinase 4 (*CDK4*) gene amplifications and cyclin-dependent kinase inhibitor 2A (*CDKN2A*) gene deletions, and the prognosis of these patients is unfavorable [12]. *IDH* wild-type glioblastomas that cluster with proneural gene expression include two glioblastoma subtypes that affect children and adolescents almost exclusively and that are characterized by G34 and K27 mutations of histone H3 (*H3F3A*). Mutations in *IDH* and *H3F3A* G34 or K27 are mutually exclusive, but share a strong association with mutations in the tumor suppressor gene *TP53* [54]. A third *IDH* wild-type glioblastoma subtype with proneural gene expression and unfavorable prognosis was termed receptor tyrosine kinase (RTK) I and is associated with high expression levels of the gene encoding platelet-derived growth factor receptor alpha (*PDGFRA*) and with gene deletion of *CDKN2A* [54]. The RTKI subtype may occur at any age. Furthermore, two non-proneural subtypes with unfavorable outcome have been defined, and these cluster with (i) the classical gene expression subtype characterized by *EGFR* amplifications and *CDKN2A* deletions (designated RTKII), and (ii) the molecularly more heterogenous mesenchymal gene expression subtype [54].

Other molecular markers in glioblastoma include activating mutations in the promoter region of telomerase reverse transcriptase (*TERT*) and a specific deletion in the ligand-binding domain of *EGFR* designated *EGFRvIII* or *delta-EGFR* yielding ligand-independent receptor activity. *TERT* promoter mutations are associated with older age and particularly poor prognosis in *IDH* wild-type glioblastoma [94, 95]. The *EGFRvIII* deletion is present in approximately half of all RTKII (classical) subtype glioblastomas with *EGFR* amplifications [96] and is thought to confer poor prognosis by interacting with cells that bear amplified wild-type *EGFR* [97], but immunologic targeting of *EGFRvIII* utilizing a peptide vaccine directed against *EGFRvIII* failed to improve survival in the double-blinded phase III trial ACT-IV (NCT01480479). Despite such drawbacks and the fact that treatment choices are not affected by the detailed molecular characterization of individual tumors, the ongoing segregation of glioblastoma subtypes will eventually yield more personalized approaches to improve the outcome of glioblastoma patients, as discussed in more detail in Chap. 3.

Standard First-Line Therapy

Surgery

Tissue for establishing the diagnosis of glioblastoma is indispensible, and therefore, surgery is the first step in the therapeutic cascade for suspected glioblastoma. Complete microsurgical resection of contrast-enhancing tumor (CRET) is the standard of care whenever safely possible, but biopsies are performed in multifocal disease or if major disability upon tumor resection is expected due to tumor location in functionally vulnerable areas of the brain [77]. Biopsies are mostly performed stereotactically, but open biopsies may be preferred in cases where the tumor is well accessible, because a larger amount of tissue can be obtained for molecular diagnostics and because the risk of sampling errors is lower.

Whether surgery for mere reduction of tumor volume rather than aiming at complete resection improves outcome is under debate, because no prospectively collected data support that the higher risk of open surgery compared to stereotactic or open biopsies pays off in terms of overall survival. Various retrospective cohorts do, however, indicate benefit from incomplete tumor resection, including one cohort comprising 500 consecutive patients from a single institution, which identified a threshold of approximately 80% reduction of tumor volume for survival benefit from surgery [38], but such estimates are rarely applied in clinical practice for pragmatic reasons, and all these uncontrolled series have been criticized for major biasses.

In contrast, the therapeutic value of CRET is well documented and clinically applicable for both planning surgery and estimating the patients' postoperative prognosis. In a randomized controlled phase III trial that was designed to assess the value of 5-aminolevulinc acid to improve the extent of resection in 322 patients with suspected anaplastic glioma or glioblastoma, a prespecified stratification by extent of resection demonstrated that CRET improved overall survival compared to patients with residual contrast-enhancing tumor on postoperative MRI (17.9 months [95% CI 14.3–19.4] vs. 12.9 months [95% CI 10.6–14.0]) [39]. CRET was also associated with improved outcome among the 371 elderly patients with anaplastic astrocytoma ($N = 40$) or glioblastoma ($N = 331$) that were treated in the phase III NOA-08 trial. Besides extent of resection, the prespecified survival model controlled for age, histology, *MGMT* promoter status, and study treatment discussed further below, i.e., postoperative radiotherapy or chemotherapy with temozolomide [85]. Means to improve the extent of resection are discussed in more detail in Chaps. 4–6.

Chemoradiotherapy

The standard postoperative therapy regimen for patients with newly diagnosed glioblastoma in good general condition is radiotherapy (30×2 Gy = 60 Gy of the involved field) plus daily concomitant temozolomide at 75 mg/m^2, followed by an interval of approximately 4 weeks without therapy and up to 6 cycles of temozolomide at 150–200 mg/m^2 on 5 out of 28 days [77]. The randomized phase III trial establishing this regimen was a transatlantic cooperative effort of the European Organisation for Research and Treatment of Cancer (EORTC) and the National Cancer Institute of Canada (NCIC) and demonstrated improvement of median overall survival from the adjunct of temozolomide to radiotherapy alone by 2.5 months (hazard ratio [HR] 0.63, 95% CI 0.52–0.75) [98], but benefit from temozolomide among patients without *MGMT* promoter hypermethylation was only marginal [84]. Furthermore, patients aged 66–70 years appeared not to benefit from the adjunct of temozolomide to radiotherapy in post hoc analyses (HR 0.78, 95% CI 0.50–1.25, $p = 0.29$) [99], and patients aged older than 70 years were not included in this trial [98]. The efficacy of combined chemoradiotherapy versus radiotherapy alone in elderly patients with newly diagnosed glioblastoma in good general condition will be defined by the recently completed NCIC CE6 phase III trial (NCT00482677), but to date combined chemoradiotherapy should probably only be considered in fit elderly patients with a methylated MGMT promoter [77]. Furthermore, two phase III trials in 811 patients with newly diagnosed glioblastoma [100] and in 223 patients with recurrent anaplastic astrocytoma or glioblastoma [101], respectively, failed to demonstrate benefit from a dose-intensified temozolomide regimen utilizing 80–100 mg/m^2 on 21 out of 28 days compared to standard temozolomide dosing at 150–200 mg/m^2 on 5 out of 28 days, but more toxicity was observed with the dose-intensified regimen in both trials, thus making dose-escalation strategies obsolete [77].

Therapeutic Approach in Elderly Patients

Radiotherapy

A randomized controlled trial that included 83 patients aged 70 years or older with newly diagnosed glioblastoma ($N = 81$) or anaplastic astrocytoma ($N = 2$) demonstrated that postoperative radiotherapy in elderly patients improves overall survival compared to best supportive care alone (median overall survival: 29.1 vs. 16.9 weeks, $p = 0.002$) without detrimental effects on quality of life or cognition [40], and a population-based retrospective analysis of almost three thousand patients with glioblastoma aged 71–98 years (median age 76.9 years) further supports these results (HR 0.43, 95% CI 0.38–0.49) [102]. In consideration that daily traveling to receive radiotherapy is too much of a burden for some of the sometimes clinically severely affected elderly patients, a randomized trial in 95 patients aged 60 years or older compared the standard radiotherapy regimen (30 × 2 Gy = 60 Gy) with hypofractionated radiotherapy (15 × 2.66 Gy = 40 Gy) and demonstrated comparable activity of both regimens (HR 0.90, 95% CI 0.60–1.35, $p = 0.61$) [41]. The rationale for this study was further underpinned by results from the intention to treat population of the three-armed randomized Nordic trial, which included a standard radiotherapy arm with numerically even inferior survival compared to a hypofractionated radiotherapy arm with 10 × 3.4 Gy = 34 Gy (overall survival 7.0 vs. 5.2 months, $p = 0.02$), probably because standard radiotherapy was discontinued prematurely by 22 of 94 patients, compared to only 2 of 119 patients who discontinued hypofractionated radiotherapy [86].

Chemotherapy

Two randomized phase III trials, the Nordic trial and the NOA-08 trial, established postoperative chemotherapy with temozolomide as an alternative to radiotherapy in elderly glioblastoma patients with hypermethylation of the *MGMT* promoter [85, 86]. The NOA-08 trial randomized 412 patients aged 65 years or older with primary diagnosis of glioblastoma or anaplastic astrocytoma, out of which 373 patients received at least one dose of standard radiotherapy or temozolomide at a dose-dense schedule of 100 mg/m^2 given on days 1–7 every other week (1 week on/1 week off) to be included in efficacy analyses and demonstrated non-inferiority of temozolomide to standard radiotherapy after adjustment for histological diagnosis, extent of resection, age, and *MGMT* promoter methylation status (HR 1.09, 95% CI 0.84–1.42) [85]. The Nordic trial randomized 342 patients aged 60 years or older with primary diagnosis of glioblastoma to receive one of two radiotherapy regimens or temozolomide dosed at 150–200 mg/m^2 on 5 out of 28 days. Survival analyses of the intention to treat population demonstrated similar efficacy of temozolomide ($N = 93$) versus hypofractionated radiotherapy ($N = 98$) (HR 0.82, 96% CI 0.63–

1.06) after adjustment for age, type of surgery (biopsy versus resection), and WHO performance score [86]. In consideration that dose-intensified temozolomide regimens yield higher toxicity at similar efficacy in glioblastoma (see above), temozolomide at 150–200 mg/m^2 on 5 of 28 days is the standard dosing regimen that should be applied in patients with newly diagnosed or recurrent glioblastoma [77].

Management at Recurrence

To date, no standard of care has been defined for recurrent glioblastoma [77] and treatment options are overall limited [103]. The choice of treatment depends not only on previously administered therapies, but is substantially influenced by tumor characteristics, availability, and local preferences. The efficacy of any established treatments for recurrent glioblastoma is modest, particularly in consideration that patients recruited to randomized controlled trials for recurrent glioblastoma comprise a preselected population with more favorable prognosis, excluding a substantial fraction of patients that are already heavily impaired at first progression. Therefore, best supportive care focusing on the amelioration of symptoms including psycho-oncological interventions may be adequate in many patients already at first progression [77].

Disease Monitoring

MRI, typically performed every 2–3 months, is the standard method for the diagnosis of recurrent disease. Unimodal response assessment based on contrast enhancement was the standard for almost two decades [104], but pseudoresponse, i.e., rapid normalization of contrast enhancement under anti-angiogenic treatment, and pseudoprogression, i.e., an increase in size of contrast-enhancing lesions after radiotherapy, challenge MRI-based response assessment in glioblastoma [105]. Therefore, multidimensional criteria defined by the Response Assessment in Neuro-Oncology (RANO) working group, which incorporate time and type of treatment, T2/FLAIR, corticosteroid use, and clinical characteristics, have been widely adopted [106] and emphasize the requirement of interdisciplinary boards for treatment decisions in glioblastoma patients (Chap. 1). More recent developments suggest that O-(2-[18F]fluoroethyl)-L-tyrosine positron emission tomography (FET-PET) may overcome some of the limitations of MRI [107–109], but FET-PET is not part of the standard work-up of glioblastoma.

Surgery

The role of repeat surgery is under debate because of a lack of randomized controlled clinical trials, availability of subgroup analyses of only few prospectively collected datasets, and high probability of selection bias for surgery among patients included in retrospective analyses. The largest available dataset was derived from a prospective registry study including 764 patients with glioblastoma diagnosed and treated 2004–2010, among which repeat surgery was performed in approximately one-third of patients. No association of repeat surgery with overall survival was noted in this cohort (HR 1.02, 95% CI 0.77–1.34) [110]. Similarly, a pooled analysis of 300 patients with recurrent glioblastoma treated in 8 phase I and II trials conducted by the EORTC brain tumor group found no association of repeat surgery with survival [111]. However, no stratified analyses and annotation of clinical predictors of survival, additional therapies or tumor volume were included in these reports.

The randomized controlled DIRECTOR trial, designed to explore the efficacy of two different dose-intensified temozolomide regimens at primary recurrence after standard first-line chemoradiotherapy, included 72 out of 105 randomized patients that underwent surgery at primary recurrence in 16 neurosurgical centers. No difference in the efficacy of both temozolomide regimens at recurrence was noted, thus providing a homogenous cohort that was well suited for the assessment of potential benefit from neurosurgery in subgroups of patients in a well-controlled setting [87]. In line with previous prospective datasets, surgery per se was not linked to improved post-recurrence survival ($P = 0.633$). However, post-recurrence survival was almost twofold longer in patients with complete resection of contrast-enhancing tumor (12.9 months, 95% CI 11.5–18.2), compared to patients with incomplete tumor resection (6.5 months, 95% CI 3.6–9.9), yielding a hazard ratio of 0.42 (95% CI 0.21–0.85) in a survival model adjusting for age, *MGMT* promoter methylation status, Karnofsky performance score (KPS), and steroid use at study entry. Despite the relatively small number of patients included in this trial, a strong trend toward inferior outcome upon incomplete resection became apparent, compared to patients not undergoing surgery (6.5 vs. 9.8 months, $P = 0.052$), thus indicating that repeat surgery should only be offered to patients where total resection of contrast-enhancing tumor seems possible [112]. Validation of these results may be achieved by the phase II RESURGE trial, which will randomize a total of 120 patients with recurrent glioblastoma in which complete resection of contrast-enhancing tumor is deemed safely feasible to receive surgery prior to systemic therapy, or systemic therapy alone (NCT02394626). Generally, tumor resections should be followed by systemic therapies, because infiltrating tumor cells beyond the radiographic tumor margin will generally remain and can drive tumor progression rapidly.

Radiotherapy

Elderly patients with *MGMT* methylated glioblastoma do commonly not receive first-line radiotherapy, and therefore, hypofractionated radiotherapy is the first-choice treatment at recurrence in this population [77]. The role of repeat radiotherapy in the remainder population of glioblastoma patients is less clear, because randomized controlled trials are lacking and due to the risk of iatrogenic harm from radiation necrosis. Reports from retrospective data analyses and uncontrolled trials suggest some activity of repeat radiotherapy in glioblastoma, particularly in patients with smaller tumor volumes, younger age, better general condition, and an interval of at least 6–12 months after first radiotherapy [113–115]. Typical dosing schedules that have been used are in the range of 30–36 Gy in 2–3.5 Gy fractions, usually applied as stereotactic radiotherapy. Hypofractionated regimens are also used. Radiosurgery and proton irradiation are rarely performed in glioblastoma, in part because the high precision of dose application that is the key characteristic of these techniques does not match the requirements of a diffusely infiltrating disease process.

The combination of repeat radiotherapy with alkylating or anti-angiogenic agents is supported by little or no evidence [103]. Novel agents continue to be explored. In a phase II trial of 91 patients with recurrent glioblastoma randomized in a 2:1 fashion to receive either repeat radiotherapy in combination with a fusion protein designed to target the cell surface death receptor CD95 (APG101), or repeat radiotherapy alone, the adjunct of APG101 showed a strong trend toward prolonged post-recurrence survival when adjusting for tumor size (HR 0.60, 95% CI 0.36–1.01), and hypomethylation in the promoter region of the gene encoding the CD95 ligand *CD95L* was associated with improved response to APG101 (HR 0.19, 95% CI 0.06–0.58) [116]. Whether the drug will be further developed remains uncertain.

Chemotherapy

Most patients are treated with single agent systemic treatments at recurrence of glioblastoma. Options that are usually well tolerated include CCNU/lomustine, temozolomide, and bevacizumab [117]. The alkylating agent lomustine is commonly utilized as a control in clinical trials for recurrent glioblastoma. Oral administration at longer time intervals (90–110 mg/m^2 every 6 weeks) is advantageous in patients with impaired general condition, but progression-free survival rates at 6 months do not exceed 19–25%

in clinical trial populations [118, 119]. Re-challenge with temozolomide is associated with longer post-recurrence survival, particularly in patients with apparent benefit from first-line temozolomide after a temozolomide-free interval [120]. Such patients bare mostly tumors with hypermethylation of the *MGMT* promoter [84, 87]. As outlined in the above section on first-line chemotherapy, dose-intensified temozolomide regimens are obsolete since more toxicity, but no survival difference was noted in two phase III trials directly comparing standard and dose-intensified temozolomide regimens in newly diagnosed and recurrent glioblastoma [100, 101]. Alternative chemotherapy agents such as procarbazine and carboplatin have also been used in the treatment of patients with recurrent glioblastoma, but no randomized data are available to support the efficacy of these approaches, whereas severe adverse effects can accompany their application. Systemic approaches to recurrent glioblastoma that are still under debate are discussed further below.

Molecularly Targeted Therapies and Future Directions

The histology-based definition of glioblastoma of the WHO classification of 2007 [78] has been increasingly complemented by the assessment of molecular markers, including *IDH*, *MGMT* and *TERT* status, as discussed in more detail in Chaps. 2 and 3. In prospect of a more personalized treatment of glioblastoma, molecular markers will be included in the revised WHO classification of 2016. However, a major challenge of decoding mechanisms of resistance is posed by temporal and intratumoral heterogeneity [121, 122]. Tumor progression and particularly failure of initially effective therapy regimens are accompanied by molecular adaptions due to clonal selection, acquisition of additional genomic alterations, epigenetic adaptions, and alterations in gene expression. For example, temozolomide chemotherapy can induce a hypermutation phenotype [123], and radiotherapy of proneural glioblastoma can induce rapid changes toward a mesenchymal gene expression pattern [124]. Yet, compared to the profound molecular landscapes generated of newly diagnosed glioblastoma, knowledge of the molecular patterns that underly glioblastoma progression and therapy resistance is only marginal and requires further joint efforts of the scientific community in order to develop effective molecularly targeted therapeutic approaches with durable efficacy.

Targeting Aberrant Signaling Pathways

Initial molecularly targeted treatments of glioblastoma and other cancers utilized small molecules to inhibit aberrant signaling pathways. RTK are the key mediators of extracellular signal transduction in glioblastoma, as outlined in more detail in Chap. 9.

RTK contain an extracellular receptor domain, which induces a conformational change upon ligand binding to initiate intracellular adenosine-triphosphate (ATP)-dependent tyrosine phosphorylation signals. The biological functions of RTK overlap widely and the convergence of downstream signals as well as crucial roles of RTK in healthy tissues complicate the development of tumor-specific RTK inhibition. However, the RTK inhibitor imatinib, designed to specifically fit the ATP-binding pouch of a cancer-specific tyrosine kinase derived from the *BCR-ABL* fusion gene, was found to offer a well tolerated, highly effective treatment for chronic myeloic leukemia [125]. This provided the incentive to develop personalized drug treatment, in particular RTK inhibition, in many cancers including glioblastoma.

Small molecule inhibitors of the RTK EGFR yielded disappointing results in glioblastoma, but *EGFR* amplification was not monitored in these trials, and blood–brain barrier penetration of all tested compounds was suboptimal [126].

Inhibition of the downstream RTK convergence molecule mammalian target of rapamycine (mTOR) utilizing temsirolimus (CCI-779) raised expectations in an uncontrolled phase II trial of

65 patients with recurrent glioblastoma: The radiographic response rate was 36% and high levels of phosphorylation of the mTOR target S6-kinase was associated with radiographic response and improved survival upon treatment with temsirolimus [127]. However, these results were not followed by a controlled trial to further explore the efficacy of temsirolimus in recurrent glioblastoma and a more recent randomized controlled phase II study of temsirolimus as an adjunct to standard chemoradiotherapy in patients with newly diagnosed, *MGMT* unmethylated glioblastoma failed to demonstrate improved survival (HR 1.16, 95% CI 0.77–1.76) [128].

A simple but key lesson from these and other clinical trials in the early days of personalized medicine for glioblastoma is the importance of a preselection of patients based on biomarker profiles that support the rationale of the tested targeted therapies. Several ongoing clinical trials utilizing small molecules to inhibit aberrant signaling in glioblastoma apply such molecular entry controls. Examples include the assessment of rare activating fibroblast growth factor receptor (FGFR) mutations and fusion proteins prior to inclusion in an uncontrolled phase II trial that assesses the safety of an FGFR-inhibitor in newly diagnosed glioblastoma (NCT01975701), or early-phase trials exploring the inhibition of the RTK signaling convergence molecule phosphatidyl inositol 3-kinase (PI3K) alone or in combination with different anti-angiogenic agents in patients with recurrent glioblastoma (NCT01339052, NCT01870726, NCT01349660).

Anti-angiogenic Therapy

Microvascular proliferation is one of the defining histopathological features of glioblastoma [78]. The concept of cutting off nutrient supply by targeting angiogenesis appeared reasonable and was intensely studied. The vascular endothelial growth factor (VEGF) is a key driver of angiogenesis in glioblastoma and other cancers and is therefore one of the most intensely studied molecules in cancer research [129–132].

The anti-angiogenic monoclonal antibody bevacizumab, commonly dosed at 10 mg/kg bodyweight, i.e., every other week, directly binds to VEGF and thereby inhibits its signaling. Severe complications associated with the administration of bevacizumab are rare and include thromboembolic events, complications of wound heeling, hemorrhage, congestive heart failure, and gastrointestinal perforations. Arterial hypertension from bevacizumab is more common and usually well manageable with common antihypertensive drugs. Overall, bevacizumab is well tolerated without significant side effects by the vast majority of patients.

Bevacizumab obtained accelerated, conditional approval for the treatment of recurrent glioblastoma by the United States Food and Drug Administration (FDA) and in various other countries. However, approval was based on durable objective response rates observed in two uncontrolled phase II trials [133, 134] in an era when radiographic pseudoresponse, i.e., the reduction of contrast enhancement due to blood vessel normalization, was not yet taken into account as a radiographic phenomenon under anti-angiogenic therapy that does not reflect tumor volume (for details, refer to Chaps. 1 and 11). More recently, the open label phase III EORTC 26101 trial randomized 437 patients with first recurrence of glioblastoma in a 2:1 fashion to receive a combination of lomustine plus bevacizumab ($N = 288$) versus lomustine alone ($N = 149$), and there was no post-recurrence survival benefit for the adjunct of bevacizumab (HR 0.95, 95% CI 0.74–1.21) despite promising gain in progression-free survival (HR 0.49, 95% CI 0.39–0.61) [135]. These data are in line with two phase III trials utilizing the small molecule inhibitors of VEGF signaling cediranib and enzastaurin, which failed to improve post-recurrence survival compared to lomustine, too [118, 119]. Furthermore, the EORTC 26101 trial rebutted results of the non-comparative randomized phase II BELOB trial, which suggested an overall survival benefit from the combination of lomustine plus bevacizumab compared to either lomustine or bevacizumab alone (median post-recurrence survival: 12 vs. 8 vs. 8 months) [136]. Thus, the conditional approval of bevacizumab for recurrent glioblastoma in some parts of the world is under debate and currently opposed only by the clinical experience of subjective benefit of sometimes heavily impaired patients.

In contrast to recurrent glioblastoma, bevacizumab is not FDA approved for the treatment of newly diagnosed glioblastoma. Two placebo-controlled phase III trials evaluating the adjunct of bevacizumab to standard first-line chemoradiotherapy (RTOG 0825 and AVAglio) noted no overall survival benefit despite prolonged progression-free survival [137, 138]. The RTOG 0825 trial even reported neurocognitive decline and stronger impairment of quality of life with the adjunct of bevacizumab [137], but this may reflect a lack of measures to detect pseudoresponse: Radiologic progression in the RTOG 0825 trial was defined based on contrast enhancement and could therefore have missed early tumor progression, and these patients could have distorted measures of quality of life and neurocognition [129]. The RANO criteria, outlined in more detail in the above section on disease monitoring and in Chap. 1, take pseudoresponse into account [106] and were applied in the AVAglio trial, which noted preserved general condition and quality of life as well as less corticosteroid use as additional benefits from bevacizumab [138]. Improved overall survival with the adjunct of bevacizumab to standard chemoradiotherapy was reported from subgroup analyses of the AVAglio trial for patients with *IDH* wild-type tumors that clustered with the proneural gene expression pattern in a survival model controlling for age, corticosteroid use, extent of resection, general condition, *MGMT*, cognitive functioning, and gender (HR 0.42, 95% CI 0.25–0.71) [139].

Despite this promising subgroup analysis, further efficacy studies of anti-angiogenic treatments in glioblastoma became unlikely after a series of three negative phase III trials in newly diagnosed glioblastoma and three negative phase III trials in recurrent glioblastoma (Table 18.1). Overall, the available evidence is unlikely to maintain the conditional approval of bevacizumab in recurrent glioblastoma and does indeed not support the administration of anti-angiogenic therapies as first-line therapy or at recurrence, but there is some rational for the coadministration of anti-angiogenic agents to improve effects of immunotherapy, as discussed in Chaps. 11 and 12.

Immunotherapy

The drainage of brain lymphatic vessels to cervical lymph nodes connects the brain directly to cellular immunity [140]. Lymphocytes readily cross the blood–brain barrier in the healthy brain and in various central nervous system diseases including glioblastoma [141], but local immunosuppression is a hallmark of cancer that prevents clearance of tumor cells by the immune system [142]. Attempts to overcome immunosuppression and reprogram the cellular immune system to specifically attack glioblastoma cells include (i) drugs that target specific T-cell receptors to overcome inhibitory signals, (ii) transfer of T cells that were boosted in vitro or that were genetically engineered to target tumor cells with high avidity, or to activate T cells, and (iii) the so-called tumor vaccines, i.e., peptides or antigen-presenting cells pre-exposed to peptides utilized to boost an antitumor immune response [141]. The molecular background of these immunotherapy approaches is discussed in more detail in Chap. 12.

The activation of cellular immune responses utilizing monoclonal antibodies that are directed against T-cell receptors that mediate immunosuppression has translated into clinical practice in the treatment of metastatic melanoma [143–145] and non-small cell lung cancer [146, 147]. Commercially available antibodies that are approved by the FDA and EMA are directed against the programmed death protein (PD)1 (nivolumab, pembrolizumab) or the cytotoxic T-lymphocyte antigen (CTLA) 4 (ipilimumab), but several reagents directed against other immune checkpoint targets such as programmed cell death 1 ligand 1 (PDL1), lymphocyte

Table 18.1 Phase III trials of anti-angiogenic agents in glioblastoma

Trial	Study population	Treatment	Hazard ratio for overall survival (95% confidence interval)	Reference
RTOG 0825	Newly diagnosed glioblastoma	Standard chemoradiotherapy[a] plus bevacizumab 10 mg/kg every 2 weeks versus standard chemoradiotherapy[a] plus placebo	1.13 (0.93–1.37)	Gilbert et al. [137]
AVAglio	Newly diagnosed glioblastoma	Standard chemoradiotherapy[a] plus bevacizumab 10 mg/kg every 2 weeks versus standard chemoradiotherapy[a] plus placebo	0.88 (0.76–1.02)	Chinot et al. [138]
			Proneural *IDH* wild type: 0.43 (0.26–0.73)	Sandman et al. [139]
CENTRIC (EORTC 26071-22072)	Newly diagnosed glioblastoma with *MGMT* promoter hypermethylation	Standard chemoradiotherapy[a] plus cilengitide 2000 mg twice weekly versus standard chemoradiotherapy[a] alone	1.02 (0.81–1.29)	Stupp et al. [166]
EORTC 26101	Recurrent glioblastoma	Lomustine 90 mg/m^2 every 6 weeks plus bevacizumab 10 mg/kg every 2 weeks versus lomustine 110 mg/m^2 every 6 weeks	0.95 (0.74–1.21)	Wick et al. [135]
Enzastaurin versus Lomustine in Glioblastoma	Recurrent glioblastoma	Enzastaurin 500 mg/days versus lomustine 100-130 mg/m^2 every 6 weeks	1.20 (0.88–1.65)	Wick et al. [118]
REGAL	Recurrent glioblastoma	Cediranib 30 mg/days versus cediranib 20 mg/days plus lomustine 110 mg/m^2 every 6 weeks versus lomustine 110 mg/m^2 plus placebo	Cediranib alone versus lomustine alone: 1.05 (0.74–1.50)	Batchelor et al. [119]
			Cediranib plus lomustine versus lomustine alone: 0.76 (0.53–1.08)	

[a]Radiotherapy of the involved field (30 × 2 = 60 Gy) plus daily concomitant temozolomide at 75 mg/m^2, followed by 6 cycles of temozolomide at 150–200 mg/m^2 on 5 of 28 days [98]

activation gene 3 (LAG-3), or killer-cell immunoglobulin-like receptors (KIR) are currently tested in early-phase trials for different cancers, including glioblastoma [148]. The efficacy of nivolumab in recurrent glioblastoma is currently being evaluated in comparison with bevacizumab in the phase III trial CheckMate 143 (NCT02017717, results expected in 2017).

Despite the apparent disruption of the blood–brain barrier in glioblastoma, there are, however, concerns regarding the pharmacokinetics of macromolecules such as monoclonal antibodies. This limitation is circumvented by genetically engineered chimeric antigen receptor T cells, which are reprogrammed to express binding domains of monoclonal antibodies linked to intracellular signaling domains that trigger T-cell activation upon tumor antigen binding [149]. In glioblastoma, a phase I/II trial targeting the tumor-specific antigen of the *EGFRvIII* deletion mutant is exploring this approach (NCT01454596). The tumor-specific *EGFRvIII* peptide sequence was also deemed an ideal target for vaccination, but monthly intradermal injections of the 13-amino-acid peptide rindopepimut, which comprises the EGFRvIII-specific antigen, failed to improve survival in combination with granulocyte–monocyte colony stimulating factor (GM-CSF) as an adjunct to standard chemoradiotherapy in the placebo-controlled, double-blind phase III ACT-IV trial (NCT01480479).

Vaccination against such tumor-specific antigens, i.e., peptide sequences that are present exclusively in tumor cells due to mutations such as *EGFRvIII*, is tempting because in theory non-tumor cells are spared from T-cell responses, but the extent of immune responses is limited when only one stimulatory peptide is utilized. This limitation may be overcome by targeting tumor-associated antigens, i.e., peptide sequences of proteins that are highly, but not specifically expressed by tumor cells. Utilizing tumor-associated antigens enables vaccination against a whole set of antigens that may be adapted depending on the expression profile of single tumors to elicit a more profound immune response, but immune tolerance against such physiologically occurring peptides may limit the T-cell response elicited from vaccination.

Tumor-associated antigens are commonly utilized for in vitro pulsing of antigen-presenting cells. In most clinical trials following this strategy, dendritic cells are isolated from the patients' peripheral blood for this purpose, as is the case in two double-blind phase III clinical trials in newly diagnosed glioblastoma that are currently evaluating the efficacy of autologous dendritic cell therapies as an adjunct to standard chemoradiotherapy: The partially undisclosed DCVax platform technology utilizes the patient's tumor lysate for in vitro dendritic cell pulsing (NCT00045968) and the ICT-107 trial utilizes epitopes from six glioblastoma-associated proteins (NCT02546102). Of note, the ICT-107 trial will include only HLA-A2 positive patients, because in a preceding phase II trial that included 124 patients randomized in a 2:1 fashion to receive ICT-107 or placebo as an adjunct to standard postoperative chemoradiotherapy, benefit appeared to be restricted to HLA-A2 positive patients. Overall, the adjunct of ICT-107 was safe and prolonged progression-free survival for 2.4 months in the per protocol group of this initial ICT-107 phase II trial (HR 0.54, $P = 0.006$) [150]. A similar vaccine consisting of 11 tumor-associated antigens designated IMA950 is currently evaluated for intracutaneous injection in a phase I/II trial of newly diagnosed glioblastoma alongside standard chemotherapy (NCT01403285 and NCT01920191).

Another potential target for adaptive immunotherapy that has evoked an antitumor response in preclinical studies is the tumor-specific epitope of mutant *IDH* [151]. Furthermore, the viral CMV antigen pp65 triggered a dendritic cell-mediated, anti-glioblastoma T-cell response in 12 patients, and the adjunct of tetanus/diphtheria toxoid has facilitated this immune response [152], calling for further exploration. However, clinical trial design is challenged by the fact that reprogrammed immune cells will most likely not suffice to induce a durable response in larger tumors and that cytotoxic therapies and steroids may suppress immune-mediated antitumor responses, thus dampening the expectations posed to ongoing and future immunotherapy approaches [36].

Tumor-Treating Fields

Based on a phase III trial in newly diagnosed glioblastoma, a device for the application of "tumor-treating fields" (TTF) via skin electrodes was proposed as a novel standard of care for newly diagnosed glioblastoma [154]. TTF are 200 kHz alternating electric fields that are supposed to be delivered through the shaved scalp. Trial design, proactive data interpretation and uniformity of benefit from the device throughout subgroups were accompanied by significant skepticism of the scientific community [155]. The place of TTF in clinical practice remains to be defined.

Outlook

Increasing the understanding of the molecular background of glioblastoma has not yet translated into survival benefit. A more thorough patient selection for clinical trials that investigate novel-targeted therapies and combination treatments based on molecular profiles of individual tumors may ultimately yield improved outcome.

However, several issues will need to be addressed in the future, including a more profound understanding of therapy-induced molecular alterations that drive resistance and tumor progression in order to design clinical trials that include combinations that anticipate such escape mechanisms.

Furthermore, the understanding of heterogeneity of glioblastoma on the cellular level must be evolved further. It is of note that the gene expression-based definition of different glioblastoma subtypes also applies to single cells within the same tumor, but the significance of these findings is yet unclear [121]. A subpopulation of cells deemed to mediate resistance to chemo- and radiotherapy was defined based on molecular marker profiles and specific features observed in vitro and upon propagation in the brains of immune-compromised mice [156]. These cells were termed glioblastoma stem cells (Box 18.2) for sharing features with neural stem cells, but the definite identification of such a subpopulation was not achieved by single-cell RNA sequencing in freshly dissected human glioblastomas [121] and attempts to target signaling cascades that are deemed specific for glioblastoma stem cells were disappointing in early clinical trials [157]. Another surprising biological characteristic of glioblastoma is the capability to transduce signals and exchange molecules in between cells even over large distances through membrane protrusions and connexins [158], thereby challenging targeted therapy approaches that aim to interrupt intercellular signaling by neutralizing cytokines or membrane bound receptors, but the actual clinical significance of these findings remains to be determined.

Box 18.2. Glioblastoma Stem Cells

Glioblastoma growth and cellular diversity is driven by similar molecular mechanisms such as embryonic and fetal neurogenesis. The term glioblastoma stem cells (GSC) refers to a subpopulation of glioblastoma cells that share features of neural stem cells and that have the capacity to grow tumors that resemble micro-anatomically the original tumors when transplanted into the brains of immunocompromised mice [159]. Other terms have been applied to GSC, particularly with referral to their stem-like features such as self-renewal and the capacity to differentiate along multiple neuroglial lineages. The existence of GSC has evoked hope for drug development, because a role of GSC in mediating resistance against conventional chemoradiotherapy has been suggested based on preclinical models [160, 161]. Experimental targeting of GSC prolongs survival [162], but therapeutic approaches that aim at targeting GSC have not been successful in clinical trials. Plasticity of glioblastoma cells allows them to switch between a non-GSC and GSC phenotype, probably via a continuum of cellular states [121]. Such cellular states are influenced by the tumor microenvironment and specific anatomical GSC niches promote the GSC phenotype.

Various cell surface markers, including CD44, CD15, CD133, integrin alpha 6, and others, have been utilized to enrich GSC experimentally [156]. However, molecular signatures of the GSC and non-GSC subpopulations are derived from genome-wide microarrays that require the expansion of freshly dissected glioblastoma cells under non-physiologic in vitro conditions that artificially alter gene expression [121] and that select for subpopulations of cells with particular epigenetic [163] and genetic features [164, 165].

Cells that proliferate slowly and subpopulations with low frequencies are likely not characterized with these approaches.

References

1. Ostrom QT, Gittleman H, Fulop J, Liu M, Blanda R, Kromer C, et al. CBTRUS statistical report: primary brain and central nervous system tumors diagnosed in the United States in 2008–2012. Neuro Oncol. 2015;17 Suppl 4:iv1–iv62.
2. Barnholtz-Sloan JS, Sloan AE, Davis FG, Vigneau FD, Lai P, Sawaya RE. Incidence proportions of brain metastases in patients diagnosed (1973 to 2001) in the Metropolitan Detroit Cancer Surveillance System. J Clin Oncol. 2004;22 (14):2865–72.
3. Wirsching HG, Happold C, Roth P, Weller M. Management of diffusely infiltrating glioma in the elderly. Curr Opin Oncol. 2015;27(6):502–9.
4. Ohgaki H, Kim YH, Steinbach JP. Nervous system tumors associated with familial tumor syndromes. Curr Opin Neurol. 2010;23(6):583–91.
5. Goodenberger ML, Jenkins RB. Genetics of adult glioma. Cancer Genet. 2012;205(12):613–21.
6. Hemminki K, Tretli S, Sundquist J, Johannesen TB, Granstrom C. Familial risks in nervous-system tumours: a histology-specific analysis from Sweden and Norway. Lancet Oncol. 2009;10(5):481–8.
7. Shete S, Lau CC, Houlston RS, Claus EB, Barnholtz-Sloan J, Lai R, et al. Genome-wide high-density SNP linkage search for glioma susceptibility loci: results from the Gliogene Consortium. Cancer Res. 2011;71(24):7568–75.
8. Walsh KM, Anderson E, Hansen HM, Decker PA, Kosel ML, Kollmeyer T, et al. Analysis of 60 reported glioma risk SNPs replicates published GWAS findings but fails to replicate associations from published candidate-gene studies. Genet Epidemiol. 2013;37(2):222–8.
9. Ostrom QT, Bauchet L, Davis FG, Deltour I, Fisher JL, Langer CE, et al. The epidemiology of glioma in adults: a "state of the science" review. Neuro Oncol. 2014;16(7):896–913.
10. Walsh KM, Rice T, Decker PA, Kosel ML, Kollmeyer T, Hansen HM, et al. Genetic variants in telomerase-related genes are associated with an older age at diagnosis in glioma patients: evidence for distinct pathways of gliomagenesis. Neuro Oncol. 2013;15(8):1041–7.
11. Ozawa T, Riester M, Cheng YK, Huse JT, Squatrito M, Helmy K, et al. Most human non-GCIMP glioblastoma subtypes evolve from a common proneural-like precursor glioma. Cancer Cell. 2014;26(2):288–300.
12. Ceccarelli M, Barthel FP, Malta TM, Sabedot TS, Salama SR, Murray BA, et al. Molecular profiling reveals biologically discrete subsets and pathways of progression in diffuse glioma. Cell. 2016;164 (3):550–63.
13. Sanai N, Alvarez-Buylla A, Berger MS. Neural stem cells and the origin of gliomas. N Engl J Med. 2005;353(8):811–22.
14. Sanai N, Tramontin AD, Quinones-Hinojosa A, Barbaro NM, Gupta N, Kunwar S, et al. Unique astrocyte ribbon in adult human brain contains neural stem cells but lacks chain migration. Nature. 2004;427(6976):740–4.
15. Nunes MC, Roy NS, Keyoung HM, Goodman RR, McKhann G 2nd, Jiang L, et al. Identification and isolation of multipotential neural progenitor cells from the subcortical white matter of the adult human brain. Nat Med. 2003;9(4):439–47.
16. Eriksson PS, Perfilieva E, Bjork-Eriksson T, Alborn AM, Nordborg C, Peterson DA, et al. Neurogenesis in the adult human hippocampus. Nat Med. 1998;4(11):1313–7.
17. Ostrom QT, Gittleman H, Liao P, Rouse C, Chen Y, Dowling J, et al. CBTRUS statistical report: primary brain and central nervous system tumors diagnosed in the United States in 2007–2011. Neuro Oncol. 2014;16 Suppl 4:iv1–63.
18. Linos E, Raine T, Alonso A, Michaud D. Atopy and risk of brain tumors: a meta-analysis. J Natl Cancer Inst. 2007;99(20):1544–50.
19. Schwartzbaum JA, Xiao Y, Liu Y, Tsavachidis S, Berger MS, Bondy ML, et al. Inherited variation in immune genes and pathways and glioblastoma risk. Carcinogenesis. 2010;31(10):1770–7.
20. Wainwright DA, Balyasnikova IV, Chang AL, Ahmed AU, Moon KS, Auffinger B, et al. IDO expression in brain tumors increases the recruitment of regulatory T cells and negatively impacts survival. Clin Cancer Res: Official J Am Assoc Cancer Res. 2012;18(22):6110–21.
21. Wainwright DA, Chang AL, Dey M, Balyasnikova IV, Kim CK, Tobias A, et al. Durable therapeutic efficacy utilizing combinatorial blockade against IDO, CTLA-4, and PD-L1 in mice with brain tumors. Clin Cancer Res: Official J Am Assoc Cancer Res. 2014;20(20):5290–301.
22. Preston DL, Ron E, Tokuoka S, Funamoto S, Nishi N, Soda M, et al. Solid cancer incidence in atomic bomb survivors: 1958–1998. Radiat Res. 2007;168(1):1–64.
23. Neglia JP, Robison LL, Stovall M, Liu Y, Packer RJ, Hammond S, et al. New primary neoplasms of the central nervous system in survivors of childhood cancer: a report from the Childhood Cancer Survivor Study. J Natl Cancer Inst. 2006;98(21):1528–37.

24. Ron E, Modan B, Boice JD Jr, Alfandary E, Stovall M, Chetrit A, et al. Tumors of the brain and nervous system after radiotherapy in childhood. N Engl J Med. 1988;319(16):1033–9.
25. Sadetzki S, Chetrit A, Freedman L, Stovall M, Modan B, Novikov I. Long-term follow-up for brain tumor development after childhood exposure to ionizing radiation for tinea capitis. Radiat Res. 2005;163(4):424–32.
26. Pearce MS, Salotti JA, Little MP, McHugh K, Lee C, Kim KP, et al. Radiation exposure from CT scans in childhood and subsequent risk of leukaemia and brain tumours: a retrospective cohort study. Lancet. 2012;380(9840):499–505.
27. Davis F, Il'yasova D, Rankin K, McCarthy B, Bigner DD. Medical diagnostic radiation exposures and risk of gliomas. Radiat Res. 2011;175(6):790–6.
28. Mathews JD, Forsythe AV, Brady Z, Butler MW, Goergen SK, Byrnes GB, et al. Cancer risk in 680,000 people exposed to computed tomography scans in childhood or adolescence: data linkage study of 11 million Australians. BMJ. 2013;346: f2360.
29. Interphone Study Group. Brain tumour risk in relation to mobile telephone use: results of the INTERPHONE international case-control study. Int J Epidemiol. 2010;39(3):675–94.
30. Roosli M, Lortscher M, Egger M, Pfluger D, Schreier N, Lortscher E, et al. Leukaemia, brain tumours and exposure to extremely low frequency magnetic fields: cohort study of Swiss railway employees. Occup Environ Med. 2007;64(8):553–9.
31. Koeman T, van den Brandt PA, Slottje P, Schouten LJ, Goldbohm RA, Kromhout H, et al. Occupational extremely low-frequency magnetic field exposure and selected cancer outcomes in a prospective Dutch cohort. Cancer Causes Control. 2014;25(2):203–14.
32. Turner MC, Benke G, Bowman JD, Figuerola J, Fleming S, Hours M, et al. Occupational exposure to extremely low-frequency magnetic fields and brain tumor risks in the INTEROCC study. Cancer Epidemiol Biomark Prev. 2014;23(9):1863–72.
33. Dziurzynski K, Chang SM, Heimberger AB, Kalejta RF, McGregor Dallas SR, Smit M, et al. Consensus on the role of human cytomegalovirus in glioblastoma. Neuro Oncol. 2012;14(3):246–55.
34. Wick W, Platten M. CMV infection and glioma, a highly controversial concept struggling in the clinical arena. Neuro Oncol. 2014;16(3):332–3.
35. Vernooij MW, Ikram MA, Tanghe HL, Vincent AJ, Hofman A, Krestin GP, et al. Incidental findings on brain MRI in the general population. N Engl J Med. 2007;357(18):1821–8.
36. Weller M, Wick W, Aldape K, Brada M, Berger M, Pfister SM, et al. Glioma. Nat Rev Dis Primers. 2015.
37. Stummer W, Reulen HJ, Meinel T, Pichlmeier U, Schumacher W, Tonn JC, et al. Extent of resection and survival in glioblastoma multiforme: identification of and adjustment for bias. Neurosurgery. 2008;62(3):564–76; discussion-76.
38. Sanai N, Polley MY, McDermott MW, Parsa AT, Berger MS. An extent of resection threshold for newly diagnosed glioblastomas. J Neurosurg. 2011;115(1):3–8.
39. Stummer W, Pichlmeier U, Meinel T, Wiestler OD, Zanella F, Reulen HJ, et al. Fluorescence-guided surgery with 5-aminolevulinic acid for resection of malignant glioma: a randomised controlled multicentre phase III trial. Lancet Oncol. 2006;7(5):392–401.
40. Keime-Guibert F, Chinot O, Taillandier L, Cartalat-Carel S, Frenay M, Kantor G, et al. Radiotherapy for glioblastoma in the elderly. N Engl J Med. 2007;356(15):1527–35.
41. Roa W, Brasher PM, Bauman G, Anthes M, Bruera E, Chan A, et al. Abbreviated course of radiation therapy in older patients with glioblastoma multiforme: a prospective randomized clinical trial. J Clin Oncol. 2004;22(9):1583–8.
42. Gallego Perez-Larraya J, Ducray F, Chinot O, Catry-Thomas I, Taillandier L, Guillamo JS, et al. Temozolomide in elderly patients with newly diagnosed glioblastoma and poor performance status: an ANOCEF phase II trial. J Clin Oncol. 2011;29(22):3050–5.
43. Taphoorn MJ, Stupp R, Coens C, Osoba D, Kortmann R, van den Bent MJ, et al. Health-related quality of life in patients with glioblastoma: a randomised controlled trial. Lancet Oncol. 2005;6(12):937–44.
44. Djalilian HR, Shah MV, Hall WA. Radiographic incidence of multicentric malignant gliomas. Surg Neurol. 1999;51(5):554–7; discussion 7–8.
45. Yuile P, Dent O, Cook R, Biggs M, Little N. Survival of glioblastoma patients related to presenting symptoms, brain site and treatment variables. J Clin Neurosci: Official J Neurosurg Soc Australasia. 2006;13(7):747–51.
46. Chaichana KL, Parker SL, Olivi A, Quinones-Hinojosa A. Long-term seizure outcomes in adult patients undergoing primary resection of malignant brain astrocytomas: clinical article. J Neurosurg. 2009;111(2):282–92.
47. Wick W, Menn O, Meisner C, Steinbach J, Hermisson M, Tatagiba M, et al. Pharmacotherapy of epileptic seizures in glioma patients: who, when, why and how long? Onkologie. 2005;28(8–9):391–6.
48. Kerkhof M, Dielemans JC, van Breemen MS, Zwinkels H, Walchenbach R, Taphoorn MJ, et al. Effect of valproic acid on seizure control and on survival in patients with glioblastoma multiforme. Neuro Oncol. 2013;15(7):961–7.
49. van Breemen MS, Rijsman RM, Taphoorn MJ, Walchenbach R, Zwinkels H, Vecht CJ. Efficacy of anti-epileptic drugs in patients with gliomas and seizures. J Neurol. 2009;256(9):1519–26.

50. Weller M, Gorlia T, Cairncross JG, van den Bent MJ, Mason W, Belanger K, et al. Prolonged survival with valproic acid use in the EORTC/NCIC temozolomide trial for glioblastoma. Neurology. 2011;77(12):1156–64.
51. Happold C, Gorlia T, Chinot O, Gilbert MR, Nabors LB, Wick W, et al. Does valproic acid or levetiracetam improve survival in glioblastoma? A pooled analysis of prospective clinical trials in newly diagnosed glioblastoma. J Clin Oncol. 2016;34(7):731–9.
52. Roth P, Wick W, Weller M. Steroids in neurooncology: actions, indications, side-effects. Curr Opin Neurol. 2010;23(6):597–602.
53. Simpson JR, Horton J, Scott C, Curran WJ, Rubin P, Fischbach J, et al. Influence of location and extent of surgical resection on survival of patients with glioblastoma multiforme: results of three consecutive Radiation Therapy Oncology Group (RTOG) clinical trials. Int J Radiat Oncol Biol Phys. 1993;26(2):239–44.
54. Sturm D, Witt H, Hovestadt V, Khuong-Quang DA, Jones DT, Konermann C, et al. Hotspot mutations in H3F3A and IDH1 define distinct epigenetic and biological subgroups of glioblastoma. Cancer Cell. 2012;22(4):425–37.
55. Ellingson BM, Lai A, Harris RJ, Selfridge JM, Yong WH, Das K, et al. Probabilistic radiographic atlas of glioblastoma phenotypes. AJNR Am J Neuroradiol. 2013;34(3):533–40.
56. Lacroix M, Abi-Said D, Fourney DR, Gokaslan ZL, Shi W, DeMonte F, et al. A multivariate analysis of 416 patients with glioblastoma multiforme: prognosis, extent of resection, and survival. J Neurosurg. 2001;95(2):190–8.
57. Herrlinger U, Forschler H, Kuker W, Meyermann R, Bamberg M, Dichgans J, et al. Leptomeningeal metastasis: survival and prognostic factors in 155 patients. J Neurol Sci. 2004;223(2):167–78.
58. Erlich SS, Davis RL. Spinal subarachnoid metastasis from primary intracranial glioblastoma multiforme. Cancer. 1978;42(6):2854–64.
59. Arita N, Taneda M, Hayakawa T. Leptomeningeal dissemination of malignant gliomas. Incidence, diagnosis and outcome. Acta Neurochir (Wien). 1994;126(2–4):84–92.
60. Awad I, Bay JW, Rogers L. Leptomeningeal metastasis from supratentorial malignant gliomas. Neurosurgery. 1986;19(2):247–51.
61. Grabb PA, Albright AL, Pang D. Dissemination of supratentorial malignant gliomas via the cerebrospinal fluid in children. Neurosurgery. 1992;30(1):64–71.
62. Lindsay A, Holthouse D, Robbins P, Knuckey N. Spinal leptomeningeal metastases following glioblastoma multiforme treated with radiotherapy. J Clin Neurosci: Official J Neurosurg Soc Australasia. 2002;9(6):725–8.
63. Korshunov A, Sycheva R, Golanov A, Pronin I. Gains at the 1p36 chromosomal region are associated with symptomatic leptomeningeal dissemination of supratentorial glioblastomas. Am J Clin Pathol. 2007;127(4):585–90.
64. Ostrom QT, de Blank PM, Kruchko C, Petersen CM, Liao P, Finlay JL, et al. Alex's Lemonade Stand Foundation infant and childhood primary brain and central nervous system tumors diagnosed in the United States in 2007–2011. Neuro Oncol. 2015;16(Suppl 10):x1–36.
65. Schweitzer T, Vince GH, Herbold C, Roosen K, Tonn JC. Extraneural metastases of primary brain tumors. J Neurooncol. 2001;53(2):107–14.
66. Watson CJ, Roberts R, Wright KA, Greenberg DC, Rous BA, Brown CH, et al. How safe is it to transplant organs from deceased donors with primary intracranial malignancy? An analysis of UK Registry data. Am J Transplant: Official J Am Soc Transplant Am Soc Transplant Surg. 2010;10(6):1437–44.
67. Warrens AN, Birch R, Collett D, Daraktchiev M, Dark JH, Galea G, et al. Advising potential recipients on the use of organs from donors with primary central nervous system tumors. Transplantation. 2012;93(4):348–53.
68. Collignon FP, Holland EC, Feng S. Organ donors with malignant gliomas: an update. Am J Transplant: Official J Am Soc Transplant Am Soc Transplant Surg. 2004;4(1):15–21.
69. Abhinav K, Yeh FC, Mansouri A, Zadeh G, Fernandez-Miranda JC. High-definition fiber tractography for the evaluation of perilesional white matter tracts in high-grade glioma surgery. Neuro Oncol. 2015;17(9):1199–209.
70. Law M, Yang S, Wang H, Babb JS, Johnson G, Cha S, et al. Glioma grading: sensitivity, specificity, and predictive values of perfusion MR imaging and proton MR spectroscopic imaging compared with conventional MR imaging. AJNR Am J Neuroradiol. 2003;24(10):1989–98.
71. Weber MA, Zoubaa S, Schlieter M, Juttler E, Huttner HB, Geletneky K, et al. Diagnostic performance of spectroscopic and perfusion MRI for distinction of brain tumors. Neurology. 2006;66(12):1899–906.
72. Kono K, Inoue Y, Nakayama K, Shakudo M, Morino M, Ohata K, et al. The role of diffusion-weighted imaging in patients with brain tumors. AJNR Am J Neuroradiol. 2001;22(6):1081–8.
73. Kickingereder P, Wiestler B, Sahm F, Heiland S, Roethke M, Schlemmer HP, et al. Primary central nervous system lymphoma and atypical glioblastoma: multiparametric differentiation by using diffusion-, perfusion-, and susceptibility-weighted MR imaging. Radiology. 2014;272(3):843–50.
74. Ellingson BM, Zaw T, Cloughesy TF, Naeini KM, Lalezari S, Mong S, et al. Comparison between intensity normalization techniques for dynamic susceptibility contrast (DSC)-MRI estimates of cerebral blood volume (CBV) in human gliomas. J Magn Reson Imaging: JMRI. 2012;35(6):1472–7.

75. Andronesi OC, Kim GS, Gerstner E, Batchelor T, Tzika AA, Fantin VR, et al. Detection of 2-hydroxyglutarate in IDH-mutated glioma patients by in vivo spectral-editing and 2D correlation magnetic resonance spectroscopy. Sci Transl Med. 2012;4(116):116ra4.
76. Albert NL, Weller M, Suchorska B, Galldiks N, Soffietti R, Kim MM, et al. Response Assessment in Neuro-Oncology (RANO) Working Group and European Association for Neuro-Oncology (EANO) recommendations for the clinical use of PET imaging in gliomas. Neuro Oncol. 2016.
77. Weller M, van den Bent M, Hopkins K, Tonn JC, Stupp R, Falini A, et al. EANO guideline for the diagnosis and treatment of anaplastic gliomas and glioblastoma. Lancet Oncol. 2014;15(9):e395–403.
78. Louis DN, Ohgaki H, Wiestler OD, Cavenee WK, Burger PC, Jouvet A, et al. The 2007 WHO classification of tumours of the central nervous system. Acta Neuropathol. 2007;114(2):97–109.
79. Temme A, Geiger KD, Wiedemuth R, Conseur K, Pietsch T, Felsberg J, et al. Giant cell glioblastoma is associated with altered aurora b expression and concomitant p53 mutation. J Neuropathol Exp Neurol. 2010;69(6):632–42.
80. Kozak KR, Moody JS. Giant cell glioblastoma: a glioblastoma subtype with distinct epidemiology and superior prognosis. Neuro Oncol. 2009;11(6):833–41.
81. Kozak KR, Mahadevan A, Moody JS. Adult gliosarcoma: epidemiology, natural history, and factors associated with outcome. Neuro Oncol. 2009;11(2):183–91.
82. Korshunov A, Capper D, Reuss D, Schrimpf D, Ryzhova M, Hovestadt V, et al. Histologically distinct neuroepithelial tumors with histone 3 G34 mutation are molecularly similar and comprise a single nosologic entity. Acta Neuropathol. 2015.
83. Karsy M, Gelbman M, Shah P, Balumbu O, Moy F, Arslan E. Established and emerging variants of glioblastoma multiforme: review of morphological and molecular features. Folia Neuropathol (Association of Polish Neuropathologists and Medical Research Centre, Polish Academy of Sciences). 2012;50(4):301–21.
84. Hegi ME, Diserens AC, Gorlia T, Hamou MF, de Tribolet N, Weller M, et al. MGMT gene silencing and benefit from temozolomide in glioblastoma. N Engl J Med. 2005;352(10):997–1003.
85. Wick W, Platten M, Meisner C, Felsberg J, Tabatabai G, Simon M, et al. Temozolomide chemotherapy alone versus radiotherapy alone for malignant astrocytoma in the elderly: the NOA-08 randomised, phase 3 trial. Lancet Oncol. 2012;13(7):707–15.
86. Malmstrom A, Gronberg BH, Marosi C, Stupp R, Frappaz D, Schultz H, et al. Temozolomide versus standard 6-week radiotherapy versus hypofractionated radiotherapy in patients older than 60 years with glioblastoma: the Nordic randomised, phase 3 trial. Lancet Oncol. 2012;13(9):916–26.
87. Weller M, Tabatabai G, Kastner B, Felsberg J, Steinbach JP, Wick A, et al. MGMT promoter methylation is a strong prognostic biomarker for benefit from dose-intensified temozolomide rechallenge in progressive glioblastoma: the DIRECTOR trial. Clin Cancer Res: Official J Am Assoc Cancer Res. 2015;21(9):2057–64.
88. Parsons DW, Jones S, Zhang X, Lin JC, Leary RJ, Angenendt P, et al. An integrated genomic analysis of human glioblastoma multiforme. Science. 2008;321(5897):1807–12.
89. Yan H, Parsons DW, Jin G, McLendon R, Rasheed BA, Yuan W, et al. IDH1 and IDH2 mutations in gliomas. N Engl J Med. 2009;360(8):765–73.
90. Capper D, Zentgraf H, Balss J, Hartmann C, von Deimling A. Monoclonal antibody specific for IDH1 R132H mutation. Acta Neuropathol. 2009;118(5):599–601.
91. Verhaak RG, Hoadley KA, Purdom E, Wang V, Qi Y, Wilkerson MD, et al. Integrated genomic analysis identifies clinically relevant subtypes of glioblastoma characterized by abnormalities in PDGFRA, IDH1, EGFR, and NF1. Cancer Cell. 2010;17(1):98–110.
92. Turcan S, Rohle D, Goenka A, Walsh LA, Fang F, Yilmaz E, et al. IDH1 mutation is sufficient to establish the glioma hypermethylator phenotype. Nature. 2012;483(7390):479–83.
93. Noushmehr H, Weisenberger DJ, Diefes K, Phillips HS, Pujara K, Berman BP, et al. Identification of a CpG island methylator phenotype that defines a distinct subgroup of glioma. Cancer Cell. 2010;17(5):510–22.
94. Eckel-Passow JE, Lachance DH, Molinaro AM, Walsh KM, Decker PA, Sicotte H, et al. Glioma groups based on 1p/19q, IDH, and TERT promoter mutations in tumors. N Engl J Med. 2015;372(26):2499–508.
95. Labussiere M, Di Stefano AL, Gleize V, Boisselier B, Giry M, Mangesius S, et al. TERT promoter mutations in gliomas, genetic associations and clinico-pathological correlations. Br J Cancer. 2014;111(10):2024–32.
96. Aldape KD, Ballman K, Furth A, Buckner JC, Giannini C, Burger PC, et al. Immunohistochemical detection of EGFRvIII in high malignancy grade astrocytomas and evaluation of prognostic significance. J Neuropathol Exp Neurol. 2004;63(7):700–7.
97. Fan QW, Cheng CK, Gustafson WC, Charron E, Zipper P, Wong RA, et al. EGFR phosphorylates tumor-derived EGFRvIII driving STAT3/5 and progression in glioblastoma. Cancer Cell. 2013;24(4):438–49.
98. Stupp R, Mason WP, van den Bent MJ, Weller M, Fisher B, Taphoorn MJ, et al. Radiotherapy plus concomitant and adjuvant temozolomide for glioblastoma. N Engl J Med. 2005;352(10):987–96.
99. Laperriere N, Weller M, Stupp R, Perry JR, Brandes AA, Wick W, et al. Optimal management of

elderly patients with glioblastoma. Cancer Treat Rev. 2013;39(4):350–7.
100. Gilbert MR, Wang M, Aldape KD, Stupp R, Hegi ME, Jaeckle KA, et al. Dose-dense temozolomide for newly diagnosed glioblastoma: a randomized phase III clinical trial. J Clin Oncol. 2013;31 (32):4085–91.
101. Brada M, Stenning S, Gabe R, Thompson LC, Levy D, Rampling R, et al. Temozolomide versus procarbazine, lomustine, and vincristine in recurrent high-grade glioma. J Clin Oncol. 2010;28 (30):4601–8.
102. Scott J, Tsai YY, Chinnaiyan P, Yu HH. Effectiveness of radiotherapy for elderly patients with glioblastoma. Int J Radiat Oncol Biol Phys. 2011;81(1):206–10.
103. Seystahl K, Wick W, Weller M. Therapeutic options in recurrent glioblastoma—an update. Crit Rev Oncol Hematol. 2016;99:389–408.
104. Macdonald DR, Cascino TL, Schold SC Jr, Cairncross JG. Response criteria for phase II studies of supratentorial malignant glioma. J Clin Oncol. 1990;8(7):1277–80.
105. Brandsma D, van den Bent MJ. Pseudoprogression and pseudoresponse in the treatment of gliomas. Curr Opin Neurol. 2009;22(6):633–8.
106. Wen PY, Macdonald DR, Reardon DA, Cloughesy TF, Sorensen AG, Galanis E, et al. Updated response assessment criteria for high-grade gliomas: response assessment in neuro-oncology working group. J Clin Oncol. 2010;28(11):1963–72.
107. Suchorska B, Jansen NL, Linn J, Kretzschmar H, Janssen H, Eigenbrod S, et al. Biological tumor volume in 18FET-PET before radiochemotherapy correlates with survival in GBM. Neurology. 2015;84(7):710–9.
108. Kebir S, Fimmers R, Galldiks N, Schafer N, Mack F, Schaub C, et al. Late pseudoprogression in glioblastoma: diagnostic value of dynamic O-(2-[18F]fluoroethyl)-L-Tyrosine PET. Clin Cancer Res: Official J Am Assoc Cancer Res. 2015.
109. Galldiks N, Dunkl V, Stoffels G, Hutterer M, Rapp M, Sabel M, et al. Diagnosis of pseudoprogression in patients with glioblastoma using O-(2-[18F]fluoroethyl)-L-tyrosine PET. Eur J Nucl Med Mol Imaging. 2015;42(5):685–95.
110. Nava F, Tramacere I, Fittipaldo A, Bruzzone MG, Dimeco F, Fariselli L, et al. Survival effect of first- and second-line treatments for patients with primary glioblastoma: a cohort study from a prospective registry, 1997–2010. Neuro Oncol. 2014;16 (5):719–27.
111. Gorlia T, Stupp R, Brandes AA, Rampling RR, Fumoleau P, Dittrich C, et al. New prognostic factors and calculators for outcome prediction in patients with recurrent glioblastoma: a pooled analysis of EORTC Brain Tumour Group phase I and II clinical trials. Eur J Cancer. 2012;48(8):1176–84.
112. Suchorska B, Weller M, Tabatabai G, Senft C, Hau P, Sabel M, et al. Complete resection of contrast-enhancing tumor volume is associated with improved survival in recurrent glioblastoma results from the DIRECTOR trial. Neurosurgery. 2015;62 (Suppl 1):209.
113. Combs SE, Debus J, Schulz-Ertner D. Radiotherapeutic alternatives for previously irradiated recurrent gliomas. BMC Cancer. 2007;7:167.
114. Grosu AL, Weber WA, Franz M, Stark S, Piert M, Thamm R, et al. Reirradiation of recurrent high-grade gliomas using amino acid PET (SPECT)/CT/MRI image fusion to determine gross tumor volume for stereotactic fractionated radiotherapy. Int J Radiat Oncol Biol Phys. 2005;63(2):511–9.
115. Combs SE, Edler L, Rausch R, Welzel T, Wick W, Debus J. Generation and validation of a prognostic score to predict outcome after re-irradiation of recurrent glioma. Acta Oncol. 2013;52(1):147–52.
116. Wick W, Fricke H, Junge K, Kobyakov G, Martens T, Heese O, et al. A phase II, randomized, study of weekly APG101+ reirradiation versus reirradiation in progressive glioblastoma. Clin Cancer Res: Official J Am Assoc Cancer Res. 2014;20(24):6304–13.
117. Weller M, Cloughesy T, Perry JR, Wick W. Standards of care for treatment of recurrent glioblastoma—are we there yet? Neuro Oncol. 2013;15(1):4–27.
118. Wick W, Puduvalli VK, Chamberlain MC, van den Bent MJ, Carpentier AF, Cher LM, et al. Phase III study of enzastaurin compared with lomustine in the treatment of recurrent intracranial glioblastoma. J Clin Oncol. 2010;28(7):1168–74.
119. Batchelor TT, Mulholland P, Neyns B, Nabors LB, Campone M, Wick A, et al. Phase III randomized trial comparing the efficacy of cediranib as monotherapy, and in combination with lomustine, versus lomustine alone in patients with recurrent glioblastoma. J Clin Oncol. 2013;31(26):3212–8.
120. Perry JR, Belanger K, Mason WP, Fulton D, Kavan P, Easaw J, et al. Phase II trial of continuous dose-intense temozolomide in recurrent malignant glioma: RESCUE study. J Clin Oncol. 2010;28 (12):2051–7.
121. Patel AP, Tirosh I, Trombetta JJ, Shalek AK, Gillespie SM, Wakimoto H, et al. Single-cell RNA-seq highlights intratumoral heterogeneity in primary glioblastoma. Science. 2014;344 (6190):1396–401.
122. Sottoriva A, Spiteri I, Piccirillo SG, Touloumis A, Collins VP, Marioni JC, et al. Intratumor heterogeneity in human glioblastoma reflects cancer evolutionary dynamics. Proc Natl Acad Sci USA. 2013;110(10):4009–14.
123. Hunter C, Smith R, Cahill DP, Stephens P, Stevens C, Teague J, et al. A hypermutation phenotype and somatic MSH6 mutations in recurrent human malignant gliomas after alkylator chemotherapy. Cancer Res. 2006;66(8):3987–91.
124. Halliday J, Helmy K, Pattwell SS, Pitter KL, LaPlant Q, Ozawa T, et al. In vivo radiation

response of proneural glioma characterized by protective p53 transcriptional program and proneural-mesenchymal shift. Proc Natl Acad Sci USA. 2014;111(14):5248–53.
125. Druker BJ, Talpaz M, Resta DJ, Peng B, Buchdunger E, Ford JM, et al. Efficacy and safety of a specific inhibitor of the BCR-ABL tyrosine kinase in chronic myeloid leukemia. N Engl J Med. 2001;344(14):1031–7.
126. Hegi ME, Rajakannu P, Weller M. Epidermal growth factor receptor: a re-emerging target in glioblastoma. Curr Opin Neurol. 2012;25(6):774–9.
127. Galanis E, Buckner JC, Maurer MJ, Kreisberg JI, Ballman K, Boni J, et al. Phase II trial of temsirolimus (CCI-779) in recurrent glioblastoma multiforme: a North Central Cancer Treatment Group Study. J Clin Oncol. 2005;23(23):5294–304.
128. Wick W, Gorlia T, van den Bent M, Vecht CJ, Steuve J, Brandes AA, et al. Radiation therapy and concurrent plus adjuvant temsirolimus (CCI-779) versus chemoirradiation with temozolomide in newly diagnosed glioblastoma without methylation of the MGMT gene promoter. J Clin Oncol. 2014;32:5s.
129. Batchelor TT, Reardon DA, de Groot JF, Wick W, Weller M. Antiangiogenic therapy for glioblastoma: current status and future prospects. Clin Cancer Res: Official J Am Assoc Cancer Res. 2014;20 (22):5612–9.
130. Folkman J. Tumor angiogenesis: therapeutic implications. N Engl J Med. 1971;285(21):1182–6.
131. Ellis LM, Hicklin DJ. VEGF-targeted therapy: mechanisms of anti-tumour activity. Nat Rev Cancer. 2008;8(8):579–91.
132. Grothey A, Galanis E. Targeting angiogenesis: progress with anti-VEGF treatment with large molecules. Nat Rev Clin Oncol. 2009;6(9):507–18.
133. Kreisl TN, Kim L, Moore K, Duic P, Royce C, Stroud I, et al. Phase II trial of single-agent bevacizumab followed by bevacizumab plus irinotecan at tumor progression in recurrent glioblastoma. J Clin Oncol. 2009;27(5):740–5.
134. Friedman HS, Prados MD, Wen PY, Mikkelsen T, Schiff D, Abrey LE, et al. Bevacizumab alone and in combination with irinotecan in recurrent glioblastoma. J Clin Oncol. 2009;27(28):4733–40.
135. Wick W, Brandes AA, Gorlia T, Bendszus M, Sahm F, Taal W, et al. Phase III trial exploring the combination of bevacizumab and lomustine in patients with first recurrence of a glioblastoma: the EORTC 26101 trial. Neuro Oncol. 2015;17:v1-v1.
136. Taal W, Oosterkamp HM, Walenkamp AM, Dubbink HJ, Beerepoot LV, Hanse MC, et al. Single-agent bevacizumab or lomustine versus a combination of bevacizumab plus lomustine in patients with recurrent glioblastoma (BELOB trial): a randomised controlled phase 2 trial. Lancet Oncol. 2014;15(9):943–53.
137. Gilbert MR, Dignam JJ, Armstrong TS, Wefel JS, Blumenthal DT, Vogelbaum MA, et al. A randomized trial of bevacizumab for newly diagnosed glioblastoma. N Engl J Med. 2014;370 (8):699–708.
138. Chinot OL, Wick W, Mason W, Henriksson R, Saran F, Nishikawa R, et al. Bevacizumab plus radiotherapy-temozolomide for newly diagnosed glioblastoma. N Engl J Med. 2014;370(8):709–22.
139. Sandmann T, Bourgon R, Garcia J, Li C, Cloughesy T, Chinot OL, et al. Patients with proneural glioblastoma may derive overall survival benefit from the addition of bevacizumab to first-line radiotherapy and temozolomide: retrospective analysis of the AVAglio trial. J Clin Oncol. 2015.
140. Stupp R, Hegi ME, Gorlia T, Erridge SC, Perry J, Hong YK, et al. Cilengitide combined with standard treatment for patients with newly diagnosed glioblastoma with methylated MGMT promoter (CENTRIC EORTC 26071-22072 study): a multicentre, randomised, open-label, phase 3 trial. Lancet Oncol. 2014;15(10):1100–8.
141. Louveau A, Smirnov I, Keyes TJ, Eccles JD, Rouhani SJ, Peske JD, et al. Structural and functional features of central nervous system lymphatic vessels. Nature. 2015;523(7560):337–41.
142. Reardon DA, Freeman G, Wu C, Chiocca EA, Wucherpfennig KW, Wen PY, et al. Immunotherapy advances for glioblastoma. Neuro Oncol. 2014;16(11):1441–58.
143. Hanahan D, Weinberg RA. Hallmarks of cancer: the next generation. Cell. 2011;144(5):646–74.
144. Wolchok JD, Kluger H, Callahan MK, Postow MA, Rizvi NA, Lesokhin AM, et al. Nivolumab plus ipilimumab in advanced melanoma. N Engl J Med. 2013;369(2):122–33.
145. Hodi FS, O'Day SJ, McDermott DF, Weber RW, Sosman JA, Haanen JB, et al. Improved survival with ipilimumab in patients with metastatic melanoma. N Engl J Med. 2010;363(8):711–23.
146. Ribas A, Kefford R, Marshall MA, Punt CJ, Haanen JB, Marmol M, et al. Phase III randomized clinical trial comparing tremelimumab with standard-of-care chemotherapy in patients with advanced melanoma. J Clin Oncol. 2013;31(5):616–22.
147. Brahmer J, Reckamp KL, Baas P, Crino L, Eberhardt WE, Poddubskaya E, et al. Nivolumab versus docetaxel in advanced squamous-cell non-small-cell lung cancer. N Engl J Med. 2015;373(2):123–35.
148. Rizvi NA, Mazieres J, Planchard D, Stinchcombe TE, Dy GK, Antonia SJ, et al. Activity and safety of nivolumab, an anti-PD-1 immune checkpoint inhibitor, for patients with advanced, refractory squamous non-small-cell lung cancer (CheckMate 063): a phase 2, single-arm trial. Lancet Oncol. 2015;16(3):257–65.
149. Preusser M, Lim M, Hafler DA, Reardon DA, Sampson JH. Prospects of immune checkpoint modulators in the treatment of glioblastoma. Nat Rev Neurol. 2015;11(9):504–14.
150. Gilham DE, Debets R, Pule M, Hawkins RE, Abken H. CAR-T cells and solid tumors: tuning T

cells to challenge an inveterate foe. Trends Mol Med. 2012;18(7):377–84.
151. Wen P, Reardon D, Phuphanich S, Aiken R, Landolfi J, Curry W, et al. A randomized double blind placebo-controlled phase 2 trial of dendritic cell (DC) vaccine ICT-107 following standard treatment in newly diagnosed patients with GBM. Neuro Oncol. 2014;16:v8–22.
152. Schumacher T, Bunse L, Pusch S, Sahm F, Wiestler B, Quandt J, et al. A vaccine targeting mutant IDH1 induces antitumour immunity. Nature. 2014;512(7514):324–7.
153. Mitchell DA, Batich KA, Gunn MD, Huang MN, Sanchez-Perez L, Nair SK, et al. Tetanus toxoid and CCL3 improve dendritic cell vaccines in mice and glioblastoma patients. Nature. 2015;519(7543):366–9.
154. Stupp R, Wong E, Scott C, Taillibert S, Kanner A, Kesari S, et al. Interim analysis of the EF-14 trial: a prospective, multi-center trial of NovoTTF-100A together with temozolomide compared to temozolomide alone in patients with newly diagnosed GBM. Neuro Oncol. 2014;16:v167.
155. Wick W. TTFields: where does all the skepticism come from? Neuro Oncol. 2016;18(3):303–5.
156. Lathia JD, Mack SC, Mulkearns-Hubert EE, Valentim CL, Rich JN. Cancer stem cells in glioblastoma. Genes Dev. 2015;29(12):1203–17.
157. Thomas AA, Brennan CW, DeAngelis LM, Omuro AM. Emerging therapies for glioblastoma. JAMA Neurol. 2014;71(11):1437–44.
158. Osswald M, Jung E, Sahm F, Solecki G, Venkataramani V, Blaes J, et al. Brain tumour cells interconnect to a functional and resistant network. Nature. 2015;528(7580):93–8.
159. Singh SK, Hawkins C, Clarke ID, Squire JA, Bayani J, Hide T, et al. Identification of human brain tumour initiating cells. Nature. 2004;432(7015):396–401.
160. Bao S, Wu Q, McLendon RE, Hao Y, Shi Q, Hjelmeland AB, et al. Glioma stem cells promote radioresistance by preferential activation of the DNA damage response. Nature. 2006;444(7120):756–60.
161. Chen J, Li Y, Yu TS, McKay RM, Burns DK, Kernie SG, et al. A restricted cell population propagates glioblastoma growth after chemotherapy. Nature. 2012;488(7412):522–6.
162. Liu HK, Wang Y, Belz T, Bock D, Takacs A, Radlwimmer B, et al. The nuclear receptor tailless induces long-term neural stem cell expansion and brain tumor initiation. Genes Dev. 2010;24(7):683–95.
163. Bhat KP, Balasubramaniyan V, Vaillant B, Ezhilarasan R, Hummelink K, Hollingsworth F, et al. Mesenchymal differentiation mediated by NF-kappaB promotes radiation resistance in glioblastoma. Cancer Cell. 2013;24(3):331–46.
164. Emlet DR, Gupta P, Holgado-Madruga M, Del Vecchio CA, Mitra SS, Han SY, et al. Targeting a glioblastoma cancer stem-cell population defined by EGF receptor variant III. Cancer Res. 2014;74(4):1238–49.
165. Piaskowski S, Bienkowski M, Stoczynska-Fidelus E, Stawski R, Sieruta M, Szybka M, et al. Glioma cells showing IDH1 mutation cannot be propagated in standard cell culture conditions. Br J Cancer. 2011;104(6):968–70.

Index

Note: Page numbers followed by *f* and *t* indicate figures and tables, respectively

J. Moliterno Günel et al. (eds.), *Malignant Brain Tumors*,
DOI 10.1007/978-3-319-49864-5

K

L

M

R

S